HOW NOT TO DIE

HOW NOT TO DIE

DISCOVER THE FOODS
SCIENTIFICALLY PROVEN TO PREVENT
AND REVERSE DISEASE

Michael Greger, M.D.

with Gene Stone

FLATIRON
BOOKS
NEW YORK

HOW NOT TO DIE. Copyright © 2015 by Michael Greger with Gene Stone. All rights reserved. Printed in the United States of America. For information, address Flatiron Books, 175 Fifth Avenue, New York, N.Y. 10010.

www.flatironbooks.com

Figure 3 illustration on page 120 by Vance Lehmkuhl.

Designed by Steven Seighman

The Library of Congress Cataloging-in-Publication Data is available upon request.

ISBN 978-1-250-06611-4 (hardcover)
ISBN 978-1-250-06612-1 (e-book)

Our books may be purchased in bulk for promotional, educational, or business use. Please contact your local bookseller or the Macmillan Corporate and Premium Sales Department at (800) 221-7945, extension 5442, or by e-mail at MacmillanSpecialMarkets@macmillan.com.

First Edition: December 2015

20   19   18   17   16   15   14   13   12

To my grandma
Frances Greger

Contents

PART 2

Preface

It all started with my grandmother.

I was only a kid when the doctors sent her home in a wheelchair to die. Diagnosed with end-stage heart disease, she had already had so many bypass operations that the surgeons essentially ran out of plumbing—the scarring from each open-heart surgery had made the next more difficult until they finally ran out of options. Confined to a wheelchair with crushing chest pain, her doctors told her there was nothing else they could do. Her life was over at age sixty-five.

I think what sparks many kids to want to become doctors when they grow up is watching a beloved relative become ill or even die. But for me, it was watching my grandma get better.

Soon after she was discharged from the hospital to spend her last days at home, a segment aired on *60 Minutes* about Nathan Pritikin, an early lifestyle medicine pioneer who had been gaining a reputation for reversing terminal heart disease. He had just opened a new center in California, and my grandmother, in desperation, somehow made the cross-country trek to become one of its first patients. This was a live-in program where everyone was placed on a plant-based diet and then started on a graded exercise regimen. They wheeled my grandmother in, and she walked out.

I'll never forget that.

She was even featured in Pritikin's biography *Pritikin: The Man Who Healed America's Heart*. My grandma was described as one of the "death's door people":

Frances Greger, from North Miami, Florida, arrived in Santa Barbara at one of Pritikin's early sessions in a wheelchair. Mrs. Greger had heart disease, angina, and claudication; her condition was so bad she could no longer walk without great pain in her chest and legs. Within three weeks, though, she was not only out of her wheelchair but was walking ten miles a day.[1]

When I was a kid, that was all that mattered: I got to play with Grandma again. But over the years, I grew to understand the significance of what had happened. At that time, the medical profession didn't even think it was possible to reverse heart disease. Drugs were given to try to slow the progression, and surgery was performed to circumvent clogged arteries to try to relieve symptoms, but the disease was expected to get worse and worse until you died. Now, however, we know that as soon as we stop eating an artery-clogging diet, our bodies can start healing themselves, in many cases opening up arteries without drugs or surgery.

My grandma was given her medical death sentence at age sixty-five. Thanks to a healthy diet and lifestyle, she was able to enjoy another thirty-one years on this earth with her six grandchildren. The woman who was once told by doctors she only had weeks to live didn't die until she was ninety-six years old. Her near-miraculous recovery not only inspired one of those grandkids to pursue a career in medicine but granted her enough healthy years to see him graduate from medical school.

By the time I became a doctor, giants like Dean Ornish, M.D., president and founder of the nonprofit Preventive Medicine Research Institute, had already proven beyond a shadow of a doubt what Pritikin had shown to be true. Using the latest high-tech advances—cardiac PET scans,[2] quantitative coronary arteriography,[3] and radionuclide ventriculography[4]—Dr. Ornish and his colleagues showed that the lowest-tech approach—diet and lifestyle—can undeniably reverse heart disease, our leading killer.

Dr. Ornish and his colleagues' studies were published in some of the most prestigious medical journals in the world. Yet medical practice hardly changed. Why? Why were doctors still prescribing drugs and using Roto-Rooter-type procedures to just treat the symptoms of heart disease and to try to forestall what they chose to believe was the inevitable—an early death?

This was my wake-up call. I opened my eyes to the depressing fact that there are other forces at work in medicine besides science. The U.S. health care system runs on a fee-for-service model in which doctors get paid for the pills and procedures they prescribe, rewarding quantity over quality. We don't get reimbursed for time spent counseling our patients about the benefits of healthy eating. If doctors were instead paid for performance, there would be a financial incentive to treat the lifestyle causes of disease. Until the model of reimbursement changes, I don't expect great changes in medical care or medical education.[5]

Only a quarter of medical schools appear to offer a single dedicated course on nutrition.[6] During my first interview for medical school, at Cornell University, I remember the interviewer emphatically stating, "Nutrition is superfluous to human health." And he was a pediatrician! I knew I was in for a long road ahead. Come to think of it, I think the only medical professional who ever asked me about a family member's diet was our veterinarian.

I was honored to be accepted by nineteen medical schools. I chose Tufts because they boasted the most nutrition training—twenty-one hours' worth, although this was still less than 1 percent of the curriculum.

During my medical training, I was offered countless steak dinners and fancy perks by Big Pharma representatives, but not once did I get a call from Big Broccoli. There is a reason you hear about the latest drugs on television: Huge corporate budgets drive their promotion. The same reason you'll probably never see a commercial for sweet potatoes is the same reason breakthroughs on the power of foods to affect your health and longevity may never make it to the public: There's little profit motive.

In medical school, even with our paltry twenty-one hours of nutrition training, there was no mention of using diet to treat chronic disease, let alone reverse it. I was only aware of this body of work because of my family's personal story.

The question that haunted me during training was this: If the cure to our number-one killer could get lost down the rabbit hole, what else might be buried in the medical literature? I made it my life's mission to find out.

Most of my years in Boston were spent scouring the dusty stacks in the basement of Harvard's Countway Library of Medicine. I started practicing medicine, but no matter how many patients I saw in the clinic every day, even when I was able to change the lives of entire families at a time, I knew it was just a drop in the bucket, so I went on the road.

With the help of the American Medical Student Association, my goal was to speak at every medical school in the country every two years to influence an entire generation of new doctors. I didn't want another doctor to graduate without this tool—the power of food—in her or his toolbox. If my grandma didn't have to die from heart disease, perhaps no one's grandparent did.

There were periods where I was giving forty talks a month. I'd roll into town to give a breakfast talk at a Rotary Club, give a presentation at the medical school over lunch, and then speak to a community group in the evening. I was living out of my car, one key on my keychain. I ended up giving more than a thousand presentations around the world.

Not surprisingly, life on the road was not sustainable. I lost a marriage over it. With more speaking requests than I could accept, I started putting all my annual research findings into a DVD series, *Latest in Clinical Nutrition*. It's hard to believe I'm almost up to volume 30. Every penny I receive from those DVDs, then and now, goes directly to charity, as does the money from my speaking engagements and book sales, including the book you're reading now.

As corrupting an influence as money is in medicine, it appears to me even worse in the field of nutrition, where it seems everyone has his or her own brand of snake-oil supplement or wonder gadget. Dogmas are entrenched and data too often cherry-picked to support preconceived notions.

True, I have biases of my own to rein in. Although my original motivation was health, over the years, I've grown into quite the animal lover. Three cats and a dog run our household, and I've spent much of my professional life proudly serving the Humane Society of the United States as the charity's public health director. So, like many people, I care about the welfare of the animals we eat, but first and foremost, I am a physician. My primary duty has always been to care for my patients, to accurately provide the best available balance of evidence.

In the clinic, I could reach hundreds; on the road, thousands. But this life-or-death information needed to reach millions. Enter Jesse Rasch, a Canadian philanthropist who shared my vision of making evidence-based nutrition freely accessible and available to all. The foundation he and his wife, Julie, set up put all my work online—thus, NutritionFacts.org was born. I can now reach more people while working from home in my pajamas than I ever could when I was traveling the world.

Now a self-sustaining nonprofit organization itself, NutritionFacts.org has more than a thousand bite-sized videos on nearly every conceivable nutrition topic, and I post new videos and articles every day. Everything on the website is free for all, for all time. There are no ads, no corporate sponsorships. It's just a labor of love.

When I started this work more than a decade ago, I thought the answer was to train the trainers, educate the profession. But with the democratization of information, doctors no longer hold a monopoly as gatekeepers of knowledge about health. When it comes to safe, simple lifestyle prescriptions, I'm realizing it may be more effective to empower individuals directly. In a recent national survey of doctor office visits, only about one in five smokers were told to quit.[7] Just as you don't have to wait for your physician to tell you to stop smoking, you don't have to wait to start eating healthier. Then together we can show my medical colleagues the true power of healthy living.

Today, I live within biking distance of the National Library of Medicine, the largest medical library in the world. Last year alone, there were more than twenty-four thousand papers published in the medical literature on nutrition, and I now have a team of researchers, a wonderful staff, and an army of volunteers who help me dig through the mountains of new information. This book is not just another platform through which I can share my findings but a long-awaited opportunity to share practical advice about how to put this life-changing, life-*saving* science into practice in our daily lives.

I think my grandma would be proud.

Introduction

PREVENTING, ARRESTING, AND REVERSING OUR LEADING KILLERS

There may be no such thing as dying from old age. From a study of more than forty-two thousand consecutive autopsies, centenarians—those who live past one hundred—were found to have succumbed to diseases in 100 percent of the cases examined. Though most were perceived, even by their physicians, to have been healthy just prior to death, not one "died of old age."[1] Until recently, advanced age had been considered to be a disease itself,[2] but people don't die as a consequence of maturing. They die from disease, most commonly heart attacks.[3]

Most deaths in the United States are preventable, and they are related to what we eat.[4] Our diet is the number-one cause of premature death and the number-one cause of disability.[5] Surely, diet must also be the number-one thing taught in medical schools, right?

Sadly, it's not. According to the most recent national survey, only a quarter of medical schools offer a *single* course in nutrition, down from 37 percent thirty years ago.[6] While most of the public evidently considers doctors to be "very credible" sources of nutrition information,[7] six out of seven graduating doctors surveyed felt physicians were inadequately trained to counsel patients about their diets.[8] One study found that people off the street sometimes know more about basic nutrition than their doctors, concluding "physicians should be more knowledgeable about nutrition than their patients, but these results suggest that this is not necessarily true."[9]

To remedy this situation, a bill was introduced in the California State Legislature to mandate physicians get at least twelve hours of nutrition training any time over the next four years. It might surprise you to learn that the California

Medical Association came out strongly *opposed* to the bill, as did other mainstream medical groups, including the California Academy of Family Physicians.[10] The bill was amended from a mandatory minimum of twelve hours over four years down to seven hours and then doctored, one might say, down to zero.

The California medical board does have one subject requirement: twelve hours on pain management and end-of-life care for the terminally ill.[11] This disparity between prevention and mere mitigation of suffering could be a metaphor for modern medicine. A doctor a day may keep the apples away.

Back in 1903, Thomas Edison predicted that the "doctor of the future will give no medicine, but will instruct his patient in the care of [the] human frame in diet and in the cause and prevention of diseases."[12] Sadly, all it takes is a few minutes watching pharmaceutical ads on television imploring viewers to "ask your doctor" about this or that drug to know that Edison's prediction hasn't come true. A study of thousands of patient visits found that the average length of time primary-care doctors spend talking about nutrition is about ten seconds.[13]

But hey, this is the twenty-first century! Can't we eat whatever we want and simply take meds when we begin having health problems? For too many patients and even my physician colleagues, this seems to be the prevailing mind-set. Global spending for prescription drugs is surpassing $1 trillion annually, with the United States accounting for about one-third of this market.[14] Why do we spend so much on pills? Many people assume that our manner of death is preprogrammed into our genes. High blood pressure by fifty-five, heart attacks at sixty, maybe cancer at seventy, and so on. . . . But for most of the leading causes of death, the science shows that our genes often account for only 10–20 percent of risk at most.[15] For instance, as you'll see in this book, the rates of killers like heart disease and major cancers differ up to a hundred-fold among various populations around the globe. But when people move from low- to high-risk countries, their disease rates almost always change to those of the new environment.[16] New diet, new diseases. So, while a sixty-year-old American man living in San Francisco has about a 5 percent chance of having a heart attack within five years, should he move to Japan and start eating and living like the Japanese, his five-year risk would drop to only 1 percent. Japanese Americans in their forties can have the same heart attack risk as Japanese in their sixties. Switching to an American lifestyle in effect aged their hearts a full twenty years.[17]

The Mayo Clinic estimates that nearly 70 percent of Americans take at least one prescription drug.[18] Yet despite the fact that more people in this country are on medication than aren't, not to mention the steady influx of ever newer and more expensive drugs on the market, we aren't living much longer than others. In terms of life expectancy, the United States is down around twenty-seven or twenty-eight out of the thirty-four top free-market democracies. People in Slovenia live longer than we do.[19] And the extra years we are living aren't necessarily healthy or vibrant. Back in 2011, a disturbing analysis of mortality and morbidity was published in the *Journal of Gerontology*. Are Americans living longer now compared to about a generation ago? Yes, technically. But are those extra years necessarily healthy ones? No. And it's worse than that: We're actually living fewer healthy years now than we once did.[20]

Here's what I mean: A twenty-year-old in 1998 could expect to live about fifty-eight more years, while a twenty-year-old in 2006 could look forward to fifty-nine more years. However, the twenty-year-old from the 1990s might live ten of those years with chronic disease, whereas now it's more like thirteen years with heart disease, cancer, diabetes, or a stroke. So it feels like one step forward, three steps back. The researchers also noted that we're living two fewer functional years—that is, for two years, we're no longer able to perform basic life activities, such as walking a quarter of a mile, standing or sitting for two hours without having to lie down, or standing without special equipment.[21] In other words, we're living longer, but we're living *sicker*.

With these rising disease rates, our children may even die sooner. A special report published in the *New England Journal of Medicine* entitled "A Potential Decline in Life Expectancy in the United States in the 21st Century" concluded that "the steady rise in life expectancy observed in the modern era may soon come to an end and the youth of today may, on average, live less healthy and possibly even shorter lives than their parents."[22]

In public health school, students learn that there are three levels of preventive medicine. The first is primary prevention, as in trying to prevent people at risk for heart disease from suffering their first heart attack. An example of this level of preventive medicine would be your doctor prescribing you a statin drug for high cholesterol. Secondary prevention takes place when you already have the disease and are trying to prevent it from becoming worse, like having a second heart attack. To do this, your doctor may add an aspirin or other drugs to your regimen. At the third level of preventive medicine, the focus is on helping people manage long-term health problems, so your doctor, for example, might prescribe a cardiac rehabilitation program that aims to prevent further physical deterioration and pain.[23] In 2000, a fourth level was proposed. What could this new "quaternary" prevention be? Reduce the complications from all the drugs and surgery from the first three levels.[24] But people seem to forget about a fifth concept, termed primordial prevention, that was first introduced by the World Health Organization back in 1978. Decades later, it's finally being embraced by the American Heart Association.[25]

Primordial prevention was conceived as a strategy to prevent whole societies from experiencing epidemics of chronic-disease risk factors. This means not just preventing chronic disease but preventing the risk factors that lead to chronic disease.[26] For example, instead of trying to prevent someone with high cholesterol from suffering a heart attack, why not help prevent him or her from getting high cholesterol (which leads to the heart attack) in the first place?

With this in mind, the American Heart Association came up with "The Simple 7" factors that can lead to a healthier life: not smoking, not being overweight, being "very active" (defined as the equivalent of walking at least twenty-two minutes a day), eating healthier (for example, lots of fruits and vegetables), having below-average cholesterol, having normal blood pressure, and having normal blood sugar levels.[27] The American Heart Association's goal is to reduce heart-disease deaths by 20 percent by 2020.[28] If more than 90 percent of heart attacks may be avoided with lifestyle changes,[29] why so modest an aim? Even 25 percent was "deemed unrealistic."[30] The AHA's pessimism may have something to do with the frightening reality of the average American diet.

An analysis of the health behaviors of thirty-five thousand adults across the United States was published in the American Heart Association journal. Most of the participants didn't smoke, about half reached their weekly exercise goals, and about a third of the population got a pass in each of the other categories—except diet. Their diets were scored on a scale from zero to five to see if they met a bare minimum of healthy eating behaviors, such as meeting recommended targets for fruit, vegetable, and whole-grain consumption or drinking fewer than three cans of soda a week. How many even reached four out of five on their Healthy Eating Score? About 1 percent.[31] Maybe if the American Heart Association achieves its goal of an "aggressive"[32] 20 percent improvement by 2020, we'll get up to 1.2 percent.

Medical anthropologists have identified several major eras of human disease, starting with the Age of Pestilence and Famine, which largely ended with the Industrial Revolution, or the stage we're in now, the Age of Degenerative and Man-Made Diseases.[33] This shift is reflected in the changing causes of death over the last century. In 1900 in the United States, the top-three killers were infectious diseases: pneumonia, tuberculosis, and diarrheal disease.[34] Now, the killers are largely lifestyle diseases: heart disease, cancer, and chronic lung disease.[35]

Is this simply because antibiotics have enabled us to live long enough to suffer from degenerative diseases? No. The emergence of these epidemics of chronic disease was accompanied by dramatic shifts in dietary patterns. This is best exemplified by what's been happening to disease rates among people in the developing world over the last few decades as they've rapidly Westernized their diets.

In 1990 around the world, most years of healthy life were lost to undernutrition, such as diarrheal diseases in malnourished children, but now the greatest disease burden is attributed to high blood pressure, a disease of overnutrition.[36] The pandemic of chronic disease has been ascribed in part to the near-universal shift toward a diet dominated by animal-sourced and processed foods—in other words, more meat, dairy, eggs, oils, soda, sugar, and refined grains.[37] China is perhaps the best-studied example. There, a transition away from the country's traditional, plant-based diet was accompanied by a sharp rise in diet-related chronic diseases, such as obesity, diabetes, cardiovascular diseases, and cancer.[38]

Why do we suspect these changes in diet and disease are related? After all, rapidly industrializing societies undergo multitudes of changes. How are scientists able to parse out the effects of specific foods? To isolate the effects of different dietary components, researchers can follow the diets and diseases of large groups of defined individuals over time. Take meat, for example. To see what effect an increase in meat consumption might have on disease rates, researchers studied lapsed vegetarians. People who once ate vegetarian diets but then started to eat meat at least once a week experienced a 146 percent increase in odds of heart disease, a 152 percent increase in stroke, a 166 percent increase in diabetes, and a 231 percent increase in odds for weight gain. During the twelve years after the transition from vegetarian to omnivore, meat-eating was associated with a 3.6 year decrease in life expectancy.[39]

Even vegetarians can suffer high rates of chronic disease, though, if they eat a lot of processed foods. Take India, for example. This country's rates of diabetes, heart disease, obesity, and stroke have increased far faster than might have been expected given its relatively small increase in per capita meat consumption. This has been blamed on the decreasing "whole plant food content of their diet," including a shift from brown rice to white and the substitution of other refined carbohydrates, packaged snacks, and fast-food products for India's traditional staples of lentils, fruits, vegetables, whole grains, nuts, and seeds.[40] In general, the dividing line between health-promoting and disease-promoting foods may be less plant- versus animal-sourced foods and more whole plant foods versus most everything else.

To this end, a dietary quality index was developed that simply reflects the percentage of calories people derive from nutrient-rich, unprocessed plant foods[41] on a scale of zero to one hundred. The higher people score, the more body fat they may lose over time[42] and the lower their risk may be of abdominal obesity,[43] high blood pressure,[44] high cholesterol, and high triglycerides.[45] Comparing the diets of 100 women with breast cancer to 175 healthy women, researchers concluded that scoring higher on the whole plant food diet index (greater than about thirty compared to less than about eighteen) may reduce the odds of breast cancer more than 90 percent.[46]

Sadly, most Americans hardly make it past a score of ten. The standard American diet rates eleven out of one hundred. According to estimates from the U.S. Department of Agriculture, 32 percent of our calories comes from animal foods, 57 percent comes from processed plant foods, and only 11 percent comes from whole grains, beans, fruits, vegetables, and nuts.[47] That means on a scale of one to ten, the American diet would rate about a one.

We eat almost as if the future doesn't matter. And, indeed, there are actually data to back that up. A study entitled "Death Row Nutrition: Curious Conclusions of Last Meals" analyzed the last meal requests of hundreds of individuals executed in the United States during a five-year period. It turns out that the nutritional content didn't differ much from what Americans normally eat.[48] If we continue to eat as though we're having our last meals, eventually they will be.

What percentage of Americans hit all the American Heart Association's "Simple 7" recommendations? Of 1,933 men and women surveyed, most met two or three, but hardly any managed to meet all seven simple health components. In fact, just a single individual could boast hitting all seven recommendations.[49] One person out of nearly two thousand. As a recent past president of the American Heart Association responded, "That should give all of us pause."[50]

The truth is that adhering to just four simple healthy lifestyle factors can have a strong impact on the prevention of chronic diseases: not smoking, not being obese, getting a half hour of exercise a day, and eating healthier—defined as consuming more fruits, veggies, and whole grains and less meat. Those four factors alone were found to account for 78 percent of chronic disease risk. If you start from scratch and manage to tick off all four, you may be able to wipe out more than 90 percent of your risk of developing diabetes, more than 80 percent of your risk of having a heart attack, cut by half your risk of having a stroke, and reduce your overall cancer risk by more than one-third.[51] For some cancers, like our number-two cancer killer, colon cancer, up to

71 percent of cases appear to be preventable through a similar portfolio of simple diet and lifestyle changes.[52]

Maybe it's time we stop blaming genetics and focus on the more than 70 percent that is directly under our control.[53] We have the power.

Does all this healthy living translate into a longer life as well? The Centers for Disease Control and Prevention (CDC) followed approximately eight thousand Americans aged twenty years or older for about six years. They found that three cardinal lifestyle behaviors exerted an enormous impact on mortality: People can substantially reduce their risk for early death by not smoking, consuming a healthier diet, and engaging in sufficient physical activity. And the CDC's definitions were pretty laid-back: By not smoking, the CDC just meant not *currently* smoking. A "healthy diet" was defined merely as being in the top 40 percent in terms of complying with the wimpy federal dietary guidelines, and "physically active" meant averaging about twenty-one minutes or more a day of at least moderate exercise. People who managed at least *one* of the three had a 40 percent lower risk of dying within that six-year period. Those who hit two out of three cut their chances of dying by more than half, and those who scored all three behaviors reduced their chances of dying in that time by 82 percent.[54]

Of course, people sometimes fib about how well they eat. How accurate can these findings really be if they're based on people's self-reporting? A similar study on health behaviors and survival didn't just take people's own word for how healthy they were eating; the researchers measured how much vitamin C participants had in their bloodstreams. The level of vitamin C in the blood was considered a "good biomarker of plant food intake" and hence was used as a proxy for a healthy diet. The conclusions held up. The drop in mortality risk among those with healthier habits was equivalent to being fourteen years younger.[55] It's like turning back the clock fourteen years—not with a drug or a DeLorean but just by eating and living healthier.

Let's talk a little more about aging. In each of your cells, you have forty-six strands of DNA coiled into chromosomes. At the tip of each chromosome, there's a tiny cap called a telomere, which keeps your DNA from unraveling and fraying. Think of it as the plastic tips on the end of your shoelaces. Every time your cells divide, however, a bit of that cap is lost. And when the telomere is completely gone, your cells can die.[56] Though this is an oversimplification,[57] telomeres have been thought of as your life "fuse": They can start shortening as soon as you're born, and when they're gone, you're gone. In fact, forensic scientists can take DNA from a bloodstain and roughly estimate how old the person was based on how long their telomeres are.[58]

Sounds like fodder for a great scene in *CSI*, but is there anything you can do to slow the rate at which your fuses burn? The thought is that if you can slow down this ticking cellular clock, you may be able to slow down the aging process and live longer.[59] So what would you have to do if you wanted to prevent this telomere cap from burning away? Well, smoking cigarettes is associated with triple the rate of telomere loss,[60] so the first step is simple: Stop smoking. But the food you eat every day may also have an impact on how fast you lose your telomeres. The consumption of fruits,[61] vegetables,[62] and other antioxidant-rich foods[63] has been associated with longer protective telomeres. In contrast, the consumption of refined grains,[64] soda,[65] meat (including fish),[66] and dairy[67] has been linked to shortened telomeres. What if you ate a diet composed of whole plant foods and stayed away from processed foods and animal foods? Could cellular aging be slowed?

The answer lies in an enzyme found in Methuselah. That's the name given to a bristlecone pine tree growing in the White Mountains of California, which, at the time, happened to be the oldest recorded living being and is now nearing its 4,800th birthday. It was already hundreds of years old before construction of the pyramids in Egypt began. There's an enzyme in the roots of bristlecone pines that appears to peak a few thousand years into their life span, and it actually rebuilds telomeres.[68] Scientists named it telomerase. Once they knew what to look for, researchers discovered the enzyme was present in human cells too. The question then became, how can we boost the activity of this age-defying enzyme?

Seeking answers, the pioneering researcher Dr. Dean Ornish teamed up with Dr. Elizabeth Blackburn, who was awarded the 2009 Nobel Prize in Medicine for her discovery of telomerase. In a study funded in part by the U.S. Department of Defense, they found that three months of whole-food, plant-based nutrition and other healthy changes could significantly boost telomerase activity, the only intervention ever shown to do so.[69] The study was published in one of the most prestigious medical journals in the world. The accompanying editorial concluded that this landmark study "should encourage people to adopt a healthy lifestyle in order to avoid or combat cancer and age-related diseases."[70]

So were Dr. Ornish and Dr. Blackburn able to successfully slow down aging with a healthy diet and lifestyle? A five-year follow-up study was recently published in which the lengths of the study subjects' telomeres were measured.

In the control group (the group of participants who did not change their life-styles), their telomeres predictably shrank with age. But for the healthy-living group, not only did their telomeres shrink less, they *grew*. Five years later, their telomeres were even longer on average than when they started, suggesting a healthy lifestyle can boost telomerase enzyme activity and *reverse* cellular aging.[71]

Subsequent research has shown that the telomere lengthening wasn't just because the healthy-living group was exercising more or losing weight. Weight loss through calorie restriction and an even more vigorous exercise program failed to improve telomere length, so it appears that the active ingredient is the quality, not quantity, of the food eaten. As long as people were eating the same diet, it didn't appear to matter how small their portions were, how much weight they lost, or even how hard they exercised; after a year, they saw no benefit.[72] In contrast, individuals on the plant-based diet exercised only half as much, enjoyed the same amount of weight loss after just three months,[73] and achieved significant telomere protection.[74] In other words, it wasn't the weight loss and it wasn't the exercise that reversed cell aging—it was the food.

Some people have expressed concern that boosting telomerase activity could theoretically increase cancer risk, since tumors have been known to hijack the telomerase enzyme and use it to ensure their own immortality.[75] But as we'll see in chapter 13, Dr. Ornish and his colleagues have used the same diet and lifestyle changes to halt and apparently *reverse* the progression of cancer in certain circumstances. We will also see how the same diet can reverse heart disease too.

What about our other leading killers? It turns out a more plant-based diet may help prevent, treat, or reverse *every single one* of our fifteen leading causes of death. In this book, I'll go through this list, with a chapter on each:

MORTALITY IN THE UNITED STATES

	Annual Deaths
1. Coronary heart disease[76]	375,000
2. Lung diseases (lung cancer,[77] COPD, and asthma[78])	296,000
3. You'll be surprised! (see chapter 15)	225,000
4. Brain diseases (stroke[79] and Alzheimer's[80])	214,000

continued

5. Digestive cancers (colorectal, pancreatic, and esophageal)[81]	106,000
6. Infections (respiratory and blood)[82]	95,000
7. Diabetes[83]	76,000
8. High blood pressure[84]	65,000
9. Liver disease (cirrhosis and cancer)[85]	60,000
10. Blood cancers (leukemia, lymphoma, and myeloma)[86]	56,000
11. Kidney disease[87]	47,000
12. Breast cancer[88]	41,000
13. Suicide[89]	41,000
14. Prostate cancer[90]	28,000
15. Parkinson's disease[91]	25,000

Certainly there are prescription medications that can help with some of these conditions. For example, you can take statin drugs for your cholesterol to lower risk of heart attacks, pop different pills and inject insulin for diabetes, and take a slew of diuretics and other blood pressure medications for hypertension. But there is only one unifying diet that may help prevent, arrest, or even reverse each of these killers. Unlike with medications, there isn't one kind of diet for optimal liver function and a different diet to improve our kidneys. A heart-healthy diet is a brain-healthy diet is a lung-healthy diet. The *same* diet that helps prevent cancer just so happens to be the same diet that may help prevent type 2 diabetes and every other cause of death on the top-fifteen list. Unlike drugs—which only target specific functions, can have dangerous side effects, and may only treat the symptoms of disease—a healthy diet can benefit all organ systems at once, has *good* side effects, and may treat the underlying cause of illness.

That one unifying diet found to best prevent and treat many of these chronic diseases is a whole-food, plant-based diet, defined as an eating pattern that encourages the consumption of unrefined plant foods and discourages meats, dairy products, eggs, and processed foods.[92] In this book, I don't advocate for a vegetarian diet or a vegan diet. I advocate for an evidence-based diet, and the best available balance of science suggests that the more whole plant foods we eat, the better—both to reap their nutritional benefits and to displace less healthful options.

Most doctor visits are for lifestyle-based diseases, which means they're preventable diseases.[93] As physicians, my colleagues and I were trained not to treat the root cause but rather the consequences by giving a lifetime's worth of medications to treat risk factors like high blood pressure, blood sugar, and cholesterol. This approach has been compared to mopping up the floor around an overflowing sink instead of simply turning off the faucet.[94] Drug companies are more than happy to sell you a new roll of paper towels every day for the rest of your life while the water continues to gush. As Dr. Walter Willett, the chair of nutrition at Harvard University's School of Public Health, put it: "The inherent problem is that most pharmacologic strategies do not address the underlying causes of ill health in Western countries, which are not drug deficiencies."[95]

Treating the cause is not only safer and cheaper but it can work better. So why don't more of my medical colleagues do it? Not only were they not trained how, doctors don't get paid for it. No one profits from lifestyle medicine (other than the patient!), so it's not a major part of medical training or practice.[96] That's just how the current system works. The medical system is set up to financially reward prescribing pills and procedures, not produce. After Dr. Ornish proved that heart disease could be reversed without drugs or surgery, he thought that his studies would have a meaningful effect on the practice of mainstream medicine. After all, he effectively found a cure for our number-one killer! But he was mistaken—not about his critically important findings regarding diet and disease reversal but about how much influence the business of medicine has on the practice of medicine. In his words, Dr. Ornish "realized reimbursement is a much more powerful determinant of medical practice than research."[97]

Though there are vested interests, such as the processed food and pharmaceutical industries, which fight hard to maintain the status quo, there is one corporate sector that actually benefits from keeping people healthy—namely, the insurance industry. Kaiser Permanente, the largest managed-care organization in the country, published a nutritional update for physicians in their official medical journal, informing their nearly fifteen thousand physicians that healthy eating may be "best achieved with a plant-based diet, which we define as a regimen that encourages whole, plant-based foods and discourages meats, dairy products, and eggs as well as all refined and processed foods."[98]

"Too often, physicians ignore the potential benefits of good nutrition and quickly prescribe medications instead of giving patients a chance to correct their disease through healthy eating and active living. . . . Physicians should consider recommending a plant-based diet to all their patients, especially those with high blood pressure, diabetes, cardiovascular disease, or obesity."[99] Physicians should give their patients a chance to first correct their disease themselves with plant-based nutrition.

The major downside Kaiser Permanente's nutritional update describes is that this diet may work a little too well. If people begin eating plant-based diets while still taking medications, their blood pressure or blood sugar could actually drop so low that physicians may need to adjust medications or eliminate them altogether. Ironically, the "side effect" of the diet may be not having to take drugs anymore. The article ends with a familiar refrain: Further research is needed. In this case, though, "Further research is needed to find ways to make plant-based diets the new normal. . . ."[100]

We're a long way off from Thomas Edison's 1903 prediction, but it is my hope that this book can help you understand that most of our leading causes of death and disability are more preventable than inevitable. The primary reason diseases tend to run in families may be that *diets* tend to run in families.

For most of our leading killers, nongenetic factors like diet can account for at least 80 or 90 percent of cases. As I noted before, this is based on the fact that the rates of cardiovascular disease and major cancers differ fivefold to a hundredfold around the world. Migration studies show this is not just genetics. When people move from low- to high-risk areas, their disease risk nearly always shoots up to match the new setting.[101] As well, dramatic changes in disease rates within a single generation highlight the primacy of external factors. Colon cancer mortality in Japan in the 1950s was less than one-fifth that of the United States (including Americans of Japanese ancestry).[102] But now colon cancer rates in Japan are as bad as they are in the United States, a rise that has been attributed in part to the fivefold increase in meat consumption.[103]

Research has shown us that identical twins separated at birth will get different diseases based on how they live their lives. A recent American Heart Association–funded study compared the lifestyles and arteries of nearly five hundred twins. It found that diet and lifestyle factors clearly trumped genes.[104] You share 50 percent of your genes with each of your parents, so if one parent dies of a heart attack, you know you've inherited some of that susceptibility. But even among identical twins who have the exact same genes, one could die early of a heart attack and the other could live a long, healthy life with clean arteries depending on what she ate and how she lived. Even if *both* your parents died with heart disease, you should be able to eat your way to a healthy heart. Your family history does not have to become your personal destiny.

Just because you're born with bad genes doesn't mean you can't effectively turn them off. As you'll see in the breast cancer and Alzheimer's disease chapters, even if you're born with high-risk genes, you have tremendous control over your medical destiny. Epigenetics is the hot new field of study that deals with this control of gene activity. Skin cells look and function a lot differently from bone cells, brain cells, or heart cells, but each of our cells has the same complement of DNA. What makes them act differently is that they each have different genes turned on or off. That's the power of epigenetics. Same DNA, but different results.

Let me give you an example of how striking this effect can be. Consider the humble honeybee. Queen bees and worker bees are genetically identical, yet queen bees lay up to two thousand eggs a day, while worker bees are functionally sterile. Queens live up to three years; workers may live only three weeks.[105] The difference between the two is diet. When the hive's queen is dying, a larva is picked by nurse bees to be fed a secreted substance called royal jelly. When the larva eats this jelly, the enzyme that had been silencing the expression of royal genes is turned off, and a new queen is born.[106] The queen has the exact same genes as any of the workers, but because of what she ate, different genes are expressed, and her life and life span are dramatically altered as a result.

Cancer cells can use epigenetics against us by silencing tumor-suppressor genes that could otherwise stop the cancer in its tracks. So even if you're born with good genes, cancer can sometimes find a way to turn them off. A number of chemotherapy drugs have been developed to restore our bodies' natural defenses, but their use has been limited due to their high toxicity.[107] There are, however, a number of compounds distributed widely throughout the plant kingdom—including beans, greens, and berries—that appear to have the same effect naturally.[108] For example, dripping green tea on colon, esophageal, or prostate cancer cells has been shown to reactivate genes silenced by the cancer.[109] This hasn't just been demonstrated in a petri dish, though. Three hours after eating a cup of broccoli sprouts, the enzyme that cancers use to help silence our defenses is suppressed in your bloodstream[110] to an extent equal to or greater than the chemotherapy agent specifically designed for that purpose,[111] without the toxic side effects.[112]

What if we ate a diet chock-full of plant foods? In the Gene Expression Modulation by Intervention with Nutrition and Lifestyle (GEMINAL) study, Dr. Ornish and colleagues took biopsies from men with prostate cancer before and after three months of intensive lifestyle changes that included a whole-food, plant-based diet. Without any chemotherapy or radiation, beneficial changes in gene expression for five hundred different genes were noted. Within just a few months, the expression of disease-preventing genes was boosted, and oncogenes that promote breast and prostate cancer were suppressed.[113]

Whatever genes we may have inherited from our parents, what we eat can affect how those genes affect our health. The power is mainly in our hands and on our plates.

This book is divided into two parts: the "why" and the "how." In part 1—the "why" to eat healthfully section—I will explore the role diet can play in the prevention, treatment, and reversal of the fifteen leading causes of death in the United States. I'll then take a closer look at more practical aspects of healthy eating in the "how" to eat healthfully section presented in part 2. For example, we'll see in part 1 *why* beans and greens are among the healthiest foods on earth. Then, in part 2, we'll take a look at *how* best to eat them—we'll explore such issues as how many greens to eat every day and whether they're best cooked, canned, fresh, or frozen. We'll see in part 1 why it's important to eat at least nine servings of fruits and vegetables daily, and then part 2 will help you decide whether to buy organic or conventional produce. I'll try to answer all the common questions I receive daily and then offer real-world tips for grocery shopping and meal planning to make it as easy as possible to best feed yourself and your family.

Besides writing more books, I intend to keep lecturing at medical schools and speaking at hospitals and conferences for as long as I can. I'm going to keep trying to ignite the spark that led my colleagues into the healing profession in the first place: to help people get better. There are tools missing from too many doctors' medical toolboxes, powerful interventions that can make many of our patients well again instead of merely slowing their decline. I'll keep working on trying to change the system, but you, the reader, don't have to wait. You can start now by following the recommendations within the following chapters. Eating healthier is easier than you think, it's inexpensive, and it might just save your life.

PART 1

CHAPTER 1

How Not to Die from Heart Disease

Imagine if terrorists created a bioagent that spread mercilessly, claiming the lives of nearly four hundred thousand Americans every year. That is the equivalent of one person every eighty-three seconds, every hour, around the clock, year after year. The pandemic would be front-page news all day, every day. We'd marshal the army and march our finest medical minds into a room to figure out a cure for this bioterror plague. In short, we'd stop at nothing until the terrorists were stopped.

Fortunately, we're not actually losing hundreds of thousands of people each year to a preventable threat . . . are we?

Actually, we are. This particular biological weapon may not be a germ released by terrorists, but it kills more Americans every few years than have all our past wars combined. It can be stopped not in a laboratory but right in our grocery stores, kitchens, and dining rooms. As far as weapons go, we don't need vaccines or antibiotics. A simple fork will do.

So what's going on here? If this epidemic is present on such a massive scale, yet so preventable, why aren't we doing more about it?

The killer I'm talking about is coronary heart disease, and it's affecting nearly everyone raised on the standard American diet.

Our Top Killer

America's number-one killer is a different kind of terrorist: fatty deposits in the walls of your arteries called atherosclerotic plaque. For most Americans raised on a conventional diet, plaque accumulates inside the coronary arteries—the blood vessels that crown the heart (hence "coronary") and supply it with oxygen-rich blood. This buildup of plaque, known as atherosclerosis, from the Greek words *athere* (gruel) and *sklerosis* (hardening), is the hardening of the arteries by pockets of cholesterol-rich gunk that builds up within the inner linings of the blood vessels. This process occurs over decades, slowly bulging into the space inside the arteries, narrowing the path for blood to flow. The restriction of blood circulation to the heart muscle can lead to chest pain and pressure, known as angina, when people try to exert themselves. If the plaque ruptures, a blood clot can form within the artery. This sudden blockage of blood flow can cause a heart attack, damaging or even killing part of the heart.

When you think about heart disease, you may think of friends or loved ones who suffered for years with chest pain and shortness of breath before they finally succumbed. However, for the majority of Americans who die suddenly from heart disease, the very first symptom may be their last.[1] It's called "sudden cardiac death." This is when death occurs within an hour of symptom onset. In other words, you may not even realize you're at risk until it's too late. You could be feeling perfectly fine one moment, and then an hour later, you're gone forever. That's why it's critical to prevent heart disease in the first place, before you even necessarily know you have it.

My patients often asked me, "Isn't heart disease just a consequence of getting old?" I can see why this is a common misconception. After all, your heart pumps literally billions of times during the average life span. Does your ticker just conk out after a while? No.

A large body of evidence shows there were once enormous swaths of the world where the epidemic of coronary heart disease simply didn't exist. For instance, in the famous China-Cornell-Oxford Project (known as the China Study), researchers investigated the eating habits and incidence of chronic disease among hundreds of thousands of rural Chinese. In Guizhou province, for example, a region comprising half a million people, over the course of three years, not a single death could be attributed to coronary artery disease among men under sixty-five.[2]

During the 1930s and 1940s, Western-trained doctors working throughout an extensive network of missionary hospitals in sub-Saharan Africa noticed that many of the chronic diseases laying waste to populations in the so-called developed world were largely absent across most of the continent. In Uganda, a country of millions in eastern Africa, coronary heart disease was described as "almost non-existent."[3]

But were the people of these nations simply dying early of other diseases, never living long enough to come down with heart disease? No. The doctors compared autopsies of Ugandans to autopsies of Americans who had died at the same age. The researchers found that out of 632 people autopsied in Saint Louis, Missouri, there had been 136 heart attacks. But in 632 age-matched Ugandans? A single heart attack. The Ugandans experienced more than one hundred times fewer heart attacks than the Americans. The doctors were so blown away that they examined another 800 deaths in Uganda. Out of more than 1,400 Ugandans autopsied, researchers found just one body with a small, healed lesion of the heart, meaning the attack wasn't even fatal. Then and now, in the industrialized world, heart disease is a leading killer. In central Africa, heart disease was so rare it killed fewer than one in a thousand.[4]

Immigration studies show that this resistance to heart disease is not just something in the Africans' genes. When people move from low-risk to high-risk areas, their disease rates skyrocket as they adopt the diet and lifestyle habits of their new homes.[5] The extraordinarily low rates of heart disease in rural China and Africa have been attributed to the extraordinarily low cholesterol levels among these populations. Though Chinese and African diets are very different, they share commonalities: They are both centered on plant-derived foods, such as grains and vegetables. By eating so much fiber and so little animal fat, their total cholesterol levels averaged under 150 mg/dL,[6,7] similar to people who eat contemporary plant-based diets.[8]

So what does all of this mean? It means heart disease may be a choice.

If you looked at the teeth of people who lived more than ten thousand years before the invention of the toothbrush, you'd notice they had almost no cavities.[9] They never flossed a day in their lives, yet no cavities. That's because candy bars hadn't been invented yet. The reason people get cavities now is that the pleasure they derive from sugary treats may outweigh the cost and discomfort of the dentist's chair. I certainly enjoy the occasional indulgence—I've got a good dental plan! But what if instead of the dental plaque on our teeth, we're talking about the atherosclerotic plaque building up in our arteries? We're not just talking about scraping tartar anymore. We're talking about life and death.

Heart disease is the number-one reason we and most of our loved ones will die. Of course, it's up to each of us to make our own decisions as to what to eat and how to live, but shouldn't we try to make these choices consciously by educating ourselves about the predictable consequences of our actions? Just as we could avoid sugary foods that rot our teeth, we can avoid the trans fat, saturated fat, and cholesterol-laden foods that clog up our arteries.

Let's take a look at the progression of coronary heart disease throughout life and learn how simple dietary choices at any stage may prevent, stop, and even reverse heart disease before it's too late.

Is Fish Oil Just Snake Oil?

Thanks in part to the American Heart Association's recommendation that individuals at high risk for heart disease should ask their physicians about omega-3 fish oil supplementation,[10] fish oil pills have grown into a multibillion-dollar industry. We now consume more than one hundred thousand tons of fish oil every year.[11]

But what does the science say? Are the purported benefits of fish oil supplementation for the prevention and treatment of heart disease just a fish tale? A systematic review and meta-analysis published in the *Journal of the American Medical Association* looked at all the best randomized clinical trials evaluating the effects of omega-3 fats on life span, cardiac death, sudden death, heart attack, and stroke. These included studies not only on fish oil supplements but also studies on the effects of advising people to eat more oily fish. What did they find? Overall, the researchers found no protective benefit for overall mortality, heart disease mortality, sudden cardiac death, heart attack, or stroke.[12]

What about for someone who had already had a heart attack and is trying to prevent another? Still no benefit was found.[13]

Where did we even get this idea that the omega-3 fats in fish and fish oil supplements are good for you? There was a notion that Eskimos were protected from heart disease, but that appears to be a complete myth.[14] Some early studies, however, looked promising. For example, the famous DART trial from the 1980s involving two thousand men found that those advised to eat fatty fish had a 29 percent reduction in mortality.[15] That's impressive, so it's no wonder the study got a lot of attention. But people seem to have forgotten about the sequel, the DART-2 trial, which found the exact opposite. Run by the same group of researchers, the DART-2 trial was an even bigger study—three thousand men—but this time, participants advised to eat oily fish and particularly those who were supplied with fish oil capsules had a *higher* risk of cardiac death.[16,17]

After putting all the studies together, researchers concluded that there was no longer justification for the use of omega-3s in everyday clinical practice.[18] What should doctors do when their patients follow the American Heart Association's advice and inquire about fish oil supplements? As the director of Lipids and Metabolism at Mount Sinai's cardiovascular institute put it: "Given this and other negative meta-analyses, our job [as doctors] should be to stop highly marketed fish oil supplementation to all our patients . . ."[19]

Heart Disease Starts in Childhood

In 1953, a study published in the *Journal of the American Medical Association* radically changed our understanding of the development of heart disease. Researchers conducted a series of three hundred autopsies on American casualties of the Korean War, with an average age of around twenty-two. Shockingly, 77 percent of soldiers already had visible evidence of coronary atherosclerosis. Some even had arteries that were blocked off 90 percent or more.[20] The study "dramatically showed that atherosclerotic changes appear in the coronary arteries years and decades before the age at which coronary heart disease (CHD) becomes a clinically recognized problem."[21]

Later studies of accidental death victims between the ages of three and twenty-six found that fatty streaks—the first stage of atherosclerosis—were found in nearly all American children by age ten.[22] By the time we reach our twenties and thirties, these fatty streaks can turn into full-blown plaques like those seen in the young American GIs of the Korean War. And by the time we're forty or fifty, they can start killing us off.

If there's anyone reading this over the age of ten, the question isn't whether or not you want to eat healthier to *prevent* heart disease but whether or not you want to *reverse* the heart disease you very likely already have.

Just how early do these fatty streaks start to appear? Atherosclerosis may start even before birth. Italian researchers looked inside arteries taken from miscarriages and premature newborns who died shortly after birth. It turns out that the arteries of fetuses whose mothers had high LDL cholesterol levels were more likely to contain arterial lesions.[23] This finding suggests that atherosclerosis may not just start as a nutritional disease of childhood but one during pregnancy.

It's become commonplace for pregnant women to avoid smoking and drinking alcohol. It's also never too early to start eating healthier for the next generation.

According to William C. Roberts, the editor in chief of the *American Journal of Cardiology*, the only critical risk factor for atherosclerotic plaque buildup is cholesterol, specifically elevated LDL cholesterol in your blood.[24] Indeed, LDL is called "bad" cholesterol, because it's the vehicle by which cholesterol is deposited into your arteries. Autopsies of thousands of young accident victims have shown that the level of cholesterol in the blood was closely correlated with the amount of atherosclerosis in their arteries.[25] To drastically reduce LDL cholesterol levels, you need to drastically reduce your intake of three things: trans fat, which comes from processed foods and naturally from meat and dairy; saturated fat, found mainly in animal products and junk foods; and to a lesser extent dietary cholesterol, found exclusively in animal-derived foods, especially eggs.[26]

Notice a pattern here? The three boosters of bad cholesterol—the number-one risk factor for our number-one killer—all stem from eating animal products and processed junk. This likely explains why populations living on traditional diets revolving around whole plant foods have largely remained free from the epidemic of heart disease.

It's the Cholesterol, Stupid!

Dr. Roberts hasn't only been editor in chief of the *American Journal of Cardiology* for more than thirty years; he's the executive director of the Baylor Heart and Vascular Institute and has authored more than a thousand scientific publications and written more than a dozen textbooks on cardiology. He knows his stuff.

In his editorial "It's the Cholesterol, Stupid!," Dr. Roberts argued (as noted earlier) that there is only one true risk factor for coronary heart disease: cholesterol.[27] You could be an obese, diabetic, smoking couch potato and *still* not develop atherosclerosis, he argues, as long as the cholesterol level in your blood is low enough.

The optimal LDL cholesterol level is probably 50 or 70 mg/dL, and apparently, the lower, the better. That's where you start out at birth, that's the level seen in populations largely free of heart disease, and that's the level at which the progression of atherosclerosis appears to stop in cholesterol-lowering trials.[28] An LDL around 70 mg/dL corresponds to a total cholesterol reading of about 150, the level below which no deaths from coronary heart disease were reported in the famous Framingham Heart Study, a generations-long project to identify risk factors for heart disease.[29] The population target should therefore be a total cholesterol level under 150 mg/dL. "If such a goal was created," Dr. Roberts wrote, "the great scourge of the Western world would be essentially eliminated."[30]

The average cholesterol for people living in the United States is much higher than 150 mg/dL; it hovers around 200 mg/dL. If your blood test results came back with a total cholesterol of 200 mg/dL, your physician might reassure you that your cholesterol is normal. But in a society where it's normal to die of heart disease, having a "normal" cholesterol level is probably not a good thing.

To become virtually heart-attack proof, you need to get your LDL cholesterol at least under 70 mg/dL. Dr. Roberts noted that there are only two ways to achieve this for our population: to put more than a hundred million Americans on a lifetime of medications or to recommend they all eat a diet centered around whole plant foods.[31]

So: drugs or diet. All health plans cover cholesterol-lowering statin drugs, so why change your diet if you can simply pop a pill every day for the rest of your life? Unfortunately, as we'll see in chapter 15, these drugs don't work nearly as well as people think, and they may cause undesirable side effects to boot.

Want Fries with That Lipitor?

The cholesterol-lowering statin drug Lipitor has become the best-selling drug of all time, generating more than $140 billion in global sales.[32] This class of drugs garnered so much enthusiasm in the medical community that some U.S. health authorities reportedly advocated they be added to the public water supply like fluoride is.[33] One cardiology journal even offered the tongue-in-cheek suggestion for fast-food restaurants to offer "McStatin" condiments along with ketchup packets to help neutralize the effects of unhealthy dietary choices.[34]

For those at high risk for heart disease who are unwilling or unable to bring down their cholesterol levels naturally with dietary changes, the benefits of statins generally outweigh the risks. These drugs do have side effects, though, such as the potential for liver or muscle damage. The reason some doctors routinely order regular blood tests for patients on these drugs is to monitor for liver toxicity. We can also test the blood for the presence of muscle breakdown products, but biopsies reveal that people on statins can show evidence of muscle damage even if their blood work is normal and they exhibit no symptoms of muscle soreness or weakness.[35] The decline in muscular strength and performance sometimes associated with these drugs may not be such a big deal for younger individuals, but they can place our seniors at increased risk for falls and injury.[36]

More recently, other concerns have been raised. In 2012, the U.S. Food and Drug Administration announced newly mandated safety labeling on statin drugs to warn doctors and patients about their potential for brain-related side effects, such as memory loss and confusion. Statin drugs also appeared to increase the risk of developing diabetes.[37] In 2013, a study of several thousand breast cancer patients reported that long-term use of statins may as much as double a woman's risk of invasive breast cancer.[38] The primary killer of women is heart disease, not cancer, so the benefits of statins may still outweigh the risks, but why accept any risk at all if you can lower your cholesterol naturally?

Plant-based diets have been shown to lower cholesterol just as effectively as first-line statin drugs, but without the risks.[39] In fact, the "side effects" of healthy eating tend to be good—*less* cancer and diabetes risk and *protection* of the liver and brain, as we'll explore throughout the rest of this book.

Heart Disease Is Reversible

It's never too early to start eating healthfully, but is it ever too late? Such lifestyle medicine pioneers as Nathan Pritikin, Dean Ornish, and Caldwell Esselstyn Jr. took patients with advanced heart disease and put them on the kind of plant-based diet followed by Asian and African populations who didn't suffer from heart disease. Their hope was that a healthy enough diet would stop the disease process and keep it from progressing further.

But instead, something miraculous happened.

Their patients' heart disease started to reverse. These patients were getting *better*. As soon as they stopped eating an artery-clogging diet, their bodies were able to start dissolving away some of the plaque that had built up. Arteries opened up without drugs or surgery, even in some cases of patients with severe triple-vessel heart disease. This suggests their bodies wanted to heal all along but were just never given the chance.[40]

Let me share with you what has been called the "best kept secret in medicine":[41] Given the right conditions, the body heals itself. If you whack your shin really hard on a coffee table, it can get red, swollen, and painful. But your shin will heal naturally if you just stand back and let your body work its magic. But what if you kept whacking it in the same place three times a day—say, at breakfast, lunch, and dinner? It would never heal.

You could go to your doctor and complain that your shin hurts. "No problem," he or she might say, whipping out a pad to write you a prescription for painkillers. You'd go back home, still whacking your shin three times a day, but the pain pills would make it feel *so* much better. Thank heavens for modern medicine! That's what happens when people take nitroglycerin for chest pain. Medicine can offer tremendous relief, but it's not doing anything to treat the underlying cause.

Your body wants to regain its health if you let it. But if you keep reinjuring yourself three times a day, you interrupt the healing process. Consider smoking and lung cancer risk: One of the most amazing things I learned in medical school was that within about fifteen years of stopping smoking, your lung-cancer risk approaches that of a lifelong nonsmoker.[42] Your lungs can clear out all that tar buildup and, eventually, it's almost as if you never smoked at all.

Your body wants to be healthy. And every night of your smoking life, as you fall asleep, that healing process is restarted until . . . *bam!*—you light up your first cigarette the next morning. Just as you can reinjure your lungs with every puff, you can reinjure your arteries with every bite. You can choose moderation and hit yourself with a *smaller* hammer, but why beat yourself up at all? You can choose to stop damaging yourself, get out of your own way, and let your body's natural healing process bring you back toward health.

Endotoxins Crippling Your Arteries

Unhealthy diets don't just affect the structure of your arteries; an unhealthy diet can also affect their functioning. Your arteries are not merely inert pipes through which blood flows. They are dynamic, living organs. We've known for nearly two decades that a single fast-food meal—Sausage and Egg Mc-Muffins were used in the original study—can stiffen your arteries within hours, cutting in half their ability to relax normally.[43] And just as this inflammatory state starts to calm down five or six hours later—lunchtime! You may once again whack your arteries with another load of harmful food, leaving many Americans stuck in a danger zone of chronic, low-grade inflammation. Unhealthy meals don't just cause internal damage decades down the road but right here and now, within hours of going into your mouth.

Originally, researchers blamed the animal fat or animal protein, but attention has recently shifted to bacterial toxins known as "endotoxins." Certain foods, such as meats, appear to harbor bacteria that can trigger inflammation dead or alive, even when the food is fully cooked. Endotoxins are not destroyed by cooking temperatures, stomach acid, or digestive enzymes, so after a meal of animal products, these endotoxins may end up in your intestines. They are then thought to be ferried by saturated fat across the gut wall into your bloodstream, where they can trigger the inflammatory reaction in your arteries.[44]

This may help explain the remarkable speed at which cardiac patients can experience relief when placed on a diet composed primarily of plant foods, including fruits, vegetables, whole grains, and beans. Dr. Ornish reported a 91 percent reduction in angina attacks within just a few weeks in patients placed on a plant-based diet both with[45] or without[46] exercise. This rapid resolution in chest pain occurred well before their bodies could have cleared the plaque from their arteries, suggesting plant-based diets don't just help clean out arteries but also improve their day-to-day function. In contrast, control-group patients who were instead told to follow the advice of their doctors had a 186 percent *increase* in angina attacks.[47] It's no surprise their conditions worsened, given that they continued to eat the same diet that crippled their arteries in the first place.

We've known about the dramatic power of dietary changes for decades. For example, there was a paper entitled "Angina and Vegan Diet" published in the *American Heart Journal* back in 1977. Vegan diets are exclusively plant based, avoiding meat, dairy, and eggs. Doctors described cases like that of Mr. F. W. (initials are often used to protect patient confidentiality), a sixty-five-year-old man with angina so severe he had to stop every nine or ten steps. He couldn't even make it to the mailbox. He was started on a vegan diet, and his pain improved within days. Within months, he was reportedly climbing mountains with no pain at all.[48]

Not ready to start eating healthier? Well, there is a new class of antiangina drugs, such as ranolazine (sold as Ranexa). A drug company executive suggested its product be used for people not "able to comply with the substantial dietary changes required to achieve a vegan diet."[49] The medication costs more than $2,000 a year, but the side effects are relatively minor, and it does work . . . technically speaking. At the highest dose, Ranexa was able to prolong exercise duration by 33.5 seconds.[50] More than half a minute! It doesn't look like those choosing the drug route will be climbing mountains anytime soon.

Brazil Nuts for Cholesterol Control?

Can a single serving of Brazil nuts bring down your cholesterol levels faster than statin drugs and keep them down even a month after that single meal?

It was one of the craziest findings I'd ever seen. Researchers from— where else?—Brazil gave ten men and women a single meal containing between one and eight Brazil nuts. Amazingly, compared to the control group who ate no nuts at all, just a single serving of four Brazil nuts almost immediately improved cholesterol levels. LDL—the "bad"—cholesterol levels were a staggering twenty points lower just nine hours after eating the Brazil nuts.[51] Even drugs don't work nearly that fast.[52]

Here's the truly insane part: The researchers went back and measured the study participants' cholesterol thirty days later. Even a month after ingesting a single serving of Brazil nuts, their cholesterol levels stayed down.

Normally, when a study comes out in the medical literature showing some too-good-to-be-true result like this, doctors wait to see the results replicated before they change their clinical practice and begin recommending something new to their patients, particularly when the study is done on only ten subjects, and especially when the findings seem too incredible to believe. But when the intervention is cheap, easy, harmless, and healthy—we're talking just four Brazil nuts per month—then in my opinion, the burden of proof is somewhat reversed. I think the reasonable default position is to do it until proven otherwise.

More is not better, however. Brazil nuts are so high in the mineral selenium that eating four every *day* may actually bump you up against the tolerable daily limit for selenium. Nevertheless, this is not something you have to worry about if you're only eating four Brazil nuts a month.

Follow the Money

Research showing that coronary heart disease can be reversed with a plant-based diet—with or without other healthy lifestyle changes—has been published for decades in some of the most prestigious medical journals in the world. Why hasn't this news translated into public policy yet?

In 1977, the U.S. Senate Committee on Nutrition and Human Needs tried to do just that. Known as the McGovern Committee, they released *Dietary Goals for the United States*, a report advising Americans to cut down on animal-based foods and increase their consumption of plant-based foods. As a founding member of Harvard University's nutrition department recalls, "The meat, milk and egg producers were very upset."[53] That's an understatement. Under industry pressure, not only was the goal to "decrease meat consumption" removed from the report but the entire Senate nutrition committee was disbanded. Several prominent senators reputedly lost their election bids as a result of supporting the report.[54]

In more recent years, it was uncovered that many members of the U.S. Dietary Guidelines Advisory Committee had financial ties to everything from candy bar companies to entities like McDonald's Council on Healthy Lifestyles and Coca-Cola's Beverage Institute for Health and Wellness. One committee member even served as "brand girl" for cake-mix maker Duncan Hines and then as the official Crisco "brand girl" before going on to help write the official *Dietary Guidelines for Americans*.[55]

As one commentator noted in the *Food and Drug Law Journal*, historically, the Dietary Guidelines Advisory Committee reports contained:

No discussion at all of the scientific research on the health consequences of eating meat. If the Committee actually discussed this research, it would be unable to justify its recommendation to eat meat, as the research would show that meat increases the risks of chronic diseases, contrary to the purposes of the Guidelines. Thus, by simply ignoring that research, the Committee is able to reach a conclusion that would otherwise look improper.[56]

What about the medical profession, though? Why haven't my colleagues fully embraced this research demonstrating the power of good nutrition? Sadly, the history of medicine holds many examples of the medical establishment rejecting sound science when it goes against the prevailing conventional wisdom. There's even a name for it: the "Tomato Effect." The term was coined in the *Journal of the American Medical Association* in reference to the fact that tomatoes were once considered poisonous and were shunned for centuries in North America, despite overwhelming evidence to the contrary.[57]

It's bad enough that most medical schools don't even require a single course on nutrition,[58] but it's even worse when mainstream medical organizations actively lobby *against* increased nutrition education for physicians.[59] When the American Academy of Family Physicians (AAFP) was called out on their proud new corporate relationship with Coca-Cola to support patient education on healthy eating, an executive vice president of the academy tried to quell protests by explaining that this alliance was not without precedent. After all, they'd had relationships with PepsiCo and McDonald's for some time.[60] Even before that, they had financial ties to cigarette maker Philip Morris.[61]

This argument didn't seem to placate the critics, so the AAFP executive quoted them the American Dietetic Association's policy statement that "[t]here are no good or bad foods, just good or bad diets." No bad foods? Really? The tobacco industry used to broadcast a similar theme: Smoking per se wasn't bad, only "excess" smoking.[62] Sound familiar? Everything in moderation.

The American Dietetic Association (ADA), which produces a series of nutrition fact sheets with guidelines on maintaining a healthy diet, also has its own corporate ties. Who writes these fact sheets? Food industry sources pay the ADA $20,000 per fact sheet to explicitly take part in the drafting process. So we can learn about eggs from the American Egg Board and about the benefits of chewing gum from the Wrigley Science Institute.[63]

In 2012, the American Dietetic Association changed its name to the Academy of Nutrition and Dietetics but didn't appear to change its policies. It continues to take millions of dollars every year from processed junk food, meat, dairy, soda, and candy bar companies. In return, the academy lets them offer official educational seminars to teach dietitians what to say to their clients.[64] When you hear the title "registered dietitian," this is the group they are registered through. Thankfully, a movement within the dietitian community, exemplified by the formation of the organization Dietitians for Professional Integrity, has started to buck this trend.

What about individual doctors, though? Why aren't all my colleagues telling their patients to lay off the Chick-fil-A? Insufficient time during office visits is a common excuse physicians cite, but the top reason doctors give for not counseling patients with high cholesterol to eat healthier is that they think patients may "fear privations related to dietary advice."[65] In other words, doctors perceive that patients would feel deprived of all the junk they're eating. Can you imagine a doctor saying, "Yeah, I'd like to tell my patients to stop smoking, but I know how much they love it"?

Neal Barnard, M.D., president of the Physicians Committee for Responsible Medicine, recently wrote a compelling editorial in the American Medical Association's journal of ethics, describing how doctors went from being bystanders—or even enablers—of smoking to leading the fight against tobacco. Doctors realized they were more effective at counseling patients to quit smoking if they no longer had tobacco stains on their own fingers.

Today, Dr. Barnard says, "Plant-based diets are the nutritional equivalent of quitting smoking."[66]

CHAPTER 2

How Not to Die from Lung Diseases

The worst death I ever witnessed was that of a man dying of lung cancer. I was interning at a public health hospital in Boston. Evidently, people dying behind bars looked bad for prison statistics, so terminally ill prisoners were shipped to my hospital for their final days, even if there was little we could do for them.

It was summer, and the prisoners' ward had no air-conditioning, at least for the inmates. We doctors could retreat to the chilled confines of the nursing station, but the inmates, handcuffed to their beds, just lay prostrate in the heat on that top floor of the tall, brick building. When they were shuffled down the hall in front of us, ankles chained together, they left a trail of sweat.

The night the man died, I was on one of my thirty-six-hour shifts. We worked 117-hour workweeks back then. It's amazing we didn't kill more people ourselves. Overnight, there were only two of us—myself and a moonlighting doctor who preferred to sleep for his $1,000 paycheck. So most of the time I was on my own to cover the hundreds of patients there, some of the sickest of the sick. It was on one of those nights that, staggering through a sleep-deprived haze, I got the call.

Up until then, all the deaths I had seen were those in which the patient was either dead on arrival or had died during cardiac "codes," when we try desperately, and nearly always unsuccessfully, to resuscitate.

This man was different.

He was wide-eyed, gasping for air, his cuffed hands clawing at the bed. The cancer was filling up his lungs with fluid. He was being drowned by lung cancer.

While he thrashed desperately, pleading, my mind was in medical mode, all protocols and procedures, but nothing much could be done. The man needed morphine, but that was held on the other side of the ward, and I'd never get to it in time, let alone back to him. I was not popular on the prison floor. I had once reported a guard for beating a sick inmate and was rewarded with death threats. There was no way they'd let me through the gates fast enough. I begged the nurse to try to get some, but she didn't make it back in time.

The man's coughing turned to gurgling. "Everything's going to be okay," I said. Immediately, I thought, *What a stupid thing to say to someone choking to death.* Just another lie in probably a long line of condescension from other authority figures throughout his life. Helpless, I turned from doctor back to human being. I took his hand in my own, which he then gripped with all his might, tugging me toward his tear-streaked, panic-stricken face. "I'm here," I said. "I'm right here." Our gaze remained locked as he suffocated right in front of me. It felt like watching someone being tortured to death.

Take a deep breath. Now imagine what it would feel like not to be able to breathe. We all need to take care of our lungs.

America's number-two killer, lung disease, claims the lives of about 300,000 people each year. And like our number-one domestic killer, heart disease, it's largely preventable. Lung disease can come in many forms, but the three types that kill the most people are lung cancer, chronic obstructive pulmonary disease (COPD), and asthma.

Lung cancer is our number-one cancer killer. Most of the 160,000 lung cancer deaths every year are the direct result of smoking. However, a healthy diet may help mitigate the DNA-damaging effects of tobacco smoke, as well as perhaps help prevent lung cancer from spreading.

COPD kills approximately 140,000 people annually, from either damage to the walls of tiny air sacs in the lungs (emphysema) or from inflamed and thickened airways plugged with thick mucus (chronic bronchitis). Although there is no cure for the permanent lung scarring that COPD causes, a diet rich in fruits and vegetables may help slow the progression of the disease and improve lung function for its thirteen million sufferers.

Finally, asthma, which claims 3,000 lives each year, is one of the most common chronic diseases among children, yet it may be largely preventable with a healthier diet. Research suggests a few extra daily servings of fruits and vegetables can reduce both the number of cases of asthma during childhood and the number of asthma attacks among people with the disease.

LUNG CANCER

Lung cancer is diagnosed about 220,000 times each year in the United States and causes more deaths annually than the next three cancers combined— those of the colon, breast, and pancreas.[1] At any given moment, nearly 400,000 Americans are living under lung cancer's dark shadow.[2] Unlike with heart disease, which has yet to be fully acknowledged as the direct result of an artery-clogging diet, there is widespread recognition that tobacco is by far the most common cause of lung cancer. According to the American Lung Association, smoking tobacco contributes to up to 90 percent of all lung cancer deaths. Men who smoke are twenty-three times more likely and women thirteen times more likely to develop lung cancer than nonsmokers. And smokers aren't just harming themselves; thousands of deaths each year have been attributed to secondhand smoke. Nonsmokers have a 20–30 percent higher risk of developing lung cancer if they're regularly exposed to cigarette smoke.[3]

Those warning labels on cigarette packs are everywhere now, but for a long time, the link between smoking and lung cancer was suppressed by powerful interest groups—much as the relationship between certain foods and other leading killers is suppressed today. For example, in the 1980s, Philip Morris, the nation's leading cigarette manufacturer, launched the notorious Whitecoat Project. The corporation hired doctors to publish ghostwritten studies purporting to negate links between secondhand smoke and lung disease. These papers cherry-picked various scientific reports to conceal and distort the damning evidence of the dangers of secondhand smoke. This whitewashing, coupled with the tobacco industry's clever marketing campaigns, including cartoonlike ads, helped hook generations of Americans onto their products.[4]

If, despite all the evidence and warnings, you're currently a smoker, the most important step you can take is to stop. Now. Please. The benefits of quitting are immediate. According to the American Cancer Society, just twenty minutes after quitting, your heart rate and blood pressure drop. Within a few weeks, your blood circulation and lung function improve. Within a few months, the sweeper cells that help clean the lungs, remove mucus, and reduce the risk of infection start to regrow. And within a year of quitting, your smoking-related risk of coronary heart disease becomes half that of current smokers.[5] As we saw in chapter 1, the human body possesses a miraculous ability to heal itself as long as we don't keep reinjuring it. Simple dietary changes may help to roll back the damage wrought by the carcinogens in tobacco smoke.

Load Up on Broccoli

First, it's important to understand the toxic effects of cigarettes on the lungs. Tobacco smoke contains chemicals that weaken the body's immune system, making it more susceptible to disease and handicapping its ability to destroy cancer cells. At the same time, tobacco smoke can damage cell DNA, increasing the chance for cancer cells to form and flourish in the first place.[6]

To test the power of dietary interventions to prevent DNA damage, scientists often study chronic smokers. Researchers rounded up a group of longtime smokers and asked them to consume twenty-five times more broccoli than the average American—in other words, a single stalk a day. Compared to broccoli-avoiding smokers, the broccoli-eating smokers suffered 41 percent fewer DNA mutations in their bloodstream over ten days. Is that just because the broccoli boosted the activity of the detoxifying enzymes in their livers, which helped clear carcinogens before they even made it to the smokers' cells? No, even when DNA was extracted from the subjects' bodies and exposed to a known DNA-damaging chemical, the genetic material from the broccoli eaters showed significantly less damage, suggesting that eating vegetables like broccoli may make you more resilient at a subcellular level.[7]

Now, don't think this means that eating a stalk of broccoli before smoking a pack of Marlboro Reds is going to completely erase the cancer-causing effects of cigarette smoke. It won't. But as you're trying to quit, such vegetables as broccoli, cabbage, and cauliflower may help prevent further damage.

The benefits of broccoli-family (cruciferous) vegetables may not stop there. While breast cancer is the most common internal cancer among American women, lung cancer is actually their number-one killer. About 85 percent of women with breast cancer are still alive five years after diagnosis, but the numbers are reversed when it comes to lung cancer: 85 percent of women die within five years of a lung cancer diagnosis. Ninety percent of those deaths are due to metastasis, the spread of the cancer to other parts of the body.[8]

Certain compounds in broccoli may have the potential to suppress this metastatic spread. In a 2010 study, scientists laid down a layer of human lung cancer cells in a petri dish and cleared a swath down the middle. Within twenty-four hours, the cancer cells had crept back together, and within thirty hours, the gap had closed completely. But when the scientists dripped some cruciferous-vegetable compounds onto the cancer cells, the cancer creep was stunted.[9] Whether or not eating broccoli will help prolong survival in cancer patients has yet to be tested in clinical trials, but the nice thing about healthy dietary interventions is that since they have no downsides, they can be added to whatever other treatments one chooses.

Smoking Versus Kale

Researchers have found that kale—that dark-green, leafy vegetable dubbed the "queen of greens"—might help control cholesterol levels. Researchers took thirty men with high cholesterol and had them consume three to four shots of kale juice a day for three months. That's like eating thirty pounds' worth of kale, or the amount the average American consumes in about a century. So what happened? Did they turn green and start to photosynthesize?

No. What the kale did do was substantially lower their bad (LDL) cholesterol and boost their good (HDL) cholesterol[10] as much as running three hundred miles.[11] By the end of the study, the antioxidant activity in the blood of most participants had shot up. But curiously, the antioxidant activity in a minority remained flat. Sure enough, these were the smokers. The free radicals created by the cigarettes were thought to have actively depleted the body of antioxidants. When your smoking habit erases the antioxidant-boosting effects of eight hundred cups of kale, you know it's time to quit.

Carcinogen-Blocking Effects of Turmeric

The Indian spice turmeric, which gives curry powder its characteristic golden color, may also help prevent some of the DNA damage caused by smoking. Since 1987, the National Cancer Institute has tested more than a thousand different compounds for "chemopreventive" (cancer-preventing) activity. Only a few dozen have made it to clinical trials, but among the most promising is curcumin, the bright-yellow pigment in turmeric.[12]

Chemopreventive agents can be classified into different subgroups based on which stage of cancer development they help to fight: Carcinogen blockers and antioxidants help prevent the initial triggering DNA mutation, and antiproliferatives work by keeping tumors from growing and spreading. Curcumin is special in that it appears to belong to all three groups, meaning it may potentially help prevent and/or arrest cancer cell growth.[13]

Researchers have investigated the effects of curcumin on the DNA-mutating ability of various carcinogens and found that curcumin was indeed an effective antimutagen against several common cancer-causing substances.[14] But these experiments were done in vitro, meaning effectively in a laboratory test tube. After all, it wouldn't be ethical to expose humans to nasty carcinogens to observe whether they got cancer. However, someone got the bright idea of finding a group of people who already, of their own accord, had carcinogens coursing through their veins. Smokers!

One way to measure the level of DNA-mutating chemicals in peoples' bodies is dripping their urine on bacteria growing in a petri dish. Bacteria, like all life on Earth, share DNA as a common genetic language. Unsurprisingly, scientists who tried this experiment found that the urine from nonsmokers caused far fewer DNA mutations—after all, they had a lot fewer carcinogens flowing through their systems. But when the smokers were given turmeric, the DNA-mutation rate dropped by up to 38 percent.[15] They weren't given curcumin pills; they merely got less than a teaspoon a day of just the regular turmeric spice you'd find at the grocery store. Of course, turmeric can't completely mitigate the effects of smoking. Even after the participants ate turmeric for a month, the DNA-damaging ability of the smokers' urine still exceeded that of the nonsmokers'. But smokers who make turmeric a staple of their diets may help lessen some of the damage.

The anticancer effects of curcumin extend beyond its ability to potentially prevent DNA mutations. It also appears to help regulate programmed cell death. Your cells are preprogrammed to die naturally to make way for fresh cells through a process known as apoptosis (from the Greek *ptosis*, falling, and *apo*, away from). In a sense, your body is rebuilding itself every few months[16] with the building materials you provide it through your diet. Some cells, however, overstay their welcome—namely, cancer cells. By somehow disabling their own suicide mechanism, they don't die when they're supposed to. Because they continue to thrive and divide, cancer cells can eventually form tumors and potentially spread throughout the body.

So how does curcumin affect this process? It appears to have the ability to reprogram the self-destruct mechanism back into cancer cells. All cells contain so-called death receptors that trigger the self-destruction sequence, but cancer cells can disable their own death receptors. Curcumin, however, appears able to reactivate them.[17] Curcumin can also kill cancer cells directly by activating "execution enzymes" called caspases inside cancer cells that destroy them from within by chopping up their proteins.[18] Unlike most chemotherapy drugs, against which cancer cells can develop resistance over time, curcumin affects several mechanisms of cell death simultaneously, making it potentially harder for cancer cells to avoid destruction.[19]

Curcumin has been found to be effective against a variety of other cancer cells in vitro, including those of the breast, brain, blood, colon, kidney, liver, lungs, and skin. For reasons not fully understood, curcumin seems to leave non-cancerous cells alone.[20] Unfortunately, turmeric has yet to be tested in clinical trials for the prevention or treatment of lung cancer, but with no downsides at culinary doses, I'd suggest trying to find ways to incorporate the spice into your diet. I offer a number of suggestions in part 2.

Dietary Secondhand Smoke

Though the majority of lung cancer is attributed to smoking, approximately a quarter of all cases occur in people who've never smoked.[21] Although some of these cases are due to secondhand smoke, another contributing cause may be another potentially carcinogenic plume: fumes from frying.

When fat is heated to frying temperatures, whether it be animal fat, such as lard, or plant fat, such as vegetable oil, toxic volatile chemicals with mutagenic properties (those able to cause genetic mutations) are released into the air.[22] This happens even before the "smoke point" temperature is reached.[23] If you do fry at home, good ventilation in the kitchen may reduce lung cancer risk.[24]

Cancer risk may also depend on what's being fried. A study of women in China found that smokers who stir-fried meat every day had nearly three times the odds of lung cancer compared to smokers who stir-fried foods other than meat on a daily basis.[25] This is thought to be because of a group of carcinogens called heterocyclic amines that are formed when muscle tissue is subjected to high temperatures. (We'll talk more about these in chapter 11.)

The effects of meat fumes can be hard to separate from the effects of eating the meat itself, but a recent study on pregnant women and barbecuing attempted to tease them out. When meat is grilled, polycyclic aromatic hydrocarbons (PAHs) are also produced, one of the probable carcinogens in cigarette smoke. The researchers discovered that not only was the ingestion of grilled meat in the third trimester associated with smaller birth weights, mothers merely exposed to the fumes tended to give birth to babies with a birth weight deficit. Exposure to the fumes was also associated with a smaller head size, an indicator of brain volume.[26] Air pollution studies suggest prenatal exposure to polycyclic aromatic hydrocarbons may then translate into adverse effects on children's future cognitive development (as manifested by a significantly lower IQ).[27]

Even just living next to a restaurant may pose a health hazard. Scientists estimated the lifetime cancer risk among those residing near the exhaust outlets at Chinese restaurants, American restaurants, and barbecue joints. While exposure to fumes from all three types of restaurants resulted in exposure to unsafe levels of PAHs, the Chinese restaurants proved to be the worst. This is thought to be due to the amount of fish being cooked,[28] as the fumes from pan-fried fish have been found to contain high levels of PAHs capable of damaging the DNA of human lung cells.[29] Given the excess cancer risk, the researchers concluded that it wouldn't be safe to live near the exhaust of a Chinese restaurant for more than a day or two a month.[30]

What about that enticing aroma of sizzling bacon? The fumes produced by frying bacon contain a class of carcinogens called nitrosamines.[31] Although all meat may release potentially carcinogenic fumes, processed meat like bacon may be the worst: A UC-Davis study found that bacon fumes cause about four times more DNA mutations than the fumes from beef patties fried at similar temperatures.[32]

What about tempeh bacon? Tempeh is a fermented soybean product used to make a variety of meat substitutes. Researchers compared the DNA-mutating effects of the fumes from frying bacon and beef to tempeh. The bacon and burger fumes were mutagenic, but the tempeh fumes were not. Nevertheless, it's still not a good idea to eat fried foods. Though no DNA changes were detected after exposure to tempeh smoke, the fried tempeh itself did cause some DNA mutations (though 45 times fewer than the beef and 346 times fewer than the bacon). The researchers proposed that these findings might account for the higher incidence of respiratory diseases and lung cancer among cooks and lower incidence overall among vegetarians.[33]

If you do need to be around frying bacon or eggs, it would be safer to limit your exposure by using a backyard grill. Studies show that the number of particles deposited into the lungs increases by a factor of ten when frying indoors versus outdoors.[34]

CHRONIC OBSTRUCTIVE PULMONARY DISEASE

Chronic obstructive pulmonary disease (COPD), such as emphysema and chronic bronchitis, is a condition that makes it difficult to breathe and gets worse and worse over time. In addition to shortness of breath, COPD can cause severe coughing, excess mucus production, wheezing, and chest tightness. The disease affects more than twenty-four million Americans.[35]

Smoking is far and away the leading cause of COPD, but other factors can contribute, such as prolonged exposure to air pollution. Unfortunately, there is no cure for COPD, but there is some good news: A healthy diet may help to prevent COPD and help keep it from getting worse.

Data going back fifty years show that a high intake of fruits and vegetables is positively associated with good lung function.[36] Just one extra serving of fruit each day may translate into a 24 percent lower risk of dying from COPD.[37] On the other hand, a twin pair of studies from Columbia and Harvard Universities found that consumption of cured meat—like bacon, bologna, ham, hot dogs, sausage, and salami—may increase the risk of COPD.[38,39] It's thought to be due to the nitrite preservatives in meat, which may mimic the lung-damaging properties of the nitrite by-products of cigarette smoke.[40]

What if you already have the disease? Can the same foods that appear to help prevent COPD be used to treat it? We didn't know until a landmark study was published in 2010. More than a hundred COPD patients were randomized into two groups—half were instructed to boost their fruit and vegetable consumption, while the others remained on their normal diet. Over the next three years, the standard-diet subjects became progressively worse, as expected. In contrast, the disease progression was halted in the group consuming more fruits and veggies. Not only did their lung function not get worse, it actually *improved* a little. The researchers suggested this could be due to a combination of the antioxidant and anti-inflammatory effects of the fruits and vegetables, along with a potential reduction in the consumption of meat, which is thought to act as a pro-oxidant.[41]

Regardless of the mechanism, a diet with more whole plant foods may help both prevent and arrest the progression of this leading killer.

ASTHMA

Asthma is an inflammatory disease characterized by recurring attacks of narrowed, swollen airways, causing shortness of breath, wheezing, and coughing. Asthma can start at any age, but it usually emerges during childhood. One of the most common chronic diseases in kids, asthma's prevalence has been increasing year after year.[42] In the United States, twenty-five million people suffer from asthma, and seven million of them are children.[43]

A groundbreaking study recently demonstrated that the rates of asthma vary dramatically around the world. The *International Study of Asthma and Allergies in Childhood* followed more than a million children in nearly one hundred countries, making it the most comprehensive survey ever undertaken of this disease. The study found a twentyfold to sixtyfold difference in the prevalence of

asthma, allergies, and eczema.[44] Why does the prevalence of rhinoconjunctivitis (itchy eyes and runny nose) range from 1 percent of children in parts of
India, for instance, to as much as 45 percent elsewhere?[45] While such factors as
air pollution and smoking rates may play a role, the most significant associations
were not with what was going into their lungs but what was going into their
stomachs.[46]

Adolescents living in areas where more starchy foods, grains, vegetables,
and nuts were consumed were significantly less likely to exhibit chronic symptoms of wheezing, allergic rhinoconjunctivitis, and allergic eczema.[47] Boys
and girls eating two or more servings of vegetables a day appear to have only
half the odds of suffering from allergic asthma.[48] In general, the prevalence of
asthma and respiratory symptoms reportedly appears to be lower among
populations eating more foods of plant origin.[49]

Foods of animal origin have been associated with increased asthma risk. A
study of more than one hundred thousand adults in India found that those who
consumed meat daily, or even occasionally, were significantly more likely to
suffer from asthma than those who excluded meat and eggs from their diets altogether.[50] Eggs (along with soda) have also been associated with asthma attacks
in children, along with respiratory symptoms, such as wheezing, shortness of
breath, and exercise-induced coughing.[51] Removing eggs and dairy from the diet
has been shown to improve asthmatic children's lung function in as few as eight
weeks.[52]

The mechanism by which diet affects airway inflammation may lie with the
thin coating of fluid that forms the interface between your respiratory-tract lining and the outside air. Using the antioxidants obtained from the fruits and vegetables you eat, this fluid acts as your first line of defense against the free radicals
that contribute to asthmatic airway hypersensitivity, contraction, and mucus
production.[53] Oxidation by-products can be measured in exhaled breath and
are significantly lowered by shifting toward a more plant-based diet.[54]

So if asthmatics eat fewer fruits and vegetables, does their lung function
decline? Researchers out of Australia tried removing fruits and vegetables from
asthma patients' diets to see what would happen. Within two weeks, asthma
symptoms grew significantly worse. Interestingly, the low-fruit, low-vegetable
diet used in the study—a restriction to no more than one serving of fruit
and two servings of vegetables per day—is typical of Western diets. In other
words, the diet they used experimentally to impair people's lung function and
worsen their asthma was effectively the standard American diet.[55]

What about improving asthma by adding fruits and vegetables? Researchers repeated the experiment, but this time increased fruit and vegetable

consumption to seven servings a day. This simple act of adding a few more fruits and vegetables to their daily diet ended up successfully cutting the study subjects' exacerbation rate in half.[56] That's the power of eating healthfully.

If it's the antioxidants, why not just take an antioxidant supplement? After all, popping a pill is easier than eating an apple. The reason is simple: Supplements don't appear to work. Studies have repeatedly shown that antioxidant supplements have no beneficial effects on respiratory or allergic diseases, underscoring the importance of eating whole foods rather than trying to take isolated components or extracts in pill form.[57] For example, the Harvard Nurses' Health Study found that women who obtained high levels of vitamin E from a nut-rich diet appeared to have nearly half the risk of asthma of those who didn't, but those who took vitamin E supplements saw no benefit at all.[58]

Who do you think did better? A group of asthma patients who ate seven servings a day of fruits and vegetables, or a group who ate three servings plus fifteen "serving equivalents" in pill form? Sure enough, the pills didn't seem to help at all. Improvements in lung function and asthma control were evident only after subjects increased their *actual* fruit and vegetable intake, strongly suggesting that consuming whole foods is paramount.[59]

If adding a few daily servings of fruits and vegetables can have such a significant effect, what if asthma sufferers were put on a diet composed entirely of plant foods? Researchers in Sweden decided to test out a strictly plant-based diet on a group of severe asthmatics who weren't getting better despite the best medical therapies—thirty-five patients with long-established, physician-verified asthma, twenty of whom had been admitted to hospitals for acute attacks during the previous two years. One patient had received emergency intravenous infusions a total of twenty-three times, another reported he'd been hospitalized more than a hundred times, and one subject had even suffered a cardiac arrest after an attack and had to be revived and placed on a ventilator.[60] These were some pretty serious cases.

Of the twenty-four patients who stuck with the plant-based diet, 70 percent improved after four months, and 90 percent improved within one year. And these were all people who had experienced no improvement in their conditions at all in the year prior to switching to a plant-based diet.[61]

Within just one year of eating healthier, all but two patients were able to drop their dose of asthma medication or get off their steroids and other drugs altogether. Objective measures like lung function and physical working capacity improved; meanwhile, subjectively, some patients said their improvement was so considerable that they felt like "they had a new life."[62]

There was no control group, so the placebo effect may have accounted for some of the improvement, but the nice thing about a healthier diet is that there are only good side effects. In addition to improvements in their asthma control, the study subjects lost an average of eighteen pounds, and their cholesterol and blood pressures got better. From a risk-benefit standpoint, then, it's definitely worth giving a plant-based diet a try.

The most lethal lung diseases vary widely in presentation and prognosis. As noted, smoking is far and away the leading cause of lung cancer and COPD, but diseases like asthma typically develop during childhood and can be associated with a range of contributing factors, such as low birth weight and frequent respiratory infections. While quitting smoking remains the most effective way to ward off the worst kinds of lung disease, we can also help the body bolster its defenses by eating a diet rich in protective plant foods. The same kind of diet that appears to help severe asthmatics may also help prevent all three diseases from occurring in the first place.

If you're one of the millions of Americans who already suffer from lung disease, quitting smoking and changing your diet can still make a difference. It's never too late to start living and eating healthier. The restorative powers of the human body are remarkable, but your body needs your help. By including foods that contain cancer-fighting compounds and loading up on antioxidant-rich fruits and veggies, you may be able to strengthen your respiratory defenses and breathe easier.

In my clinical practice, whenever I've felt under too much time pressure to address a patient's smoking or bad dietary habits, I stop and think back to the hideous death of that man in Boston. No one deserves to die like that. I'd like to think no one has to.

CHAPTER 3

How Not to Die from Brain Diseases

My mom's father died of a stroke, and her mother died of Alzheimer's disease.

As a kid, I loved going to see my grandma in Long Island. We lived out west, so I got to fly on a plane—sometimes all by myself! She was the perfect—and perfectly doting—grandmother. She'd want to take me to toy stores, but, geeky me, I just wanted to go to the library. When we'd get back to the house, my arms filled with borrowed books, she'd let me sit way back on her big couch—shoes off, of course—and read and draw pictures. Then she'd bring me blueberry muffins she made with a big mechanical mixer that took up half the kitchen counter.

Later in life, my grandma started to lose her mind. By then, I was in medical school, but my newfound knowledge was useless. She had turned. My previously sweet and stately grandmother? Now she threw things at people. She cursed. Her caretaker showed me the teeth marks on her arm where my once kind, loving grandma had bitten her.

That's the horror of brain disease. Unlike a problem with your foot or your back or even another vital organ, brain disease can attack your *self*.

The two most serious brain diseases are stroke, which kills nearly 130,000 Americans each year,[1] and Alzheimer's disease, which kills nearly 85,000.[2] Most strokes can be thought of as "brain attacks"—like heart attacks, but the rupturing plaques in your arteries cut off blood flow to parts of the brain rather than to parts of the heart. Alzheimer's is more like a mind attack.

Alzheimer's disease is one of the most physically and emotionally burdensome diseases, for both sufferers and caregivers. Unlike stroke, which can kill instantly and without any warning, Alzheimer's involves a slower, more subtle decline over months or years. Instead of cholesterol-filled plaques in your arteries, plaques made of a substance called amyloid develop in the brain tissue itself, associated with the loss of memory and, eventually, loss of life.

While the pathology of stroke and Alzheimer's are different, one key factor unites them: Mounting evidence suggests that a healthy diet may help prevent them both.

STROKE

In about 90 percent of strokes,[3] blood flow to part of the brain gets cut off, depriving it of oxygen and killing off the part fed by the clogged artery. That's called an ischemic stroke (from the Latin *ischaemia*, meaning "stopping blood"). A small minority of strokes are hemorrhagic strokes, which are caused by bleeding into the brain when a blood vessel bursts. The damage wrought by a stroke depends on which area of the brain was deprived of oxygen (or where bleeding occurred) and for how long the deprivation lasted. People who experience a brief stroke might only need to contend with arm or leg weakness, while those who suffer a major stroke can develop paralysis, lose the ability to speak, or, as is too often the case, die.

Sometimes the blood clot lasts only a moment—not long enough to notice but still long enough to kill off a tiny portion of your brain. These so-called silent strokes can multiply and slowly reduce cognitive function until full-blown dementia develops.[4] The goal is to reduce the risk of both the massive strokes that can kill you instantly and the ministrokes that kill you over the course of years. Just as with heart disease, a healthy diet can reduce stroke risk by reducing cholesterol and blood pressure while improving blood flow and antioxidant capacity.

Fiber! Fiber! Fiber!

In addition to its well-known effects on bowel health, high fiber intake appears to reduce the risk of cancers of the colon[5] and breast,[6] diabetes,[7] heart disease,[8] obesity,[9] and premature death in general.[10] A number of studies now show that high fiber intake may also help ward off stroke.[11] Unfortunately, less than 3 percent of Americans meet the minimum daily recommendation for fiber.[12] This means about 97 percent of Americans eat fiber-deficient diets. Fiber is naturally concentrated in only one place: whole plant foods. Processed foods have less, and animal-derived foods have no fiber at all. Animals have bones to hold them up; plants have fiber.

It apparently doesn't take much fiber to cut stroke risk. Increasing fiber intake by just seven grams a day may be associated with a 7 percent risk reduction.[13] Different strokes for different folks—depending, evidently, on how much fiber they ate. An additional seven grams of fiber is easy to add to your diet; it's the equivalent of a bowl of oatmeal with berries or a serving of baked beans.

How does fiber protect the brain? We're not exactly sure. We do know that fiber helps control your cholesterol[14] and blood sugar levels,[15] which can help reduce the amount of artery-clogging plaque in your brain's blood vessels. High-fiber diets may also lower blood pressure,[16] which reduces the risk of brain bleeds. But scientists don't have to know the exact mechanism before you act on this knowledge. As the biblical passage goes: "A man scatters seed on the ground . . . the seed sprouts and grows, though he does not know how." Had the farmer from scripture postponed his sowing until he understood the biology of seed germination, he wouldn't have lasted very long. So why not go ahead and reap the benefits of eating fiber by eating more unprocessed plant foods?

It's never too early to start eating healthier. Though stroke is considered an older person's disease—only about 2 percent of stroke deaths occur before the age of forty-five[17]—the risk factors may begin accumulating in childhood. In a remarkable study published recently, hundreds of children were followed for a period of twenty-four years, from junior high school to adulthood. Researchers found that low fiber intake early on was associated with stiffening of the arteries leading up to the brain—a key risk factor for stroke. By the time these adolescents were only fourteen, clear differences in arterial health were found for those consuming different amounts of fiber in their daily diets.[18]

Again, it did not appear to take much. One more apple, an extra quarter cup of broccoli, or just two tablespoons of beans a day during childhood could translate into a meaningful effect on artery health later in life.[19] If you *really* want to be proactive, the best available science[20] suggests you can minimize stroke risk by eating a minimum of 25 grams a day of soluble fiber (fiber that dissolves in water, typically found in beans, oats, nuts, and berries) *and* 47 daily grams of insoluble fiber (fiber that does not dissolve in water, found primarily in whole grains, such as brown rice and whole wheat). Granted, you'd have to eat an extraordinarily healthy diet to attain this level of fiber intake, far beyond what is arbitrarily determined as adequate by most health authorities.[21] Rather than patronizing you with what they think is "achievable"[22] by the masses, though, I wish these authorities would just tell you what the science says and let you make up your own mind.

Potassium

Take a plant, any plant, and burn it to ash. Throw that ash in a pot of water, boil it, skim off the ashes, and eventually you'll be left with a white residue known as potash ("pot ash"). Potash has been used for millennia for making everything from soap and glass to fertilizer and bleach. It wasn't until 1807 that an English chemist figured out that this "vegetable alkali" contained an undiscovered element, which he called pot-ash-ium—that is, potassium.

I mention this simply to emphasize the primary source of potassium in your diet—namely, plants. Every cell in your body requires potassium to function, and you need to get it from your diet. For much of human history, we ate so many plants that we got upward of 10,000 mg of potassium every day.[23] Nowadays, less than *2 percent* of Americans even reach the recommended daily intake of 4,700 mg.[24]

The major reason is simple: We don't eat enough unprocessed plant foods.[25] What does potassium have to do with stroke? A review of all the best studies on the relationship between potassium and our top-two killers, heart disease and stroke, determined that a 1,640 mg increase per day in potassium intake was associated with a 21 percent reduction in stroke risk.[26] That isn't enough to bring the average American's potassium levels to where they should be, but it's still enough to substantially reduce the risk of stroke. Imagine how much lower your risk would be if you doubled or tripled your intake of whole plant foods.

Bananas, although they've been marketed for their potassium content, aren't actually particularly rich in the mineral. According to the current U.S. Department of Agriculture database, bananas don't even make the list of the top-thousand foods with the highest levels of potassium; in fact, they come in at number 1,611, right after Reese's Pieces.[27] You'd have to eat a dozen bananas a day just to get the bare minimum recommended amount of potassium.

What are some of the truly potassium-rich foods? The healthiest common whole-food sources are probably greens, beans, and sweet potatoes.[28]

Citrus

Good news for all you orange lovers: Citrus fruit intake has been associated with reduced stroke risk—even more so than apples.[29] Say I can't compare them? I just did! The key may lie with a citrus phytonutrient called hesperidin, which appears to increase blood flow throughout the body, including the brain. Using a machine known as a doppler fluximeter, scientists can measure blood flow through the skin using a laser beam. If we hook people up to this machine and give them a solution containing the amount of hesperidin found in two cups of orange juice, blood pressure decreases and overall blood flow increases. When subjects drank straight orange juice instead of the hesperidin solution, their blood flow was even better. In other words, the stroke-reducing effects of oranges extend beyond just the hesperidin.[30] When it comes to food, the whole is often greater than the sum of its parts.

The positive effects of citrus fruits on blood flow don't require a machine to measure them. In one study, scientists recruited women who suffered from sensitivity to cold weather due to poor blood flow—women with chronically cold hands, feet, and toes—and placed them in a highly air-conditioned room. The women in the experimental group drank a solution containing actual citrus phytonutrients, while another (control) group drank a placebo (an artificially flavored orange drink). The placebo drinkers got colder and colder. Because of decreased blood flow, the temperature of their fingertips dropped nearly 9 degrees Fahrenheit during the course of the study. The fingertips of the women who drank real citrus, meanwhile, cooled less than half as fast, because their blood flow remained steadier. (The researchers also had both groups of women plunge their hands into icy water and saw the citrus drinkers recover about 50 percent faster than the control group.)[31]

So eating a few oranges before snowboarding may help keep your fingers and toes from getting as chilly. But while warm digits are nice, the reduced stroke risk associated with higher citrus intake is even nicer.

Optimal Sleep Duration and Stroke

Lack of sleep, or even too much of it, is associated with increased stroke risk.[32] But how much sleep may be too little? How much too much?

Scientists in Japan were the first to take a major stab at this question. They followed nearly 100,000 middle-aged men and women for fourteen years. Compared with people who slept an average of seven hours per night, subjects who got four hours of sleep or less, or ten hours or more, had roughly a 50 percent greater likelihood of dying from a stroke.[33]

A recent study of 150,000 Americans was able to examine the issue more thoroughly. Higher stroke rates were found among individuals sleeping six hours or less, or nine hours or more. Those at lowest risk got around seven or eight hours of sleep a night.[34] Large studies in Europe,[35] China,[36] and elsewhere[37] have confirmed that seven or eight hours appears to be associated with the lowest risk. We're not sure if the relationship is cause and effect, but until we know more, why not aim for that range? Sleep well!

Antioxidants and Stroke

Awarded the National Medal of Science, the highest honor for scientific achievement in this country, revered biochemist Earl Stadtman was quoted as saying, "Aging is a disease. The human lifespan simply reflects the level of free radical damage that accumulates in cells. When enough damage accumulates, cells can't survive properly anymore and they just give up."[38]

First proposed in 1972,[39] this concept—now called the mitochondrial theory of aging—suggests that free radical damage to your cells' power source, known as mitochondria, leads to a loss of cellular energy and function over time. This process may be a little like charging your iPod battery over and over—each time, its capacity gets less and less.

But what exactly are free radicals, and what can we do about them?

Here's my best attempt to simplify the quantum biology of oxidative phosphorylation: Plants get their energy from the sun. You take a plant and place it in the sun, and through a process called photosynthesis, the chlorophyll in the leaves harnesses the sun's energy and transfers it to tiny building blocks of matter called electrons.

The plant starts out with low-energy electrons and, using the energy of the sun, charges them up into high-energy electrons. In this way, plants store the sun's energy. When you then eat the plant (or the animals who ate the plant), these electrons (in the form of carbohydrates, protein, and fat) are delivered to all your cells. Then your mitochondria take the plant's power-packed electrons and use them as an energy source—that is, as fuel—and slowly release their energy. Mind you, this process has to occur in a precise, tightly controlled manner, because these electrons are packed with energy and are therefore volatile, like gasoline.

In fact, gasoline, petroleum, oil, and charcoal aren't called fossil fuels for nothing. The tanks of our SUVs are filled with mostly prehistoric plant matter that stored the energy of the sun that shone millions of years ago as high-energy electrons.

And just as it would be dangerous to toss a match into a can of gasoline and release all its energy at once, your body has to be cautious. That's why your cells take these same high-energy electrons from the plants you eat and release their energy in a controlled manner, like a gas stove—just a little at a time until the energy is used up. Your body then passes these used-up electrons to an all-important molecule you may have heard of: oxygen. In fact, the way poisons like cyanide kill you is by preventing your body from giving up these spent electrons to oxygen.

Fortunately, oxygen loves electrons, although maybe a little too much. While your body is taking its sweet time, slowly releasing the electrons' energy, the oxygen is waiting impatiently at the end of the line. Oxygen would love to get its grubby little hands on one of those high-energy electrons, but your body says, "Hold on. We've got to do this slowly, so wait your turn and let it cool off first. We'll give you your electron, but only after we've removed the energy so it's safe to play with."

Then the oxygen molecule gets all huffy and exclaims, "I could handle one of them souped-up electrons any day!" Pouting, it spies a stray high-energy electron sitting out in the open. Oxygen looks left, looks right, and then pounces on it. Your body isn't perfect; it can't keep an eye on oxygen all the time. About 1–2 percent[40] of all high-energy electrons that pass through your cells leak out where oxygen can grab them.

When oxygen gets its hands on a high-energy electron, it basically turns into the Hulk, changing from lowly oxygen into what's called superoxide, a type of free radical. A free radical is what it sounds like—a molecule that can be unstable, out of control, and violently reactive. The superoxide is just pumped up with energy and can start smashing around the cell, knocking stuff over and tripping over your DNA.

When superoxide comes in contact with DNA, it can damage your genes, which, if not repaired, can cause mutations in your chromosomes that may lead to cancer.[41] Thankfully, the body calls in its defense squad, known as *antioxidants*. They arrive at the scene and say, "Drop that electron!"

The superoxide fights back. "You want a piece of me, Mr. Vitamin C? Bring it!"

So the antioxidants proceed to jump the superoxide and wrestle the super-charged electron away from it, leaving behind poor little oxygen and its ripped jeans.

In scientific circles, the phenomenon by which oxygen molecules grab stray electrons and go crazy is called oxidant, or oxidative, stress. According to the theory, the resulting cellular damage is what essentially causes aging. Aging and disease have been thought of as the oxidation of the body. Those brown age spots on the back of your hands? They're just oxidized fat under the skin. Oxidant stress is thought to be why we all get wrinkles, why we lose some of our memory, why our organ systems break down as we get older. Basically, the theory goes, we're rusting.

You can slow down this oxidant process by eating foods containing lots of antioxidants. You can tell whether a food is rich in antioxidants by slicing it open, exposing it to air (oxygen), and then seeing what happens. If it turns brown, it's oxidizing. Think about our two most popular fruits: apples and bananas. They turn brown quickly, which means there aren't a lot of antioxidants inside them. (Most of the antioxidants in apples are in the peels.) Cut open a mango and what happens? Nothing happens, because there are lots of antioxidants in there. How do you keep fruit salad from turning brown? By adding lemon juice, which contains the antioxidant vitamin C. Antioxidants can keep your food from oxidizing, and they may do the same inside your body.

One of the diseases antioxidant-rich foods may help prevent is stroke. Swedish researchers followed more than thirty thousand older women over a period of a dozen years and found that those who ate the most antioxidant-rich foods had the lowest stroke risk.[42] Similar findings were reported in a younger cohort of men and women in Italy.[43] As with lung disease,[44] antioxidant *supplements* don't appear to help.[45] Mother Nature's powers cannot be stuffed into a pill.

Knowing this, scientists set out to find the most antioxidant-rich foods. Sixteen researchers spanning the globe published a database of the antioxidant power of more than a whopping three thousand foods, beverages, herbs, spices, and supplements. They tested everything from Cap'n Crunch cereal to the crushed dried leaves of the African baobab tree. They tested dozens of brands of beer to see which has the most antioxidants. (Santa Claus beer from Eggenberg, Austria, tied for first place.)[46] Sadly, beer represents Americans' fourth-largest source of dietary antioxidants.[47] You can check out the list to see where your favorite foods and beverages rank at this link: http://bit.ly/antioxidantfoods.

No need to post the 138-page chart on your fridge, though. Here's the simple rule: On average, plant foods contain *sixty-four times* more antioxidants than animal foods. As the researchers put it, "[A]ntioxidant rich foods originate from the plant kingdom while meat, fish and other foods from the animal kingdom are low in antioxidants."[48] Even the least healthy plant food I can think of, good old American iceberg lettuce (which is 96 percent water![49]), contains 17 units (daµmol using a modified FRAP assay) of antioxidant power. Some berries have more than 1,000 units, to give you some perspective, making iceberg look pretty pathetic. But compare iceberg lettuce's 17 units to fresh salmon, which has only 3 units. Chicken? As few as 5 units of antioxidant power. Skim milk or a hard-boiled egg? Just 4 units, and Egg Beaters has a big old goose egg—0 units. "Diets comprised mainly of animal-based foods are thus low in antioxidant content," concluded the research team, "while diets based mainly on a variety of plant-based foods are antioxidant rich, due to the thousands of bioactive antioxidant phytochemicals found in plants which are conserved in many foods and beverages."[50]

There is no need to necessarily cherry-pick individual foods to boost your antioxidant intake (though cherries do have up to 714!); you can simply strive to include a variety of fruits, vegetables, herbs, and spices at every meal. This way, you can continuously flood your body with antioxidants to help ward off stroke and other age-related diseases.

Antioxidants, in a Pinch

The food category that averages the most antioxidants is herbs and spices.

Let's say you prepare a nice healthy bowl of whole-wheat pasta with marinara sauce. Together, they may achieve a score of about 80 units of antioxidant power (approximately 20 units from the pasta and 60 from the sauce). Add in a handful of steamed broccoli florets, and you may end up with a delicious 150-unit meal. Not bad. Now sprinkle on a single teaspoonful of dried oregano or marjoram, oregano's sweeter and milder twin. That alone could double your meal's antioxidant power, up to more than 300 units.[51]

How about a bowl of oatmeal for breakfast? By adding just a half-teaspoon of cinnamon, you could bring the antioxidant power of your meal from 20 units to 120 units. And if you can stand the punch, adding even a pinch of cloves could bring your unassuming breakfast up to an antioxidant score of 160 units.

Plant-based meals tend to be rich in antioxidants on their own, but taking a moment to spice up your life may make your meal even healthier.

Antioxidant-rich diets appear to protect against stroke by preventing the circulation of oxidized fats in the bloodstream that can damage the sensitive walls of small blood vessels in the brain.[52] They can also help decrease artery stiffness,[53] prevent blood clots from forming,[54] and lower blood pressure[55] and inflammation. Free radicals can disfigure proteins in our bodies to the extent they become unrecognizable by our immune systems.[56] The inflammatory response this triggers can be prevented by saturating our bodies with sufficient antioxidants. Whereas all whole plant foods may have anti-inflammatory effects,[57] some plants are better than others. High-antioxidant fruits and vegetables, such as berries and greens, have been found to douse systemic inflammation significantly better than the same number of servings of more common low-antioxidant fruits and veggies, such as bananas and lettuce.[58]

The foods we choose make a difference.

ALZHEIMER'S DISEASE

In my clinical practice, the one diagnosis I dreaded giving more than cancer was Alzheimer's. It wasn't just because of the psychological toll to come for the patient but because of the emotional toll that would be placed on loved ones. The Alzheimer's Foundation estimates that fifteen million friends and family members supply more than fifteen billion unpaid hours annually caring for loved ones who may not even recognize them.[59]

Despite the billions of dollars spent on research, there is still neither a cure nor an effective treatment for the disease, which invariably progresses to death. In short, Alzheimer's is reaching a state of crisis—emotionally, economically, and even scientifically. Over the past two decades, more than seventy-three thousand research articles have been published on the disease. That's about a hundred papers a day. Yet very little clinical progress has been made in treating or even understanding it. And a total cure is likely impossible, given that lost cognitive function in Alzheimer's patients may never be regained due to fatally damaged neuronal networks. Dead nerve cells cannot be brought back to life. Even if drug companies can figure out how to halt the disease's progression, for many patients, the damage has already been done, and the individual's personality may be forever lost.[60]

The good news, as a senior scientist at the Center for Alzheimer's Research entitled a review article, is that "Alzheimer's Disease Is Incurable but Preventable."[61] Diet and lifestyle changes could potentially prevent millions of cases a year.[62] How? There is an emerging consensus that "what is good for our hearts is also good for our heads,"[63] because clogging of the arteries inside of the brain with atherosclerotic plaque is thought to play a pivotal role in the development of Alzheimer's disease.[64] It is not surprising, then, that the dietary centerpiece of the 2014 "Dietary and Lifestyle Guidelines for the Prevention of Alzheimer's Disease," published in the journal *Neurobiology of Aging*, was: "Vegetables, legumes (beans, peas, and lentils), fruits, and whole grains should replace meats and dairy products as primary staples of the diet."[65]

Is Alzheimer's a Vascular Disorder?

In 1901, a woman named Auguste was taken to an insane asylum in Frankfurt, Germany, by her husband. She was described as a delusional, forgetful, disoriented woman who "could not carry out her homemaking duties."[66] She was seen by a Dr. Alzheimer and was to become the subject of the case that made Alzheimer a household name.

On autopsy, Alzheimer described the plaques and tangles in her brain that would go on to characterize the disease. But lost in the excitement of discovering a new disease, a clue may have been overlooked. He wrote, *"Die größeren Hirngefäße sind arteriosklerotisch verändert,"* which translates to "The larger cerebral vessels show arteriosclerotic change." He was describing the hardening of arteries inside his patient's brain.[67]

We generally think of atherosclerosis as a condition of the heart, but it's been described as "an omnipresent pathology that involves virtually the entire human organism."[68] You have blood vessels in every one of your organs, including your brain. The concept of "cardiogenic dementia," first proposed in the 1970s, suggested that because the aging brain is highly sensitive to a lack of oxygen, lack of adequate blood flow may lead to cognitive decline.[69] Today, we have a substantial body of evidence strongly associating atherosclerotic arteries with Alzheimer's disease.[70]

Autopsies have shown repeatedly that Alzheimer's patients tend to have significantly more atherosclerotic plaque buildup and narrowing of the arteries within the brain.[71,72,73] Normal resting cerebral blood flow—the amount of blood circulating to the brain—is typically about a quart per minute. Starting in adulthood, people appear to naturally lose about half a percent of blood flow per year. By age sixty-five, this circulating capacity could be down by as much as 20 percent.[74] While such a drop alone may not be sufficient to impair brain function, it can put you close to the edge. The clogging of the arteries inside, and leading to, the brain with cholesterol-filled plaque can drastically reduce the amount of blood—and therefore oxygen—your brain receives. Supporting this theory, autopsies have demonstrated that Alzheimer's patients had particularly significant arterial blockage in the arteries leading to the memory centers of their brains.[75] In light of such findings, some experts have even suggested that Alzheimer's be reclassified as a vascular disorder.[76]

There are limitations to how much we can glean from autopsy studies, however. For example, perhaps a person's dementia led to his or her poor diet rather than vice versa. To further assess the role of clogged brain arteries in the development of Alzheimer's, researchers followed about four hundred people who were just starting to lose their mental faculties, which is called mild cognitive impairment. Special brain-artery scans were employed to evaluate the amount of arterial blockage in each patient's brain. The researchers found that the cognition and daily functioning of those with the least narrowing of the arteries in their heads remained stable over the course of the four-year study. Meanwhile, subjects with more arterial blockage lost significant brain function, and those with the worst cases of plaque buildup declined rapidly, doubling their likelihood of progressing to full-blown Alzheimer's. The researchers concluded: "An inefficient blood supply to the brain has very grave consequences on brain function."[77]

A study of three hundred Alzheimer's patients found that treating vascular risk factors, such as high cholesterol and blood pressure, may even slow the progression of the disease but not stop it.[78] That's why prevention is the key. Cholesterol doesn't just help generate atherosclerotic plaques within your brain arteries; it may help seed the amyloid plaques that riddle the brain tissue of Alzheimer's victims.[79] Cholesterol is a vital component of your cells, which is why your body makes all that you need. Consuming excess cholesterol, and especially trans and saturated fats, can raise your blood cholesterol level.[80] Too much cholesterol in your blood is not only considered the primary risk factor for heart disease[81] but is also unanimously recognized as a risk factor for Alzheimer's disease.[82]

Autopsies have revealed that Alzheimer's brains have significantly more cholesterol buildup than normal brains.[83] We used to think that the pool of cholesterol in the brain was separate from the cholesterol circulating in the blood, but there is growing evidence to the contrary.[84] Excess cholesterol in the blood can lead to excess cholesterol in the brain, which may then help trigger the clumping of amyloid seen in Alzheimer's brains. Under an electron microscope, we can see the clustering of amyloid fibers on and around tiny crystals of cholesterol.[85] And indeed, advanced brain imaging techniques, such as PET scans, have shown a direct correlation between the amount of LDL ("bad") cholesterol in the blood and amyloid buildup in the brain.[86] Drug companies have hoped to capitalize on this connection to sell cholesterol-lowering statin drugs to prevent Alzheimer's, but statins themselves can cause cognitive impairment, including short- and long-term memory loss.[87] For people unwilling to change their diets, the benefits of statins outweigh the risks,[88] but it's better to lower your cholesterol levels naturally by eating healthier to help preserve your heart, brain, and mind.

Genetics or Diet?

This dietary concept may be surprising, because most of the popular press today treats Alzheimer's as a genetic disease. They say it's your genes, rather than your lifestyle choices, that determine whether or not you'll succumb. However, when you examine the distribution of Alzheimer's disease around the world, that argument begins to crumble.

The rates of Alzheimer's vary tenfold around the world, even taking into account that some populations live longer than others.[89] For example, in rural Pennsylvania, if you knew one hundred senior citizens, it is likely that an average of nineteen of them would develop Alzheimer's disease within the next decade. However, that number would probably be closer to just three out of one hundred if you lived in rural Ballabgarh, in India.[90] How do we know some populations aren't just more genetically susceptible? Because of migration studies, in which disease rates within the same ethnic group are compared between their current locale and their homeland. For example, the Alzheimer's rates among Japanese men living in the United States are significantly higher than those of Japanese men living in Japan.[91] The Alzheimer's rates among Africans in Nigeria are up to four times lower than those of African Americans in Indianapolis.[92]

Why does living in the United States increase dementia risk?

The balance of evidence suggests that the answer lies in the American diet. Of course, in our new global world, you don't have to move to the West to adopt a Western diet. In Japan, the prevalence of Alzheimer's has shot up over the past few decades, thought to be due to the shift from a traditional rice-and-vegetable-based diet to one featuring triple the dairy and six times the meat. The closest correlation researchers found between diet and dementia was animal fat consumption; animal fat intake shot up nearly 600 percent between 1961 and 2008.[93] A similar trend linking diet and dementia was found in China.[94] With diets Westernizing globally, Alzheimer's rates are expected to continue to increase, writes one researcher in the *Journal of Alzheimer's Disease*, "unless dietary patterns change to those with less reliance on animal products. . . ."[95]

The lowest validated rates of Alzheimer's disease in the world are found in rural India,[96] where people eat traditional, plant-based diets centered on grains and vegetables.[97] In the United States, those who don't eat meat (including poultry and fish) appear to cut their risk of developing dementia in half. And the longer meat is avoided, the lower dementia risk may fall. Compared to those eating meat more than four times a week, those who have eaten vegetarian diets for thirty years or more had three times lower risk of becoming demented.[98]

Surely genetic factors play some part? They do. Back in the 1990s, scientists discovered a gene variant called apolipoprotein E4, or ApoE4, that makes you more susceptible to getting Alzheimer's. Everyone has some form of ApoE, but about one in seven people have a copy of the E4 gene that is linked to the disease. It's been shown that if you inherit one ApoE4 gene from your mother or father, your risk of getting Alzheimer's may triple. If you get the ApoE4 gene from both parents—which about one in fifty people do—you might end up with nine times the risk.[99]

What does the ApoE gene do? It makes the protein that's the principal cholesterol carrier in the brain.[100] The E4 variant may lead to an abnormal accumulation of cholesterol within brain cells, which could trigger Alzheimer's pathology.[101] This mechanism may explain the so-called Nigerian paradox. The highest frequency of the ApoE4 variant occurs in Nigerians,[102] who surprisingly also have some of the lowest rates of Alzheimer's.[103] Wait a second. The population with the highest rate of the "Alzheimer's gene" has one of the lowest rates of Alzheimer's disease? This contradiction may be explained by Nigerians' extremely low blood-cholesterol levels, thanks to a diet low in animal fat[104] and consisting mainly of grains and vegetables.[105] So, it seems, diet can trump genetics.

Consider that in one study of a thousand people over a period of two decades, the presence of the ApoE4 gene, unsurprisingly, was found to more than double the odds of Alzheimer's. But in those same subjects, high blood cholesterol was found to nearly *triple* the odds. The researchers suspect that controlling such risk factors as high blood pressure and cholesterol could substantially reduce the risk of Alzheimer's, dropping the odds from up around ninefold with the dreaded, double-barreled ApoE4 down to just twice the risk.[106]

Too often, doctors and patients have a fatalistic approach to chronic degenerative diseases, and Alzheimer's is no exception.[107] "It's all in your genes," they say, "and what will happen will happen." Research shows that although you might have been dealt some poor genetic cards, you may be able to reshuffle the deck with diet.

Preventing Alzheimer's with Plant Foods

Alzheimer's manifests as a disease of the elderly, but like heart disease and most cancers, it's a disease that may take decades to develop. At the risk of sounding like a broken record (or should I say an MP3 glitch?), it's never too early to start eating healthier. Dietary decisions you make now may directly influence your health much later in life, including the health of your brain.

Most Alzheimer's sufferers aren't diagnosed until they're in their seventies,[108] but we now know that their brains began deteriorating long before that. Based on thousands of autopsies, pathologists seemed to detect the first silent stages of Alzheimer's disease—what appear to be tangles in the brain—in half of people by age fifty and even 10 percent of those in their twenties.[109] The good news is that the clinical manifestation of Alzheimer's disease—like heart disease, lung disease, and stroke—may be preventable.

Plant-based diets are recommended in Alzheimer's prevention guidelines because of which foods they tend to accentuate and which they tend to reduce.[110] The Mediterranean diet, for example, which is higher in vegetables, beans, fruits, and nuts, and lower in meats and dairy products, has been associated with slower cognitive decline and lower risk of Alzheimer's.[111] When researchers tried to tease out the protective components, the critical ingredients appeared to be the diet's high vegetable content and lower ratio of saturated to unsaturated fats.[112] This conclusion aligns with that of the Harvard Women's Health Study, which found that higher saturated fat intake (sourced predominantly from dairy, meat, and processed foods) was associated with a significantly worse trajectory of cognition and memory. Women with the highest saturated fat intake had a 60–70 percent greater chance of cognitive deterioration over time. Women with the lowest saturated fat intake had the brain function, on average, of women six years younger.[113]

The benefits of a plant-based diet may also be due to the plants themselves. Whole plant foods contain thousands of compounds with antioxidant properties,[114] some of which can traverse the blood-brain barrier and may provide neuroprotective effects[115] by defending against free radicals (see page 48)—that is, protecting against the "rusting" of the brain. Your brain is only about 2 percent of your body weight but may consume up to 50 percent of the oxygen you breathe, potentially releasing a firestorm of free radicals.[116] Special antioxidant pigments in berries[117] and dark-green leafies[118] may make them the brain foods of the fruit and vegetable kingdom.

The first human study to show that blueberries improve memory abilities in older adults exhibiting early cognitive deterioration was published in 2010.[119] Then, in 2012, Harvard University researchers actually quantified these findings by using data from the Nurses' Health Study, in which the diets and health of sixteen thousand women were followed starting in 1980. They found that women who consumed at least one serving of blueberries and two servings of strawberries each week had slower rates of cognitive decline—by as much as two and a half years—compared with those who didn't eat berries. These results suggest that simply eating a handful of berries every day, one easy and delicious dietary tweak, may slow your brain's aging by more than two years.[120]

Even just drinking fruit and vegetable juices may be beneficial. A study that followed nearly two thousand people for about eight years found that people who drank fruit and vegetable juices regularly appeared to have a 76 percent lower risk of developing Alzheimer's disease. "Fruit and vegetable juices may play an important role in delaying the onset of Alzheimer's disease," the researchers concluded, "particularly among those who are at high risk for the disease."[121]

The researchers suspect the active ingredient may be a class of powerful brain-accessing antioxidants called polyphenols. If that's the case, Concord (purple) grape juice may be the best choice,[122] although whole fruits are generally preferable to juices.[123] Concord grapes aren't always in season, though, so look for cranberries, which are also packed with polyphenols[124] and can typically be found frozen year-round. (Later in this book, I offer my Pink Juice recipe for a whole-food cranberry cocktail with twenty-five times fewer calories and at least eight times the phytonutrient content of store-bought cranberry "juice." See page 151.)

Beyond their antioxidant activity, polyphenols have been shown to protect nerve cells in vitro by inhibiting the formation of the plaques[125] and tangles[126] that characterize Alzheimer's brain pathology. In theory, they could also "pull out"[127] metals that accumulate in certain brain areas and may play a role in the development of Alzheimer's and other neurodegenerative diseases.[128] Polyphenols are one of the reasons I make specific recommendations for berries and green tea in part 2.

Treating Alzheimer's with Saffron

Despite the billions poured into Alzheimer's research, there is no effective treatment to reverse the progression of the disease. There are medications that can help manage the symptoms, though, and so can something found right in your grocery store.

Although some remarkable benefits have been reported in anecdotal case studies with the spice turmeric,[129] the best data we have on spice-based interventions for Alzheimer's is for saffron. A spice derived from the flower of *Crocus sativus*, saffron was found in a double-blind trial to help diminish the symptoms of Alzheimer's disease. In a sixteen-week study, Alzheimer's patients with mild to moderate dementia who took saffron capsules displayed significantly better cognitive function on average than a group of patients who took a placebo.[130]

continued

How about putting saffron head-to-head against one of the most popular Alzheimer's drugs on the market: donepezil (commonly marketed under the brand name Aricept)? A twenty-two-week double-blind study (meaning that neither the researchers nor the subjects knew who was on the drug and who was on the spice until the study's conclusion) found that saffron appears just as effective at treating Alzheimer's symptoms as the leading drug.[131] Unfortunately, working just as well as medication isn't saying much,[132] but at least a person doesn't have to risk the drug's side effects, most typically nausea, vomiting, and diarrhea.[133]

While there is no proven way to halt the progression of Alzheimer's, if you do know anyone suffering from the disease, regularly cooking him or her saffron-spiced paella may help.

Gerontotoxins

Each of us contains tens of billions of miles of DNA—enough for one hundred thousand round trips to the moon if you uncoiled each strand and placed them end to end.[134] How do our bodies keep it from all getting tangled up? Enzymes known as sirtuins keep our DNA wrapped up nice and neat around spool-like proteins.

Although they were only discovered recently, sirtuins represent one of the most promising areas of medicine, as they appear to be involved in promoting healthy aging and longevity.[135] Autopsy studies show the loss of sirtuin activity is closely associated with the hallmarks of Alzheimer's disease—namely, the accumulation of plaques and tangles in the brain.[136] Suppression of this key host defense is considered a central feature of Alzheimer's.[137] The pharmaceutical industry is trying to come up with drugs to increase sirtuin activity, but why not just prevent its suppression in the first place? You may be able to do this by reducing your dietary exposure to advanced glycation end products, or AGEs.[138]

AGE is an appropriate acronym, as they are considered "gerontotoxins,"[139] meaning aging toxins (from the Greek *geros*, meaning "old age," as in "geriatric"). AGEs are thought to accelerate the aging process by cross-linking proteins together, causing tissue stiffness, oxidative stress, and inflammation. This process may play a role in cataract formation and macular degeneration in the eye, as well as damage to the bones, heart, kidneys, and liver.[140] They may also impact the brain, appearing to accelerate the slow shrinkage of your brain as you age[141] and suppressing your sirtuin defenses.[142]

Older adults with high levels of AGEs in their blood[143] or urine[144] appear to suffer an accelerated loss of cognitive function over time. Elevated levels of AGEs are also found in the brains of Alzheimer's victims.[145] Where are these AGEs coming from? Some are produced and detoxified naturally in your body,[146] but other than cigarette smoke,[147] major sources are "meat and meat-derived products" exposed to dry-heat cooking methods.[148] AGEs are formed primarily when fat- and protein-rich foods are exposed to high temperatures.[149]

More than five hundred foods have been tested for AGE content, everything from Big Macs and Hot Pockets to coffee and Jell-O. In general, meat, cheese, and highly processed foods had the highest AGE content, and grains, beans, breads, vegetables, fruits, and milk had the least.[150]

The top-twenty most AGE-contaminated products per serving tested were various brands of:

1. BBQ chicken	11. Pan-fried turkey burger
2. Bacon	12. BBQ chicken
3. Broiled hot dog	13. Oven-fried fish
4. Roasted chicken thigh	14. McDonald's Chicken McNuggets
5. Roasted chicken leg	
6. Pan-fried steak	15. Broiled chicken
7. Oven-fried chicken breast	16. Pan-fried turkey burger
8. Deep-fried chicken breast	17. Baked chicken
9. Stir-fried steak strips	18. Pan-fried turkey burger
10. McDonald's Chicken Selects breast strips	19. Boiled hot dog
	20. Broiled steak[151]

You get the idea.

Yes, cooking methods matter. A baked apple has three times more AGEs than a raw apple, and a broiled hot dog has more than a boiled hot dog. But the source is what matters most: a baked apple has 45 units of AGEs compared to a raw apple's 13 units, while a broiled hot dog has 10,143 units compared to a boiled hot dog's 6,736. The researchers recommend cooking meat using moist-heat cooking methods, such as steaming or stewing, but even boiled fish has more than 10 times more AGEs than a sweet potato roasted for an hour. Meat averages about 20 times more AGEs than highly processed foods like breakfast cereals and about 150 times more than fresh fruits and vegetables. Poultry was the worst, containing about 20 percent more AGEs than beef. The researchers concluded that even a modest reduction in meat intake could realistically cut daily AGE intake in half.[152]

Because sirtuin suppression is both preventable and reversible by AGE reduction, avoiding high-AGE foods is seen as potentially offering a new strategy to combat the Alzheimer's epidemic.[153]

Halting Cognitive Decline with Exercise?

There is exciting news for people on the verge of losing their mental faculties. In a 2010 study published in the *Archives of Neurology,* researchers took a group of people with mild cognitive impairment—those who are starting to forget things, for example, or regularly repeating themselves—and had them engage in aerobic exercise for forty-five to sixty minutes a day, four days a week, for six months. The control group was instructed to simply stretch for the same time periods.[154]

Memory tests were performed before and after the study. Researchers found that in the control (stretching) group, cognitive function continued to decline. But the exercising group not only didn't get worse, they got *better.* The exercisers got more test answers correct after six months, indicating their memory had improved.[155]

Subsequent studies using MRI scans found that aerobic exercise can actually reverse age-related shrinkage in the memory centers of the brain.[156] No such effect was found in the stretching and toning control groups or a nonaerobic strength-training group.[157] Aerobic exercise can help improve cerebral blood flow, improve memory performance, and help preserve brain tissue.

Let's face it: A life without memories is not much of a life. Whether those memories are lost all at once from a massive stroke, chipped away by ministrokes that leave little holes in the brain, or destroyed from within by degenerative diseases like Alzheimer's, eating and living healthier can help eliminate some of the worst risk factors for the most serious brain diseases.

But the key is starting early. High cholesterol and high blood pressure may begin hurting your brain as early as your twenties. By your sixties and seventies, when the damage can become apparent, it may already be too late.

Like so many other organs, the brain possesses a miraculous ability to heal itself, to forge new synaptic connections around old ones, to learn and relearn. That is, however, if you don't keep damaging it three times a day. A wholesome diet and exercise may offer your best hope for remaining sharp and healthy into your twilight years.

Thankfully, I can conclude this chapter on a happier note than how it began. Despite our family history, both my mom and my brother, Gene, now eat a healthy, plant-based diet, and my mom shows no signs of succumbing to the same fate of brain disease that claimed the lives of her parents. Although Gene and I know that one day we'll eventually lose her, given her new healthy diet, our hope is that we won't lose our mom before she is gone.

CHAPTER 4

How Not to Die from Digestive Cancers

Every year, Americans lose more than five million years of life from cancers that may have been prevented.[1] Only a small percentage of all human cancers are attributable to purely genetic factors. The rest involve external factors, particularly our diet.[2]

Your skin covers about twenty square feet. Your lungs, if you were to flatten out all the tiny air pockets, could cover hundreds of square feet.[3] And your intestines? Counting all the little folds, some scientists estimate that your gut would blanket thousands of square feet,[4] vastly more expansive than your skin and lungs combined. What you eat may very well be your primary interface with the outside world. This means that regardless of the carcinogens that could be lurking in the environment, your greatest exposure may be through your diet.

Three of the most common cancers of the digestive tract kill approximately one hundred thousand Americans each year. Colorectal (colon and rectal) cancer, which claims fifty thousand lives annually,[5] ranks among the most commonly diagnosed of all cancers. Thankfully, it is also among the most treatable if caught early enough. Pancreatic cancer, on the other hand, is virtually a death sentence for the approximately forty-six thousand people who develop it every year.[6] Few survive beyond a year after diagnosis, which means prevention is paramount. Esophageal cancer, which affects the tube between your mouth and stomach, is also frequently fatal for its eighteen thousand annual victims.[7] The foods you eat can indirectly affect cancer risk, for example, by exacerbating acid reflux, a risk factor for esophageal cancer, or through direct contact with the lining of the digestive tract.

COLORECTAL CANCER

The average person has about a one-in-twenty chance of developing colorectal cancer over the course of his or her lifetime.[8] Fortunately, it is among the most treatable cancers, as regular screening has enabled doctors to detect and remove the cancer before it spreads. There are more than one million colorectal cancer survivors in the United States alone, and, among those diagnosed before the cancer has spread beyond the colon, the five-year survival rate is about 90 percent.[9]

But, in its early stages, colorectal cancer rarely causes symptoms. If the cancer is not caught until later stages, treatment is more difficult and less effective. Starting at age fifty until age seventy-five, you should either get stool testing every year, stool testing every three years plus a sigmoidoscopy every five years, or a colonoscopy every ten years.[10] For more on the risks and benefits of these options, see chapter 15. While regular screenings are certainly sensible to detect colorectal cancer, preventing it in the first place is even better.

Turmeric

India's gross domestic product (GDP) is about eight times less than that of the United States,[11] and about 20 percent of its population lives below the poverty line,[12] yet cancer rates in India are much lower than in the United States. Women in the United States may have ten times more colorectal cancer than women in India, seventeen times more lung cancer, nine times more endometrial cancer and melanoma, twelve times more kidney cancer, eight times more bladder cancer, and five times more breast cancer. Men in the United States appear to have eleven times more colorectal cancer than men in India, twenty-three times more prostate cancer, fourteen times more melanoma, nine times more kidney cancer, and seven times more lung and bladder cancer.[13] Why such a discrepancy? The regular use of the spice turmeric in Indian cooking has been proposed as one possible explanation.[14]

In chapter 2, we saw how curcumin, the yellow pigment in the spice turmeric, may be effective against cancer cells in vitro. Very little of the curcumin you eat gets absorbed into your bloodstream, however, so it may never come in sufficient contact with tumors outside the digestive tract.[15] But what doesn't get absorbed into your blood ends up in your colon, where it could impact the cells lining your large intestine where cancerous polyps develop.

The emergence of colorectal cancer can be broken up into three stages. The first sign may be what are called "aberrant crypt foci," or abnormal clusters of cells along the lining of the colon. Next come polyps that grow from that inner surface. The final stage is thought to occur when a benign polyp transforms into a cancerous one. The cancer can then eat through the wall of the colon and spread throughout the body. To what degree can curcumin block each stage of colorectal cancer?

Studying smokers, who tend to have a lot of aberrant crypt foci, investigators found that curcumin consumption could reduce the number of those cancer-associated structures in their rectums up to nearly 40 percent, from eighteen down to eleven, within just thirty days. The only reported side effect was a yellow tint to their stools.[16]

What if polyps have already developed? Six months of curcumin, along with another phytonutrient called quercetin, which is found naturally in such fruits and vegetables as red onions and grapes, were found to decrease the number and size of polyps by more than half in patients with a hereditary form of colorectal cancer. Again, virtually no side effects were reported.[17]

What if the polyps have already transformed into cancer? In a last-ditch attempt to save the lives of fifteen patients with advanced colorectal cancer who didn't respond to any of the standard chemotherapy agents or radiation, oncologists started them on a turmeric extract. In the two to four months of treatment, it appeared to help stall the disease in one-third of the patients, five out of fifteen.[18]

If we were talking about some new kind of chemotherapy drug that only helped one in three people, you'd have to weigh that against all the serious side effects. But when it's just some plant extract shown to be remarkably safe, even if it just helped one in a hundred, it would be worth considering. With no serious downsides, a one-in-three potential benefit for end-stage cancer seems like it would spark further research, right? But who's going to pay for a study of something that can't be patented?[19]

The low cancer rate in India may be due in part to the spices they use, but it may also stem from the types of foods they are putting those spices on. India is one of the world's largest producers of fruits and vegetables, and only about 7 percent of the adult population eats meat on a daily basis. What most of the population does eat every day are dark-green, leafy vegetables and legumes,[20] such as beans, split peas, chickpeas, and lentils, which are packed with another class of cancer-fighting compounds called phytates.

Stool Size Matters

The bigger and more frequent your bowel movements are, the healthier you may be. Based on a study of twenty-three populations across a dozen countries, the incidence of colon cancer appears to skyrocket as the average daily stool weight drops below about a half a pound. Populations dropping quarter pounders appear to have three times the rate of colon cancer. You can measure the weight of your stools with a simple bathroom scale. No, not that way—by weighing yourself before and after you "go."

The link between stool size and colon cancer may be related to "intestinal transit time," the number of hours it takes for food to travel from mouth to toilet. The larger the stool, the quicker the transit time, as it's easier for your intestines to move things along.[21] People don't realize you can have daily bowel movements and still effectively be constipated; what you're flushing today you may have eaten last week.

How long it takes food to get from one end to the other can depend on gender and dietary habits. Food goes through men eating plant-based diets in just a day or two, but this transit time takes as long as five or more days among those eating more conventional diets. Women eating plant-based diets also average a day or two, but the average intestinal transit time in most women eating conventional diets may be four days.[22] So you can be regular but four days late. You can measure your own oral-anal transit time by eating some beets and noting when your stools turn pink. If that takes less than twenty-four to thirty-six hours, you're probably meeting the healthy half-pound target.[23]

Constipation is the most common gastrointestinal complaint in the United States, leading to millions of doctor visits each year.[24] But beyond just the discomfort, the straining associated with trying to pass small, firm stools may play a role in a host of health problems, including hiatal hernia, varicose veins, hemorrhoids,[25] and painful conditions with names like anal fissure.[26]

Constipation can be considered a nutrient-deficiency disease, and that nutrient is fiber.[27] Just as you can get scurvy if you don't get enough vitamin C, you can get constipation if you don't get enough fiber. Since fiber is found only in plant foods, it's no surprise that the more plants you eat, the less likely you are to be constipated. For example, a study comparing thousands of omnivores, vegetarians, and vegans found that those eating strictly plant-based diets are three times more likely to have daily bowel movements.[28] Looks like vegans are just regular people.

Phytates

Colorectal cancer is the second-leading cause of cancer-related death in the United States,[29] yet in some parts of the world, it's practically unheard of. The highest rates have been recorded in Connecticut, and the lowest in Kampala, Uganda.[30] Why is colorectal cancer so much more prevalent in Western cultures? Seeking answers to this question, renowned surgeon Denis Burkitt spent twenty-four years in Uganda. Many of the Ugandan hospitals Dr. Burkitt visited had never even seen a case of colon cancer.[31] He eventually came to the conclusion that fiber intake was the key,[32] as most Ugandans consumed diets centered around whole plant foods.[33]

Subsequent research has suggested that dietary prevention of cancer may involve something other than just fiber. For instance, colorectal cancer rates are higher in Denmark than in Finland,[34] yet Danes consume slightly more dietary fiber than Finns.[35] What other protective compounds might explain the low cancer rates among plant-based populations? Well, fiber isn't the only thing found in whole plant foods that's missing from processed and animal-based foods.

The answer might lie in natural compounds called phytates, which are found in the seeds of plants—in other words, in all whole grains, beans, nuts, and seeds. Phytates have been shown to detoxify excess iron in the body, which otherwise can generate a particularly harmful kind of free radical called hydroxyl radicals.[36] The standard American diet may therefore be a double whammy when it comes to colorectal cancer: Meat contains the type of iron (heme) particularly associated with colorectal cancer[37] but lacks, as do refined plant foods, the phytates to extinguish these iron-forged free radicals.

For many years, phytates were maligned as inhibitors of mineral absorption, which is why you might have heard advice to roast, sprout, or soak your nuts to get rid of the phytates. In theory, this would allow you to absorb more minerals, such as calcium. This belief stemmed from a series of laboratory experiments on puppies from 1949 that suggested that phytates had a bone-softening, anticalcifying effect,[38] as well as from subsequent studies with similar findings on rats.[39] But more recently, in light of actual human data, phytates' image has undergone a complete makeover.[40] Those who eat more high-phytate foods actually tend to have a greater bone mineral density,[41] less bone loss, and fewer hip fractures.[42] Phytates appear to protect bone in a manner similar to that of antiosteoporosis drugs like Fosamax,[43] but without the risk of osteonecrosis (bone rot) of the jaw, a rare, potentially disfiguring side effect associated with that class of drugs.[44]

Phytates may also help protect against colorectal cancer. A six-year study of about thirty thousand Californians found that higher meat consumption was associated with higher risk of colon cancer. Unexpectedly, white meat appeared to be worse. Indeed, those who ate red meat at least once each week had about double the risk of developing colon cancer; that risk appeared to triple, however, for those who ate chicken or fish once or more a week.[45] Eating beans, an excellent source of phytates, was found to help mediate some of that risk, so your colon cancer risk may be determined by your meat-to-vegetable ratio.

There may be as much as an eightfold difference in colorectal cancer risk between the two extremes—high-vegetable, low-meat diets and low-vegetable, high-meat diets.[46] So it may not be enough to just cut down on how much meat is in your diet; you also need to eat more plants. The National Cancer Institute's Polyp Prevention Trial found that those who increased their bean consumption by even less than one-quarter cup a day appeared to cut their odds of precancerous colorectal polyp recurrence by up to 65 percent.[47]

Of all the wonderful nutrients in beans, why do we credit the phytates with reduced risk? Petri-dish studies have shown that phytates inhibit the growth of virtually all human cancer cells tested so far—including cancers of the colon, breast, cervix, prostate, liver, pancreas, and skin[48]—while leaving normal cells alone.[49] This is the mark of a good anticancer agent, the ability to discriminate between tumor cells and normal tissue. When you eat whole grains, beans, nuts, and seeds, phytates are rapidly absorbed into the bloodstream and readily taken up by tumor cells. Tumors concentrate these compounds so efficiently that phytate scans can be used to trace the spread of cancer within the body.[50]

Phytates target cancer cells through a combination of antioxidant, anti-inflammatory, and immune-enhancing activities. Besides affecting the cancer cells directly, phytates have been found to boost the activity of natural killer cells, which are white blood cells that form your first line of defense by hunting down and disposing of cancer cells.[51] Phytates can also play a role in your last line of defense, which involves starving tumors of their blood supply. There are many phytonutrients in plant foods that can help block the formation of new blood vessels that feed tumors, but phytates also appear able to disrupt existing tumor supply lines.[52] Similarly, many plant compounds appear able to help slow down and even stop cancer cell growth,[53] but phytates can sometimes also cause cancer cells to apparently revert back to their normal state—in other words, to stop behaving like cancer. This cancer cell "rehabilitation" has been demonstrated in vitro in colon cancer cells,[54] as well as in cancer cells of the breast,[55] liver,[56] and prostate.[57]

Phytates do have side effects, but they all appear to be good. High phytate intake has been associated with less heart disease, less diabetes, and fewer kidney stones. In fact, some researchers have suggested that phytates be considered an essential nutrient. Like vitamins, phytates participate in important biochemical reactions in the body. Your levels fluctuate with dietary intake, and insufficient consumption is associated with diseases that can be moderated by eating adequate amounts. Maybe phytates should be considered "Vitamin P."[58]

Reversing Rectal Polyps with Berries?

There are many ways the healthfulness of different fruits and vegetables can be compared, such as by nutrient content or antioxidant activity. Ideally, we would use a measure involving actual biological activity. One way to do this is by measuring the suppression of cancer cell growth. Eleven common fruits were tested by dripping their extracts on cancer cells growing in a petri dish. The result? Berries came out on top.[59] Organically grown berries in particular may suppress cancer cell growth better than those grown conventionally.[60] But a laboratory is different from real life. These findings are only applicable if the active components of the food are absorbed into your system and manage to find their way to budding tumors. Colorectal cancer, however, grows out of the inner lining of your intestines, so what you eat may have a direct effect regardless. So researchers decided to give berries a try.

Familial adenomatous polyposis is an inherited form of colorectal cancer caused by a mutation in your tumor-suppression genes. People who are affected develop hundreds of polyps in their colons, some of which inevitably turn cancerous. Treatment can involve prophylactic colectomy, where the colon is removed early in life as a preventive step. There was a drug that appeared able to cause polyps to regress, but it was pulled from the market after it killed tens of thousands of people.[61] Could berries also cause polyps to retreat without the fatal side effects? Yes. After nine months of daily treatment with black raspberries, the polyp burden of fourteen patients with familial adenomatous polyposis was cut in half.[62]

Normally, polyps would have to be surgically removed, but the berries seemed to have made them disappear naturally. The method by which the berries were administered, though, was anything but natural. The researchers used a shortcut, giving the berries as suppositories. Don't try this at home! After they inserted the equivalent of eight pounds of raspberries into patients' rectums over those nine months, some of the patients suffered from torn anuses.[63] The hope is that research will one day show similar cancer-fighting effects of berries taken the old-fashioned way—through the mouth.

Too Much Iron?

In 2012, the results from two major Harvard University studies were published. The first, known as the Nurses' Health Study, began following the diets of about 120,000 women aged thirty to fifty-five starting back in 1976; the second, the Health Professionals Follow-Up Study, followed about 50,000 men aged forty to seventy-five. Every four years, researchers checked in with the study participants to keep track of their diets. By 2008, a total of about 24,000 subjects had died, including approximately 6,000 from heart disease and 9,000 from cancer.[64]

After the results were analyzed, the researchers found that the consumption of both processed and unprocessed red meat was associated with an increased risk of dying from cancer and heart disease and shortened life spans overall. They reached this conclusion even after controlling for (factoring in) age, weight, alcohol consumption, exercise, smoking, family history, caloric intake, and even the intake of whole plant foods, such as whole grains, fruits, and vegetables. In other words, the study subjects apparently weren't dying early because they ate less of some beneficial compound like phytates in plants. The findings suggest there may be something harmful in the meat itself.

Imagine the logistics of following more than 100,000 people for decades. Now imagine a study five times that size. The largest study of diet and health in history is the NIH-AARP study, cosponsored by the National Institutes of Health and the American Association of Retired Persons. Over the course of a decade, researchers followed about 545,000 men and women aged fifty to seventy-one in the largest study of meat and mortality ever conducted. The scientists came to the same conclusion as the Harvard researchers: Meat consumption was associated with increased risk of dying from cancer, dying from heart disease, and dying prematurely in general. Again, this was after controlling for other diet and lifestyle factors, effectively excluding the possibility that people who ate meat also smoked more, exercised less, or failed to eat their fruits and veggies.[65] The accompanying editorial in the American Medical Association's *Archives of Internal Medicine* (titled "Reducing Meat Consumption Has

Multiple Benefits for the World's Health") called for a "major reduction in total meat intake."[66]

What does meat contain that may raise the risk of premature death? One of the possibilities is heme iron, the form of iron found predominantly in blood and muscle. Because iron can generate cancer-causing free radicals by acting as a pro-oxidant,[67] iron can be considered a double-edged sword—too little of it and you risk anemia, too much and you may increase risk of cancer and heart disease.

The human body has no specific mechanism to rid itself of excess iron.[68] Instead, humans have evolved to tightly regulate the amount of iron absorbed. If you don't have enough iron circulating in your body, your intestines begin boosting iron absorption; if you have too much iron in circulation, your intestines decrease absorption. But this thermostat-like system only works effectively with the primary source of iron in the human diet: the nonheme iron variety found predominantly in plant foods. Once you have a sufficient amount of iron in your blood, your body is about five times more effective at blocking the absorption of excess iron from plant foods than from animal foods.[69] This may be why heme iron is associated with cancer[70] and heart disease risk.[71] Similarly, heme iron is associated with higher risk of diabetes, but nonheme iron is not.[72]

If we remove iron from people's bodies, can we decrease cancer rates? Studies have found that people randomized to give regular blood donations to reduce their iron stores appear to cut their risk of getting and dying from new gut cancers by about half over a five-year period.[73] The findings were so remarkable that an editorial in the *Journal of the National Cancer Institute* responded that "these results almost seem too good to be true."[74]

Donating blood is great, but we should also try to prevent the excess buildup of iron in the first place. The meat industry is working on coming up with additives that "suppress the toxic effects of heme iron,"[75] but a better strategy may be to emphasize plant sources in your diet, which your body can better manage.

Getting Enough Iron on a Plant-Based Diet

Compared with people who eat meat, vegetarians tend to consume more iron (as well as more of most nutrients),[76] but the iron in plant foods is not absorbed as efficiently as the heme iron in meat. While this can be an advantage in preventing iron overload, about one in thirty menstruating women in the United States lose more iron than they take in, which can lead to anemia.[77] Women who eat plant-based diets do not appear to have higher rates of iron deficiency anemia than women who eat a lot of meat,[78] but all women of childbearing age need to ensure adequate iron intake.

Those diagnosed with iron deficiency should talk with their doctors about first trying to treat it with diet, as iron supplements have been shown to increase oxidative stress.[79] The healthiest sources of iron are whole grains, legumes, nuts, seeds, dried fruits, and green, leafy vegetables. Avoid drinking tea with meals, as that can inhibit iron absorption. Consuming vitamin C–rich foods can improve iron absorption. The amount of vitamin C in a single orange can enhance iron absorption as much as three- to sixfold, so those trying to boost their iron absorption should reach for some fruit instead of a cup of tea.[80]

PANCREATIC CANCER

My grandfather died of pancreatic cancer. By the time the first symptom arose—a dull ache in his gut—it was too late. That's why we need to prevent it in the first place.

Pancreatic cancer is among the most lethal forms of cancer, with just 6 percent of patients surviving five years after diagnosis. Thankfully, it's relatively rare, killing only about forty thousand Americans each year.[81] As many as 20 percent of pancreatic cancer cases may be a result of tobacco smoking.[82] Other modifiable risk factors include obesity and heavy alcohol consumption.[83] As we'll see, specific dietary factors may also play a significant role in the development of this deadly disease.

For instance, how the fat in one's diet may contribute to pancreatic cancer risk has long been a subject of debate. The inconsistency of research findings on the impact of total fat intake may be partly because different fats affect risk differently. The previously mentioned NIH-AARP study was large enough to be able to tease out what kind of fat was most associated with pancreatic cancer. It was the first to separate out the role of fats from plant sources, such as those found in nuts, seeds, avocados, and olive and vegetable oils, versus all animal sources, including meats, dairy products, and eggs. The consumption of fat from all animal sources was significantly associated with pancreatic cancer risk, but no correlation was found with the consumption of plant fats.[84]

Chicken and Pancreatic Cancer Risk

Starting in the early 1970s, a series of laws have restricted the use of asbestos, yet thousands of Americans continue to die every year from exposure to it. The Centers for Disease Control and Prevention, the American Academy of Pediatrics, and the Environmental Protection Agency have estimated that over a period of thirty years, approximately one thousand cases of cancer will occur among people exposed to asbestos in school buildings as children.[85]

It all started generations ago with the asbestos workers. The first asbestos-related cancers occurred in the 1920s among miners digging up the stuff. Then came a second wave among shipbuilders and construction workers who used asbestos. We are now in the third wave of asbestos-related disease, as buildings constructed with asbestos are beginning to deteriorate.[86]

As the history of asbestos shows, to see if something causes cancer, scientists first study those who have the greatest exposure to it. That's how we're now learning about the potential cancer-causing effects of poultry viruses. There has been long-standing concern about the possibility that wart-causing chicken cancer viruses are being transmitted to the general population through the handling of fresh or frozen chicken.[87] These viruses are known to cause cancer in the birds, but their role in human cancers is unknown. This concern arises out of studies that show that people who work in poultry slaughtering and processing plants have increased risk of dying from certain cancers.

The most recent, a study of thirty thousand poultry workers, was designed specifically to test whether "exposure to poultry cancer-causing viruses that widely occurs occupationally in poultry workers—not to mention the general population—may be associated with increased risks of deaths from liver and pancreatic cancers." The study found that those who slaughter chickens have about *nine times* the odds of both pancreatic cancer and liver cancer.[88] To put this result in context, the most carefully studied risk factor for pancreatic cancer is cigarette smoking. But even if you smoked for fifty years, you'd have "only" doubled your odds of getting pancreatic cancer.[89]

What about people who eat chicken? The largest study to ever address that question is the European Prospective Investigation into Cancer and Nutrition (EPIC) study, which followed 477,000 people for about a decade. The researchers found a 72 percent increased risk of pancreatic cancer for every fifty grams of chicken consumed daily.[90] And that's not much meat, under two ounces—just about a quarter of a chicken breast.

The researchers expressed surprise that it was the consumption of poultry—not red meat—that was more closely tied to cancer. When a similar result was found for lymphomas and leukemias, the same EPIC research team acknowledged that while the growth-promoting drugs fed to chickens and turkeys could be playing a role, it might also be cancer viruses found in poultry.[91]

The reason the connection between asbestos and cancer was comparatively easy to nail down is that asbestos caused a particularly unusual cancer (mesothelioma), which was virtually unknown before widespread asbestos use.[92] But because the pancreatic cancer one might get from eating chicken is the same pancreatic cancer one might get from smoking cigarettes, it's more difficult to tease out a cause-and-effect relationship. There are diseases unique to the meat industry, such as the newly described "salami brusher's disease" that only affects people whose full-time job is to wire-brush off the white mold that naturally grows on salami.[93] But most diseases suffered by meat industry workers are more universal. So despite the compelling evidence linking poultry exposure to pancreatic cancer, don't expect an asbestos-type ban on Chick-fil-A anytime soon.

Treating Pancreatic Cancer with Curry

Pancreatic cancer is among the most aggressive forms of cancer. Untreated, most patients die two to four months after diagnosis. Unfortunately, only about 10 percent of patients appear to respond to chemotherapy, with the majority suffering severe side effects.[94]

Curcumin, the colorful component of the spice turmeric, appears able to reverse precancerous changes in colon cancer and has been shown in laboratory studies to be effective against lung cancer cells. Similar results were obtained using pancreatic cancer cells.[95] So why not try using curcumin to treat patients with pancreatic cancer? In a study funded by the National Cancer Institute and performed at the MD Anderson Cancer Center, patients with advanced pancreatic cancer were given large doses of curcumin. Of the twenty-one patients the researchers were able to evaluate, two responded positively to the treatment. One had a 73 percent reduction in his tumor size, though eventually a curcumin-resistant tumor developed in its place.

continued

The other patient, however, showed steady improvement over the course of eighteen months. The only time cancer markers bumped up was during a brief three-week period when the curcumin therapy was halted.[96] Yes, the tumors of only two out of twenty-one participants responded, but that's about the same as the chemo regimen, and zero adverse effects were reported with the curcumin treatment. As a result, I'd certainly suggest curcumin to pancreatic cancer sufferers regardless of what other treatments they choose. Given the tragic prognosis, though, prevention is critical. Until we know more, your best bet is to avoid tobacco, excess alcohol intake, and obesity and to eat a diet low in animal products, refined grains, and added sugars[97] and rich in beans, lentils, split peas, and dried fruit.[98]

ESOPHAGEAL CANCER

Esophageal cancer occurs when cancer cells develop in the esophagus, the muscular tube carrying food from your mouth to your stomach. Typically, the cancer arises in the lining of the esophagus and then invades the outer layers before metastasizing (spreading) to other organs. Early on, there may be few symptoms—if any at all. But as the cancer grows, swallowing difficulties can develop.

Every year, there are about eighteen thousand new cases of esophageal cancer and fifteen thousand deaths.[99] The primary risk factors include smoking, heavy alcohol consumption, and gastroesophageal reflux disease (GERD, also called acid reflux), in which acid from the stomach gurgles up into the esophagus, burning the inner layer and causing inflammation that can eventually lead to cancer. Besides avoiding tobacco and alcohol (even light drinking appears to increase risk),[100] the most important thing you can do to prevent esophageal cancer is to eliminate acid reflux disease—and that can often be accomplished through diet.

Acid Reflux and Esophageal Cancer

Acid reflux is one of the most common disorders of the digestive tract. The usual symptoms include heartburn as well as the regurgitation of stomach contents back up toward the throat, which can leave a sour taste in the mouth. GERD causes millions of doctor visits and hospitalizations each year and represents the highest annual cost of all digestive diseases in the United States.[101] Chronic inflammation caused by acid reflux can lead to Barrett's esophagus, a precancerous condition that involves changes in the esophageal lining.[102] To prevent adenocarcinoma, the most common type of esophageal cancer in the United States, this sequence of events must be stopped—and that means halting acid reflux in the first place.

That's a tall order in the United States. Over the past three decades, the incidence of esophageal cancer in Americans has increased sixfold[103]—an increase greater than that of breast or prostate cancer, and it may be chiefly because acid reflux is on the rise.[104] In the United States, about one in four people (28 percent) suffer at least weekly heartburn and/or acid regurgitation, compared to just 5 percent of the population in Asia.[105] This suggests that dietary factors may play a key role.

Over the past two decades, about forty-five studies have examined the link between diet, Barrett's esophagus, and esophageal cancer. The most consistent association with cancer was the consumption of meat and high-fat meals.[106] Interestingly, different meats were associated with cancers in different locations. Red meat is strongly associated with cancer in the esophagus itself, whereas poultry was more strongly associated with cancer down around the stomachesophagus border.[107]

How does this happen? Within five minutes of eating fat, your sphincter muscle at the top of your stomach—which acts like a valve to keep down food inside the stomach—relaxes, allowing acids to creep back up into the esophagus.[108] For example, in one study, volunteers consuming a high-fat meal (McDonald's sausage, egg, and cheese sandwich) experienced more acid squirting up into their esophagus than those eating a lower-fat meal (McDonald's hotcakes).[109] Part of this effect may be due to the release of a hormone called cholecystokinin, which is triggered by both meat[110] and eggs[111] and may also relax the sphincter.[112] This helps explain why those who eat meat have been found to have twice the odds of reflux-induced esophageal inflammation compared with vegetarians.[113]

Even without the cancer risk, GERD itself can cause pain, bleeding, and scar-tissue narrowing of the esophagus that can interfere with swallowing. Billions of dollars are spent on medications to alleviate heartburn and acid reflux by reducing the amount of stomach acid produced, but these drugs can contribute to nutrient deficiencies and increase the risk of pneumonia, intestinal infections, and bone fractures.[114] Perhaps the better strategy would be to just keep the acid in its place by minimizing the intake of foods that allow acid to escape.

The protection afforded by plant-based eating may not be based just on the foods that are reduced, though. Centering your diet around antioxidant-rich plant foods may cut in half your odds of esophageal cancer.[115] The most protective foods for cancer at the esophagus-stomach border appear to be red, orange, and dark-green leafy vegetables, berries, apples, and citrus fruits,[116] but all unprocessed plant foods have the advantage of containing fiber.

Fiber and Hiatal Hernia

While fat intake is associated with increased risk of reflux, fiber intake appears to decrease that risk.[117] High fiber intake may reduce the incidence of esophageal cancer by as much as one-third[118] by helping to prevent the root cause of many cases of acid reflux: the herniation of part of the stomach up into the chest cavity.

Hiatal hernia, as this condition is known, occurs when part of the stomach is pushed up through the diaphragm into the chest. More than one in five Americans suffer from hiatal hernias. In contrast, hiatal hernias are almost unheard of among populations whose diets are plant based, with rates closer to one in a thousand.[119] This is thought to be because they smoothly pass large, soft stools.[120]

People who don't eat an abundance of whole plant foods have smaller, firmer stools that can be difficult to pass. (See box on page 65.) If you regularly strain to push out stool, over time the increased pressure can push part of the stomach up and out of the abdomen, allowing acid to flow up toward the throat.[121]

This same pressure from straining on the toilet week after week can cause other problems. Similar to the way squeezing a stress ball causes a balloon bubble to pop out, the pressure from straining at the toilet may herniate outpouchings from the wall of the colon, a condition known as diverticulosis. The increased abdominal pressure may also back up blood flow in the veins around the anus, causing hemorrhoids, and even push blood flow back into the legs, resulting in varicose veins.[122] But a fiber-rich diet can relieve the pressure in both directions. Those who eat diets that revolve around whole plant foods tend to pass such effortless bowel movements that their stomachs stay where they're supposed to,[123] which can reduce the acid spillover implicated in one of our deadliest cancers.

Can Strawberries Reverse the Development of Esophageal Cancer?

Esophageal cancer joins pancreatic cancer as one of the gravest diagnoses imaginable. The five-year survival rate is less than 20 percent,[124] with most people dying within the first year after diagnosis.[125] This underscores the need to prevent, stop, or reverse the disease process as early as possible.

Researchers decided to put berries to the test. In a randomized clinical trial of powdered strawberries in patients with precancerous lesions in their esophagus, subjects ate one to two ounces of freeze-dried strawberries every day for six months—that's the daily equivalent of about a pound of fresh strawberries.[126]

All of the study participants started out with either mild or moderate precancerous disease, but, amazingly, the progression of the disease was *reversed* in about 80 percent of the patients in the high-dose strawberry group. Most of these precancerous lesions either regressed from moderate to mild or disappeared entirely. Half of those on the high-dose strawberry treatment walked away disease-free.[127]

Fiber consumption doesn't just take off the pressure. Humans evolved eating huge amounts of fiber, likely in excess of one hundred grams daily.[128] That's up to about ten times what the average person eats today.[129] Because plants don't tend to run as fast as animals, the bulk of our diet used to be made up of a lot of bulk. In addition to keeping you regular, fiber binds to toxins, such as lead and mercury, and flushes them away (pun intended!).[130] Our bodies were designed to expect an ever-flowing fiber stream, so it dumps such unwanted waste products as excess cholesterol and estrogen into the intestines, assuming they will be swept away. But if you aren't constantly filling your bowels with plant foods, the only natural source of fiber, unwanted waste products can get reabsorbed and undermine your body's attempts at detoxifying itself. Only 3 percent of Americans may even reach the recommended minimum daily intake of fiber, making it one of the most widespread nutrient deficiencies in the United States.[131]

CHAPTER 5

How Not to Die from Infections

I was still in medical school when I got a call to help defend Oprah Winfrey, who was being sued by a cattle rancher under a Texas food-disparagement law (thirteen states have so-called food-libel laws that make it illegal to make a comment that unfairly "implies that [a] perishable food product is not safe for consumption by the public"[1]).

Oprah had been talking on her television show with Howard Lyman, a former fourth-generation cattle rancher who decried the cannibalistic feeding of cow parts to other cows, a risky practice blamed for the emergence and spread of mad cow disease. Repulsed by the thought, Oprah told the viewing audience, "It has just stopped me cold from eating another burger." The next day, cattle futures tumbled, and the Texas cattleman claimed to have lost millions.

My job was to help establish that Lyman's comments were "based on reasonable and reliable scientific inquiry, facts, or data."[2] Despite the ease with which we did just that, not to mention the blatant violation of First Amendment protections inherent in the law, the Texas cattleman was able to tie Oprah up in a long and harrowing appeals process. Finally, five years later, a federal judge dismissed the case with prejudice, ending Oprah's ordeal.

In a narrow legal sense, she won. But if the meat industry is able to drag one of the country's richest and most powerful people through the courts for years and cost her a small fortune in legal fees, what kind of chilling effect does that have on others who want to speak out? Now the meat industry is trying to pass so-called ag-gag laws, which make it illegal to take pictures inside their operations. Presumably, they fear people might be less inclined to buy their products if they knew how these products are made.[3]

Thankfully, humanity dodged a bullet with mad cow disease. Nearly an entire generation in Britain was exposed to infected beef, but only a few hundred people died. We weren't as lucky with swine flu, which the CDC estimates killed twelve thousand Americans.[4] Nearly three-quarters of all emerging and reemerging human diseases arise from the animal kingdom.[5]

Humanity's dominion over animals has unleashed a veritable Pandora's ark of infectious diseases. Most modern human infectious diseases were unknown before domestication led to a mass spillover of animal disease into human populations.[6] For example, tuberculosis appears to have been originally acquired through the domestication of goats[7] but now infects nearly one-third of humanity.[8] Meanwhile, measles[9] and smallpox[10] may have arisen from mutant cattle viruses. We domesticated pigs and got whooping cough, we domesticated chickens and got typhoid fever, and we domesticated ducks and got influenza.[11] Leprosy may have come from water buffalo and the cold virus from horses.[12] How often did wild horses have the opportunity to sneeze into humans' faces until they were broken and bridled? Before then, the common cold was presumably common only to them.

Once pathogens jump the species barrier, they can then transmit person-to-person. HIV, a virus thought to have originated from the butchering of primates in Africa for the bush-meat trade,[13] causes AIDS by weakening the immune system. The opportunistic fungal, viral, and bacterial infections AIDS patients contract—but to which healthy people are resistant—demonstrate the importance of baseline immune function. Your immune system is not just active when you're lying in bed sick spiking a fever—it's involved in a daily life-or-death struggle to save your life from the pathogens that surround and live inside you.

With every breath you take, you inhale thousands of bacteria,[14] and with every bite you eat, you can ingest millions more.[15] Most of these tiny germs are completely harmless, but some can cause serious infectious diseases, occasionally making headlines with sinister-sounding names like SARS or Ebola. Although many of these exotic pathogens receive a lot of press coverage, more lives are lost to some of our most common infections. For example, such respiratory infections as influenza and pneumonia kill nearly fifty-seven thousand Americans each year.[16]

Bear in mind that you don't need to come in contact with a sick person to fall ill with an infection. There are latent infections that may exist within you, waiting to strike should your immune function falter. That is why it's not enough to just wash your hands; you have to keep your immune system healthy.

Protecting Others

To protect others when you're sick, you need to practice good respiratory etiquette by coughing or sneezing into the crook of your arm (into your bent elbow). This practice limits the dispersal of respiratory droplets and also avoids contaminating your hands. The Mayo Clinic has a slogan worth remembering: "The ten worst sources of contagion are our fingers." When you cough into your hand, you can transfer contagion to everything from elevator buttons and light switches to gas pumps and toilet handles.[17] It's no surprise that during flu season, the influenza virus can be found on more than 50 percent of common household and day-care-center surfaces.[18]

Ideally, you should sanitize your hands after every bathroom visit and handshake, before all food preparation, and before touching your eyes, nose, or mouth after coming in contact with public surfaces. The latest recommendations from the World Health Organization favor the use of alcohol-based sanitizing rubs or gels over hand washing for routine disinfection of your hands throughout the day. (Products containing between 60 and 80 percent alcohol were found to be more effective than soap in every scientific study available for review.) The only time hand washing is preferable is when they are dirty or visibly contaminated with bodily fluids. For routine decontamination—that is, for all other times—alcohol-based products are the preferred method for hand sanitation.[19]

Still, some germs will always get past your first line of defense of practicing good hand hygiene. This is why you need to keep your immune system functioning at peak performance with a healthy diet and lifestyle.

PREVENTING INFECTIOUS DISEASES WITH A HEALTHY IMMUNE SYSTEM

The term "immune system" is derived from the Latin word *immunis*, meaning untaxed or untouched, which is fitting, given that the immune system protects the body from foreign invaders. Composed of various organs, white blood cells, and proteins called antibodies that form alliances against trespassing pathogens threatening the body, the immune system, apart from the nervous system, is the most complex organ system humans possess.[20]

Your first layer of protection against intruders are physical surface barriers like your skin. Beneath that are white blood cells, such as neutrophils that attack and engulf pathogens directly, and natural killer cells that put your cells out of their misery if they become cancerous or infected with a virus. How do natural killer cells recognize pathogens and infected cells? They are often marked for destruction by antibodies, which are special proteins made by another type of white blood cell, known as B cells, that home in like smart bombs and stick to invaders.

Each B cell makes one type of antibody that's specific for one foreign molecular signature. You don't have one B cell that covers grass pollen and another that covers bacteria; instead, you have a B cell whose only job is to make antibodies against the pollen of purple Siberian onion grass and another whose only job is to make antibodies against the tail proteins of bacteria that live in the thermal vents at the bottom of the ocean. If each of your B cells produces only one type of antibody, then you'd need to have a billion different types of B cells given the incredible variety of potential pathogens on our planet. And you do!

Let's suppose one day you're walking along and suddenly get attacked by a platypus (they have poisonous spurs on their heels, you know). For your whole life up until that point, the B cell in your body that produces antibodies against duck-billed platypus venom was just hanging around, twiddling its thumbs, until that very moment. As soon as the venom is detected, this specific B cell begins dividing like crazy, and soon you have a whole swarm of clones each producing millions of antibodies against platypus poison. You fend off the toxin and live happily ever after. That is how the immune system works— aren't our bodies spectacular?

As you get older, though, your immune function declines. Is this just an inevitable consequence of aging? Or could it be because dietary quality also tends to go down in older populations? To test the theory that inadequate nutrition could help explain the loss in immune function as you age, researchers split eighty-three volunteers between sixty-five and eighty-five years old into two groups. The control group ate fewer than three daily servings of fruits and vegetables, while the experimental group consumed at least five servings a day. They were all then vaccinated against pneumonia, a practice recommended for all adults over the age of sixty-five.[21] The goal of vaccination is to prime your immune system to produce antibodies against a specific pneumonia pathogen should you ever become exposed. Compared with the control group, people eating five or more servings of fruits and vegetables had an 82 percent greater protective antibody response to the vaccine—and this was after only a few months of eating just a few extra servings of fruits and vegetables a day.[22] That is how much control the fork may exert over immune function.

Certain fruits and vegetables may give the immune function an extra boost.

Kale

Americans eat far too little kale. According to the U.S. Department of Agriculture, the average American may consume about 0.05 pounds of kale each year.[23] That's about one and a half cups per person . . . per decade.

As a dark-green, leafy vegetable, kale is not only one of the most nutrient-dense foods on the planet—it may also help fight off infection. Japanese researchers tried dripping a minute quantity of kale on human white blood cells in a petri dish, about one-millionth of a gram of kale protein. Even that miniscule quantity triggered a quintupling of antibody production in the cells.[24]

The researchers used raw kale, but the scant amounts of kale Americans consume are often cooked. Does cooking kale destroy its immune-boosting effects? It turned out that even boiling the veggies nonstop for thirty minutes did not affect antibody production. In fact, the cooked kale appeared to work even better.[25]

However, this property was discovered in a test-tube study. Even kale aficionados don't mainline it like heroin, which is presumably the only way intact kale proteins would ever come in direct contact with our blood cells. No clinical studies (that is, studies on real people) on kale have been performed to date. Big Kale, it seems, has yet to muster the research dollars. Currently, we have stronger evidence for the immune benefits of kale's less pretentious cousin, broccoli.

Broccoli

As I've mentioned, your body's greatest exposure to the outside world is through the lining of your intestines, which may cover more than two thousand square feet,[26] which is about the floor area of an average house.[27] But the lining is extremely thin—just fifty-millionths of a meter. In other words, the barrier separating your bloodstream from the world is many times thinner than a single sheet of tissue paper. This is because the body needs to absorb nutrients from food: If the gut lining were any thicker, nutrients would have trouble passing through. It's a good idea for your skin to be waterproof so you don't start leaking, but the lining of the gut has to allow for the absorption of both fluids and nutrition. With such a fragile layer between your sterile core and the chaos outside, you need to have a good defense mechanism in place to keep out the bad.

This is where the immune system comes in, specifically a special type of white blood cell called intraepithelial lymphocytes. These cells serve two functions: They condition and repair the thin intestinal lining, and they also serve as its first line of gut defense against pathogens.[28] These lymphocytes are covered with "Ah receptors" that activate the cells.[29] For years, scientists couldn't find the key that fit into the Ah receptor lock. If we could figure out how to activate these cells, we might be able to boost our immunity.[30]

It turns out that key is contained in broccoli.

You may have been taught as a kid to eat your veggies, including cruciferous ones like broccoli, kale, cauliflower, cabbage, and brussels sprouts. But your parents probably didn't tell you *why* you should eat them. Now we know that this family of vegetables contains compounds necessary for the maintenance of the body's intestinal defenses. In short, broccoli is able to rally your immune system foot soldiers.[31]

Why did our immune systems evolve to depend on certain vegetables? Well, when do we need to boost our intestinal defenses? When we eat. The body uses up a lot of energy to maintain its immune system, so why remain on high alert 24-7 when we only eat a few times a day? Why would our bodies specifically use vegetables as the bat signal to assemble the troops? We evolved over millions of years eating mostly weeds—wild plants, including dark-green, leafy vegetables (or, as they were known back then, *leaves*)—so our bodies may have evolved to equate vegetables with mealtime. Vegetables' presence in the gut works as a signal to upkeep our immune systems.[32] So if we don't eat plants with each meal, we may be undermining our bodies' strategy to protect us.

Interestingly, the immune boost provided by cruciferous vegetables like broccoli not only protects us against the pathogens found in food but also against pollutants in the environment. We're all constantly being exposed to a wide range of toxic substances—from cigarette smoke, car exhaust, furnaces, cooked meat, fish, dairy, and even from mother's milk[33] (as a consequence of what the mother was exposed to). Because some of these pollutants, such as dioxins, exert their toxic effects through the Ah receptor system, cruciferous compounds may block them.[34]

Other plants may also defend against toxic invaders. Researchers in Japan found that phytonutrients in such plant foods as fruits, vegetables, tea leaves, and beans can block the effects of dioxins in vitro. For instance, the researchers found that having phytonutrient levels in the bloodstream achieved by eating three apples a day or a tablespoon of red onion appeared to cut dioxin toxicity in half. The only catch was that these phytonutrient effects lasted only a few hours, meaning you may have to keep eating healthy foods, meal after meal, if you want to maintain your defenses against pathogens as well as pollutants.[35]

The ability to block toxins isn't limited to plant foods, however. There is one animal product that has also been shown to potentially block the cancer-causing effects of dioxins—camel urine.[36] So next time your kids don't want to eat their fruits and veggies, you can just say, "Hey, it's either the broccoli or camel pee. Your choice."

Pretty in Pee-nk

Ever noticed that your urine turns a bit pink after you eat beets? Though the color looks a little unnatural, it's a completely harmless and temporary condition called beeturia.[37] It's a vivid reminder of an important fact: When you eat plant foods, many of the pigment phytonutrients that act as antioxidants in your body (such as lycopene and beta-carotene) are absorbed into the bloodstream and bathe your organs, tissues, and cells.

In other words, beet pigments find their way into your urine because they are absorbed through the gut and then travel into the bloodstream, where they circulate throughout the body until eventually being filtered out by the kidneys. During this trip through the body, even your blood becomes a bit pinker too.

The same principle causes garlic breath. It isn't just the residue in your mouth that's scaring everyone off; it's also the health-promoting compounds that were absorbed into your bloodstream after you swallowed the garlic, which are then exhaled pungently from your lungs in your breath. Even if you just had a garlic enema, you'd *still* get garlic breath. For this reason, garlic can potentially be used as an adjunct treatment for critical cases of pneumonia, as it may help clear bacteria on its way out of the lungs.[38]

Boosting Natural Killer Cell Activity with Berries

For disease prevention, berries of all colors have "emerged as champions," according to the head of the Bioactive Botanical Research Laboratory.[39] The purported anticancer properties of berry compounds have been attributed to their apparent ability to counteract, reduce, and repair damage resulting from oxidative stress and inflammation.[40] But it wasn't known until recently that berries may also boost your levels of natural killer cells.

They may sound sinister, but natural killer cells are a type of white blood cell that's a vital member of the immune system's rapid-response team against virus-infected and cancerous cells. They're called natural killers because they don't require prior exposure to a disease to be activated, unlike some other parts of the immune system that can only respond effectively after a history of exposure, as in the case of, say, chicken pox.[41] After all, you don't want to wait until your *second* tumor appears before your immune system starts fighting.

There are about two billion of these elite, special-ops fighters patrolling the bloodstream at any one time, but research suggests that you can bolster their ranks by eating blueberries. In one study, researchers asked athletes to eat about a cup and a half of blueberries every day for six weeks to see if the berries could reduce the oxidative stress caused by long-distance running.[42] The blueberries succeeded, unsurprisingly, but a more important finding was their effect on natural killer cells. Normally, these cells decrease in number after a bout of prolonged endurance exercise, dropping by half to about one billion. But the athletes consuming blueberries actually *doubled* their killer cell counts, to more than four billion.

Blueberries can boost the number of natural killer cells, but are there any foods that can boost killer cell *activity*—that is, how effectively they fight cancer cells? Yes, it seems an aromatic spice called cardamom may be one. Researchers put some lymphoma cells in a petri dish and added natural killer cells, which were able to wipe out about 5 percent of the cancer cells. But after researchers effectively sprinkled on some cardamom, the natural killer cells became supercharged and eradicated even more cancer cells—up to about ten times more than without cardamom.[43] No clinical trials have yet been done to try this out in cancer patients.

In theory, though, cardamom-infused blueberry muffins may increase the number of circulating natural killer cells in the body, as well as boost their cancer-killing instincts.

Preventing the Common Cold with Probiotics?

Babies delivered via cesarean section appear to be at increased risk for various allergic diseases, including allergic runny nose, asthma, and perhaps even food allergies.[44] (Allergy symptoms are caused when your immune system over-reacts to normally harmless stimuli, such as tree pollen.) Normal delivery leads to the colonization of the baby's gut with the mother's vaginal bacteria. C-section babies, on the other hand, are deprived of this natural exposure. The resulting difference in gut flora may affect the way the baby's immune system develops, accounting for the difference in allergy rates. This explanation is supported by research showing that a disturbance in a mother's vaginal flora during pregnancy due, for example, to sexually transmitted infections or douching may result in higher asthma risk for the infant.[45]

These findings raise a broader question about the effects the good bacteria in the gut may have on the immune system. Some studies have shown that supplementing with good bacteria (probiotics) might have immunity-enhancing effects. The first such study demonstrated that white blood cells extracted from subjects on a probiotic regimen for a few weeks demonstrated a significantly enhanced ability to engulf and destroy potential invaders. This effect lasted for at least three weeks after the probiotics were discontinued. Natural killer cell activity against cancer cells in vitro was improved as well.[46]

Improving cell function in a petri dish is nice, but do these results translate into fewer infections? It took another ten years before a randomized, double-blind, placebo-controlled study was performed. (Considered the gold standard of research, a randomized, double-blind, placebo-controlled study is a trial in which neither the participants nor the researchers know who is receiving an experimental treatment and who is receiving a placebo until the end of the study.) The study showed that people who take probiotic supplements may indeed have significantly fewer colds, fewer sick days, and fewer overall symptoms.[47] The evidence to date suggests probiotics may reduce the risk of upper-respiratory-tract infections but is insufficient for recommending that people start popping probiotic pills.[48]

Unless you've suffered a major disruption in gut flora due to a course of antibiotics or an intestinal infection, it may be best to focus on feeding the good bacteria already living in your gut.[49] What do your friendly flora eat? Fiber and a certain type of starch concentrated in beans. These substances are called *prebiotics*. Probiotics are the good bacteria themselves, whereas prebiotics are what your good bacteria eat. So the best way to keep your good bacteria happy and well fed is to eat lots of whole plant foods.

When you eat fresh produce, you can get *both* pre- and probiotics into your gut. Fruits and veggies are covered with millions of lactic acid bacteria, some of which are the same types used in probiotic supplements. When you make sauerkraut, for example, you don't need to add a starter culture, because the bacteria are already naturally present on cabbage leaves. Including raw fruits and vegetables in your daily diet may therefore offer the best of both worlds.[50]

Boosting the Immune System with Exercise

What if there were a drug or supplement that could halve the number of sick days you take due to such upper-respiratory infections as the common cold? It would make some pharmaceutical company billions of dollars. But there is already something that can boost your immune system for free and by so much that you can achieve a 25–50 percent reduction in sick days. And it has only good side effects. What is it?

Exercise.[51]

What's more, it doesn't take much of a workout to get results. Studies find that if you let kids run around for just six minutes, the levels of immune cells circulating in their blood increases by nearly 50 percent.[52] At the other end of the life cycle, regular exercise can also help prevent age-related immune decline. One study found that while elderly, sedentary women have a 50 percent chance of getting an upper-respiratory illness during the fall season, those randomized to begin a half-hour-a-day walking program dropped their risk down to 20 percent. Among conditioned runners, though, the risk was just 8 percent.[53] Exercising appeared to make their immune systems more than five times better at fighting infection.

So what's going on here? How does the simple act of moving decrease the chance of contracting an infection? Approximately 95 percent of all infections start in the mucosal (moist) surfaces, including the eyes, nostrils, and mouth.[54] These surfaces are protected by antibodies called IgA (short for immunoglobulin, type A), which provide an immunological barrier by neutralizing and preventing viruses from penetrating into the body. The IgA in saliva, for instance, is considered the first line of defense against such respiratory-tract infections as pneumonia and influenza.[55] Moderate exercise may be all it takes to boost IgA levels and significantly reduce the chance of coming down with flu-like symptoms. Compared to a sedentary control group, those who performed aerobic exercises for thirty minutes three times a week for twelve weeks had a 50 percent increase in the levels of IgA in their saliva and reported significantly fewer respiratory infection symptoms.[56]

While regular physical activity improves immune function and lowers respiratory infection risk, sustained and intense exertion may have the opposite effect. As you go from inactive to active, infection risk declines, but at a certain point, overtraining and excessive stress can *increase* the risk of infection by impairing immune function.[57] In the weeks following marathons or ultramarathons, runners report a two- to sixfold increase in upper-respiratory-tract infections.[58] Within a day of starting an international competition, elite soccer players were found to suffer a significant drop in their IgA production.[59] This drop has been tied to upper-respiratory-tract infections during training. Other studies have found that IgA levels can drop after even just single bouts of overstrenuous exercise.[60]

What can you do, then, if you're a hard-core athlete? How can you reduce your chance of infection? Traditional sports medicine recommendations don't appear to have much to offer: They'll tell you to get a flu shot, avoid touching your eyes or picking your nose, and stay away from sick people.[61] Gee, thanks. The reason these steps may be insufficient is that respiratory infections are often triggered by reactivations of latent viruses already inside the body, such as Epstein-Barr virus, the cause of mononucleosis. So even if you never came in contact with anyone else, as soon as your immune function dips, these dormant viruses can return and make you sick.

Thankfully, a number of foods may help maintain your immunity to keep the germs at bay.

First up is chlorella, a single-celled, freshwater, green algae typically sold as a powder or compressed into tablets. Researchers in Japan were the first to show that mothers given chlorella saw increased IgA concentrations in their breast milk.[62] Although chlorella extract supplements failed to boost overall immune function,[63] there is evidence that whole algae may be effective. In a study out of Japan in 2012, researchers rounded up athletes ripe for infection during the middle of training camp. Among the control group, who received no supplements, IgA levels dropped significantly during intense exercise. But among those who were given chlorella, IgA levels remained steady.[64]

One note of caution: A disturbing case report from Omaha, Nebraska, was published recently, entitled "Chlorella-Induced Psychosis."[65] A forty-eight-year-old woman suffered a psychotic break two months after starting to take chlorella. Her physicians told her to stop it and put her on an antipsychotic drug. One week later, she was fine. Chlorella had never before been linked to psychosis, so they initially presumed it was just a fluke. In other words, the psychosis may have just coincidentally begun after the woman started taking chlorella, and the reason she felt better after stopping it may have just been due to the drug kicking in. But seven weeks later, she was still on the drug and had restarted taking chlorella—and she became psychotic again. The chlorella was stopped, and her psychosis resolved again.[66] Perhaps it wasn't the chlorella itself that triggered the episode but some toxic impurity or adulteration. We don't know. Given the scandalously ill-regulated supplement market, it's hard to know what you're getting when you try to buy "food" in supplement bottles.

Another option for athletes who want to sustain their immune function is nutritional yeast. A 2013 study reported that you may more effectively maintain your levels of white blood cells after exercise by consuming a special type of fiber found in baker's, brewer's, and nutritional yeast.[67] Brewer's yeast is bitter, but nutritional yeast has a pleasant, cheese-like flavor. It tastes particularly good on popcorn.

The study found that after two hours of intense cycling, the number of monocytes (another type of immune system white blood cell) in subjects' bloodstreams took a dip. But those who were given the equivalent of about three-quarters of a teaspoon of nutritional yeast before they exercised ended up with even higher levels of monocytes than when they started working out.[68]

That's all well and good on a lab report, but does consuming yeast fiber actually translate to fewer illnesses? Researchers put that question to the test at the Carlsbad Marathon in California.

Runners who were given the daily equivalent of about a spoonful of nutritional yeast in the four weeks after the race appeared to have just half the rates of upper-respiratory infection compared to runners consuming a placebo. Remarkably, the runners on yeast reported feeling better too. When asked how they felt on a scale of one to ten, with ten being the best, the people taking the placebo reported about a four or five. On the other hand, the subjects on the nutritional yeast consistently reported feeling better, around a six or seven. Elite athletes normally experience mood deterioration before and after a marathon, but this study revealed that a little nutritional yeast may improve a wide range of emotional states, reducing feelings of tenseness, fatigue, confusion, and anger, while at the same time increasing perceived "vigor."[69] Pass the popcorn!

Boosting Immunity with Mushrooms

Do you suffer from seasonal allergies? Runny nose, itchy eyes, sneezing? While your allergies may make you feel lousy because your immune system is busily attacking things left and right, that same heightened state of alertness may have benefits for your overall health.

Individuals suffering from allergies appear to have a decreased risk for certain cancers.[70] Yes, your immune system might be in overdrive striking

continued

out at harmless things like pollen or dust, but that same overvigilance may also take down budding tumors in the body. It would be nice if there were a way to boost the part of the immune system that fights infections while down-regulating the part that results in chronic inflammation (and all those annoying symptoms).

Mushrooms may just do the trick.

Just as algae can be thought of as single-celled plants, yeast can be thought of as single-celled mushrooms. Thousands of edible mushrooms grow naturally, with worldwide annual commercial production in the millions of tons.[71] But check the nutrition label on a carton of mushrooms and you won't see much beyond some B vitamins and minerals. Is that all mushrooms have? No. What you don't see listed is the array of unique myconutrients that may boost our immune function.[72]

Researchers in Australia split people into two groups. One group ate its regular diet, while the other ate its regular diet plus a cup of cooked white button mushrooms every day. After just a week, the mushroom eaters showed a 50 percent boost in the IgA levels in their saliva. These antibody levels remained elevated for about a week before dropping.[73] So, for sustained benefits, try to make mushrooms a steady part of your diet.

But wait. If mushrooms trigger such a dramatic rise in antibody production, shouldn't we be concerned they may worsen the symptoms of allergic or autoimmune diseases? On the contrary, it seems mushrooms may have an *anti*-inflammatory effect. In vitro studies have shown that a variety of mushrooms, including plain white button mushrooms, appear to blunt the inflammatory response, potentially offering a boost in immune and anticancer function without aggravating diseases of inflammation.[74] The first randomized, double-blind, placebo-controlled clinical study of its kind, published in 2014, confirmed an apparent antiallergy effect in children with a history of recurrent upper-respiratory-tract infections.[75]

Food Poisoning

Pathogens (from the Greek *pathos*, for "suffering," and *genes*, meaning "producer of") can also be found in what you eat. Foodborne illness, or food poisoning, is an infection caused by eating contaminated food. According to the CDC, about one in six Americans develops food poisoning every year. Roughly forty-eight million people are sickened annually—larger than the combined populations of California and Massachusetts. More than one hundred thousand of them are hospitalized, and thousands die, just because of something they ate.[76]

In terms of healthy years of life lost, the top five most devastating pathogen-food combinations are *Campylobacter* and *Salmonella* bacteria in poultry, *Toxoplasma* parasites in pork, and *Listeria* bacteria in deli meats and dairy products.[77] One of the reasons animal foods are the leading culprits is that most food-borne pathogens are fecal pathogens. Because plants don't poop, the *E. coli* you may get from spinach didn't actually originate in the spinach; *E. coli* is an intestinal pathogen, and spinach doesn't have intestines. The application of manure to crops has been found to increase the odds of *E. coli* contamination by more than fiftyfold.[78]

Eggs and *Salmonella*

The single greatest public health burden in the United States in terms of food poisoning is *Salmonella*. It's the leading cause of food poisoning–related hospitalizations, as well as the number-one cause of food poisoning–related death.[79] And it's on the rise. Over the past decade, the number of cases has increased by 44 percent, particularly among children and the elderly.[80] Within twelve to seventy-two hours after infection, the most common symptoms appear—fever, diarrhea, and severe abdominal cramps.[81] The illness typically lasts between four and seven days, but among children and the elderly, the disease can be severe enough to require hospitalization—or funeral arrangements.

Many people associate *Salmonella* with eggs—and for good reason. In 2010, for instance, more than half a billion eggs were recalled due to *Salmonella* outbreaks.[82] However, the egg industry mantra remained: Stop whining; eggs are safe. Responding to cries for a recall in an op-ed published in *USA Today*, the chairman of the industry trade group United Egg Producers insisted that "completely cooked eggs are completely safe eggs."[83] But what exactly does "completely cooked" mean?

The egg industry itself funded research on *Salmonella* and the various ways to cook eggs. What did they find? *Salmonella* in eggs can survive scrambled, over-easy, and sunny-side-up cooking methods. Sunny side up was found to be the riskiest. The industry-funded researchers bluntly concluded: "The sunny-side-up method should be considered unsafe."[84] In other words, even the egg industry itself knows that its product, prepared in a manner that millions of Americans eat on any given day all across the country, is *unsafe*. Actually, we've known this for some time. Twenty years ago, Purdue University researchers determined that *Salmonella* can survive in cooked omelets and french toast.[85] *Salmonella* may even survive in eggs boiled up to eight minutes.[86]

Given all of this, it should come as no surprise that, according to the Food and Drug Administration (FDA), an estimated 142,000 Americans are sickened each year by *Salmonella*-tainted eggs.[87] That's an egg-borne epidemic each year in the United States. But eggs are "only" number ten on the worst pathogen-food combination list.

Poultry and *Salmonella*

Eating chickens, not their eggs, is actually the most common source of *Salmonella* poisoning.[88] A nationwide outbreak of a particularly virulent strain of the bacteria was linked to our sixth-largest poultry producer, Foster Farms. It lasted from March 2013 until July 2014.[89] Why did the outbreak last so long? It was largely because the company continued to churn out contaminated chicken despite repeated warnings from the CDC.[90] Though the official tally of cases numbered only in the hundreds, the CDC estimates that for every confirmed case of *Salmonella*, another thirty-eight slip through the cracks.[91] This means Foster Farms' chicken may have sickened more than ten thousand people. When U.S. Department of Agriculture officials went in to investigate, they found that 25 percent of the chickens they sampled were contaminated with the same strain of *Salmonella*, likely the result of fecal matter found on the chicken carcasses.[92]

Mexico banned the importation of Foster Farms' chicken, but in the United States, it remained available throughout the country.[93] When a car manufacturer's brakes malfunction, it announces a recall due to safety concerns. Why hasn't *Salmonella*-tainted chicken been recalled? The U.S. Department of Agriculture once tried to shut down a company found to be repeatedly violating *Salmonella* standards. The company sued and won. "Because normal cooking practices for meat and poultry destroy the *Salmonella* organism," the judges in the case concluded, "the presence of *Salmonella* in meat products does not render them 'injurious to health.'"[94]

If proper cooking kills the bug, then why do hundreds of thousands of Americans continue to be sickened by *Salmonella*-contaminated poultry every year? It's not like *E. coli* and medium-rare hamburgers—who undercooks chicken? The problem here is cross-contamination. Between the time the fresh or frozen bird is picked up from the store and when it's slid into the oven, the germs on the chicken can contaminate hands, utensils, and kitchen surfaces.

Studies have shown that up to 80 percent of the time, placing fresh chicken on a cutting board for a few minutes can transfer disease-causing bacteria.[95] Then, if you put cooked chicken back on the same cutting board, there's about a 30 percent chance that the meat will become recontaminated.[96]

Foster Farms' tone-deaf response to the outbreak may actually prove the most foresighted: "It is not unusual for raw poultry from any producer to have *Salmonella* bacteria," they quoted in a press release. "Consumers must use proper preparation, handling and cooking practices."[97] In other words, it should be considered normal for chicken to be contaminated with *Salmonella*. Eat at your own risk.

Why are American consumers placed at such high risk? Some European countries have gotten *Salmonella* contamination in poultry down as low as 2 percent. How? Because it's illegal to sell chicken tainted with *Salmonella*. What a concept! They don't allow the sale of fowl fouled with a pathogen that sickens more than a million Americans a year.[98] In a meat industry trade publication, an Alabama poultry science professor explained why we don't have such a "heavy handed" policy: "The American consumer is not going to pay that much. It's as simple as that." If the industry had to pay to make it safer, the price would go up. "The fact," he said, "is that it's too expensive not to sell salmonella-positive chicken."[99]

Fecal Bacteria on Meat

The contamination problem extends far beyond a single poultry producer. In a 2014 issue of *Consumer Reports*, researchers published a study on the true cost of cheap chicken. They discovered that 97 percent of chicken breasts found in retail stores were contaminated with bacteria that could make people sick.[100] Thirty-eight percent of the *Salmonella* they found was resistant to multiple antibiotics; the CDC considers such pathogens to be a serious public health threat.[101]

As the Mayo Clinic rather indelicately put it, "Most people are infected with *Salmonella* by eating foods that have been contaminated by feces."[102] How does it get there? In slaughter plants, birds are typically gutted by a metal hook, which too often punctures their intestines and can expel feces onto the flesh itself. According to the latest national FDA retail-meat survey, about 90 percent of retail chicken showed evidence of contamination with fecal matter.[103]

Using the presence of bugs like *E. faecalis* and *E. faecium* as markers of fecal contamination, 90 percent of chicken parts, 91 percent of ground turkey, 88 percent of ground beef, and 80 percent of pork chops are tainted on the retail level nationally.[104]

While outbreaks of *Salmonella* infection have increased, *E. coli* infection from fecal matter in beef has decreased.[105] Why is beef getting safer but chicken getting riskier?[106] One likely factor is that the government was able to enact a ban on the sale of beef contaminated with a particularly dangerous strain of *E. coli*. But why is it illegal to sell beef known to be contaminated with a potentially deadly pathogen but perfectly legal to sell contaminated chicken? After all, *Salmonella* in chicken kills far more people than *E. coli* in beef.[107]

The problem dates back to a famous case in 1974 when the American Public Health Association sued the U.S. Department of Agriculture for putting its stamp of approval on meat contaminated with *Salmonella*. Defending the meat industry, the USDA pointed out that because "there are numerous sources of contamination which might contribute to the overall problem," it would be "unjustified to single out the meat industry and ask that the [USDA] require it to identify its raw products as being hazardous to health."[108] In other words, because *Salmonella* has also been linked to dairy and eggs, it wouldn't be fair to force only the meat industry to make their products safer. That's like the tuna industry arguing there's no need to label cans of tuna with mercury warnings because you could also get exposed by eating a thermometer.

The Washington, D.C., Circuit Court of Appeals upheld the meat industry's position, asserting that the USDA can allow potentially deadly *Salmonella* in meat because "American housewives and cooks normally are not ignorant or stupid and their methods of preparing and cooking of food do not ordinarily result in salmonellosis."[109] That's like saying minivans don't need airbags or seat belts, and kids don't need car seats, because soccer moms don't *ordinarily* crash into things.

Avoiding Chicken to Avoid Urinary Tract Infections

Where do bladder infections come from? Back in the 1970s, studies of women over time found that movement of bacteria from the rectum into the vaginal area preceded the appearance of bladder infections.[110] It took another twenty-five years, though, before DNA fingerprinting techniques proved that *E. coli* strains residing in the gut serve as the reservoir for urinary tract infections (UTIs).[111]

Another fifteen years passed before scientists tracked down the ultimate culprit, the original source of some of the UTI-associated bacteria in the rectum: chicken. McGill University researchers were able to capture UTI-causing *E. coli* at the slaughter plants, tracing them to the meat supply and, eventually, to urinary specimens obtained from infected women.[112] As a result, we now have direct proof that bladder infections can be a zoonosis—an animal-to-human disease.[113] This is a critical discovery, since UTIs affect more than ten million women each year in the United States at the cost of more than $1 billion.[114] Even worse, it turns out that many of the strains of E. coli in chicken that cause UTIs are now resistant to some of our most powerful antibiotics.[115]

Can't we solve this crisis by simply distributing meat thermometers and making sure people cook chicken thoroughly? No—because of the cross-contamination issue. Studies have shown that handling raw chicken can lead to intestinal colonization even if you don't eat any of it.[116] In that case, it doesn't matter how well you cook your chicken. You could incinerate it to ash and still walk away infected. After infection, the drug-resistant chicken bacteria was then found to multiply to the point of becoming a major part of the research subject's gut flora.[117]

The reason most people have more fecal bacteria in their kitchen sinks than their toilet seats[118] is likely because they prepare their chickens in the kitchen, not the bathroom. But what if you're really careful? A landmark study, published as "The Effectiveness of Hygiene Procedures for Prevention of Cross-Contamination from Chicken Carcasses in the Domestic Kitchen," put this question to the test. Researchers visited five dozen homes, gave each family a raw chicken, and asked them to cook it. After the bird was cooked, researchers returned to find bacteria from chicken feces—Salmonella and Campylobacter, both serious human pathogens—all over the families' kitchens: on the cutting board, utensils, cupboard, the refrigerator handle, the oven handle, the door-knob, and so on.[119]

Obviously, people didn't know what they were doing, so the researchers then repeated the experiment, but this time gave the families specific instructions. After they cooked the chicken, the subjects were told to wash these surfaces with hot water and detergent, specifically the cutting board, utensils, cupboard, handles, and knobs. Yet the researchers still found pathogenic fecal bacteria all over.[120]

Reading the study, you could tell the researchers were getting a bit exasperated. Finally, they insisted the subjects use bleach. The dishcloth used to clean up was to first be immersed in bleach disinfectant, and then the subjects were to spray a bleach solution on all surfaces and let it sit for five minutes. However, the researchers returned to still find Salmonella and Campylobacter on some utensils, a dishcloth, the counter around the sink, and the cupboards.[121] The extent of the kitchen contamination was much less, but still, it appears that unless you treat your kitchen like a biohazard laboratory, the only way to guarantee you're not going to leave fecal pathogens around the kitchen is to not bring them into your house in the first place.

There is some good news: It's not as if you eat chicken once and your gut is colonized for life. In the study in which volunteers became infected after just handling the meat, the chicken bacteria that tried to take over their gut only seemed to last about ten days.[122] The good bacteria in their guts seemed able to muscle the bad guys out of the way. The problem, unfortunately, is that people tend to eat chicken more than once every ten days, so they may be constantly reintroducing these chicken bugs into their systems.

Yersinia in Pork

Nearly one hundred thousand Americans are sickened each year by *Yersinia* bacteria.[123] In every outbreak for which a source has been found, the culprit was contaminated pork.[124]

In most cases, *Yersinia* food poisoning leads to little more than acute gastroenteritis, but the symptoms can become severe and mirror appendicitis, resulting in unnecessary emergency surgeries.[125] Long-term consequences of *Yersinia* infection include chronic inflammation of the eyes, kidneys, heart, and joints.[126] Studies have found that within a year of contracting *Yersinia* food poisoning, victims appear forty-seven times more likely to come down with autoimmune arthritis,[127] and the bacteria may also play a role in triggering an autoimmune thyroid condition known as Graves' disease.[128]

How contaminated are U.S. pork products? *Consumer Reports* magazine tested nearly two hundred samples from cities across the country and found that more than two-thirds of the pork was contaminated with *Yersinia*.[129] This may be because of the intensification and overcrowding that characterizes most of today's industrial pig operations.[130] As noted in an article in *National Hog Farmer* entitled "Crowding Pigs Pays," pork producers can maximize their profits by confining each pig to a six-square-foot space. This basically means cramming a two-hundred-pound animal into an area equivalent to about two feet by three feet. The authors acknowledged that overcrowding presents problems, including inadequate ventilation and increased health risks, but they concluded that sometimes, "crowding pigs a little tighter will make you more money."[131]

Unfortunately, this situation is not expected to change anytime soon. Why? *Yersinia* bacteria do not cause clinical disease in pigs.[132] In other words, it's a public health problem, not an animal production problem. It doesn't affect the industry's bottom line. So instead of giving these animals a little more breathing room, the pork industry just largely passes along to society the estimated $250 million cost of sickening tens of thousands of Americans every year.[133]

C. Difficile Superbugs in Meat

There's a new superbug in town: *Clostridium difficile*. *C. diff*, as it's commonly known, is one of our most urgent bacterial threats, infecting an estimated quarter-million Americans annually and killing thousands at a cost of $1 billion a year.[134] It causes a condition called pseudomembranous colitis, which manifests as painful, crampy diarrhea. *C. diff* has traditionally been considered a hospital-acquired infection—something you pick up in health care settings—but it was recently discovered that only about one-third of *C. diff* cases can be linked to contact with an infected patient.[135] What's going on?

Well, another source of infection may be meat. The CDC found that 42 percent of packaged meat products sold at three national chain grocery stores sampled contained toxin-producing *C. diff* bacteria.[136] The United States, it turns out, has the highest reported levels of *C. diff* meat contamination in the world.[137]

C. diff has also been found in chicken, turkey, and beef, but pork contamination has received the greatest attention from health officials, as it most closely matches the same strain found in non-hospital-related human infections.[138] Since 2000, *C. diff* has increasingly been reported as one of the leading causes of intestinal infections among baby piglets.[139] Carcass contamination with this diarrheal pathogen at the time of slaughter is considered the most likely source of the contamination of retail pork.[140]

Normally, *C. diff* won't do anything to you. Even if it gets into your gut, your good bacteria can usually muscle it into submission. It can lie in wait, though, until the good guys are out of the way. The next time you have to take an antibiotic that disrupts your normal gut flora, *C. diff* can rear its ugly head and cause a range of inflammatory bowel conditions, including a life-threatening condition that's as bad as it sounds: toxic megacolon.[141] (It carries a mortality rate as high as a flip of a coin.)[142]

Doesn't cooking wipe out most bugs? Well, *C. diff* isn't like most bugs. For most meat, 71 degrees Celsius is the recommended internal cooking temperature. But *C. diff* can survive two hours of cooking at that temperature.[143] In other words, you could grill chicken at the recommended cooking thermometer temperature for two hours straight and still not kill the bug.

You've probably seen advertisements for those alcohol-based hand sanitizers that advertise they kill 99.99 percent of all germs. Well, *C. diff* falls into that 0.01 percent. They don't call it a superbug for nothing. Residual spores of the pathogen have been shown to be readily transmitted with a handshake even after using hand sanitizer.[144] As one of the lead researchers who discovered another superbug in the U.S. meat supply, MRSA,[145] has advised,[146] people who handle raw meat may want to wear gloves.

Facing a Post-Antibiotic Age

Dr. Margaret Chan, Director-General of the World Health Organization, recently warned that we may be facing a future in which many of our miracle drugs no longer work. She stated, "A post-antibiotic era means, in effect, an end to modern medicine as we know it. Things as common as strep throat or a child's scratched knee could once again kill."[147] We may soon be past the age of miracles.

The director-general's prescription to avoid this catastrophe included a global call to "restrict the use of antibiotics in food production to therapeutic purposes." In other words, only use antibiotics in agriculture to treat sick animals. But that isn't happening. In the United States, meat producers feed millions of pounds of antibiotics each year to farm animals just to promote growth or prevent disease in the often cramped, stressful, and unhygienic conditions of industrial animal agriculture. Yes, physicians overprescribe antibiotics as well, but the FDA estimates that 80 percent of the antimicrobial drugs sold in the United States every year now go to the meat industry.[148]

Antibiotic residues can then end up in the meat you eat. Studies have revealed that traces of such antibiotics as Bactrim, Cipro, and Enrofloxacin have been found in the urine of people eating meat—even though none of them was taking those drugs. The researchers concluded: "Consumption amounts of beef, pork, chicken, and dairy products could explain the daily excretion amount of several antibiotics in urine."[149] These antibiotic levels can be lowered, however, after merely five days of removing meat from the diet.[150]

Nearly every major medical and public health institution has come out against the dangerous practice of feeding antibiotics to farm animals by the ton just to fatten them faster.[151] Yet the combined political might of agribusiness and the pharmaceutical industries that profit from the sales of these drugs has effectively thwarted any effective legislative or regulatory action, all to save the industry less than a penny per pound of meat.[152]

Healthy living may help protect you against both airborne and foodborne illnesses. Eating more fruits and vegetables and exercising more frequently can boost your immune system to help you fight off respiratory infections like the common cold. And sticking to mostly plant foods can help prevent you from becoming another food poisoning statistic by reducing your exposure to some of the deadliest fecal pathogens.

Six years after I helped defend Oprah against her meat-defamation lawsuit, I received my own legal threat. The Atkins corporation accused me of "defamatory" statements in my book *Carbophobia: The Scary Truth About America's Low-Carb Craze.* Their lawyer claimed my words "continue to harm Atkins' reputation and cause injury to Atkins." My book certainly couldn't have caused more injury to Dr. Atkins than his own diet. You see, he died the year before, overweight and—according to his autopsy report—suffering from a history of heart attack, congestive heart failure, and hypertension.[153]

However, the lawyers were talking about damage to Atkins Nutritionals, Inc. Rather than let them shut me up, I posted their legal threat online with a point-by-point rebuttal.[154] Thankfully, under the law, the truth is considered an absolute defense against defamation.

Atkins's attorneys never made good on their threat. Within four months of my book's publication, the Atkins corporation filed for bankruptcy.

CHAPTER 6

How Not to Die from Diabetes

A few years ago, Millan, a member of the NutritionFacts.org community, was kind enough to share her story with me. When she was thirty years old, she was diagnosed with type 2 diabetes. Millan had struggled with obesity all her life and suffered through the highs and lows of years of yo-yo dieting. She had tried nearly every fad diet she could find but, not surprisingly, would quickly gain back whatever weight she'd lost. Diabetes wasn't a stranger to her. Millan's parents, brothers, and aunt were all diabetic, so she figured that her own diagnosis was inevitable. It's age related. It's genetic. There was nothing she could do. Or so she thought.

Millan's initial diagnosis was back in 1970, and she lived as a diabetic for two decades. Then, in the 1990s, she switched to an entirely plant-based diet and completely turned her life around. Today, her energy levels are better than ever, she looks and feels younger, and she's finally been able to maintain a healthy weight. More than four decades after being diagnosed as a diabetic, Millan, now in her seventies, is fit as a fiddle. She even teaches high-intensity Zumba classes! She didn't find some wonder drug or trademarked diet. She simply decided to eat healthier food.

The disease called diabetes mellitus comes from two words: *diabetes* (Greek for "to pass through or siphon") and *mellitus* (Latin for "honey sweet"). Diabetes mellitus is characterized by chronically elevated levels of sugar in your blood. This is because either your pancreas gland isn't making enough insulin (the hormone that keeps your blood sugar in check) or because your body becomes resistant to insulin's effects. The insulin-deficiency disease is called type 1 diabetes, and the insulin-resistance disease is called type 2 diabetes. If too much sugar builds up in your blood, it can overwhelm the kidneys and spill into your urine.

How did people test urine before they had modern laboratory techniques? They tasted it. Diabetic urine can evidently taste as sweet as honey. Hence the name.

Type 2 diabetes has been called the "Black Death of the twenty-first century" in terms of its exponential spread around the world and its devastating health impacts. Instead of the bubonic plague, though, the pathological agents in obesity and type 2 diabetes are identified as "high-fat and high-calorie diets," and instead of fleas and rodents, the causes are "advertisements and inducements to poor lifestyle."[1] More than twenty million Americans are currently diagnosed with diabetes, a tripling of cases since 1990.[2] At this rate, the CDC predicts that one in three Americans will be diabetic by midcentury.[3] Currently in the United States, diabetes causes about 50,000 cases of kidney failure, 75,000 lower extremity amputations, 650,000 cases of vision loss,[4] and about 75,000 deaths every year.[5]

Your digestive system breaks down the carbohydrates you eat into a simple sugar called glucose, which is the primary fuel powering all the cells in your body. To get from the bloodstream into your cells, glucose requires insulin. Think of insulin as the key that unlocks the doors to your cells to allow glucose to enter. Every time you eat a meal, insulin is released by your pancreas to help shuttle the glucose into your cells. Without insulin, your cells can't accept glucose, and, as a result, the glucose builds up in your blood. Over time, this extra sugar can damage the blood vessels throughout the body. That's why diabetes can lead to blindness, kidney failure, heart attacks, and stroke. High blood sugar can also damage your nerves, creating a condition known as neuropathy that can cause numbness, tingling, and pain. Because of the damage to their blood vessels and nerves, diabetics may also suffer from poor circulation and lack of feeling in the legs and feet, which can lead to poorly healing injuries that can, in turn, end as amputations.

Type 1 diabetes, previously called juvenile-onset diabetes, represents approximately 5 percent of all diagnosed diabetes cases.[6] In most people with type 1 diabetes, the immune system mistakenly destroys the insulin-producing beta cells in the pancreas. Without insulin, blood sugar rises to unsafe levels. Type 1 diabetes is therefore treated with injections of insulin, a type of hormone-replacement therapy, to make up for the lack of production. The exact cause of type 1 diabetes is unknown, though a genetic predisposition combined with exposure to such environmental triggers as viral infection and/or cow's milk may play a role.[7]

Type 2 diabetes, previously known as adult-onset diabetes, accounts for 90–95 percent of diabetes cases.[8] In type 2 diabetes, the pancreas can make insulin, but it doesn't work as well. The accumulation of fat inside the cells of your muscles and liver interferes with the action of insulin.[9] If insulin is the key that unlocks the doors to your cells, saturated fat is what appears to gum up the locks. With glucose denied entry into your muscles, the primary consumer of such fuel, sugar levels can rise to damaging levels in your blood. The fat inside these muscle cells can come from the fat you eat or the fat you wear (i.e., your body fat). The prevention, treatment, and reversal of type 2 diabetes therefore depends on diet and lifestyle.

The CDC estimates that more than twenty-nine million Americans are living with diagnosed or undiagnosed diabetes—that's about 9 percent of the U.S. population. Out of one hundred people you know, chances are six of them already know they are diabetic and about three have diabetes but haven't yet been diagnosed. More than one million new cases of type 2 diabetes are diagnosed each year.[10]

The good news: Type 2 diabetes is almost always preventable, often treatable, and sometimes even reversible through diet and lifestyle changes. Like other leading killers—especially heart disease and high blood pressure—type 2 diabetes is an unfortunate consequence of your dietary choices. But even if you already have diabetes and its complications, there is hope. Through lifestyle changes, you may be able to achieve a complete remission of type 2 diabetes, even if you've been suffering with the disease for decades. In fact, by switching to a healthy diet, you can start improving your health within a matter of hours.

What Causes Insulin Resistance?

The hallmark of type 2 diabetes is insulin resistance in your muscles. As we've learned, insulin normally enables blood sugar to enter the cells, but when the cells are resistant and don't respond to insulin as they should, it can lead to dangerous levels of sugar remaining in the bloodstream.

What causes insulin resistance in the first place?

Studies dating back nearly a century note a striking finding. In 1927, researchers divided healthy young medical students into multiple groups to test out the effects of different diets. Some were given a fat-rich diet composed of olive oil, butter, egg yolks, and cream; others were given a carbohydrate-rich diet of sugar, candy, pastry, white bread, baked potatoes, syrup, bananas, rice, and oatmeal. Surprisingly, insulin resistance skyrocketed in the fat-rich diet group; within a matter of days, their blood sugar levels doubled in response to a sugar challenge, far more than those on the sugar and starch diet.[11] It took scientists another seven decades to unravel the mystery of why this happened, but the answer would provide the key to what causes type 2 diabetes.

To understand the role of diet, we must first understand how the body stores fuel. When athletes talk about "carb loading" before a competition, they're referring to the need to build a fuel supply in their muscles. Carb loading is a more extreme version of what you do every day: Your digestive system breaks down the starch you eat into glucose, which enters your circulatory system as blood sugar and is then stored in your muscles to be used for energy as needed.

Blood sugar, though, is a little like a vampire: It needs an invitation to come into your cells. And that invitation is insulin, the key that unlocks the front door of your muscle cells so glucose can enter. When insulin attaches to insulin receptors on a cell, it activates a series of enzymes that escort in the glucose. Without insulin, blood glucose is stuck out in the bloodstream, banging on your cells' front door, unable to enter. Blood sugar levels then rise, damaging vital organs in the process. In type 1 diabetes, the body destroys the insulin-producing beta cells of the pancreas, so very little insulin is present to let blood sugar enter your cells. But with type 2 diabetes, insulin production isn't the problem. The key is there, but something has gummed up the lock. This is called insulin resistance. Your muscle cells become resistant to the effect of insulin.

So what's jamming up the door locks on your muscle cells, preventing insulin from letting glucose enter? Fat—more specifically, intramyocellular lipid, the fat inside your muscle cells.

Fat in your bloodstream, either from your own fat stores or from your diet, can build up inside your muscle cells, where it can create toxic breakdown products and free radicals that block the insulin-signaling process.[12] No matter how much insulin you produce, your fat-compromised muscle cells can't effectively use it.

This mechanism by which fat interferes with insulin function has been demonstrated by either infusing fat into people's bloodstreams and watching insulin resistance shoot up[13] or by removing fat from people's blood and seeing insulin resistance drop.[14] We can now even visualize the amount of fat in the muscles using MRI technology.[15] Researchers are now able to track the fat going from the blood into the muscles and watch insulin resistance rise.[16] One hit of fat, and within 160 minutes, the absorption of glucose into your cells becomes compromised.[17]

Researchers don't have to give their study subjects fat through an IV, though. All they have to do is feed them.

Even among healthy individuals, a high-fat diet can impair the body's ability to handle sugar. But you can lower your insulin resistance by lowering your fat intake. Research has clearly shown that as the amount of fat in your diet becomes increasingly lower, insulin works increasingly better.[18] Unfortunately, given the current diets of American children, we're seeing both obesity and type 2 diabetes occur earlier and earlier in life.

Prediabetes in Children

Prediabetes is defined by elevated blood sugar levels that are not yet high enough to reach the official diabetes threshold. Commonly found among those who are overweight and obese, in the past, prediabetes was regarded as a high-risk state that presaged diabetes, but it was not thought to be a disease in itself. However, we now know that prediabetic individuals may already be experiencing organ damage.

Prediabetics may already have sugar damage to their kidneys, eyes, blood vessels, and nerves even before diabetes is diagnosed.[19] Evidence from numerous studies suggests that chronic complications of type 2 diabetes begin occurring during the prediabetic state.[20] To prevent diabetic damage, therefore, we need to prevent prediabetes—and the earlier, the better.

Thirty years ago, virtually all diabetes in children was assumed to be type 1. But since the mid-1990s, we've started to see an increase in type 2 diabetes among kids.[21] What was once called "adult-onset diabetes" is now known as type 2 diabetes because children as young as eight are developing the disease.[22] This trend can have devastating consequences: A fifteen-year follow-up study of children who were diagnosed with type 2 diabetes found an alarming prevalence of blindness, amputation, kidney failure, and death by the time these kids had reached young adulthood.[23]

Why the dramatic rise in childhood diabetes? It's likely due to the dramatic rise in childhood obesity.[24] Over recent decades, the number of American children considered to be overweight has increased by more than 100 percent.[25] Children who are obese at age six are more likely than not to stay that way, and 75–80 percent of obese adolescents will remain obese as adults.[26]

Childhood obesity is a powerful predictor of adult disease and death. For example, being overweight as a teenager was found to predict disease risk fifty-five years later. Such individuals may end up with twice the risk of dying from heart disease and a higher incidence of other diseases, including colorectal cancer, gout, and arthritis. Researchers have found that being overweight as a teen could be an even more powerful predictor of disease risk than being overweight as an adult.[27]

To prevent childhood diabetes, we need to prevent childhood obesity. How do we do that?

In 2010, the chair of the nutrition department at Loma Linda University published a paper suggesting that giving up meat entirely is an effective way to combat childhood obesity, pointing to population studies demonstrating that people eating plant-based diets are consistently thinner than those who eat meat.[28]

To study body weight, we usually rely on body mass index (BMI), which is a measure of weight that also takes height into account. For adults, a BMI over 30 is considered obese. Between 25 and 29.9 is considered overweight, and a BMI between 18.5 and 24.9 is considered "ideal weight." In the medical profession, we used to call a BMI of under 25 "normal weight." Sadly, that's no longer normal.

What's your BMI? Visit one of the scores of online BMI calculators or grab a calculator and multiply your weight in pounds by 703. Then divide that twice by your height in inches. For example, if you weigh 200 pounds and are 71 inches tall (five foot eleven), that would be $(200 \times 703) \div 71 \div 71 = 27.9$, a BMI indicating that you would be, unfortunately, significantly overweight.

The largest study ever to compare the obesity rates of those eating plant-based diets was published in North America. Meat eaters topped the charts with an average BMI of 28.8—close to being obese. Flexitarians (people who ate meat more on a weekly basis rather than daily) did better at a BMI of 27.3, but were still overweight. With a BMI of 26.3, pesco-vegetarians (people who avoid all meat except fish) did better still. Even U.S. vegetarians tend to be marginally overweight, coming in at 25.7. The only dietary group found to be of ideal weight were the vegans, whose BMI averaged 23.6.[29]

So why aren't more parents feeding their kids plant-based diets? There's a common misconception in America that their growth will be stunted. However, the opposite may be true. Loma Linda University researchers found that children who eat vegetarian diets not only grow up leaner than kids who eat meat but taller, too, by about an inch.[30] In contrast, meat intake is associated more with horizontal growth: The same researchers found a strong link between consumption of animal foods and increased risk of being overweight.[31]

Developing diabetes in childhood appears to cut life expectancy by about twenty years.[32] Who among us wouldn't go to the ends of the earth to enable our kids to live two decades longer?

THE FAT YOU EAT AND THE FAT YOU WEAR

Carrying excess body fat is the number-one risk factor for type 2 diabetes; up to 90 percent of those who develop the disease are overweight.[33] What's the connection? In part, a phenomenon known as the spillover effect.

Interestingly, the number of individual fat cells in your body doesn't change much in adulthood, no matter how much weight you gain or lose. They just swell up with fat as the body gains weight, so when your belly gets bigger, you're not necessarily creating new fat cells; rather, you're just cramming more fat into existing ones.[34] In overweight and obese people, these cells can get so bloated that they actually spill fat back into the bloodstream, potentially causing the same clogging of insulin signaling one would experience from eating a fatty meal.

Doctors can actually measure the level of freely floating fat in the bloodstream. Normally, it's between about one hundred and five hundred micromoles per liter. But people who are obese have blood levels between roughly six hundred and eight hundred. People eating low-carb, high-fat diets can reach the same elevated levels. Even a trim person eating a high-fat diet can average eight hundred, so that sky-high number isn't exclusive to obese patients. Because those eating high-fat diets are absorbing so much fat into their bloodstreams from their digestive tract, the level of free fat in their blood is as high as someone who's grossly obese.[35]

Similarly, being obese can be like gorging on bacon and butter all day even if you are actually eating healthfully. That's because an obese person's body may be constantly spilling fat into the bloodstream, regardless of what goes into the mouth. No matter the *source* of fat in your blood, as fat levels rise, your ability to clear sugar from the blood drops due to insulin resistance—the cause of type 2 diabetes.

People who eat a plant-based diet, on the other hand, have just a small fraction of the rate of diabetes seen in those who regularly eat meat. As you can see in figure 1, as diets become increasingly plant based, there appears to be a stepwise drop in diabetes rates.[36] Based on a study of eighty-nine thousand Californians, flexitarians appear to cut their rate of diabetes by 28 percent, good news for those who eat meat maybe once a week rather than every day. Those who cut out all meat except fish appear to cut their rates in half. What about those eliminating all meat, including fish? They appear to eliminate 61 percent of their risk. And those who go a step farther and drop eggs and dairy foods too? They may drop their diabetes rates 78 percent compared with people who eat meat on a daily basis.

Why would this be?

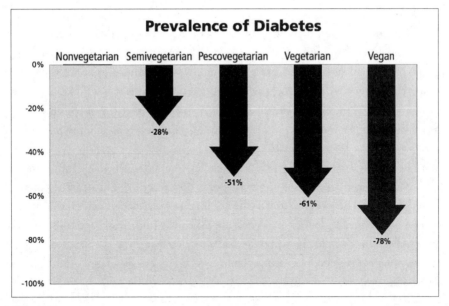

Figure 1

Is it just because people eating plant-based diets are better able to control their weight? Not entirely. Even at the same weight as regular omnivores, vegans appear to have less than half the risk of diabetes.[37] The explanation may lie in the difference between plant fats and animal fats.

Saturated Fat and Diabetes

Not all fats affect our muscle cells in the same way. For example, palmitate, the kind of saturated fat found mostly in meat, dairy, and eggs, causes insulin resistance. On the other hand, oleate, the monounsaturated fat found mostly in nuts, olives, and avocados, may actually protect against the detrimental effects of the saturated fat.[38] Saturated fats can wreak all sorts of havoc in muscle cells and may result in the accumulation of more toxic breakdown products (such as ceramide and diacylglycerol)[39] and free radicals and can cause inflammation and even mitochondrial dysfunction—that is, interference with the little power plants (mitochondria) within our cells.[40] This phenomenon is known as lipotoxicity (*lipo* meaning fat, as in liposuction).[41] If we take muscle biopsies from people, saturated fat buildup in the membranes of their muscle cells correlates with insulin resistance.[42] Monounsaturated fats, however, are more likely to be detoxified by the body or safely stored away.[43]

This discrepancy may explain why individuals eating plant-based diets are better protected from diabetes. Researchers have compared the insulin resistance and muscle-fat content of vegans versus omnivores. Because people eating plant-based diets have the advantage of being so much slimmer on average, the researchers recruited omnivores who weighed the same as the vegans they were studying so that they could see whether plant-based diets had a direct effect beyond the indirect benefit of pulling fat out of the muscles by helping people to lose weight.

The result? There was significantly less fat trapped in the deep calf muscles of vegans than in those of comparably slim omnivores.[44] Those eating plant-based diets have been found to have better insulin sensitivity, better blood sugar levels, better insulin levels,[45] and even significantly improved function of their beta cells—the cells in the pancreas that produce insulin in the first place.[46]

In other words, people eating plant-based diets appear to be better at both producing and using insulin.

Preventing Diabetes by Eating More

Many population studies have shown that people who eat significant amounts of legumes (e.g., beans, split peas, chickpeas, and lentils) tend to weigh less. They also have slimmer waists, less obesity, and lower blood pressure compared to people who don't eat many legumes.[47] But couldn't these benefits be due not to the legumes themselves but to the fact that people who eat more legumes may eat a healthier diet in general? To tease out the connection, researchers used the most powerful tool in nutrition research: the interventional trial. Instead of just observing what people eat, you change their diets to see what happens. In this case, they put legumes to the test by comparing extra legume consumption head-to-head against calorie restriction.

Reducing belly fat may be the best way to prevent prediabetes from turning into full-blown diabetes. Though calorie cutting has been the cornerstone of most weight-loss strategies, evidence suggests that the majority of individuals who lose weight by portion control eventually regain it. Starving ourselves almost never works long term. So wouldn't it be great if instead we could find a way to eat more food to get the same weight-loss benefit?

The researchers divided overweight subjects into two groups. The first group was asked to eat five cups a week of lentils, chickpeas, split peas, or navy beans—but not to change their diets in any other way. The second group was asked to simply cut out five hundred calories a day from their diets. Guess who got healthier? The group directed to eat *more* food. Eating legumes was shown to be just as effective at slimming waistlines and improving blood sugar control as calorie cutting. The legume group also gained additional benefits in the form of improved cholesterol and insulin regulation.[48] This is encouraging news for overweight individuals at risk for type 2 diabetes. Instead of just eating smaller portions and reducing the quantity of the food they eat, they can also improve the *quality* of their food by eating legume-rich meals.

Saturated fats may also be toxic to the cells in the pancreas that produce insulin. At around age twenty, the body stops making new insulin-producing beta cells. After that, if they are lost, they may be lost for good.[49] Autopsy studies have shown that by the time type 2 diabetes is diagnosed later in life, you may have already killed off half your beta cells.[50]

The toxicity of saturated fats can be demonstrated directly. If we expose beta cells to saturated fat[51] or to LDL ("bad") cholesterol in a petri dish, the beta cells begin to die.[52] The same effect is not observed with the monounsaturated fats concentrated in fatty plant foods, such as nuts.[53] When you eat saturated fat, both insulin action and insulin secretion are impaired within hours.[54] The more saturated fat you have in your blood, the higher your risk may be for developing type 2 diabetes.[55]

Of course, just as everyone who smokes doesn't develop lung cancer, everyone who eats excessive saturated fat doesn't develop diabetes. There is a genetic component. But for those who already have a genetic predisposition, a diet with too many calories and rich in saturated fat is considered a cause of type 2 diabetes.[56]

Losing Weight with a Plant-Based Diet

As noted earlier, even if you don't eat extra fat, the extra fat you *wear* may cause the spillover effect—the tendency for overstretched fat cells to spill fat into the bloodstream. The advantage of a whole-food, plant-based approach to weight loss is that there may be no need for portion control, skipping meals, or counting calories, because most plant foods are naturally nutrient dense and low in calories.

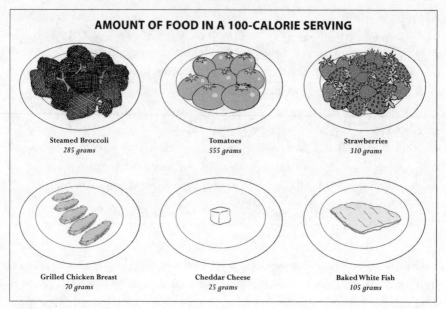

AMOUNT OF FOOD IN A 100-CALORIE SERVING

Steamed Broccoli
285 grams

Tomatoes
555 grams

Strawberries
310 grams

Grilled Chicken Breast
70 grams

Cheddar Cheese
25 grams

Baked White Fish
105 grams

Figure 2

Fruits and vegetables, on average, contain about 80–90 percent water. Just as fiber can bulk up the volume of foods without adding calories, so can water. Experiments have shown that people tend to eat the same amount of food at a meal, regardless of calorie count—probably because stretch receptors in the stomach send signals to the brain after a certain volume of food has been ingested. When much of that volume is a zero-calorie component like fiber or water, that means you can eat more food but gain less weight.[57]

Figure 2 shows the amounts of broccoli, tomatoes, and strawberries that contain one hundred calories, compared with the quantities of one hundred calories of chicken, cheese, and fish. You'll notice that even though the calorie content is the same, the volume of these foods is different. So it makes sense that one hundred calories of the plants would be more likely to fill you up, while the same one hundred calories from animal or processed foods may leave you half-empty.

That's why whole-food, plant-based diets are great for people who like to eat, since you can basically eat as much as you want without worrying about counting calories.

A head-to-head randomized clinical trial found that a plant-based diet beat out the American Diabetes Association's recommended diet for weight loss. This occurred without restricting portions the subjects ate and without requiring calorie or carb counting.[58] Moreover, a review of similar studies found that, in addition to weight loss, individuals consuming plant-based meals ex-

perienced improved blood sugar control as well as reduced risk of cardiovascular disease compared with people who followed diets that included more
animal products.[59] Such are the benefits of a plant-based diet.

Diabetics are more likely to suffer from strokes and heart failure.[60] In fact,
diabetic patients without a history of coronary heart disease may have the same
risk of heart attack as nondiabetic individuals with confirmed heart disease.[61]
In addition to improving insulin sensitivity better than conventional diabetic
diets, the plant-based approach can also lead to a significant drop in LDL cholesterol, thereby reducing risk of the number-one killer of diabetics, heart disease.[62] But how do people feel about making such a major shift in their diets? As
Dr. Dean Ornish has quipped, are we all going to live longer, or is it just going
to *seem* longer?[63]

Apparently, most people who switch to a plant-based diet are happy they did.
One of the reasons there's been such great compliance with plant-based dietary
interventions is that people not only tend to get measurably better, they also tend
to *feel* much better. In a recent randomized, clinical weight-loss trial, diabetics
were split into two groups. Half were put on the conventional diabetic diet as
recommended by diabetes organizations; the other half were prescribed a plant-
based diet consisting mostly of vegetables, grains, legumes, fruits, and nuts. At
the end of six months, the plant-based group reported both a significantly better quality of life and significantly higher mood scores than those assigned to the
conventional diet. Patients consuming the plant-based diet also felt less con-
strained than those consuming the conventional diet. Moreover, disinhibition decreased, meaning patients eating vegetarian food were less likely to binge, and
the plant-based folks tended to feel less hungry as well—both of which could help
these subjects sustain this way of eating in the long run.[64] So not only do plant-
based diets appear to work better but they may be easier to adopt long term. And
with the improvement in mood they seem to bring, there may be benefits for
both physical and mental health. (See chapter 12 for more on this topic.)

When it comes to maximally lowering diabetes risk, does it matter if you
eat just a little meat? Researchers in Taiwan sought to answer that question.
Traditionally, Asian populations have enjoyed very low rates of diabetes. In recent years, however, diabetes has emerged on a near-epidemic scale, coincid-
ing with the Westernization of Asian diets. Rather than compare vegetarians
to modern-day omnivores, these researchers compared vegetarians to those
eating a traditional Asian diet, which customarily included very little fish and
other meat. The women ate the equivalent of just a single serving of meat
each week, while the men had a serving every few days.[65]

Both the vegetarian and traditional Asian diet groups were following healthy diets, avoiding soda, for example. Despite the similarities in diet among the four thousand study subjects and after accounting for weight, family history, exercise, and smoking, the researchers found that the vegetarian men had only half the odds of diabetes as the occasional meat eaters. The vegetarian women had 75 percent lower odds of diabetes. Those who avoided meat altogether appeared to have significantly lower risk of both prediabetes and diabetes than those who ate plant-based diets with an occasional serving of meat, including fish. The researchers were unable to compare the diabetes rates of the more than one thousand vegetarians in the study to the sixty-nine vegans in the group, however, because the prevalence of diabetes among those eating strictly plant-based was zero.[66]

Diabetes-Promoting Pollutants

The dramatic rise in obesity has been blamed squarely on overeating and inactivity. But could there be something else about the food we're eating that's plumping us up? Scientists have begun identifying "obesogenic" chemical pollutants released into the environment that may disrupt your metabolism and predispose you to obesity. Contaminated food is the main source of exposure to these chemicals, and 95 percent of that exposure may come through the consumption of animal fat.[67] What's the big deal? A nationwide study found that people with the highest levels of pollutants in their bloodstreams had an astounding thirty-eight times the odds of diabetes.[68] Harvard University researchers identified one chemical in particular, hexachlorobenzene, as a potent risk factor for the disease.[69]

Where is this toxin found? Apparently, at the grocery store. In a supermarket survey of a variety of foods, canned sardines were found to be the most heavily tainted with hexachlorobenzene, though salmon was found to be the most contaminated food overall. Two dozen pesticides were detected in the salmon fillets.[70] Farmed salmon may be the worst, containing ten times more of a class of toxic chemicals called PCBs than wild-caught salmon.[71]

Industrial toxins like hexachlorobenzene and PCBs were largely banned decades ago. So how could they account for any of our increasing rates of diabetes? The answer to this paradox may be our obesity epidemic. The association between these toxic chemicals and diabetes was much stronger among obese subjects than in lean subjects studied, raising the possibility that your own fat stores are acting as reservoirs for these pollutants.[72] Overweight individuals may be effectively carrying around a personal toxic waste dump on their hips. Without significant weight loss, people whose bodies contain salmon pollutants may take between fifty to seventy-five years to clear the chemicals from their bodies.[73]

Do those who avoid meat completely get enough nutrients? To find out, researchers looked at a day in the life of thirteen thousand people all across America. They compared the nutrient intake of those who ate meat to those who didn't. The study found that, calorie for calorie, those eating vegetarian diets were getting higher intakes of nearly every nutrient: more fiber, more vitamin A, more vitamin C, more vitamin E, more of the B vitamins thiamin, riboflavin, and folate, as well as more calcium, magnesium, iron, and potassium. Furthermore, many of the nutrients that are so rich in plant-based diets are among the very ones that most Americans normally don't get enough of— namely, vitamins A, C, E, not to mention fiber, calcium, magnesium, and potassium. At the same time, people who avoided meat also ingested fewer harmful substances, such as sodium, saturated fat, and cholesterol.[74]

In terms of weight management, those eating meat-free diets consumed an average of 364 fewer calories daily.[75] That's about what most people on traditional weight-loss programs strive to cut out, meaning a meatless diet could be considered an all-you-care-to-eat version of a calorie-restricted weight-loss diet, without having to count calories or restrict portion intake.

Those who eat plant-based diets may even have an 11 percent higher resting metabolic rate.[76] That means vegetarians could be burning more calories even in their sleep. Why? This could be because vegetarians have a higher gene expression of a fat-burning enzyme called carnitine palmitoyltransferase, which effectively shovels fat into the mitochondrial furnaces in your cells.[77]

So a calorie may not be a calorie when it comes to meat. A massive study with an equally massive name, the European Prospective Investigation into Cancer–Physical Activity, Nutrition, Alcohol, Cessation of Smoking, Eating Out of Home, and Obesity—commonly known as EPIC-PANACEA—was comprised of hundreds of thousands of men and women who were followed for years. It's the largest study ever to investigate eating meat and body weight, and it found that meat consumption was associated with significant weight gain even after adjusting for calories. This means that if you had two people eating the *same* number of calories, it appears the person eating more meat would, on average, gain significantly more weight.[78]

REVERSING DIABETES

What About Drugs and Surgery?

As noted earlier, those with type 2 diabetes are at elevated risk for such serious health problems as heart disease, premature death, blindness, kidney failure, and amputations, as well as fractures, depression, and dementia. And the higher people's blood sugar levels, the more heart attacks and strokes they tend to have, the shorter their life spans are, and the higher their risk of complications are. To see if these outcomes could be averted, a study was performed in which ten thousand diabetics were randomized into one of two groups, the standard therapy group (in which the goal was just to lower blood sugar levels) and an intensive blood-sugar-lowering group (in which the researchers put the diabetics on up to five different classes of oral drugs at the same time) with or without insulin injections. The goal was not just to drive down blood sugars, as is the case with standard therapy, but to drive them down consistently into the normal range.[79]

Considering that type 2 diabetes is a disease of insulin resistance, high blood sugar is just a symptom of that disease, not the disease itself. So even by artificially forcing down blood sugars by any means necessary, we aren't actually treating the cause—just like blood pressure–lowering drugs aren't actually treating the cause. By lowering one of the disease's effects, however, scientists hoped they could prevent some of its devastating complications.

The results of this study, published in the *New England Journal of Medicine*, sent shock waves through the medical community. The intensive blood-sugar-lowering therapy actually *increased* subjects' mortality, requiring the researchers to halt the study prematurely for safety reasons.[80] The drug combinations may have been more dangerous than the high blood sugars they were trying to treat.[81]

Insulin treatments themselves may accelerate aging, worsen diabetic vision loss, and promote cancer, obesity, and atherosclerosis.[82] Insulin can promote inflammation in the arteries, which may help explain the increased death rate in the intensively treated group.[83] So rather than trying to overcome insulin resistance by brute force—just pumping in more and more insulin—isn't it better to treat the disease itself by eliminating the unhealthy diet that caused it? That reminds me of people who undergo bypass surgery for clogged arteries. If they keep eating unhealthfully, their bypasses will eventually get clogged too. It's better to treat the cause than the symptoms.

How about surgery for diabetes? Gastric bypass surgery—which effectively reduces the size of the stomach by 90 percent or more—is one of the most successful treatment methods for type 2 diabetes, with reported long-term remission rates of up to 83 percent. These results had led to the suggestion that gastric bypass surgery improves diabetes by somehow altering digestive hormones, but this interpretation ignores the fact that patients are placed on a severely limited diet for up to two weeks following the procedure to recover from the surgery. Extreme calorie restriction alone can reverse diabetes. So is the success of surgery the result of the operation itself or due to the restrictive diet?

Once again, researchers designed a study to uncover the answer.[84] They compared diabetics placed on the same postoperative diet before and after they actually had the surgery. Amazingly, they found that the diet alone worked *better* than the surgery even in the same group of patients: The subjects' blood sugar control was better in the absence of the operation. This means the benefits of major surgery may be obtained without you ever having to go under the knife and getting your internal organs rearranged.[85]

The bottom line: Blood sugar levels can normalize within a week of eating six hundred calories daily, because fat is pulled out of the muscles, liver, and pancreas, allowing them to function normally again.[86]

This reversal of diabetes can be accomplished either by voluntary calorie restriction[87] or involuntarily, by having most of your stomach removed, a form of compulsory food restriction. Undergoing surgery may be easier than starving yourself, but major surgery carries major risks, both during the operation and afterward. These risks include bleeding, leakage, infections, erosions, herniation, and severe nutritional deficiencies.[88]

Surgery or starvation? There's got to be a better way, and, in fact, there is. Instead of changing the quantity of food you eat, it's possible to reverse diabetes by changing the *quality* of that food.

Does Eating Obesity Cause Obesity?

The EPIC-PANACEA study, which found that meat consumption is associated with weight gain even independent of calories, identified poultry as potentially the most fattening meat,[89] a finding that has since been confirmed in another study. Men and women eating even a single ounce of chicken a day (think two chicken nuggets) had a significantly greater gain in body mass index over the fourteen-year follow-up period than those who consumed no chicken at all.[90] Perhaps this news shouldn't be surprising,

continued

considering how fat chickens themselves are now genetically manipulated to become.

According to the U.S. Department of Agriculture, about one hundred years ago, a single serving of chicken may have contained only sixteen fat calories. Nowadays, one serving of chicken may have more than two hundred calories of fat. The fat content in poultry has ballooned from less than two grams per serving a century ago to up to twenty-three grams today. That's ten times more fat. Chicken now contains two to three times more calories from fat than from protein, leading nutrition researchers to ask, "Does eating obesity cause obesity in the consumer?"[91] As the beef industry is proud of pointing out, even skinless chicken can have more fat, and more artery-clogging saturated fat, than a dozen different cuts of steak.[92]

Reversing Diabetes with Food

We've known since the siege of Paris in 1870 that type 2 diabetes can be reversed by an extreme reduction in food intake. Parisian doctors documented how glucose disappeared from their patients' urine after people went weeks without food.[93] Diabetes specialists have long known that iron-willed patients who are able to lose up to one-fifth of their body weight can reverse their diabetes and bring their metabolic function back to normal.[94]

Instead of starving by eating less food, though, what if diabetics just ate better food, as in a 90 percent or more plant-based diet of all-you-can-eat greens, lots of other vegetables and beans, whole grains, fruits, nuts, and seeds? In a pilot study, thirteen diabetic men and women were told to eat at least one big salad every day, as well as veggie-bean soup, a handful of nuts and seeds, fruit at every meal, a pound of cooked greens, and some whole grains; to restrict their animal product consumption; and to eliminate refined grains, junk food, and oil. Then, the researchers measured their hemoglobin A1c levels, considered the best measure of how poorly blood sugars have been controlled over time.

At the onset of the study, the diabetics had A1c levels averaging 8.2. An A1c level under 5.7 is considered normal, between 5.7 and 6.4 is considered prediabetic, and above 6.5 is considered diabetic. However, the American Diabetes Association's target is just to get most diabetics down below 7.0.[95] (Recall that intensive blood-sugar-lowering trials using drugs, which tried to push A1c levels under 6.0, unfortunately ended up pushing many diabetics six feet under.)

After about seven months of eating a diet centered on whole plant foods, the subjects' A1c levels dropped to a nondiabetic 5.8—and this was after they were able to stop taking most of their medications.[96] We've known diabetes can be reversed with an extremely low-calorie diet.[97] Now we know that it can also be reversed with an extremely healthy diet, but is that because it was also low in calories? The study subjects lost about as much weight on the vegetable-packed, plant-based diet as people who went on semistarvation diets based on liquid meal replacements.[98] But even if this type of diabetes reversal was just about calorie restriction, which would be healthier? Subsisting on mostly diet shakes made out of sugar, powdered milk, corn syrup, and oil, or eating a plant-based diet where you can enjoy real food and lots of it?

Surprisingly, even participants who temporarily didn't lose weight on the plant-based diet, or who actually gained weight, still appeared to improve their diabetes. In other words, the beneficial effects of plant-based diets may extend beyond weight loss.[99] However, the study described just a handful of people, had no control group, and included only those who could stick to the eating plan. To prove plant-based diets could actually improve diabetes independent of weight loss, researchers would need to design a study in which they switched people to a healthy diet but forced them to eat so much that they didn't lose any weight.

Just such a study was published more than thirty-five years ago. Type 2 diabetics were placed on a plant-based diet and weighed every day. If they started losing any weight, they were made to eat more food—so much that some of the participants actually had trouble eating it all! The result: Even with no weight loss, subjects on the plant-based diet saw their insulin requirements cut by about 60 percent, meaning the amount of insulin these diabetics had to inject dropped by more than half. Furthermore, half of the diabetics were able to get off insulin altogether, despite no change in body weight—just by eating a healthier diet.[100]

This wasn't over the course of months or years, either. This was after eating a plant-based diet for an average of only sixteen days. Some of the subjects had been diabetic for two decades and had been injecting twenty units of insulin a day. Yet within two weeks of eating a plant-based diet, they were off insulin altogether. One patient was on thirty-two units of insulin per day at the onset of the study. After eighteen days, his blood sugar levels plummeted so low that insulin injections were no longer necessary. Even at approximately the same body weight, he had lower blood sugars on a plant-based diet using no insulin than when he had been on a regular diet using thirty-two units of insulin daily.[101] That's the power of plants.

Curing Diabetic Neuropathy

Up to 50 percent of diabetics eventually develop neuropathy, or damage to their nerves.[102] Neuropathy can be very painful, and that pain is frequently resistant to conventional treatments. No medical treatment is considered effective for the condition.[103] We doctors are left with only steroids, opiates, and antidepressants to try to ease our patients' suffering. But then a remarkable study was published, entitled "Regression of Diabetic Neuropathy with Total Vegetarian (Vegan) Diet." Twenty-one diabetics who had been suffering from painful neuropathy for up to ten years were placed on a whole-food, plant-based diet. After years and years of suffering, seventeen out of the twenty-one patients reported that they felt complete relief from their pain—*within days*. Their numbness noticeably improved too. And the side effects were all good: The diabetics lost an average of ten pounds, their blood sugar levels dropped, their insulin needs dropped in half, and, in five of the patients, not only was their painful neuropathy cured, so was, apparently, their diabetes. After having been diabetic for up to twenty years, they were off all blood sugar drugs in less than a month.[104]

On top of that, the diabetics' triglyceride and cholesterol levels improved on average as well. High blood pressures dropped by so much that half of the subjects also appeared cured of their hypertension. Within three weeks, the subjects' need for high blood pressure medications dropped by 80 percent.[105] (This is why it is critically important to work with your doctor when radically improving your diet, because if they don't reduce or eliminate your medications accordingly, your blood sugar levels or blood pressure may drop too low.)

We've long known that plant-based diets can reverse diabetes[106] and hypertension,[107] but reversing nerve damage pain with diet was new.

This study involved a live-in program in which patients were provided meals. What happened after they were sent home, back into the real world? These seventeen subjects were followed for years, and in all cases but one, the relief from their painful neuropathy continued—or improved even further. How were the researchers able to achieve such a high degree of dietary compliance even in an uncontrolled setting? "Pain and ill health," the researchers wrote, "are strong motivating factors."[108] In other words: Because plant-based diets work.

Think about it. Patients walk in with one of the most painful, frustrating, and hard-to-treat conditions in all of medicine, and three-quarters of them were cured in a handful of days using a natural, nontoxic treatment—namely, a diet composed of whole plant foods. This should have been front-page news.

How could nerve damage pain be reversed so suddenly? It didn't appear to involve the improvement in blood sugar control. It took approximately ten days for the diet to control the diabetes itself, but the pain was gone in as few as four days.[109]

The most interesting speculation was that trans fats naturally found in meat and dairy could be causing an inflammatory response in the patients' bodies. The researchers found that a significant percentage of the fat under the skin of those who ate meat, or even just dairy and eggs, was composed of trans fats, whereas those who had been on a strictly whole-food, plant-based diet had no detectable trans fat in their tissues.[110]

The researchers stuck needles into the buttocks of subjects who had been eating different diets and discovered that people who had been on a whole-food, plant-based diet for nine months or more appeared to have removed all the trans fat from their bodies (or at least from their butts!).[111] But their neuropathy pain didn't take nine months to get better. It improved in closer to nine days. It's more likely that this amazing reversal was due to an improvement in blood flow.[112]

Nerves contain tiny blood vessels that may become clogged, depriving the nerves of oxygen. Indeed, biopsies of leg nerves in diabetics with severe progressive neuropathy have shown arterial disease within the sural nerve in the leg.[113] However, within days of eating healthier meals, blood flow may improve to the extent that neuropathy disappears.[114] Within an average of two years of eating a plant-based diet composed mostly of rice and fruits, even diabetic vision loss can be reversed in as many as 30 percent of patients.[115]

So why didn't I learn about any of this in medical school? There's little money to be made from prescribing plants instead of pills. The neuropathy pain reversal study was published more than twenty years ago, and the blindness reversal studies more than fifty years ago. As one commentator wrote, "The neglect of this important work by the broader medical community is little short of unconscionable."[116]

WHtR Versus BMI

The body mass index (BMI) is a better predictor of disease than body weight alone, as BMI takes height into account. But BMI has long been criticized for not considering the location or the nature of your weight. Bodybuilders, for instance, have extremely low body fat but can have off-the-chart BMIs, because muscle is heavier than fat.

continued

Today, it's generally accepted that health risks can be determined as much by the relative distribution of body fat as by its total amount.[117] What's the worst kind? Abdominal fat—the kind that builds up around your internal organs. Having a potbelly may be a strong predictor of premature death.[118]

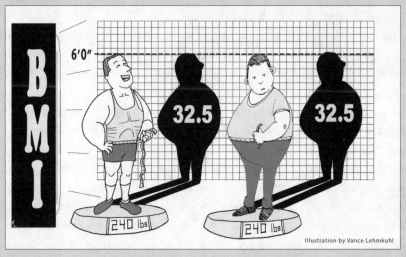

Illustration by Vance Lehmkuhl

Figure 3

Both the men in figure 3 have the same BMI, but the distribution of weight is different. People with the so-called apple shape, with body fat concentrated in the abdominal region, may have the lowest life expectancy.[119]

Fortunately, there may be an even better tool than BMI that we can use to gauge the health risks of body fat. It's called Waist-to-Height Ratio, or WHtR.[120] Instead of a scale, grab a simple measuring tape. Stand up straight and take a deep breath, exhale, and let it all hang out. The circumference of your belly (halfway between the top of your hip bones and the bottom of your rib cage) should be half your height—ideally, less. If that measurement is more than half your height, it's time to start eating healthier and exercising more regardless of your weight.[121]

Type 2 diabetes in the United States is reaching epidemic proportions. The CDC estimates that 37 percent of U.S. adults—and 51 percent of adults over sixty-five—have prediabetes. That's eighty-six million people,[122] most of whom will become full-blown diabetics.[123] But type 2 diabetes can be prevented, arrested, and even reversed with a healthy-enough diet. Unfortunately, doctors don't tend to educate their patients about diabetes prevention. Only about one in three prediabetic patients reports ever being told by their doctors to exercise or to improve their diets.[124] Possible reasons for not counseling patients include a lack of insurance reimbursement for the extra time spent, a lack of resources, a lack of time, and a lack of knowledge.[125] We're just not training doctors how to empower the people they serve.

The current medical education system has yet to adapt to the great transformation of disease from acute to chronic. Medicine is no longer about just setting broken bones or curing strep throat. Such chronic diseases as diabetes are now the principal cause of death and disability in America, consuming three-quarters of the nation's health care budget. Medical education has yet to recognize and respond to the changing nature of disease patterns, which now requires a focus on prevention and lifestyle change.[126] How far behind the times is the medical profession? A report by the Institute of Medicine on medical training concluded that the fundamental approach to medical education has not changed since 1910.[127]

Not long ago, I received an e-mail that helps sum up where we are. Tonah, a sixty-five-year-old Native American, had been on insulin for type 2 diabetes for the last twenty-seven years. He was told by his doctor that Native Americans were "genetically predisposed" to the disease. He just had to live with it, including the excruciating nerve pain, three heart stents, and erectile dysfunction. After watching my "Uprooting the Leading Causes of Death" video on NutritionFacts.org, his granddaughter convinced him to try a plant-based diet.

It wasn't easy, since the nearest store with fresh food was fifty miles away. Nevertheless, in less than two weeks, he turned his life around. His nerve pain diminished dramatically, to the point where it no longer kept him up at night. He lost thirty pounds in a matter of months and no longer needed insulin. His own doctor couldn't believe this was possible and ordered a CT scan to check for tumors. There weren't any. Now he feels better than he has in years.

"I'm grateful that my granddaughter has stopped seeing me as a sick old man," Tonah concluded his note. "I feel young again, Doc."

CHAPTER 7

How Not to Die from High Blood Pressure

The most comprehensive and systematic analysis of the causes of death ever undertaken was published recently in the *Lancet*, one of the world's leading medical journals.[1] Funded by the Bill & Melinda Gates Foundation, the Global Burden of Disease Study involved nearly five hundred researchers from more than three hundred institutions in fifty countries and examined nearly one hundred thousand data sources.[2] The results allow us to answer such questions as "How many lives could we save if people around the world cut back on soda?" The best answer? 299,521.[3] So soft drinks and their empty calories don't just fail to promote health—they actually seem to promote death. But apparently soda isn't nearly as deadly as bacon, bologna, ham, and hot dogs. Processed meat is blamed for the deaths of more than eight hundred thousand people every year. Worldwide, that's four times more people than who die from illicit drug use.[4]

The study also noted which foods, if added to the diet, might *save* lives. Eating more whole grains could potentially save 1.7 million lives a year. More vegetables? 1.8 million lives. How about nuts and seeds? 2.5 million lives. The researchers didn't look at beans, but of the foods they considered, which does the world need most? Fruit. Worldwide, if humanity ate more fruit, we might save 4.9 million lives. That's nearly 5 million lives hanging in the balance, and their salvation isn't medication or a new vaccine—it may be just more fruit.[5]

The number-one risk factor for death in the world they identified is high blood pressure.[6] Also known as hypertension, high blood pressure lays waste to nine million people worldwide every year.[7] It kills so many people because it contributes to deaths from a variety of causes, including aneurysms, heart attacks, heart failure, kidney failure, and stroke.

You've probably had your blood pressure taken at the doctor's office. The nurse reads off two numbers, say, for example, "115 over 75." The first number ("systolic") represents the pressure in your arteries as your blood pumps from the heart; the second number ("diastolic") is the pressure in your arteries while the heart is resting between beats. The American Heart Association defines "normal" blood pressure as a systolic pressure under 120 and a diastolic pressure under 80—or 120/80. Anything above 140/90 is considered hypertensive. Values in between are considered prehypertensive.[8]

Increased blood pressure puts a strain on the heart and can damage the sensitive blood vessels in your eyes and kidneys, cause bleeding in the brain, and even lead certain arteries to balloon and rupture. The fact that hypertension can damage so many organ systems and increase the risk of heart disease and stroke, two of our leading killers, explains why it is the number-one killer risk factor worldwide.

In the United States, nearly seventy-eight million people have high blood pressure—that's about one in three American adults.[9] As you age, your blood pressure tends to get higher and higher. In fact, after age sixty, 65 percent of Americans can expect to be diagnosed with the condition.[10] This has led many people, including doctors, to assume that high blood pressure, like wrinkles or gray hair, is just an inevitable consequence of getting older. However, we've known for nearly a century that this isn't true.

In the 1920s, researchers measured the blood pressure of a thousand native Kenyans who ate a low-sodium diet centered around whole plant foods—whole grains, beans, fruits, and dark, leafy greens, and other vegetables.[11] Up until age forty, the blood pressure of the rural Africans was similar to that of Europeans and Americans, about 125/80. However, as Westerners aged, their blood pressure began to surge past the Kenyans. By age sixty, the average Westerner was hypertensive, with blood pressure exceeding 140/90. What about the Kenyans? By age sixty, their average blood pressure had actually *improved* to an average of about 110/70.[12]

The 140/90 threshold for hypertension is considered an arbitrary cutoff.[13] Just like having too much cholesterol or body fat, there are benefits to having a blood pressure that is even lower than the "normal" range. So even people who start out with a so-called normal blood pressure of 120/80 appear to benefit from going down to 110/70.[14] But is it possible to do that? Look at the Kenyans—not only is it possible, it appears *typical* for people who live healthy, plant-based lifestyles.

Over a two-year period, 1,800 patients were admitted into a rural Kenyan hospital. How many cases of high blood pressure did they find? Zero. There also wasn't a single case found of America's number-one killer, atherosclerosis.[15]

High blood pressure, then, appears to be a choice. You can continue eating the artery-bursting Western diet, or you can choose to take off the pressure. The truth is that eliminating humanity's primary risk factor for death may be simple. No drugs, no scalpels. Just forks.

Sodium

The two most prominent dietary risks for death and disability in the world may be not eating enough fruit and eating too much salt. Nearly five million people appear to die every year as a result of not eating enough fruit,[16] while eating too much salt may kill up to four million.[17]

Salt is a compound made up of about 40 percent sodium and 60 percent chloride. Sodium is an essential nutrient, but vegetables and other natural foods provide the small amounts of sodium you need in your diet. If you consume too much, it can cause water retention, and your body may respond by raising your blood pressure to push the excess fluid and salt out of your system.[18]

For the first 90 percent of human evolution, we likely ate diets containing less than the equivalent of a quarter teaspoon of salt's worth of sodium a day.[19] Why? Because we likely ate mostly plants.[20] We went millions of years without saltshakers, so our bodies evolved into sodium-conserving machines. That served us well until we discovered that salt could be used to preserve foods.[21] Without refrigeration, this was a boon to human civilization. It didn't matter that the addition of salt to our food resulted in a general rise in blood pressure—the alternative was starving to death because all our food rotted away.

But where does that leave us now? After all, we no longer have to live off pickles and jerky. Humans are genetically programmed to eat ten times less sodium than we do now.[22] Many so-called low-salt diets can actually be considered high-salt diets. That's why it's critical to understand what the concept of "normal" is when it comes to sodium. Having a "normal" salt intake can lead to a "normal" blood pressure, which can contribute to us dying from all the "normal" causes, like heart attacks and strokes.[23]

The American Heart Association recommends everyone consume less than 1,500 mg of sodium daily[24]—that's about three-quarters of a teaspoon of salt. The average American adult consumes more than double that amount, about 3,500 mg daily.[25] Reducing sodium consumption by just 15 percent worldwide could save millions of lives every year.[26]

If we could cut our salt intake by about a half teaspoon a day, which is achievable by avoiding salty foods and not adding salt to our food, we might prevent 22 percent of stroke deaths and 16 percent of fatal heart attacks. That's potentially more lives saved than if we were able to successfully treat people with blood pressure pills.[27] Simply put, reducing salt is an easy at-home intervention that may be more powerful than filling a prescription from the pharmacy. Up to ninety-two thousand American lives could be saved each year simply by eating less salt.[28]

The evidence that sodium raises blood pressure is clear, including double-blind, randomized trials dating back decades.[29] If we take subjects with high blood pressure and put them on a sodium-restricted diet, their blood pressure drops. If we keep them on the low-salt diet and add a placebo, nothing happens. However, if we instead give subjects salt in the form of a time-release sodium pill, their blood pressure goes back up again.[30] The more sodium we give them secretly, the higher their blood pressure climbs.[31]

Even just a single meal can do it. If we take people with normal blood pressure and give them a bowl of soup containing the amount of salt that may be found in an average American meal,[32] their blood pressure climbs over the next three hours compared to eating the same soup without any added salt.[33] Dozens of similar studies demonstrate that if you reduce your salt intake, you reduce your blood pressure. And the greater the reduction, the greater the benefit. But if you don't cut down, chronic high salt intake can lead to a gradual increase in blood pressure throughout life.[34]

Doctors used to be taught that a "normal" systolic blood pressure is approximately 100 plus age. Indeed that's about what you're born with. Babies start out with a blood pressure around 95/60. But, as you age, that 95 can go up to 120 by your twenties. By the time you're in your forties, it can be up to 140—the official cutoff for high blood pressure—and then keep climbing as you get older.[35]

What would happen if, instead of consuming ten times more sodium than what your bodies were designed to handle, you just ate the natural amount found in whole foods? Is it possible your blood pressure would stay low your whole life? To test that theory, we'd have to find a population in modern times that doesn't use salt, eat processed food, or go out to eat. To find a no-salt culture, scientists had to go deep into the Amazon rainforest.[36]

Strangers to saltshakers, Cheetos, and KFC, the Yanomamo Indians were found to have the lowest sodium intake ever recorded—which is to say the sodium intake we evolved eating.[37] Lo and behold, researchers found that the blood pressures among older Yanomamo were the same as those of adolescents.[38] In other words, they start out with an average blood pressure of about 100/60 and stay that way for life. The researchers couldn't find a single case of high blood pressure.[39]

Why do we suspect it was the sodium? After all, the Yanomamos studied didn't drink alcohol, ate a high-fiber, plant-based diet, had lots of exercise, and were not obese.[40] An interventional trial could prove that sodium was the culprit. Imagine if we took people literally dying from out-of-control high blood pressure (known as malignant hypertension), a condition from which you go blind from bleeding into your eyes, your kidneys shut down, and your heart eventually fails. What if you put these patients on a Yanomamo-level salt intake—in other words, a normal-for-the-human-species salt intake?

Enter Dr. Walter Kempner and his rice-and-fruit diet. Without drugs, he brought patients with eye-popping blood pressures like 240/150 down to 105/80 with dietary changes alone. How could he ethically withhold medication from such seriously ill patients? Modern high-blood-pressure pills hadn't been invented yet—Dr. Kempner conducted his work back in the 1940s.[41] Back then, malignant hypertension was a death sentence, with a life expectancy of about six months.[42] Nevertheless, he was able to reverse the course of disease with diet in more than 70 percent of cases.[43] Though the diet wasn't merely extremely low sodium—it was also strictly plant-based and low in fat and protein—Dr. Kempner is now recognized as the person who established, beyond any shadow of doubt, that high blood pressure can often be lowered by a low-sodium diet.[44]

In addition to high blood pressure, salty meals can significantly impair artery function,[45] even among people whose blood pressure tends to be unresponsive to salt intake.[46] In other words, salt itself can injure our arteries independent of its impact on blood pressure. And that harm begins within thirty minutes.[47]

Using a technique called laser Doppler flowmetry, researchers are able to measure blood flow in the tiny vessels in the skin. After a high-sodium meal, there is significantly less blood flow—unless vitamin C is injected into the skin, which appears to reverse much of the sodium-induced suppression of blood vessel function. So, if an antioxidant helps block the sodium effect, then the mechanism by which salt impairs arterial function may be oxidative stress, the formation of free radicals in your bloodstream.[48] It turns out that sodium intake appears to suppress the activity of a key antioxidant enzyme in the body called superoxide dismutase,[49] which has the ability to detoxify a million free radicals per second.[50] With the action of this workhorse of an enzyme stifled by sodium, artery-crippling levels of oxidative stress can build up.

After one salty meal, not only does blood pressure increase but the arteries actually begin to stiffen.[51] This may be how we figured out thousands of years ago that too much salt was bad for us. Quoting from a translation of *The Yellow*

Emperor's Classic of Internal Medicine, an ancient Chinese medical text, "If too much salt is used in food, the pulse hardens . . ."[52] It turns out that we may not need a double-blind trial; maybe we just have to feed someone a bag of potato chips and take his or her pulse.

Unsurprisingly, the salt industry isn't thrilled about the idea of us cutting back on salt. Back in 2009, the American Heart Association quoted the chair of the U.S. Dietary Guidelines Advisory Committee as saying that Americans should reduce their sodium intake. The Salt Institute, a salt industry trade organization, accused her of having an "unhealthy prejudice" against salt, arguing that she had "pre-judged the salt issue."[53] This is like the tobacco industry complaining that people at the American Lung Association are biased against smoking. Of course, the Salt Institute wasn't the only aggrieved party. Cheese, it turns out, ranks as a leading contributor of sodium in the American diet,[54] and the National Dairy Council stood shoulder-to-shoulder with Big Salt in its condemnation of the Dietary Guidelines Advisory Committee recommendations.[55]

The salt industry has its own PR and lobbying firms to play tobacco-industry-style tactics to downplay the dangers of its product.[56] But the real villains aren't necessarily the salt-mine barons—it's the processed food industry. The trillion-dollar processed food industry uses dirt-cheap added salt and sugar to sell us their junk.[57] That's why it's not easy avoiding sodium on the typical American diet, since three-quarters of salt comes from processed foods rather than a saltshaker.[58] By hooking you on hypersweet and hypersalty foods, your taste buds get so dampened that natural foods can taste like cardboard. Indeed, the ripest fruit may not be as sweet as Froot Loops.

But there are two other major reasons the food industry adds salt to foods. If you add salt to meat, it draws in water. This way, a company can increase the weight of its product by nearly 20 percent. Since meat is sold by the pound, that's 20 percent more profits for very little added cost. Second, as everyone knows, eating salt makes us thirsty. There's a reason bars put out free baskets of salted nuts and pretzels, and it's the same reason soda conglomerates own snack-food companies. A cold drink and a salty snack go hand in hand. It may be no coincidence that Pepsi and Frito-Lay are part of the same corporation.[59]

Pop quiz! Which has been reported to contain the most sodium: a serving of beef, a serving of baked all-natural chicken, a large McDonald's french fries, or a serving of salted pretzels?

The answer? Chicken. The poultry industry commonly injects chicken carcasses with salt water to artificially inflate their weight, yet they can still be labelled "100 percent natural." *Consumer Reports* found that some supermarket chickens were pumped so full of salt that they registered a whopping

840 mg of sodium per serving—that could mean more than a full day's worth of sodium in just one chicken breast.[60]

The number-one source of sodium for American kids and teens is pizza.[61] A single slice of Pizza Hut pepperoni pizza can contain half your recommended sodium intake limit for the entire day.[62] For adults over fifty, it's bread, but between the ages of twenty and fifty, the greatest contributor of sodium to the diet is chicken—not the canned soups, pretzels, or potato chips one might expect.[63]

How can you overcome your built-in craving for salt, sugar, and fat? Just give it a few weeks, and your taste buds will start to change. When researchers put people on a low-salt diet, over time, the research subjects increasingly enjoyed the taste of salt-free soup and became turned off by the salt-heavy soup they had previously craved. As the study progressed, when the participants were allowed to salt their own soup to taste, they preferred less and less salt as their taste buds became acclimated to healthier levels.[64]

The same may be true for sugar and fat. It's likely that humans actually taste fat, just like they taste sweet, sour, and salty flavors.[65] People placed on low-fat diets start preferring low-fat foods over fatty options.[66] Your tongue may actually become more sensitive to fat, and the more sensitive your tongue becomes, the less butter, meat, dairy, and eggs you eat. On the flip side, if you eat too much of these foods, you may blunt your taste for fat, which can cause you to eat more calories and more fat, dairy, meat, and eggs and ultimately gain weight.[67] This can all happen in just a matter of weeks.[68]

There are three things you can do to shake the salt habit.[69] First, don't add salt at the table. (One out of three people may add salt to their food before even tasting it!)[70] Second, stop adding salt when cooking. The food may taste bland at first, but within two to four weeks, the salt-taste receptors in your mouth become more sensitive, and food tastes better. Believe it or not, after two weeks, you may actually *prefer* the taste of food with less salt.[71] Try any combination of such fantastic flavorings as pepper, onions, garlic, tomatoes, sweet peppers, basil, parsley, thyme, celery, lime, chili powder, rosemary, smoked paprika, curry, coriander, and lemon instead.[72] Also, it's probably a good idea to avoid eating out as much as possible. Even non-fast-food restaurants tend to pile on the salt.[73] Finally, do what you can to avoid processed foods.

In most countries studied, processed foods provide only about half of people's sodium intake, but in the United States, we consume so much sodium from processed foods that even if we completely stopped adding salt in the kitchen and dining room, we'd still only reduce our salt intake by a small fraction.[74] Try to buy foods with fewer milligrams of sodium on the label than there are grams in the serving size. For example, if it's a 100 g serving size, the product should have less than 100 mg of sodium.[75] Alternatively, you can shoot for fewer milligrams of sodium per serving than there are calories. That's a trick I learned from one of my favorite dietitians, Jeff Novick. Most people get around 2,200 calories a day, so if everything you ate had more calories than sodium, you would probably make it at least under the Dietary Guidelines for Americans' upper limit of 2,300 mg of sodium a day.[76]

Ideally, though, you'd buy mostly food without any labels at all. It is considered almost impossible to come up with a diet consisting of unprocessed natural foods that exceeds the strict 1,500 mg a day American Heart Association guidelines for sodium reduction.[77]

Whole Grains

On average, high blood pressure medications reduce the risk of heart attack by 15 percent and the risk of stroke by 25 percent.[78] But in a randomized, controlled trial, three portions of whole grains a day were able to help people achieve this blood-pressure-lowering benefit too.[79] The study revealed that a diet rich in whole grains yields the same benefits without the adverse side effects commonly associated with antihypertensive drugs, such as electrolyte disturbances in those taking diuretics (also known as water pills);[80] increased breast cancer risk for those taking calcium-channel blockers (like Norvasc or Cardizem);[81] lethargy and impotence for those on beta blockers (like Lopressor and Corgard);[82] sudden, potentially life-threatening swelling for those taking ACE inhibitors (like Vasotec and Altace);[83] and an increased risk of serious fall injuries for apparently any class of these blood pressure drugs.[84]

Whole grains do have side effects, though. Good ones! Whole-grain intake is associated with lower risks of type 2 diabetes, coronary heart disease, weight gain,[85] and colon cancer.[86] Take note of the *whole*, however. While whole grains, such as oats, whole wheat, and brown rice, have been shown to reduce your risk of developing chronic disease,[87] *refined* grains may actually increase your risk. Harvard University researchers, for example, found that while regular consumption of brown rice was associated with a lower risk of type 2 diabetes, consuming white rice was associated with higher risk. Daily servings of white rice were associated with a 17 percent greater risk of diabetes, whereas replacing one-third of a serving a day of white rice for brown rice might lead to a 16 percent *drop* in risk. And it looks like replacing white rice with oats and barley may be an even more powerful step, associated with a 36 percent drop in diabetes risk.[88]

Given the improvements in cardiac risk factors seen in interventional trials of whole grains,[89] it's not surprising to see a reduction in the progression of arterial disease among those who regularly eat them. In studies of two of the most important arteries in the body, the coronary arteries that feed the heart and the carotid arteries that feed the brain, people who ate the most whole grains had significantly slower narrowing of their arteries.[90,91] Since atherosclerotic plaque in the arteries is our leading killer, ideally, you should not just slow down the process but actually stop or even reverse it altogether. As we saw in chapter 1, this appears to require more than just whole grains; whole vegetables, whole fruits, whole beans, and other whole plant foods are needed, along with a significant reduction in your intake of trans fats, saturated fats, and cholesterol, the food components that contribute to clogging your arteries shut.

What About the DASH Diet?

What if you are among the seventy-eight million Americans who already have high blood pressure? How can you bring it down?

The American Heart Association (AHA), the American College of Cardiology (ACC), and the Centers for Disease Control and Prevention (CDC) all recommend that patients first try lifestyle modifications, such as reducing body weight, limiting sodium and alcohol intake, getting more exercise, and eating a healthier diet.[92]

However, if their recommended lifestyle changes don't work, then it's off to the pharmacy. First up is a diuretic (water pill), and before you can spell "pharmaceutical cocktail," the medications begin piling up until your blood pressure comes down. High blood pressure patients commonly end up on three different antihypertensive drugs at a time,[93] yet only about half tend to stick to even the first-line drugs.[94] (This is due in part to all their side effects, which can include erectile dysfunction, fatigue, and leg cramps.)[95] At the end of all of this, the drugs still haven't gotten to the root cause of the problem. The cause of high blood pressure isn't medication deficiency. The underlying cause is what you eat and how you live.

As we discussed earlier, the ideal blood pressure, defined as the level at which lowering it further yields no additional benefit, is probably around 110/70.[96] Can you really get it that low without medication? Remember, this was the *average* blood pressure of men more than sixty years old in rural Africa on no treatment other than their traditional, plant-based diets and lifestyles.[97] In rural China, we find similar results: 110/70 throughout life without any increase with age.[98] The reason we suspect that the plant-based nature of their diets is responsible is because, in the Western world, the only group able to routinely achieve these blood pressure readings is vegetarians.[99]

So do the AHA/ACC/CDC guidelines recommend that people with high blood pressure eat a meat-free diet? No. They recommend the DASH diet, which stands for Dietary Approaches to Stop Hypertension, an eating plan specifically designed to lower blood pressure.[100] Although it's been described as a lactovegetarian diet[101] (dairy, but no meat or eggs), that isn't accurate. The DASH diet emphasizes fruits, vegetables, and low-fat dairy, but meat is still present—you're just supposed to eat less of it.[102]

Why not recommend an even more plant-based diet? We've known for decades that "food of animal origin was highly significantly associated with systolic and diastolic B[lood] P[ressure] after the age and weight effects were removed."[103] That's a quote from a series of studies performed by renowned physician Frank Sacks and colleagues back in the 1970s, but there are studies going all the way back to the 1920s demonstrating that adding meat to a plant-based diet can significantly elevate blood pressure in a matter of days.[104]

Why isn't the DASH diet meatless? Based on the work of Dr. Sacks at Harvard University, the American Heart Association acknowledged that "[s]ome of the lowest B[lood]P[ressure]s observed in industrialized countries have been documented in strict vegetarians. . . ."[105] Were the designers of the DASH diet just not aware of Dr. Sacks's work? No, the chair of the committee that designed the diet *was* Dr. Sacks.[106]

The reason that the DASH diet was modeled explicitly after vegetarian diets but was not meat-free itself might surprise you. The primary design goal of the DASH diet was to explicitly create eating patterns "that would have the blood pressure lowering benefits of a vegetarian diet yet contain enough animal products to make them palatable to nonvegetarians. . . ."[107] Dr. Sacks had even shown that the more dairy vegetarians consumed, the higher their blood pressure appeared to rise.[108] But he figured there was no point in calling for a diet he believed few would follow. This is a recurring theme in official dietary recommendations. Instead of simply telling you what the science shows and then letting you make up your own mind, experts patronize the population by advocating what they think is practical rather than ideal. By making the decision for you, they undermine those willing to make even greater changes for optimal health.

The DASH diet does help to bring down blood pressure, but the primary effect seems to arise not from the switch to low-fat dairy and white meat or the reduction in sweets and added fats but from the added fruits and vegetables.[109] If the benefits are due to the added plant foods, why not strive to center people's diets more around these healthiest of foods in the first place?

This question is even more pointed given a 2014 meta-analysis (a compilation of many similar studies) showing that vegetarian diets may be particularly good at lowering blood pressure.[110] And the more plants, perhaps, the better. Meat-free diets in general "confer protection against cardiovascular diseases . . . some cancers and total mortality," but completely plant-based diets "seem to offer additional protection for obesity, hypertension, type-2 diabetes, and cardiovascular mortality."[111]

There appears to be a stepwise drop in hypertension rates the more plant-based foods you eat. Based on the same study of eighty-nine thousand Californians featured in chapter 6, compared with people who eat meat more than once a week, flexitarians (those who eat less meat, perhaps a few times a month) had 23 percent lower rates of high blood pressure. Those who cut out all meat except for fish had a 38 percent lower risk of high blood pressure, and those who cut out all meat had a 55 percent lower rate. People who cut out all meat, eggs, and dairy did the best, with a 75 percent reduced risk of high blood pressure. Those eating completely plant-based diets appeared to have thrown three-quarters of their risk for developing this major killer out the window.[112]

When scientists looked at diabetes and body weight, they found the same apparent progressive improvements as consumption of animal products decreased and plant foods increased. Those eating plant-based diets had just a fraction of the diabetes risk even after factoring out the weight benefits,[113] but what about hypertension? On average, those who eat completely plant-based foods are about thirty pounds lighter than those eating conventional diets.[114] Maybe they have such great blood pressure just because they're so much thinner? In other words, do omnivores who are as slim as vegans enjoy the same blood pressure?

To answer this question, researchers would have to find a group of individuals who eat the standard American diet but are also as thin as people eating plant-based diets. To find an omnivorous group that fit and trim, researchers recruited long-distance endurance athletes who had run, on average, forty-eight miles per week for twenty-one years. Running almost two marathons a week for twenty years, pretty much anyone can become as slim as a plant eater no matter what they eat! The researchers then compared these hard-core athletes to two groups: sedentary meat eaters who exercised less than an hour per week and sedentary vegans who ate mostly unprocessed, uncooked plant foods.

How did the numbers come out? Not surprisingly, the endurance runners on a standard American diet had a better blood pressure average than their sedentary, meat-eating counterparts: 122/72 compared with 132/79, which fits the definition of prehypertensive. But the sedentary vegans? They averaged an extraordinary 104/62.[115] Apparently, eating standard American fare even when running two thousand miles a year may not bring down your blood pressure as low as a being a couch-potato vegan.

Foods for Additional Hypertension Protection

A low-sodium diet centered around whole plant foods appears to be the best way to bring down high blood pressure. What if you're already eating this way but that 110/70 still eludes you? There are a few foods in particular you can try that may offer additional protection.

I've already touched on whole grains and will go into detail about flaxseeds, hibiscus tea, and nitrate-rich vegetables. Ground flaxseeds alone "induced one of the most potent blood-pressure-lowering effects ever achieved by a dietary intervention."[116] Eating just a few tablespoons a day appears to be two to three times more powerful than adopting an aerobic endurance exercise program[117] (not that you shouldn't do both—incorporate flaxseeds into your diet *and* exercise).

Consumption of both raw and cooked vegetables is associated with lower blood pressure, but raw veggies may be slightly more protective.[118] Studies have also found that loading up on beans, split peas, chickpeas, and lentils may help a little,[119] so add those to your shopping list. Red wine may help, but only nonalcoholic brands. Only wine that has had the alcohol removed appears to lower blood pressure.[120]

Watermelon appears to offer protection, which is great (and delicious) news, but you may have to eat about two pounds of it per day to achieve an effect.[121] Kiwifruits flopped, though. In a study funded by a kiwifruit company, kiwi failed to offer any protection.[122] Perhaps the kiwi industry should take a cue from the California Raisin Marketing Board, which funded a study designed to show that raisins can reduce blood pressure. To inflate the benefits of raisins, they used junk food as the control group. So the study found raisins may lower blood pressure, but only, apparently, compared to fudge cookies, Cheez-Its, and Chips Ahoy![123]

Flaxseed

In chapters 11 and 13, we will see how effective flaxseeds can be against breast and prostate cancers, but you have to be a little skeptical when scientists throw around words like "miraculous" to describe them. (One medical journal published a review titled "Flaxseed: A Miraculous Defense Against Some Critical Maladies.")[124] But a remarkable intervention trial published in the journal *Hypertension* suggests that in this case, the term "miraculous" may not be too far off.

Rarely does one see a dietary study of this caliber: It was a prospective, double-blind, placebo-controlled, randomized trial. That's hard to pull off with food. With a drug trial, a blinded study is easy: Researchers give someone a sugar pill that looks identical to the drug, so that neither the study subject nor the person giving the pill knows which one is which (hence, double-blind). But how do you do that with food? People tend to notice if you try to sneak a quarter cup of ground flaxseed into their lunch.

The researchers tried a clever tactic to overcome this problem. They created a number of recipes for common foods including muffins and pasta in which they could disguise placebo ingredients like bran and molasses to match the texture and color of the flax-laden foods. This way, they could randomize people into two groups and secretly introduce tablespoons of daily ground flaxseeds into the diets of half the participants to see if it made any difference.

After six months, those who ate the placebo foods started out hypertensive and stayed hypertensive, despite the fact that many of them were on a variety of blood pressure pills. On average, they started the study at 155/81 and ended it at 158/81. What about the hypertensives who were unknowingly eating flaxseeds every day? Their blood pressure dropped from 158/82 down to 143/75. A seven-point drop in diastolic blood pressure may not sound like a lot, but that would be expected to result in 46 percent fewer strokes and 29 percent less heart disease over time.[125]

How does that result compare with taking drugs? The flaxseeds managed to drop subjects' systolic and diastolic blood pressure by up to fifteen and seven points, respectively. Compare that result to the effect of powerful antihypertensive drugs, such as calcium-channel blockers (for example, Norvasc, Cardizem, Procardia), which have been found to reduce blood pressure by only eight and three points, respectively, or to ACE inhibitors (such as Vasotec, Lotensin, Zestril, Altace), which drop patients' blood pressure by only five and two points, respectively.[126] Ground flaxseeds may work two to three times better than these medicines, and they have only good side effects. In addition to their anticancer properties, flaxseeds have been demonstrated in clinical studies to help control cholesterol, triglyceride, and blood sugar levels; reduce inflammation, and successfully treat constipation.[127]

Hibiscus Tea for Hypertension

Hibiscus tea, derived from the flower of the same name, is also known as roselle, sorrel, jamaica, or sour tea. With a distinct tart, cranberry-like flavor and bright red color, this herbal tea is served and enjoyed both hot and cold around the world. In a comparison of the antioxidant content of 280 common beverages, hibiscus ranked number-one, beating out other heavyweights, including the oft-lauded green tea.[128] Within an hour of consumption, the antioxidant power of your bloodstream shoots up, demonstrating that the antioxidant phytonutrients in the tea are absorbed into your system.[129] What effects might this infusion have on your health?

Unfortunately, efficacy against obesity has been disappointing. After giving hibiscus tea to overweight individuals for months, researchers have only been able to show about an extra half pound of weight loss per month over a placebo.[130] Early studies on cholesterol-lowering effects looked promising, suggesting that drinking two cups of hibiscus tea a day for a month may provide as much as an 8 percent drop in cholesterol,[131] but when all such studies were put together, the results were pretty much a wash.[132] This may be because, for some reason, hibiscus tea only seemed to have an effect on about half the study subjects. If you're in the lucky half, you may be able to get as much as a 12 percent drop in cholesterol.[133]

But high blood pressure is where hibiscus really shines.[134] A double-blind, placebo-controlled study out of Tufts University that compared hibiscus tea with an artificially colored and flavored lookalike showed that three cups of hibiscus tea a day significantly lowered blood pressure in prehypertensive adults better than the placebo beverage.[135] But by how much? How does drinking hibiscus tea compare with other interventions?

The PREMIER Clinical Trial randomized hundreds of men and women with elevated blood pressure into an "advice only" control group or an active lifestyle intervention group. The control group was given a brochure and told to lose weight, reduce their salt intake, get more exercise, and eat healthier (i.e., to go on the DASH diet). The behavioral intervention group received the same instruction but also got face-to-face sessions, attended group meetings, kept food diaries, and monitored their physical activity, calories, and sodium intake.

Within six months, the intervention group achieved a four-point drop in systolic blood pressure compared with the advice-only group. That may not seem like a lot, but on a population scale, a five-point drop may lead to 14 percent fewer stroke deaths, 9 percent fewer fatal heart attacks, and 7 percent fewer deaths overall each year.[136] Meanwhile, in the Tufts study, a cup of hibiscus tea with each meal managed to lower subjects' systolic blood pressure by six points over the control group.[137]

To lower blood pressure, you should still lose weight, reduce your salt intake, get more exercise, and eat healthier, but the evidence shows that adding hibiscus tea to your daily routine may offer an additional benefit, comparable even to that provided by antihypertensive drugs. Tested head-to-head against a leading blood pressure drug, two cups of strong hibiscus tea every morning (using a total of five tea bags) was as effective in lowering subjects' blood pressure as a starting dose of the drug Captopril taken twice a day.[138]

However, there are differences: Captopril can have side effects, most commonly rash, cough, and taste impairment, and it can even, though extremely rarely, cause fatal swelling of the throat.[139] No side effects were reported for hibiscus tea, though it isn't called sour tea for nothing. If you drink it, make sure to rinse your mouth with water afterward to keep the natural acids in the tea from softening the enamel on your teeth.[140] And given the extraordinary manganese content in hibiscus tea,[141] to be on the safe side, I wouldn't recommend drinking more than a quart of it a day.

The Power of NO

Nitric oxide (NO) is a key biological messenger within the body, and its message is: "Open Sesame!" When released by your endothelium (the cells lining your arteries), it signals the muscle fibers within the walls of your arteries to relax, allowing them to open up and for more blood to flow. That's how nitroglycerin pills work: The nitroglycerin people take when they're experiencing chest pain is converted into NO, which dilates the coronary arteries, allowing more blood to flow to the heart muscle. Erectile dysfunction (ED) pills like Viagra work the same way; they boost nitric oxide signaling, which relaxes penile arteries and improves blood flow to the penis.

The ED you really need to be concerned about, though, is endothelial dysfunction, the failure of the linings of your arteries to produce enough NO to properly dilate them. Nitric oxide is produced by an enzyme called NO synthase. Its enemy is free radicals, which not only gobble up nitric oxide but can hijack NO synthase and force it to start pumping out *additional* free radicals.[142]

Without enough NO, your arteries can then stiffen, become dysfunctional, and raise your blood pressure and your risk for heart attack.

So you need to flood your body with antioxidant-rich plant foods throughout the day to extinguish the free radicals and let NO synthase get back to its job of keeping your arteries fully functional. There's an ultrasound device researchers use to measure the NO-induced dilation of your arteries. One study using this device found that if you take people following a standard Western diet and have them eat even fewer antioxidants, their artery dilation only gets a little bit worse. It seems we're already near the bottom of the barrel arterial-function-wise, so there's not much room for further decline. But put people on a high-antioxidant diet by, among many other things, switching their bananas for berries and their white chocolate for dark, and within just two weeks, they experience a significant boost in their arteries' ability to relax and dilate normally.[143]

In addition to eating antioxidant-rich foods that can boost your body's ability to produce NO, you can also eat certain vegetables, such as beets and greens, that are rich in natural nitrates, which your body can convert into nitric oxide. (For the difference between nitrates and nitrites, see chapter 10.) This process explains why researchers have been able to show a ten-point systolic blood pressure drop in volunteers within hours of their consuming beet juice—an effect that lasted throughout the day.[144]

That study was performed on a group of healthy subjects, though. Obviously, we need to test the power of beets where it counts most—in people with high blood pressure. If nitrate-rich vegetables can so powerfully modulate humanity's leading risk factor for dying, why did it take until 2015 before such a study was published? Well, who was going to fund it? Big Beet? Drug companies rake in more than $10 billion a year from blood pressure medications.[145] You can't make billions on beets. That's why we are fortunate to have charities like the British Heart Foundation, which finally funded a beet juice study involving people with high blood pressure.

Half the subjects were provided a cup of beet juice daily for four weeks, while the other half was given an indistinguishable, nitrate-free placebo drink. The researchers found that not only was systolic blood pressure reduced by about eight points in the beet-juice drinkers but the benefits grew week by week, suggesting their blood pressure might have continued to improve even further. The scientists concluded that "nitrate-rich vegetables may prove to be both cost-effective, affordable, and favorable for a public health approach to hypertension."[146]

The optimal dose appears to be one-half cup,[147] but beet juice is perishable, processed, and hard to find. A typical fifteen-ounce can of beets would provide the same dose of nitrate, but the most concentrated sources of the compound are dark-green, leafy vegetables. The following is a top-ten list of nitrate-rich foods, in ascending order. As you'll see, eight out of the top ten are greens.

TOP-TEN FOOD SOURCES OF NITRATES

10. Beets
9. Swiss chard
8. Oak leaf lettuce
7. Beet greens
6. Basil

5. Mesclun greens
4. Butter leaf lettuce
3. Cilantro
2. Rhubarb
1. Arugula

Arugula comes out on top with a whopping 480 mg of nitrate per hundred-gram serving, which is more than four times the content of beets.[148]

The healthiest way to get your nitrate fix is to eat a big salad every day. You could take nitrate- and nitric-oxide-boosting supplements, but they have questionable safety[149] and efficacy[150] records and should be avoided. What about V8 juice, which boasts both beet and spinach juice? It must not have much, because you'd have to drink nineteen quarts of it a day to reach your daily nitrate intake target.[151]

The benefits of nitrates may explain why eating your greens is associated with reduced rates of heart disease[152] and a longer life span,[153] not to mention the "veggie Viagra" effect. You read that right. There's a link between vegetable consumption and improved sexual function,[154] as well as improved blood flow to the most important organ of the body, the brain.[155] And the only side effect of beeting your brains out may be a little extra color in your life—namely, red stools and urine that is pretty in pee-nk.

Doping with Beet Juice

A Lamborghini goes faster than a lemon not because the chemistry of gasoline combustion is somehow different in a sports car from that in a beater. It's because the Lambo has a more powerful engine. Similarly, athletes may have bigger muscles and be able to get more oxygen to those muscles faster. But fundamentally, the amount of energy a body can extract from oxygen remains the same . . . or so we thought.

About five years ago, one of the gospels of sports physiology got turned on its head—all because of beet juice.

Nitrates, concentrated in green, leafy vegetables and beets, not only help deliver oxygenated blood to your muscles by helping dilate your arteries but also enable your body to extract more energy from that oxygen—something never before thought possible. For example, one little shot of beet juice has been found to allow free divers to hold their breath for a half minute longer than usual.[156] After sipping beet juice, cyclists were able to perform at the same level of intensity while consuming 19 percent less oxygen than the placebo group. Then, when they ramped up their bike resistance for an intense bout of what they called "severe cycling," the time to exhaustion was extended from 9:43 minutes to 11:15 minutes. The beet-juice-drinking group exhibited greater endurance while using less oxygen. In short, the beet juice made the bikers' bodies' energy production significantly more efficient. No drug, steroid, supplement, or intervention had ever before been shown to do what beet juice could do.[157]

This effect works with whole beets too. In another study, men and women eating one and a half cups of baked beets seventy-five minutes before running a 5K race improved their running performance while maintaining the same heart rate and even reported less exertion.[158] Faster time with less effort? Them's some block-rockin' beets!

To maximize athletic performance, the ideal dose and timing appears to be a half cup of beet juice (or three three-inch beets, or a cup of cooked spinach[159]) two to three hours before a competition.[160]

It seems sports news programs are always talking about steroids and other illegal performance-enhancing drugs. Why hasn't anyone mentioned these mighty and perfectly legit performance-enhancing vegetables? Beets me.

A blood pressure checkup is easy to ignore or postpone. Unlike the case with many of our other leading killers, the insidious consequences of hypertension may not be apparent until you're lifted into an ambulance or lowered into a grave. So go to your local pharmacy, fire station, or doctor's office and get your blood pressure checked. If it's too high, the bad news is that you'll join the one billion people living with this condition. The good news is that you *don't* have to join the millions who die from it every year. Try eating and living healthfully for even just a few weeks, and you may be amazed by the results. Here are just a few stories about people who did just that.

Every day, NutritionFacts.org gets hundreds of e-mails, many from people eager to share how their lives were turned around by taking their health into their own hands. There's Bob, for example, who once weighed 230 pounds and had a 200-plus cholesterol level and triglycerides through the roof. He was on a battery of blood pressure medications. After starting a whole-food, plant-based diet, he's now down to 175 pounds, boasts a total cholesterol of 136, and no longer takes any blood pressure meds. At sixty-five, Bob feels better now than he has in decades, not by trying a new exercise program or the latest block-buster drug—just by changing his diet.

Patricia e-mailed not long ago. Her brother had just been diagnosed with severe high blood pressure and atherosclerosis. He was nearly sixty pounds overweight, and his skin was the color of "white paper." He was so unhealthy he couldn't even get a driver's license. Patricia and her brother decided to start a plant-based diet together. Now he's fit and trim, his weight is normal, he has no more need for blood pressure drugs, and Patricia most deservedly takes the (sugar-, milk-, and egg-free) cake for best sister ever.

Then there's Dean. He "filled up" with the standard American diet and became obese. He had high blood pressure, so his doctor put him on meds. Then he got high cholesterol, so his doctor put him on more meds. Moreover, every winter, Dean would suffer from terrible respiratory infections that required antibiotics. Finally, he got fed up and adopted a plant-based diet. He's now lost fifty pounds. His blood sugar and cholesterol levels, and even his blood pressure, are all normal. And he happily spends his winters ailment-free. Dean ended his note to me with this simple pledge: "I will be on a plant-based diet for the rest of my life." Thanks to a healthy diet, that may be quite a long time.

CHAPTER 8

How Not to Die from Liver Diseases

There are some patients you never forget. On the first day of my GI rotation (GI stands for gastrointestinal, which means I was about to come face-to-face with any issues in the digestive tract from mouth to tush), I reported in and was told to go observe my team of senior doctors in one of the endoscopy rooms, where physicians use a scope to look into the GI tract for all manner of routine procedures. I expected to walk into a colonoscopy looking at a rectal polyp or maybe an upper endoscopy looking at a stomach ulcer. But I'll never forget what I saw. It fuels me to this day in my mission to help people understand the connection between lifestyle and health (or lack of it).

A sedated patient was lying on a gurney, surrounded by a team of doctors using a scope with a camera. I looked at the monitor, trying to find anatomical landmarks to understand where the scope was. It was definitely down the throat, but the esophagus was snaked with what looked like throbbing varicose veins. They were everywhere. They looked like worms trying to emerge from under the smooth surface of the esophagus. Several had eroded through the lining and were spurting blood. I watched as more blood surged out with every one of the patient's heartbeats. She was basically bleeding to death into her stomach. The doctors tried desperately to cauterize and tie off these fountains of fresh red blood, but it was like a game of Whack-A-Mole. Every time one was cut off, another sprang up.

These were known as esophageal varices—veins swollen with backed-up blood due to a cirrhotic liver. Watching this nightmare unfold, I wondered how the patient first came down with cirrhosis. Was she an alcoholic? Did she contract hepatitis? I remember thinking how devastated she must have felt when she found out she had end-stage liver disease. How was her family coping? I was jerked back from my thoughts by screeching monitor alarms. She was bleeding out.

The doctors couldn't transfuse blood faster than the patient was losing it internally. Her blood pressure fell, and her heart stopped. The staff jumped into action with chest compressions, paddles delivering shocks, and injections of adrenaline, but within minutes, she was gone.

It was my job to talk to the patient's family. I learned that her cirrhosis was not due to drinking too much or from being an IV drug user. Her liver had scarred over because she was obese and had developed a fatty liver. Everything I had just witnessed was preventable, a direct result of lifestyle choices. When people are overweight, they can suffer from social stigma, knee problems, and increased risk for metabolic disorders like diabetes, but this was the first person I saw bleed to death before my eyes.

The family cried. I cried. I swore to myself I'd do whatever was necessary to help prevent this from ever happening to anyone under my care.

You can make do with only one kidney. You can survive without a spleen or a gallbladder. You can even get by without a stomach. But you can't live without a liver, the body's largest internal organ.

What exactly does the liver do? Up to five hundred different functions have been attributed to this vital organ.[1] First and foremost, it plays the role of bouncer, keeping unwanted guests out of your bloodstream. Whatever you absorb through your digestive tract isn't immediately circulated throughout your body. The blood from your intestines first goes straight to the liver, where nutrients are metabolized and toxins are neutralized. It's no surprise, then, that what you eat can and does play a critical role in liver health and disease.

About sixty thousand Americans die of liver disease every year, and the death rates have risen each of the last five years.[2] The incidence of liver cancer alone has been rising about 4 percent every year over the last decade.[3] Liver dysfunction can run in families, like the iron-overload disease hemochromatosis. It can be caused by infections that can lead to liver cancer, or it can stem from drugs—most often inadvertent or intentional overdoses of Tylenol.[4] The most common causes, however, are drink and food: alcoholic liver disease and fatty liver disease.

ALCOHOLIC LIVER DISEASE

According to a famous series of papers in the *Journal of the American Medical Association* called the "*Actual* Causes of Death in the United States" [emphasis added], the leading killer of Americans in the year 2000 was tobacco, followed by diet and inactivity. The third-leading killer? Alcohol.[5] About half of alcohol-related deaths were due to sudden causes like motor vehicle accidents; the other half were slower, and the leading cause was alcoholic liver disease.[6]

Excessive alcohol consumption can lead to an accumulation of fat in the liver (what's known as fatty liver), which can cause inflammation and result in liver scarring and, eventually, liver failure. The CDC defines excessive drinking as the regular consumption of more than one drink a day for women and more than two a day for men. A drink is defined as 12 ounces of beer, 8 ounces of malt liquor, 5 ounces of wine, or 1.5 ounces (a "shot") of hard liquor.[7] Progression of the disease can usually be halted by stopping drinking, but sometimes it's too late.[8]

Heavy alcohol consumption can cause a fatty liver in less than three weeks,[9] but it usually resolves within four to six weeks after stopping drinking.[10] But in 5–15 percent of cases, the disease continues to progress, and the liver starts to scar despite alcohol cessation.[11]

Similarly, once alcohol-induced hepatitis (liver inflammation) is diagnosed, three-year survival rates can be as high as 90 percent among people who stop drinking after diagnosis.[12] But as many as 18 percent of them go on to develop cirrhosis, an irreparable scarring of the liver.[13]

The best strategy to avoid alcoholic liver disease is to not drink so much in the first place. But if you do drink excessively, help is available. Though most people who drink may not be alcoholics,[14] there is convincing evidence that twelve-step programs such as Alcoholics Anonymous can be effective for those who do suffer from alcohol dependence.[15]

Isn't Moderate Drinking Beneficial?

Everyone agrees that heavy drinking, drinking during pregnancy, and binge drinking are bad ideas, but what about "moderate" drinking? Yes, excessive drinkers appear to significantly shorten their lives, but so can teetotalers.[16] While smoking is bad for you and smoking a lot is worse, that logic may not

continued

hold for alcohol consumption. There actually appears to be a beneficial effect on overall mortality by drinking some alcohol—but only, it seems, for those who are not taking good care of themselves already.[17]

Moderate drinking does appear to protect against heart disease, perhaps because of a blood-thinning effect,[18] but even light drinking (less than one drink a day) has been found to increase cancer risk, as you'll see in chapter 11. How could something that increases cancer risk still prolong life? Cancer is "only" our second-leading killer disease. Because heart disease is the leading cause of death, it explains why people who drink moderately may live longer lives than those who abstain. But this advantage may be restricted only to those who fail to practice a bare modicum of healthy behaviors.[19]

To find out who might benefit from moderate alcohol consumption, researchers recruited close to ten thousand men and women and followed them for seventeen years after assessing their drinking and lifestyle habits. The results were published in a paper entitled "Who Benefits Most from the Cardioprotective Properties of Alcohol Consumption—Health Freaks or Couch Potatoes?" What constituted a "health freak"? According to the researchers' definition, anyone who exercises thirty minutes a day, doesn't smoke, and eats at least one serving of fruits or vegetables daily.[20] (What does that say about our current diets if eating a single apple means you're a "health freak"?)

One to two drinks a day did lower the risk of heart disease for the "couch potatoes," those living unhealthy lifestyles. But people who practiced even the bare minimum of healthy behaviors showed no benefit from alcohol. The lesson: Grapes, barley, and potatoes are best eaten in their nondistilled form, and Johnnie Walker is no substitute for actual walking.

NONALCOHOLIC LIVER DISEASE

The most common cause of a fatty liver is not alcohol but *nonalcoholic fatty liver disease* (NAFLD). You may remember the blockbuster documentary *Super Size Me*, in which the film's director, Morgan Spurlock, ate exclusively at McDonald's for a month. Predictably, Spurlock's weight, blood pressure, and cholesterol all went up—but so did his liver enzymes. That was a sign that his liver cells were dying and spilling their contents into his bloodstream. How was his diet causing liver damage? Let's put it this way: He was beginning to turn his liver into human foie gras (fatty liver pâté).

Some critics wrote off the film as overly sensational, but researchers in Sweden took it seriously enough to formally replicate Spurlock's one-man experiment. In their study, a group of men and women agreed to eat two fast-food meals a day. At the start, their liver enzyme levels were normal, but after just one week of this diet, more than 75 percent of the volunteers' liver function test results became pathological.[21] If an unhealthy diet can cause liver damage within just seven days, it should be no surprise that NAFLD has quietly become the most common cause of chronic liver disease in the United States, afflicting an estimated seventy million people.[22] That's about one in three adults. Nearly 100 percent of those with severe obesity may be affected.[23]

Like alcoholic fatty liver, NAFLD starts with a buildup of fat deposits in the liver that cause no symptoms. In rare cases, this can progress to inflammation and, over years, end up scarring the liver into a state of cirrhosis, resulting in liver cancer, liver failure, and even death—as I saw in that endoscopy suite.[24]

Fast food is so effective at instigating the disease because NAFLD is associated with the intake of soft drinks and meat. Drinking just one can of soda a day appears to raise the odds of getting fatty liver disease by 45 percent.[25] Meanwhile, those who eat the meat equivalent of fourteen chicken nuggets or more daily have nearly triple the rate of fatty liver disease compared to people who eat seven nuggets' worth or less.[26]

NAFLD has been characterized as a "tale of fat and sugar,"[27] but not all fat affects the liver similarly. People suffering from fatty liver inflammation were found to be consuming more animal fat (and cholesterol) but less plant fat (and fiber and antioxidants).[28] This may explain why adherence to a Mediterranean-style diet with plenty of fruits, vegetables, whole grains, and beans has been associated with less severe fatty liver disease even though it is not typically a low-fat diet.[29]

NAFLD may also be caused by cholesterol overload.[30] The dietary cholesterol found in eggs, meat, and dairy can become oxidized and then set off a chain reaction that results in excess fat in the liver.[31] When the concentration of cholesterol in your liver cells gets too high, it can crystallize like rock candy and result in inflammation. This process is similar to the way uric acid crystals cause gout (as we'll see in chapter 10).[32] Your white blood cells try to engulf the cholesterol crystals but then die in the process, spilling out inflammatory compounds. This may explain how benign fatty liver cases can turn into serious hepatitis.[33]

To explore the relationship between diet and serious liver disease, about nine thousand American adults were studied for thirteen years. The researchers noted that their most important finding may be that cholesterol consumption was a strong predictor of cirrhosis and liver cancer. Those consuming the amount of cholesterol found in two Egg McMuffins[34] or more each day appeared to double their risk of hospitalization or death.[35]

Your best bet for avoiding NAFLD, the most common cause of liver disease, may be to avoid excess calories, cholesterol, saturated fat, and sugar.

VIRAL HEPATITIS

Another common cause of liver disease is viral hepatitis, which is triggered by one or more of five different viruses: hepatitis A, B, C, D, or E. The mode of transmission and prognosis differs for each of these viruses. Hepatitis A is spread primarily through food or water that is tainted with contaminated feces. It can be prevented through vaccination, avoiding raw and undercooked shellfish, and trying to ensure that everyone who handles your food washes their hands after changing diapers or using the toilet.

While hepatitis A virus is foodborne, hepatitis B virus is bloodborne and is transmitted sexually. As with hepatitis A, an effective vaccine is available against hepatitis B that every child should get. Hepatitis D virus infection can only occur in someone who is already infected with hepatitis B and so can be prevented by preventing hepatitis B. So get vaccinated and refrain from intravenous drug use and unsafe sex.

Unfortunately, there is currently no vaccine for the hepatitis C virus, the most dreaded of liver viruses. Exposure can lead to a chronic infection that, over decades, can lead to cirrhosis and liver failure. Hepatitis C is now the leading cause of liver transplants.[36]

Chlorella and Hepatitis C

The green algae chlorella looks promising for the treatment of hepatitis C. A randomized, double-blind, placebo-controlled study found that about two teaspoons a day of chlorella boosted the activity of natural killer cells in participants' bodies, which can naturally kill hepatitis C-infected cells.[37]

A clinical study of hepatitis-C patients found that chlorella supplementation may lower the level of liver inflammation, but the study was small and uncontrolled.[38]

There is a desperate need for alternative treatments for hepatitis C, as older, less expensive therapies frequently fail due to their unbearable side effects, whereas newer, more tolerable drugs cost as much as $1,000 per pill.[39] Chlorella may help as an adjunct (additional) therapy or for those who can't tolerate or afford conventional antiviral therapy but may not be without risk (see page 88).

Hepatitis C is transmitted via blood, usually through sharing needles rather than via blood transfusions, now that the blood supply is screened for the virus. However, sharing personal-care items that can be contaminated with trace amounts of blood, such as toothbrushes and razors, may also present a risk.[40]

Although a case was once reported involving a woman who contracted hepatitis C from sharing a supermarket meat slicer with an infected coworker,[41] the virus would not naturally be present in the meat itself, as humans and chimpanzees are the only animals who appear susceptible to it.

The same cannot be said for hepatitis E virus.

Preventing Hepatitis E Through Diet

As one of the CDC's Division of Viral Hepatitis laboratory chiefs explained in a paper entitled "Much Meat, Much Malady: Changing Perceptions of the Epidemiology of Hepatitis E," hepatitis E virus is now considered a zoonotic disease, able to spread from animals to humans, and pigs may be the primary viral reservoir.[42]

The shift in thinking began in 2003, when researchers in Japan linked the hepatitis E virus (HEV) with the consumption of grilled pork liver. After testing pig livers from Japanese grocery stores, the researchers determined that nearly 2 percent of the meat tested positive for HEV.[43] In the United States, it was even worse: 11 percent of commercial pig livers purchased from grocery stores were contaminated with HEV.[44]

That's alarming, but how many people really eat pig livers? What about plain old pork?

Unfortunately, pork may harbor HEV as well. Experts suspect that much of the American population has been exposed to this virus, as there is known to be a relatively high prevalence of HEV antibodies among U.S. blood donors. This exposure may be a result of individuals consuming HEV-contaminated pork.[45]

So do more people die of liver disease in countries where pork is more popular? It appears so. The relationship between national per capita pork consumption and deaths from liver disease correlates as tightly as per capita alcohol consumption and liver fatalities. Each pork chop consumed per capita may be associated with about two beers' worth of increased liver mortality risk on a countrywide scale.[46]

Aren't viruses deactivated by cooking? Usually, but there's always the problem of cross-contaminating your hands or kitchen surfaces while handling raw meat. Once meat is in the oven, most foodborne pathogens can be destroyed by cooking the meat to proper internal cooking temperatures, with an emphasis on *proper*. Researchers at the National Institute of Health subjected the hepatitis E virus to various levels of heat and found that HEV can survive the internal temperature of meat cooked rare.[47] So if you cook pork, invest in a meat thermometer and make sure to follow proper handling techniques, including washing kitchen surfaces with a bleach solution.[48]

Though most people who develop hepatitis E recover completely, it can be deadly for pregnant women: The risk of death during the third trimester can reach as high as 30 percent.[49] If you are pregnant, please be especially careful about pork preparation. And if there are people in the household who like their pork pink in the middle, they should be sure to wash their hands thoroughly after using the bathroom.

Weight-Loss Supplements and Liver Disease

We've all seen those marketing schemes involving products espousing all sorts of health claims. And given the pyramid-like multilevel structure of those types of distribution programs—you earn money by selling products and also for recruiting others to sell—word can spread pretty fast, which is particularly troubling when PR outruns the truth.

Indeed, while the vast majority of drug-induced liver injuries are caused by conventional medications, liver damage caused by certain classes of dietary supplements can be even more serious and may lead to higher rates of liver transplants and death.[50] Multilevel marketers of products later linked to toxic reactions (such as noni juice[51] and Herbalife[52]) have pointed to scientific studies to support their health claims. However, a public health review found that such studies often seemed "deliberately created for marketing purposes" and were presented in such a way as to appear "designed to mislead potential consumers." Often, multilevel marketing study researchers didn't disclose their funding sources, but a little detective work can expose a web of financial conflicts of interest.[53]

These suspect studies were the same ones cited to provide proof of safety for their products. For example, a multilevel marketing company that sells mangosteen juice cited a study they paid for to support its assertion that their product is "safe for everyone." The study involved exposing just thirty people to their product with another ten people given a placebo. With so few people tested, the stuff could literally kill 1 or 2 percent of users and you wouldn't know.[54]

A study that the multilevel marketing company behind a supplement called Metabolife cited for safety placed thirty-five people on the stuff.[55] Metabolife has since been withdrawn from the market after being linked to heart attacks, strokes, seizures, and deaths.[56] Hydroxycitric acid, a component of such products as Hydroxycut, was studied on forty people.[57] No serious adverse effects were found, but the story ended the same way: Hydroxycut was withdrawn after dozens of verified cases of organ damage were brought to light—including massive liver failure requiring transplantation and even death.[58] Until the multibillion-dollar herbal supplement industry is better regulated, you're better off saving your money—and your health—by sticking to real food.

PROTECTING THE LIVER AT BREAKFAST

Specific plant foods have been found to be protective of the liver. For instance, starting out the day with a bowl of oatmeal and (surprisingly) coffee may help safeguard our liver function.

Oatmeal

In numerous population studies, consumption of whole grains has been associated with reduced risk for a range of chronic diseases,[59] but it's hard to tease out whether eating whole grains may just be a marker for a healthier lifestyle in general. For example, people who eat whole grains, such as oatmeal, whole wheat, and brown rice, also tend to be more physically active, smoke less, and eat more fruits, vegetables, and dietary fiber[60] than those who might prefer a breakfast of Froot Loops, for example. No wonder the former group may have lower disease risk. Fortunately, researchers can control for these factors, effectively comparing nonsmokers only to nonsmokers with similar diet and exercise habits. When that's done, whole grains still appear to be protective.[61]

In other words, the evidence seems clear that oatmeal eaters may have lower rates of disease, but that's not the same as showing that if you start eating more oatmeal, your risk will drop. To prove cause and effect, we need to put it to the test by performing an interventional trial: Change people's diets and see what happens. Ideally, researchers would randomly split people into two groups and give half of them oatmeal and the other half a placebo—a fake, similar-tasting and -looking oatmeal. Neither the study subjects nor the researchers themselves can know who's in which group until the end. This robust, double-blind method is easy to use when studying drugs, as you just give people a sugar pill that looks like the drug in question. As we've discussed, it's not as easy to make placebo food.

But in 2013, a group of researchers published the first double-blinded, randomized, placebo-controlled trial of oatmeal in overweight men and women.[62] They found a significant reduction in liver inflammation in the real oatmeal group, but that may have been because they lost so much more weight than the controls (that is, the placebo-oatmeal eaters). Nearly 90 percent of the real-oatmeal-treated subjects had lost weight, compared with no weight loss, on average, among the control group. So it may be that the benefits of whole grains on liver function are indirect.[63] A follow-up study in 2014 helped confirm the findings of a protective role for whole grains in nonalcoholic fatty liver patients in reducing the risk of liver inflammation. In this study, refined grain consumption was associated with increased risk of the disease.[64] So lay off the Wonder Bread and stick to truly wonderful whole-grain foods, including oatmeal.

Making Your Own Whole-Cranberry Cocktail

A specific class of plant compounds called anthocyanins—the purple, red, and blue pigments in such plants as berries, grapes, plums, red cabbage, and red onions—have been found to prevent fat accumulation in human liver cells in in vitro studies.[65] A single confirmatory clinical (human) trial has been published in which a purple sweet potato concoction successfully dampened liver inflammation better than a placebo.[66]

When it came to suppressing the growth of human liver cancer cells in a petri dish,[67] cranberries beat out the other most common fruits in the United States: apples, bananas, grapefruits, grapes, lemons, oranges, peaches, pears, pineapples, and strawberries. Other studies have found that cranberries are also effective in vitro against additional cancers, including those of the brain,[68] breast,[69] colon,[70] lung,[71] mouth,[72] ovary,[73] prostate,[74] and stomach.[75] Unfortunately, there have yet to be clinical studies of the effects of cranberries on cancer patients that confirm these findings.

Moreover, to the drug industry's chagrin, scientists have been unable to pin down the active ingredients involved in cranberries' special effects. Extracts concentrating individual components fail to match the anticancer effects of the cranberry as a whole,[76] which of course can't be patented. More proof that it's nearly always best to give preference to whole foods.

How do you do that with cranberries, though, since they're so tart?

It's not easy at the grocery store. Ninety-five percent of cranberries are sold in the form of processed products, such as juices and sauces.[77] In fact, to get the same amount of anthocyanins found in a single cup of fresh or frozen cranberries, you'd have to drink sixteen cups of cranberry juice cocktail, eat seven cups of dried cranberries, or make your way through twenty-six cans of cranberry sauce.[78] The ruby-red phytonutrient found in cranberries is a powerful antioxidant, but the high-fructose corn syrup added to cranberry cocktail acts as a pro-oxidant, canceling out some of the benefit.[79]

Here's a simple recipe for a whole-food version of a tasty cranberry beverage, what I call my Pink Juice:

1 handful fresh or frozen cranberries

2 cups water

8 teaspoons erythritol (a naturally derived low-calorie sweetener; read more about erythritol and other sweeteners in part 2)

Place all the ingredients in a blender and blend at high speed. Pour over ice and serve.

continued

At just twelve calories, this recipe has twenty-five times fewer calories and at least eight times more phytonutrients than typical cranberry juice drinks.[80]

For an extra boost, blend in some fresh mint leaves. You'll get a weird-looking green foam on top, but not only will it taste good, you'll be happy to know that you're chugging down berries and dark, leafy greens, two of the healthiest foods on the planet. Bottoms up!

Coffee

Back in 1986, a group of Norwegian researchers came across an unexpected finding: Alcohol consumption was associated with liver inflammation (no surprise there), but coffee consumption was associated with *less* liver inflammation.[81] These results were replicated in subsequent studies performed around the world. In the United States, a study was done with people at high risk for liver disease—for example, those who were overweight or drank too much alcohol. Subjects who drank more than two cups of coffee a day appeared to have less than half the risk of developing chronic liver problems as those who drank less than one cup.[82]

What about liver cancer, one of the most feared complications of chronic liver inflammation? It is now the third-leading cause of cancer-related death, an upsurge driven largely by increases in hepatitis C infections and nonalcoholic fatty liver disease.[83]

The news is good. A 2013 review of the best studies to date found that people who drank the most coffee had half the risk of liver cancer compared to those who drank the least.[84] A subsequent study found the consumption of four or more cups of coffee a day was associated with 92 percent lower risk among smokers dying from chronic liver disease.[85] Of course, quitting smoking would have helped as well; smoking may multiply by as much as tenfold the odds of those with hepatitis C dying from liver cancer.[86] Similarly, heavy alcohol drinkers who consume more than four cups of coffee per day appear to reduce their risk of liver inflammation—but not by nearly as much as people who cut down on alcohol.[87]

Liver cancers are among the most avoidable cancers, through hepatitis B vaccination, control of hepatitis C transmission, and reduction of alcohol consumption. These three measures could, in principle, wipe out 90 percent of liver cancers worldwide. It remains unclear whether coffee drinking has an additional role to play, but such a role would be limited compared with preventing liver damage in the first place.[88]

But what if you're already infected with hepatitis C or are among the nearly one in three American adults[89] with nonalcoholic fatty liver disease? Until relatively recently, no clinical trials had put coffee to the test. But in 2013, researchers published a study in which forty patients with chronic hepatitis C were placed into two groups: The first group consumed four cups of coffee daily for a month, while the second group drank no coffee at all. After thirty days, the groups switched. Of course, two months is not long enough to detect changes in cancer outcomes, but during that time, the researchers were able to demonstrate that coffee consumption may reduce DNA damage, increase the clearance of virus-infected cells, and slow the scarring process.[90] These results help explain the role coffee appears to play in reducing the risk of liver disease progression.

A commentary in the journal *Gastroenterology* entitled "Is It Time to Write a Prescription for Coffee?" explored the pros and cons.[91] Some insist that we must first identify the active ingredient in coffee beans that's protective. After all, more than one thousand different compounds have already been found in coffee.[92] More studies are needed, but meanwhile, moderate daily ingestion of unsweetened coffee should be considered a reasonable adjunct to medical therapy for people at high risk for liver damage, such as those with fatty liver disease.[93] Keep in mind that daily consumption of caffeinated beverages can lead to physical dependence, and caffeine withdrawal symptoms can include days of headache, fatigue, difficulty concentrating, and mood disturbances.[94] Ironically, coffee's tendency to be habit forming could turn out to be a good thing. If the liver health benefits are confirmed, then daily consumption may ultimately prove to be an advantage.[95]

With liver disease, as always, prevention is the key. All the most serious liver conditions—liver cancer, liver failure, and cirrhosis—can start with an inflamed liver. That inflammation can be caused by an infection or the buildup of fatty deposits. Liver viruses can be prevented by common-sense measures. Don't inject drugs, do get vaccinated, and do practice safe sex. Liver fat can also be prevented by common sense measures: Avoid excess consumption of alcohol, calories, cholesterol, saturated fat, and sugar.

CHAPTER 9

How Not to Die from Blood Cancers

Eleven-year-old Missy had leukemia. It was in remission, thanks in part to the yellow bags of chemo that hung from the IV pole she rolled down the hospital halls. Missy was one of my first patients in my pediatrics rotation during medical school at the Eastern Maine Medical Center in Bangor—home to Stephen King, moose-crossing signs, and billboards advertising lobster ice cream.

During this time, I was in full Patch Adams regalia, from the fuzzy pink rabbit ears on my head down to the plastic rainbow Slinkys trailing at my feet. On every button of my white doctor's coat hung a Beanie Baby, in every buttonhole was crammed a stuffed animal's foot. Missy drew a smiley face on my beanie hippo and named the rooster attached to my stethoscope "Elvis."

She loved to paint pictures for me and signed each one of them, in all caps: FROM MISSY. In these pictures, she still had her curly brown locks. In reality, though, her head was completely bald. She refused to wear a wig, which only made her smile seem brighter.

I painted her nails a pale pink, and she painted mine a lovely purplish brown.

I remember the morning after she gave me the manicure. My senior resident took me aside after rounds. "Your fingernails are getting in people's way," he said.

"Huh?" I asked.

"The attending physicians are complaining," he replied. "This is a conservative profession."

I tried to explain that I didn't paint them myself, upset that I even felt the need to explain at all. The senior resident knew that Missy had done it, but he didn't seem to care. "Medicine," he said, "is also an anti-emotion profession."

Later, the chair of the department had a talk with me. A number of the attending physicians were concerned I was "too enthusiastic," "too dramatic," and "too sensitive."

My wife remarked they probably just had Slinky envy.

The next day, head down, I walked into Missy's room.

"I'm sorry," I told her. "The doctors made me take off the nail polish."

I held up my hands to show her. She inspected them and said, with great indignation, "If you can't wear it, then I'm not going to, either!" So I helped her take off her polish, bemused and empowered by such solidarity from an eleven-year-old. (I let her paint my toenails instead.)

I remember the last note I wrote in Missy's medical chart. Hospital progress notes are written in SOAP format, a mnemonic for Subjective findings, Objective findings, Assessment, and Plan. I wrote: "Assessment: 11yo girl finishing last round of maintenance chemotherapy. Plan: Disney World."

Childhood leukemia is one of the few success stories in our war on cancer, with ten-year survival rates as high as 90 percent.[1] Yet it still affects more children than any other cancer and is ten times more likely to be diagnosed in adults, among whom current treatments are much less effective.[2]

What can we do to help prevent blood cancers in the first place?

Blood cancers are sometimes referred to as liquid tumors, since the cancer cells often circulate throughout the body rather than get concentrated in a solid mass. These cancers typically begin undetected in the bone marrow, that spongy tissue in the interior of our bones where red blood cells, white blood cells, and platelets are born. When healthy, your red blood cells deliver oxygen throughout your body, your white blood cells fight off infections, and your platelets help your blood to clot. Most blood cancers involve mutations of the white cells.

Blood cancers can be categorized into three types: leukemia, lymphoma, and myeloma. Leukemia (from the Greek roots *leukos*, or "white," and *haima*, or "blood") is a disease in which the bone marrow feverishly produces abnormal white blood cells. Unlike normal ones, these imposters aren't able to fight infection. They also impair the ability of your bone marrow to produce normal red and white cells by crowding out healthy ones, creating a diminished healthy blood cell count that can lead to anemia, infection, and, eventually, death. According to the American Cancer Society, fifty-two thousand Americans are diagnosed with leukemia, and twenty-four thousand die from it every year.[3]

Lymphoma is a blood cancer of lymphocytes, which are specialized types of white blood cells. Lymphoma cells multiply quickly and can collect in your lymph nodes, small immune organs that are spread throughout the body, including the armpits, neck, and groin. Lymph nodes help to filter your blood. Like leuke-mia, lymphoma can crowd out healthy cells and impair your ability to fight in-fections. You may have heard of non-Hodgkin's lymphoma. Hodgkin's lymphoma can strike young adults, but it's a rare and usually treatable form of lymphoma. As its name suggests, non-Hodgkin's lymphoma (NHL) includes all the other dozens of types of lymphoma. They're more common and can be harder to treat, and their risk increases with age. The American Cancer Society estimates that there are seventy thousand new cases of non-Hodgkin's lymphoma each year and about nineteen thousand deaths.[4]

Finally, myeloma is a cancer of plasma cells, which are white blood cells that produce antibodies, the proteins that stick to invaders and infected cells to neutralize or tag them for destruction. Cancerous plasma cells can displace healthy cells from your bone marrow and make abnormal antibodies that can clog the kidneys. About 90 percent of myeloma sufferers are discovered with masses of cancer cells growing in multiple bones of their bodies, hence the com-mon term for this condition, multiple myeloma. Each year, twenty-four thou-sand people are diagnosed with multiple myeloma, and eleven thousand die.[5]

Most people with multiple myeloma live for only a few years after diagno-sis. Though treatable, multiple myeloma is considered incurable. That's why prevention is key. Fortunately, dietary changes may reduce our risk of all these blood cancers.

FOODS ASSOCIATED WITH DECREASED RISK OF BLOOD CANCERS

After following more than sixty thousand people for more than a dozen years, University of Oxford researchers found that those who consume a plant-based diet are less likely to develop all forms of cancer combined. The greatest protection appeared to be against blood cancers. The incidence of leukemia, lymphoma, and multiple myeloma among those eating vegetarian diets is nearly half that of those eating meat.[6] Why is this greatly reduced risk of blood cancers associated with a more plant-based diet? The British Journal of Cancer concluded, "More research is needed to understand the mechanisms behind this."[7] While they are figuring out the reasons, why not get a head start and try adding more healthy plant foods to your plates today?

Greens and Cancer

The key to cancer prevention and treatment is to keep tumor cells from multiplying out of control while allowing healthy cells to grow normally. Chemotherapy and radiation can do a great job of wiping out cancer cells, but healthy cells can get caught in the crossfire. Some compounds in plants, though, may be more discriminating.

For instance, sulforaphane, considered one of the more active components in cruciferous vegetables, kills human leukemia cells in a petri dish while having little impact on the growth of normal cells.[8] As we've discussed, cruciferous vegetables include broccoli, cauliflower, and kale, but there are many others in this family, such as collard greens, watercress, bok choy, kohlrabi, rutabaga, turnips, arugula, radishes (including horseradish), wasabi, and all types of cabbage.

It's intriguing that dripping cabbage compounds on cancer cells affects them in a laboratory, but what really matters is whether people with blood cancers who eat lots of vegetables actually live longer than those who don't. For about eight years, Yale University researchers followed more than five hundred women with non-Hodgkin's lymphoma. Those who started out eating three or more servings of vegetables daily had a 42 percent improved survival rate over those who ate less. Green, leafy vegetables, including salad and cooked greens, and citrus fruits appeared most protective.[9] It's not clear, though, whether the survival benefit arose from helping to keep the cancer at bay or from improving patients' tolerance to the chemotherapy and radiation treatments they were receiving. The accompanying editorial in the journal *Leukemia & Lymphoma* suggested that a "lymphoma diagnosis may be an important 'teachable' moment to improve diet. . . ."[10] I would suggest you not wait until a cancer diagnosis to clean up your diet.

The Iowa Women's Health Study, which has followed more than thirty-five thousand women for decades, found that higher broccoli and other cruciferous vegetable intake was associated with lower risk of getting non-Hodgkin's lymphoma in the first place.[11] Likewise, a study at the Mayo Clinic found that those who ate about five or more servings of green, leafy vegetables a week had roughly half the odds of getting lymphoma compared with those who ate less than one serving a week.[12]

Some of the plant-based protection might have been due to the antioxidant properties of fruits and vegetables. Higher dietary intake of antioxidants is associated with significantly lower lymphoma risk. Note I said *dietary* intake, not supplementary intake. Antioxidant supplements don't appear to work.[13] For example, getting lots of vitamin C in your diet is associated with lower lymphoma risk, but taking in even more vitamin C in pill form did not seem to help. The same was found for carotenoid antioxidants like beta-carotene.[14] Apparently, pills do not have the same cancer-fighting effects as produce.

When it comes to certain other cancers, like those of the digestive tract, antioxidant supplements may even make things worse. Combinations of antioxidants like vitamin A, vitamin E, and beta-carotene in pill form were associated with increased risk of death in those who took them.[15] Supplements contain only a select few antioxidants, whereas your body relies on hundreds of them, all working synergistically to create a network to help the body dispose of free radicals. High doses of a single antioxidant may upset this delicate balance and may actually diminish your body's ability to fight cancer.[16]

When you buy antioxidant supplements, you may be doling out money to live a shorter life. Save your cash and your health by eating the real thing: food.

Açai Berries and Leukemia

Açai berries gained celebrity status in 2008 when television personality Dr. Mehmet Oz talked about them on *The Oprah Winfrey Show*. This spawned a frenzy of knockoff supplements, powders, shakes, and other dubious products bearing the açai berry label but not necessarily containing any of the actual berry.[17] Even major corporations have jumped on the açai bandwagon, including Anheuser-Busch with its 180 Blue "with Açai Energy" drink and Coca-Cola with its Bossa Nova beverage. This is an all-too-common practice in the "superfruit" supplement and beverage market, where less than a quarter of products sold may even contain the ingredients their labels claim.[18,19] The benefits of these products are suspect at best, but there is some preliminary research on real açai berries, which can be purchased as unsweetened frozen pulp.

The first study published in the medical literature on the effects of açai on human tissue was performed on leukemia cells. Researchers dripped an açai berry extract on leukemia cells taken from a thirty-six-year-old woman. It appeared to trigger self-destruct reactions in up to 86 percent of the cells.[20] Also, sprinkling some freeze-dried açai berries on immune cells called macrophages (from the Greek words *makros* and *phagein*, meaning "big eater") in a petri dish appeared to enable the cells to engulf and devour up to 40 percent more microbes than usual.[21]

Though the leukemia study was done using açai extract at the concentration one might expect to find in the bloodstream after eating the berries, no studies have yet been performed on cancer patients themselves (just cancer cells in a test tube), so more testing is needed. Indeed, the only clinical studies on açai berries published so far were two small industry-funded trials that showed modest benefit for osteoarthritis sufferers[22] and some metabolic parameters of overweight subjects.[23]

In terms of antioxidant bang for your buck, açai berries get honorable mention, beating out other superstars, such as walnuts, apples, and cranberries. The bronze for best bargain, though, goes to cloves, the silver to cinnamon, and the gold for most antioxidants per dollar—according to a USDA database of common foods—goes to purple cabbage.[24] Açai berries, however, would probably make a tastier smoothie.

Curcumin and Multiple Myeloma

As noted, multiple myeloma is one of the most dreaded cancers. It is practically incurable even with aggressive medical treatment. As myeloma cells take over the bone marrow, healthy white blood cells continue to decline in number, which increases your susceptibility to infection. Reduced levels of red blood cells can lead to anemia, and reduced platelet counts can lead to serious bleeding. Once diagnosed, most people survive fewer than five years.[25]

Multiple myeloma does not occur out of the blue. It appears to be nearly always preceded by a precancerous condition known as monoclonal gammopathy of undetermined significance, or MGUS.[26] When scientists first discovered MGUS, it was aptly named because, at that time, the significance of finding elevated levels of abnormal antibodies in someone's body was unclear. We now know it's a precursor to multiple myeloma, and about 3 percent of Caucasians over age fifty have it,[27] while the rate among African Americans may be double.[28]

MGUS causes no symptoms. You won't even know you have it unless your doctor finds it incidentally during routine blood work. The chance of MGUS progressing into myeloma is about 1 percent per year, which means many MGUS-stricken people may die of other causes before they develop myeloma.[29] However, since multiple myeloma is basically a death sentence, scientists have been desperate to find ways to stop MGUS in its tracks.

Given the safety and efficacy of the turmeric spice component curcumin against other types of cancer cells, researchers from the University of Texas collected multiple myeloma cells and put them in a petri dish. Without any intervention, the cancer cells quadrupled within a few days—that's how fast this cancer can grow. But when a little curcumin was added to the broth they were bathing in, the myeloma cells' growth was either stunted or stopped altogether.[30]

As we've discovered, stopping cancer in a laboratory is one thing. What about in people? In 2009, a pilot study found that half (five out of ten) of the subjects with MGUS who had particularly high abnormal antibody levels responded positively to curcumin supplements. None (zero out of nine) of those given a placebo experienced a similar drop in antibody levels.[31] Buoyed by this success, scientists conducted a randomized, double-blind, placebo-controlled trial and achieved similarly encouraging results in both patients with MGUS and those with "smoldering" multiple myeloma, an early stage of the disease.[32] This result suggests that a simple spice found in the grocery store might have the ability to slow or stop this horrific cancer in a certain percentage of patients, though we won't know more until longer studies are performed to see if these hopeful changes in blood-work biomarkers translate into changes in actual patient outcomes. In the meantime, it couldn't hurt to spice up your diet.

ARE ANIMAL VIRUSES INVOLVED IN HUMAN BLOOD CANCERS?

The reason people eating plant-based diets appear to have much lower rates of blood cancers[33] may be due to the foods they're choosing to eat and/or choosing to avoid. To tease out the role different animal products might play in the myriad blood cancers, we would need to conduct a very large study. Enter the aptly named EPIC study, the European Prospective Investigation into Cancer and Nutrition, which did just that. As we saw in chapter 4, researchers recruited more than four hundred thousand men and women across ten countries and followed them for about nine years. If you recall, regular chicken consumption was associated with an increased risk for pancreatic cancer. Similar findings were found for blood cancers. Of all the animal products studied (including unusual categories, such as offal, or entrails and organs), poultry tended to be associated with the greatest increased risk of non-Hodgkin's lymphoma, all grades of follicular lymphoma, and B-cell lymphomas, such as B-cell chronic lymphatic leukemia (including small lymphocytic leukemia and prolymphocytic lymphocytic leukemia).[34] The EPIC study found that risk increased between 56 percent and 280 percent for every 50 grams of poultry consumed daily. For comparison, a cooked, boneless chicken breast may weigh as much as 384 grams.[35]

Why is there so much lymphoma and leukemia risk associated with eating such relatively small amounts of poultry? The researchers suggested this result could be a fluke, or it could be due to the drugs, such as antibiotics, that are often fed to chickens and turkeys to promote their growth. Or it might be the dioxins found in some poultry meat, which have been linked to lymphoma.[36]

But dairy can also contain dioxins, and milk consumption was not linked to NHL. The researchers surmised it may be the cancer-causing viruses in poultry, given that lower risk of NHL has been associated with eating meat cooked well done instead of rare (thereby inactivating any viruses).[37] This suggestion is consistent with the results of the NIH-AARP study (see page 71), which found an association between eating just-done chicken and one type of lymphoma and *lower* risk of another blood cancer tied to greater exposure to the cooked meat carcinogen MeIQx.[38]

How could less cancer be linked to *more* carcinogen exposure? MeIQx is one of the heterocyclic amines created by cooking meat at high temperatures, such as baking, broiling, and frying.[39] If, in the case of blood cancers, one cause is a poultry virus, then the more the meat was cooked, the more likely it is that the virus was destroyed. Cancer-causing poultry viruses—including the avian herpesvirus that causes Marek's disease, several retroviruses like reticuloendotheliosis virus, the avian leukosis virus found in chickens, and the lymphoproliferative disease virus found in turkeys—may explain the higher rates of blood cancers among farmers,[40] slaughterhouse workers,[41] and butchers.[42] Viruses can cause cancer by directly inserting a cancer-causing gene into a host's DNA.[43]

Animal viruses can infect people who prepare meat with unpleasant skin diseases, such as contagious pustular dermatitis.[44] There's even a well-defined medical condition commonly known as "butchers' warts" that affects the hands of those who handle fresh meat, including poultry and fish.[45] Even the wives of butchers appear to be at higher risk for cervical cancer, a cancer definitively associated with wart-virus exposure.[46]

Workers in poultry slaughterhouses have been found to have higher rates of cancers of the mouth, nasal cavities, throat, esophagus, rectum, liver, and blood. On a public health level, the concern here is that the cancer-causing viruses present in poultry and poultry products may then be transmitted to those in the general population who handle or eat inadequately cooked chicken.[47] These results were replicated recently in the largest such investigation to date, studying more than twenty thousand workers in poultry slaughtering and processing plants. They confirmed the findings of three other studies to date: Workers in these facilities do have increased risk of dying from certain cancers, including cancers of the blood.[48]

Researchers are finally starting to connect the dots. The high levels of antibodies to avian leukosis/sarcoma viruses[49] and to reticuloendotheliosis viruses[50] recently found in poultry workers provide evidence of human exposure to these cancer-causing poultry viruses. Even line workers who simply cut up the finished product and weren't ever exposed to live birds had elevated levels of antibodies in their blood.[51] Beyond just occupational safety, the potential threat to the public, the researchers concluded, "is not trivial."[52]

Elevated blood cancer rates can even be traced back to the farm. An analysis of more than one hundred thousand death certificates found that those who grew up on a farm raising animals appeared significantly more likely to develop a blood cancer later in life, whereas growing up on a farm growing only crops was not. Worst was growing up on a poultry farm, which was associated with nearly three times the odds of developing blood cancer.[53]

Exposure to cattle and pigs has also been associated with non-Hodgkin's lymphoma.[54] A 2003 study by University of California researchers revealed that nearly three-quarters of human subjects tested positive for exposure to the bovine leukemia virus, likely through the consumption of meat and dairy products.[55] Approximately 85 percent of U.S. dairy herds have tested positive for the virus (and 100 percent on industrial-scale operations).[56]

However, just because people are exposed to a virus that causes cancer in cows does not mean that humans themselves can become actively infected with it. In 2014, researchers supported in part by the U.S. Army Breast Cancer Research Program published a remarkable report in a journal of the Centers for Disease Control and Prevention. They reported that the bovine leukemia virus DNA was found to be incorporated into normal and cancerous human breast tissue, effectively proving that people can also become infected with this cancer-causing animal virus.[57] To date, however, the role poultry and other farm animal viruses play in the development of human cancers remains unknown.

What about the *feline* leukemia virus? Thankfully, pet companionship is associated with *lower* rates of lymphoma, which is a personal relief given how many animals I've shared my life with. And the longer people have had cats or dogs in their lives, the lower their risk. In one study, the lowest risk of lymphoma was found in people who had had pets for twenty years or longer. The researchers suspect the reason is connected to the fact that having pets may have beneficial effects on the immune system.[58]

A pair of Harvard University studies suggested that diet soda consumption may increase the risk of non-Hodgkin's lymphoma and multiple myeloma,[59] but this association was only seen among men and was not confirmed in two other large studies on aspartame-sweetened soda.[60,61] Eliminating soda can't hurt, though, in addition to making the dietary changes outlined above.

Plant-based diets are associated with nearly half the risk of blood cancers, protection likely to derive both from the avoidance of foods tied to liquid tumors, such as poultry, as well as the additional consumption of fruits and vegetables. Greens may be particularly useful for non-Hodgkin's lymphoma and turmeric for multiple myeloma. The role tumor-promoting farm animal viruses play in human cancers is not known, but this should be a research priority given the potential extent of public exposure.

CHAPTER 10

How Not to Die from Kidney Disease

Letters and e-mails from patients never fail to inspire me. One note that came to mind as I was writing this chapter was from Dan, a retired NFL player. I first met him when he was forty-two. Even at that relatively young age, the former professional athlete was already taking three separate blood pressure medications. Still, his blood pressure was elevated. He was a little overweight, maybe by twenty-five pounds. He and his significant other waited around after one of my talks to see me.

Dan's physician had just told him that his kidneys were starting to show signs of damage due to his blood pressure. The first thing I asked was if he was taking his meds as prescribed, since many people skip their blood pressure medications because of their unpleasant side effects. Yes, he assured me, he was. He showed me a checklist he carried around to keep track of his meds. He asked me what supplements he could add to the list to help his kidneys.

I told him that no matter what he might have seen on the Internet, there's no such magic pill, but if he filled up his plate with lots of whole, healthy foods each day, the damage might be stopped or even reversed. Well, Dan took this advice to heart (and to kidney!), and he allowed me to share his e-mail:

Well, I went home that night and we cleaned house. Got rid of everything that didn't grow out of the ground, everything processed. And guess what, over the next year, I lost my beer belly *and* the high blood pressure. Life is so much better without those medications—they made me feel so tired all the time. And my kidney function is back to normal. It makes me mad that no one told me this sooner and that I had to feel so bad before I felt better.

It's easy to take your kidneys for granted, but they work around the clock, like a high-tech, nonstop water filter for your blood. They process up to 150 quarts of blood every twenty-four hours just to make the 1–2 quarts of urine you pee out each day.

If your kidneys do not function properly, metabolic waste products can accumulate in the blood and eventually lead to such symptoms as weakness, shortness of breath, confusion, and abnormal heart rhythms. Most people with deteriorating kidney function, however, don't experience any symptoms at all. If your kidneys fail completely, you will either need a new one (i.e., need a kidney transplant) or have to go on dialysis, a process by which a machine artificially filters the blood. But kidney donors are in short supply, and the average life expectancy of a person on dialysis is less than three years.[1] It's better to keep your kidneys healthy in the first place.

Although your kidneys can fail suddenly in response to certain toxins, infections, or urinary blockage, most kidney disease is characterized by a gradual loss of function over time. A national survey found that only 41 percent of Americans tested had normal kidney function, a drop from 52 percent about a decade earlier.[2] Approximately one in three Americans over the age of sixty-four may suffer from chronic kidney disease (CKD),[3] though three-quarters of the millions affected may not even know they have it.[4] More than half of American adults currently aged thirty to sixty-four are expected to develop chronic kidney disease during their lifetimes.[5]

Why, then, aren't millions of people on dialysis? Because kidney malfunction can be so damaging to the rest of the body that most people don't live long enough to reach that stage. In a study in which more than a thousand Americans over age sixty-four with CKD were followed for a decade, only one in twenty developed end-stage kidney failure. Most of the others had already died, with cardiovascular disease killing more than all other causes combined.[6] That's because our kidneys are so critical to proper heart function that patients under age forty-five with kidney failure can be a hundred times more likely to die of heart disease than those with working kidneys.[7]

The good news? The diets that are healthiest for our hearts—those centered around unprocessed plant foods—may be the best way to prevent and treat kidney disease as well.

Damaging Your Kidneys with Diet

Kidneys are highly vascular organs, meaning they're packed with blood vessels, which is why they look so red. We've already seen that the standard

American diet can be toxic to blood vessels in the heart and the brain—so what might it be doing to the kidneys?

Putting that question to the test, researchers at Harvard University followed thousands of healthy women, their diets, and their kidney function for more than a decade[8] to look for the presence of protein in the women's urine. Healthy kidneys work hard to retain protein and other vital nutrients, preferably filtering toxic or useless wastes out of the bloodstream via our urine. If the kidneys are leaking protein into urine, it's a sign that they may be starting to fail.

The researchers found three specific dietary components associated with this sign of declining kidney function: animal protein, animal fat, and cholesterol. Each of these is found in only one place: animal products. The researchers found no association between kidney function decline and the intake of protein or fat from plant sources.[9]

One hundred and fifty years ago, Rudolf Virchow, the father of modern pathology, first described fatty degeneration of the kidney.[10] This concept of lipid nephrotoxicity, or the idea that fat and cholesterol in the bloodstream could be toxic to the kidneys, has since been formalized,[11] based in part on studies that found plugs of fat clogging up the works in autopsied kidneys.[12]

The link between cholesterol and kidney disease has gained such momentum in the medical community that cholesterol-lowering statin drugs have been recommended to slow its progression.[13] But wouldn't it be better (not to mention safer and cheaper) to treat the underlying cause of the disease by eating healthier?

Which Type of Protein Is Better for Our Kidneys?

In the two decades between 1990 and 2010, the leading causes of death and disability remained relatively constant. As noted in chapter 1, heart disease is still the leading cause of loss of health and life. Some diseases, such as HIV/AIDS, have slid down the list, but among the diseases whose incidence has increased the most over the past generation is chronic kidney disease. The number of deaths has doubled.[14]

This has been blamed on our "meat-sweet" diet.[15] Excess table sugar and high-fructose corn syrup consumption is associated with increased blood pressure and uric acid levels, both of which can damage the kidney. The saturated fat, trans fat, and cholesterol found in animal products and junk food are also associated with impaired kidney function, and meat protein increases the acid load to the kidneys, boosting ammonia production and potentially damaging our sensitive kidney cells.[16] This is why a restriction of protein intake is often recommended to chronic kidney disease patients to help prevent further functional decline.[17]

But all protein isn't created equal. It's important to understand that not all protein has the same effect on your kidneys.

High animal protein intake can have a profound influence on normal human kidney function by inducing a state called hyperfiltration, a dramatic increase in the workload of the kidney. Hyperfiltration isn't harmful if it occurs only occasionally. We all have built-in reserve kidney function—so much so that people can live with only one kidney. The human body is thought to have evolved the capacity to handle intermittent large doses of protein from our remote hunting and scavenging days. But now many of us are ingesting large doses of animal protein day after day, forcing our kidneys to call on their reserves continuously. Over time, this unrelenting stress may explain why kidney function tends to decline as people age, predisposing even otherwise healthy people to progressive deterioration of kidney function.[18]

The reason those who eat a plant-based diet appear to have better kidney function was originally thought to be due to their lower overall protein intake.[19] However, we now know that it's more likely due to the fact that the kidneys appear to handle plant protein very differently from animal protein.[20]

Within hours of consuming meat, your kidneys rev up into hyperfiltration mode. This is true of a variety of animal proteins—beef, chicken, and fish appear to have similar effects.[21] But an equivalent amount of plant protein causes virtually no noticeable stress on the kidneys.[22] Eat some tuna, and within three hours, your kidney filtration rate can shoot up 36 percent. But eating the same amount of protein in the form of tofu doesn't appear to place any additional strain on the kidneys.[23]

Could substituting plant protein for animal protein help slow the deterioration of kidney function? Yes, half a dozen clinical trials have shown that plant protein replacement can reduce hyperfiltration and/or protein leakage,[24,25,26,27,28,29] but all these studies were short term, lasting fewer than eight weeks. It wasn't until 2014 that a six-month, double-blind, randomized, placebo-controlled clinical trial was performed examining how the kidneys process soy protein versus dairy protein. Consistent with the other studies, plant protein was found to help preserve function in ailing kidneys.[30]

Why does animal protein cause the overload reaction while plant protein doesn't? Because of the inflammation animal products can cause. Researchers discovered that after giving study subjects a powerful anti-inflammatory drug along with animal protein, the hyperfiltration response and protein spillage disappeared.[31]

Reducing Dietary Acid Load

Another reason animal protein may be so detrimental to kidney function is that it is generally more acid forming. This is because animal protein tends to have higher levels of sulfur-containing amino acids, such as methionine, which produce sulfuric acid when metabolized in the body. Fruits and vegetables, on the other hand, are generally base forming, which helps neutralize acids in our kidneys.[32]

Dietary acid load is determined by the balance of acid-inducing foods (such as meats, eggs, and cheese) and base-inducing foods (such as fruits and vegetables). A 2014 analysis of the diets and kidney function of more than twelve thousand Americans across the country found that a higher dietary acid load was associated with significantly higher risk of protein leakage into the urine, an indicator of kidney damage.[33]

Ancient human diets largely consisted of plants, so they likely produced more base than acid in the kidneys of our ancestors. Humans evolved eating these alkaline (base-forming) diets over millions of years. Most contemporary diets, on the other hand, produce acid in excess. This switch from base- to acid-forming diets may help explain our modern epidemic of kidney disease.[34] Acid-inducing diets are believed to impact the kidney through "tubular toxicity," damage to the tiny, delicate, urine-making tubes in the kidneys. To buffer the excess acid formed by your diet, kidneys produce ammonia, which is a base and can neutralize some of that acid. Counteracting the acid is beneficial in the short term, but over the long run, all the extra ammonia in the kidneys may have a toxic effect.[35] The decline in kidney function over time may be a consequence of a lifetime of ammonia overproduction.[36] Kidneys may start to deteriorate in your twenties,[37] and by the time you reach your eighties, you may be down to half capacity.[38]

The chronic, low-grade, metabolic acidosis attributed to a meat-rich diet[39] helps explain why people eating plant-based diets appear to have superior kidney function[40] and why various plant-based diets have been so successful in treating chronic kidney failure.[41,42] Under normal circumstances, a vegetarian diet alkalinizes the kidneys, whereas a nonvegetarian diet carries an acid load. This proved to be true even among vegetarians who consumed processed meat substitutes, such as veggie burgers.[43]

If people are unwilling to reduce their meat consumption, they should be encouraged to eat more fruits and vegetables to balance out that acid load.[44] "However," one kidney doctor editorialized, "many patients find it difficult to follow a diet high in fruits and vegetables and might therefore be more adherent to a supplement."[45]

So what did researchers try? Giving people baking soda (sodium bicarbonate) pills. Instead of treating the primary cause of the excess acid formation (too many animal products and too few fruits and vegetables), they preferred to treat the consequences. Too much acid? Here's some base to neutralize it. Sodium bicarbonate can effectively buffer the acid load,[46] but, rather obviously, sodium bicarbonate contains sodium, which over the long term may itself contribute to kidney damage.[47]

Unfortunately, this type of Band-Aid approach is all too typical of today's medical model. Cholesterol too high from eating a diet unnaturally high in saturated fat and cholesterol? Take a statin drug to cripple your cholesterol-making enzyme. Diet unnaturally high in acid-forming foods? Swallow some baking soda pills to balance that right out.

These same researchers also tried giving people fruits and vegetables instead of baking soda and found that they offered similar protections, with the additional advantage of lowering the subjects' blood pressure. The title of the accompanying commentary in the medical journal was telling: "The Key to Halting Progression of CKD Might Be in the Produce Market, Not in the Pharmacy."[48]

Kidney Stones

Eating a plant-based diet to alkalinize your urine may also help prevent and treat kidney stones—those hard mineral deposits that can form in your kidneys when the concentration of certain stone-forming substances in your urine becomes so high they start to crystallize. Eventually, these crystals can grow into pebble-sized rocks that block the flow of urine, causing severe pain that tends to radiate from one side of the lower back toward the groin. Kidney stones can pass naturally (and often painfully), but some become so large that they have to be removed surgically.

The incidence of kidney stones has increased dramatically since World War II[49] and even just in the last fifteen years. Approximately one in eleven Americans are affected today, compared with one in twenty less than two decades ago.[50] What accounts for this rising incidence? The first clue to an answer came in 1979 when scientists reported a striking relationship between the prevalence of kidney stones since the 1950s and increasing consumption of animal protein.[51]

As in all observational studies, though, the researchers couldn't prove cause and effect, so they decided to perform an interventional trial: They asked the subjects to add extra animal protein to their daily diets, the equivalent of about an extra can's worth of tuna fish. Within two days of eating the extra tuna, the levels of stone-forming compounds—calcium, oxalate, and uric acid—shot up such that the subjects' kidney-stone risk increased 250 percent.[52]

Note the experimental "high" animal protein diet was designed to re-create the animal protein intake of the average American,[53] suggesting that Americans could considerably lower their risk of kidney stones by lowering their meat intake.

By the 1970s, enough evidence had accumulated that researchers began to ask whether people suffering from recurrent kidney stones should stop eating meat altogether.[54] A study on the kidney stone risk of vegetarians wasn't published until 2014, though. Oxford University researchers found that subjects who didn't eat meat at all had a significantly lower risk of being hospitalized for kidney stones, and for those who did eat meat, the more they ate, the higher their associated risk.[55]

Is some meat worse than others? People who form kidney stones are commonly advised to restrict their intake of red meat, but what about chicken or fish? We didn't know until another 2014 study compared salmon and cod to chicken breasts and burgers. It found that gram for gram, fish might be slightly worse than other meat in terms of the risk of certain kidney stones, but they concluded that overall, "[s]tone formers should be counseled to limit the intake of all animal proteins."[56]

Most kidney stones are composed of calcium oxalate, which forms like rock candy when urine becomes supersaturated with calcium and oxalates. For many years, doctors assumed that because the stones are made of calcium, they should counsel their patients to simply reduce their calcium intake.[57] As with so much in medicine, clinical practice often flies blind without solid experimental support. This changed with a landmark study, published in the *New England Journal of Medicine*, which pitted the traditional, low-calcium diet against a diet low in animal protein and sodium. After five years, the study found that eating less meat and salt was about twice as effective as the conventionally prescribed low-calcium diet, cutting kidney-stone risk by half.[58]

What about cutting down on oxalates, which are concentrated in certain vegetables? Reassuringly, a recent study found there was no increased risk of stone formation with higher vegetable intake. In fact, greater intake of fruits and vegetables was associated with a reduced risk independent of other known risk factors, meaning there may be additional benefits to bulking up on plant foods above and beyond restricting animal foods.[59]

Another reason a reduction in animal protein is helpful is that it lowers uric acid buildup, which can form crystals that seed calcium stones or form stones all by itself. Indeed, uric acid stones are the second most common type of kidney stones. So it makes sense that to reduce your risk, you should try to reduce excess uric acid production. This can be accomplished either of two ways: by adding drugs or by subtracting meat.[60] Uric acid–blocking medications like allopurinol may be effective, but they can have serious side effects.[61] On the other hand, removing all meat from a standard Western diet appears to reduce the risk of uric acid crystallization by more than 90 percent within as few as five days.[62]

Bottom line: When urine is more alkaline, stones are less likely to form. This helps explain why less meat and more fruits and vegetables appear so protective. The standard American diet yields acidic urine. When people are placed on a plant-based diet, however, their urine can be alkalinized up to a near neutral pH in less than a week.[63]

Not all plant foods are alkalinizing, though, and not all animal foods are equally acidifying. The LAKE (Load of Acid to Kidney Evaluation) score takes into account both the acid load of foods and their typical serving sizes in order to help people modify their diets for the prevention of kidney stones and other acid-related diseases, such as gout. As you can see in figure 4, the single

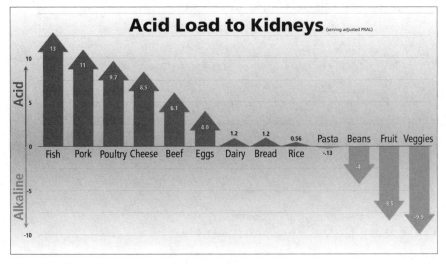

Figure 4

most acid-producing food was fish, including tuna, followed by pork, poultry, cheese, and beef. Eggs are actually more acid producing than beef, but people tend to eat fewer of them at one sitting. Some grains can be a little acid form-ing, such as bread and rice, but not pasta, interestingly. Beans are significantly acid reducing, but not as much as fruits are, with vegetables crowned the most alkaline forming of foods.[64]

Dietary changes can be so powerful they can not only help prevent kidney stones but also, in some cases, cure them without drugs or surgery. Uric acid stones can apparently be dissolved away completely with a combination of eat-ing more fruits and vegetables, restricting animal protein and salt intake, and drinking at least ten glasses of fluid a day.[65]

Testing Your "Pee-H" with Purple Cabbage

We know that the average Western diet is acid producing, while the average plant-based diet is acid reducing.[66] Eating an acid-forming diet can not only affect kidney stone risk but may also produce the systemic, chronic, low-grade metabolic acidosis[67]—excess acid in the bloodstream—that is thought to contribute to muscle breakdown as you age.[68] So what's the best way to determine how acid forming your diet really is? Perhaps the easiest (and most boring) method is to order some pH paper strips to pee on. Alterna-tively, why not use what you (should) have right now in your refrigerator's crisper: purple cabbage. Purple, or red, cabbage provides one of the single best nutritional bangs for your buck, and you can even use it to perform kitchen chemistry experiments, or in this case, bathroom chemistry.

Boil some purple cabbage until the water turns deep purple, or blend raw cabbage with some water and then strain out the solids. Pee into your toilet then take your purple-cabbage cocktail and pour it into the toilet bowl. (Low-flow toilets work best, because there's less water in the bowl.) If the liquid in the toilet bowl remains purple or, even worse, turns pink, your urine is too acidic. Blue is the target. If your pee and cabbage water turns blue, your urine is not acidic but neutral or even basic.

Preventing Excess Phosphorus Intake

Having too much phosphorus in the blood may increase the risk of kidney fail-ure, heart failure, heart attacks, and premature death. Excess phosphorus also appears to damage our blood vessels and accelerate aging and bone loss.[69] As such, elevated levels appear to be an independent risk factor for early death among the general population.[70]

Phosphorus is found in a variety of plant and animal foods. Most Americans consume about twice as much phosphorus as they need,[71] but it's not just about how much you eat but how much you absorb. By switching to a plant-based diet, you can achieve a significant drop in your blood phosphorus levels even as your intake levels of the mineral remains constant.[72] This occurs because the phosphorus in animal foods appears in the form of a compound called phosphate, which is absorbed into the bloodstream more readily than phytate, the predominant form of phosphorus in plant foods.[73] As you may remember from chapter 4, this situation is similar to the case of iron, another essential mineral of which you can get too much. Your body can better protect itself from absorbing too much plant-based iron, but it can't as effectively stop surplus muscle or blood-based (heme) iron from slipping through the intestinal wall.

The worst type of phosphorus, though, is that found in phosphate food additives. These phosphorus compounds are added to cola drinks and meat to enhance their color.[74] (Without added phosphate, Coca-Cola would be pitch black.[75]) Less than half of most plant phosphorus[76] and about three-quarters of natural animal product phosphorus gets into your bloodstream,[77] but added phosphate can be absorbed at a rate of nearly 100 percent.[78]

Phosphate additives play an especially important role in the meat industry. Chicken meat is often injected with phosphates to improve its color, to add water weight (and thus to increase profitability since chicken can be sold by the pound), and to reduce "purge," the term used to describe the liquid that seeps from meat as it ages.[79] The problem with this additive is that it can nearly double the phosphorous levels in meat.[80] Phosphate additives have been described as "a real and insidious danger" for kidney patients, since they have diminished capacity to excrete it,[81] but given what we now know about excess phosphorus, it's a concern for us all.

In the United States, eleven different types of phosphate salts are allowed to be injected into raw meat and poultry,[82] a practice that's long been banned in Europe.[83] This is because phosphates found in meat and processed foods are considered "vascular toxins,"[84] capable of impairing our arterial function within hours of consuming a high-phosphate meal.[85] In meat, there's an additional food safety concern, as adding phosphate may increase the growth of leading food poisoning bacteria *Campylobacter* in poultry purge up to a millionfold.[86]

It's easy to avoid added phosphorus in processed foods—just don't buy anything containing ingredients with the word "phosphate" in their names, including pyrophosphate and sodium triphosphate.[87] With meat, it's more difficult to determine the phosphate content, as producers aren't required to disclose injected additives. Added phosphate may be labeled as "flavorings" or "broth" or not labeled at all.[88] Meat already contains highly absorbable phosphates; adding more may just add insult to kidney injury. Chicken appears to be the worst offender: A supermarket survey found more than 90 percent of chicken products contained phosphate additives.[89]

Who Determines Whether Food Additives Are Safe?

In 2015, the U.S. Food and Drug Administration finally announced its plans to all but eliminate trans fats from processed foods,[90] citing a CDC estimate that as many as twenty thousand heart attacks each year could be prevented by eliminating partially hydrogenated oils.[91] Until June 16, 2015, trans fats enjoyed so-called GRAS status: "generally recognized as safe."

Why were these killer fats deemed safe in the first place?

Guess who makes the "generally recognized as safe" determination? It's not the government or a scientific body. It's the manufacturer. You read that right. The food maker gets to determine whether or not its own product is safe for the public, a process the FDA refers to as "GRAS self-determination." What's more, these manufacturers can legally add things to our food supply without informing the FDA.[92] An estimated one thousand food-additive safety decisions have never even been reported to the FDA or the public.[93]

But sometimes food manufacturers do notify the FDA when they introduce a new additive. Sounds responsible of them, doesn't it? Presumably they found some independent, third-party panel to evaluate the safety of their product so as to avoid a financial conflict of interest, right?

Well, not exactly.

Of all the GRAS safety determinations that were voluntarily submitted to the FDA between 1997 and 2012, 22.4 percent were made by someone directly employed by the manufacturer itself, 13.3 percent were made by someone directly employed by a firm handpicked by the manufacturer, and 64.3 percent were made by a panel either handpicked by the manufacturer or chosen by a firm hired by the manufacturer.[94] Are you doing the math? Yes, *zero* food safety decisions were made independently.

How could regulators let companies decide for themselves whether the food additives they use in their own products are safe? Follow the money. Three of Washington's largest lobbying firms reportedly now work for the food industry.[95] For example, PepsiCo alone spent more than $9 million in a single year to lobby Congress.[96] The deeper you dig, the less surprising it is that such food additives as trans fats have been allowed to kill thousands year after year.

But hey, according to the manufacturer, they're safe . . .

Can Diet Protect Against Kidney Cancer?

Each year, sixty-four thousand Americans are diagnosed with kidney cancer, and about fourteen thousand die from it.[97] Approximately 4 percent of these cases are hereditary,[98] but what about the other 96 percent?

Historically, the only accepted risk factor for kidney cancer has been tobacco use.[99] A class of carcinogens in cigarette smoke called nitrosamines are considered to be so harmful that even so-called thirdhand smoke is a concern. The risks of tobacco smoke do not end when a cigarette is extinguished, as residual smoke can stick to walls and other surfaces.[100] Around 80 percent of nitrosamines from cigarette smoke can remain in a room, even with normal ventilation,[101] so always try to choose smoke-free hotel rooms. Nitrosamines are one of the reasons you can't smoke indoors without endangering others, even if you smoke without anyone present. As one of the leading scholars in the tobacco control movement recently wrote, "Carcinogens of this strength in any other consumer product designed for human consumption would be banned immediately."[102]

Except for one: meat.

Did you know that one hot dog has as many nitrosamines (and nitrosamides, which are similar tobacco carcinogens[103]) as four cigarettes and that these carcinogens are also found in fresh meat, including beef, chicken, and pork?[104] This may help explain the rising rates of kidney cancer over the last few decades despite the falling rates of smoking.

Clearing the Confusion: Nitrates, Nitrites, and Nitrosamines

Although fresh meat also contains nitrosamines, processed or cured meat like deli slices may be particularly harmful. In Europe, the world's second-largest prospective study on diet and cancer calculated that a reduction in processed meat consumption to less than twenty grams a day—less than a small matchbook-sized portion—would prevent more than 3 percent of all deaths.[105] In the largest such investigation the NIH-AARP study of more than five hundred thousand Americans (see page 69) found the preventable fraction of deaths may be even higher. The researchers suggested, for example, that 20 percent of heart disease deaths among American women could be averted if the highest consumers of processed meat would cut down to the equivalent of less than a half strip of bacon a day.[106] No wonder the American Institute for Cancer Research recommends that you simply "avoid processed meat such as ham, bacon, salami, hot dogs and sausages."[107]

Nitrites are added to cured meat as a "color fixative" and to help prevent the growth of botulism bacteria (a rare but serious paralytic illness).[108] What about "uncured" bacon? It says right on the package: "No nitrites or nitrates added." But study the fine print and you may see a little footnote that reads something like "except those naturally occurring in celery juice." Vegetables do contain nitrates that can be fermented into nitrites, so adding fermented celery juice to bacon is just a sneaky way of adding nitrites. Even commentators in the journal *Meat Science* have realized this may be perceived by consumers as "incorrect at best or deceptive at worst."[109]

But the same fermentation that converts nitrates to nitrites can happen when you eat vegetables, thanks to bacteria on your tongue. So why are vegetable nitrates and nitrites okay but the same compounds from meat are linked to cancer?[110] Because nitrites themselves are not carcinogenic; they turn into carcinogens. Nitrites only become harmful when they turn into nitros*amines* and nitros*amides*. For them to do that, amines and amides must be present, and amines and amides are found in abundance in animal products. This transformation can happen in the meat itself or in your stomach after you eat it. In the case of plant foods, the vitamin C and other antioxidants that are found naturally in them block the formation of these carcinogens in your body.[111] This process would explain why intake of both nitrate and nitrite from processed meat has been linked to kidney cancer, but no increased risk was found for nitrate or nitrite intake from plant sources.[112]

While nitrite from animal sources—not just processed meats—was associated with an increased risk of kidney cancer, some of the highest nitrate-containing vegetables, such as arugula, kale, and collards, are associated with significantly reduced risk for kidney cancer.[113]

Kidneys are tasked with the monumental responsibility of filtering your blood all day, every day. That's a lot of work for two fist-sized organs. Kidneys are extremely resilient, but they aren't indestructible. When they begin to fail, the body can start failing too. Toxic substances that healthy kidneys would ordinarily filter out can pass through and build up in the bloodstream.

To keep your kidneys strong and your blood clean, you must carefully consider what you eat. The meat-sweet American diet can slowly damage your kidneys one meal at a time, forcing the kidneys into a state of hyperfiltration. Imagine how long your car engine would last if you always revved it near the red line? Thankfully, medical science has proven that you can reduce your kidneys' workload (and acid load) by moving toward a more plant-based diet.

CHAPTER 11

How Not to Die from Breast Cancer

"You have breast cancer."

These are among the most feared words a woman can hear, and for a good reason. Besides skin cancer, breast cancer is the most common cancer among American women. Every year, about 230,000 are diagnosed with breast cancer, and 40,000 die from it.[1]

Breast cancer does not occur overnight. That lump you feel in the shower one morning may have started forming decades ago. By the time doctors detect the tumor, it may have been present for forty years or even longer.[2] The cancer has been growing, maturing, and acquiring hundreds of new survival-of-the-fittest mutations that allow it to grow even more quickly as it tries to outmaneuver your immune system.

The scary reality is that what doctors call "early detection" is actually late detection. Modern imaging simply isn't good enough to detect cancer at its earliest stages, so it can spread long before it's even spotted. A woman is considered "healthy" until she shows signs or symptoms of breast cancer. But if she has been harboring a malignancy for two decades, can she truly be considered healthy?

People who are doing the right thing by improving their diets in hopes of preventing cancer may in fact be successfully treating it as well. Autopsy studies have shown that as many as 20 percent of women aged twenty to fifty-four who died from unrelated causes, such as car accidents, had so-called "occult" (or hidden) breast cancers growing inside them.[3] Sometimes there's nothing you can do to prevent the initiation stage of cancer, when that first normal breast cell mutates into a cancerous one. Some breast cancers may even start in the womb and be related to your mother's diet.[4] For this reason, we all need to choose a diet and lifestyle that not only prevents the initiation stage of cancer but also hampers the promotion stage, during which the cancer grows to a size large enough to pose a threat.

The good news is that no matter what your mom ate or how you lived as a child, by eating and living healthfully, you may be able to slow the growth rate of any hidden cancers. In short, you can die *with* your tumors rather than *from* them. This is how dietary cancer prevention and treatment can end up being the same thing.

One or two cancer cells never hurt anyone. But how about a billion cancer cells? That's how many may be in a tumor[5] by the time it's picked up by a mammogram.[6] Like most tumors, breast cancer starts with just one cell, which divides to become two, four, and then eight. Every time breast cancer cells divide, the tumor can effectively double in size.[7]

Let's see how many times a tiny tumor has to double to get to a billion cells. Take out a calculator. Multiply one times two. Then multiply that number by two. Keep doing that until you reach one billion. Don't worry. It won't take long. It's only thirty doublings. In just thirty doublings, a single cancer cell can turn into a billion.

The key to how quickly you'd be diagnosed with cancer, then, is the doubling time. How long does it take tumors to double once? Breast cancers can double in size in anywhere from as few as twenty-five days[8] to a thousand days or more.[9] In other words, it could be two years, or it could be more than a hundred years, before a tumor starts to cause problems.

Where you fall on that timescale—two years or a century—may depend in part on what you eat.

When I was teen, I ate a lousy diet. One of my favorite meals was—no joke—chicken-fried steak. During my youth, I may have caused one of the cells in my colon or prostate to mutate. But I've been eating much healthier for the last twenty-five years. My hope is that even if I did initiate a cancerous growth, if I don't promote it, I may be able to slow down its growth. I don't care if I get diagnosed with cancer a hundred years from now. I don't expect to be around at that point to worry about it.

Current controversy over the cost and effectiveness of mammograms[10] misses an important point: Breast cancer screening, by definition, does not prevent breast cancer. It can just pick up existing breast cancer. Based on autopsy studies, as many as 39 percent of women in their forties already have breast cancers growing within their bodies that may be simply too small to be detected by mammograms.[11] That's why you can't just wait until diagnosis to start eating and living healthier. You should start tonight.

RISK FACTORS FOR BREAST CANCER

The American Institute for Cancer Research (AICR) is considered one of the world's leading authorities on diet and cancer. Based on the best available research, it came up with ten recommendations for cancer prevention.[12] Beyond never chewing tobacco, their bottom-line dietary message was: "Diets that revolve around whole plant foods—vegetables, whole grains, fruits and beans—cut the risk of many cancers, and other diseases as well."[13]

To demonstrate how dramatically lifestyle choices can impact breast cancer risk, over the course of about seven years, researchers followed a group of about thirty thousand postmenopausal women with no history of breast cancer. Achieving just three of the ten AICR recommendations—limiting alcohol, eating mostly plant foods, and maintaining a normal body weight—was associated with a 62 percent lower risk of breast cancer.[14] Yes, three simple health behaviors appeared to cut risk by more than half.

Remarkably, eating a plant-based diet along with walking every day can improve our cancer defenses within just two weeks. Researchers dripped the blood of women before and after fourteen days of healthy living onto breast cancer cells growing in petri dishes. The blood taken after they started eating healthier suppressed cancer growth significantly better and killed 20–30 percent more cancer cells than the blood taken from the same women just two weeks before.[15] The researchers attributed this effect to a decrease in levels of a cancer-promoting growth hormone called IGF-1,[16] likely due to the reduced intake of animal protein.[17]

What kind of blood do you want in your body—what kind of immune system? The kind of blood that just rolls over when new cancer cells pop up, or blood that circulates to every nook and cranny in your body with the power to slow down and stop cancer cells in their tracks?

Alcohol

In 2010, the official World Health Organization body that assesses cancer risks formally upgraded its classification of alcohol to a definitive human breast carcinogen.[18] In 2014, it clarified its position by stating that, regarding breast cancer, no amount of alcohol is safe.[19]

But what about drinking "responsibly"? In 2013, scientists published a compilation of more than one hundred studies on breast cancer and light drinking (up to one alcoholic beverage a day). The researchers had found a small but statistically significant increase in breast cancer risk even among women who had at most one drink per day (except, perhaps, for red wine—see box below). They estimated that, every year around the world, nearly five thousand breast cancer deaths may be attributable to light drinking.[20]

The carcinogen isn't alcohol itself. The culprit is actually the toxic breakdown product of alcohol called acetaldehyde, which can form in your mouth almost immediately after you take a sip. Experiments show that even holding a single teaspoon of hard liquor in your mouth for five seconds before spitting it out results in the production of potentially carcinogenic levels of acetaldehyde that lingers for more than ten minutes.[21]

If even a single sip of alcohol might produce cancer-causing levels of acetaldehyde in the mouth, what about using mouthwash that contains alcohol? Researchers who tested the effects of a variety of retail mouthwashes and oral rinses concluded that, although the risk is slight, it is probably best to refrain from using such products if they contain alcohol.[22]

Red Wine Versus White Wine

The Harvard Nurses' Health Study found that even less than one drink a day may be associated with a small increase in breast cancer risk.[23] Interestingly, drinking only red wine was *not* associated with breast cancer risk. Why? A compound in red wine appears to suppress the activity of an enzyme called estrogen synthase, which breast tumors can use to create estrogen to fuel their own growth.[24] This compound is found in the skin of the dark-purple grapes used to make red wine, which explains why white wine appears to provide no such benefit,[25] since it's produced without the skin.

The researchers concluded that red wine may "ameliorate the elevated breast cancer risk associated with alcohol intake."[26] In other words, the grapes in red wine may help cancel out some of the cancer-causing effects of the alcohol. But you can reap the benefits without the risks associated with imbibing alcoholic beverages by simply drinking grape juice or, even better, eating the purple grapes themselves—preferably ones with seeds, as they appear to be most effective at suppressing estrogen synthase.[27]

It's good (and delicious) to know that strawberries,[28] pomegranates,[29] and plain white mushrooms[30] may also suppress the potentially cancer-promoting enzyme.

Melatonin and Breast Cancer Risk

For billions of years, life on planet Earth evolved under conditions of about twelve hours of light and twelve hours of darkness. Humans controlled fire for cooking about a million years ago, but we've only been using candles for about five thousand years and electric lights for a mere century. In other words, our ancient ancestors lived half their lives in the dark.

These days, though, because of the electric-light pollution at night, the only Milky Way your children may see is inside a candy wrapper. Electric lighting has enabled us to remain productive well into the wee hours, but might this unnatural nighttime light exposure have any adverse health effects?

In philosophy, there's a flawed argument called the appeal-to-nature fallacy, in which someone proposes that something is good merely because it's natural. In biology, however, this may hold some truth. The conditions under which our bodies were finely tuned over millions of years can sometimes give us insight into our optimal functioning. For example, we evolved running around naked in equatorial Africa. Therefore, it's not surprising that many of us modern humans become deficient in vitamin D (the "sunshine vitamin") if we live in Northern climes or in countries where the culture dictates full-body coverings for women.[31]

Could something as ubiquitous as the lightbulb be a mixed blessing? Right in the middle of your brain sits the pineal gland, your so-called third eye. It's connected to your actual eyes and has just one function: to produce a hormone called melatonin. During the day, the pineal gland is inactive. But once the sky darkens, it activates and begins pumping melatonin into your bloodstream. You start getting tired, feel less alert, and start thinking about sleep. Melatonin secretion may peak between 2:00 A.M. and 5:00 A.M. and then shuts off at daybreak, which is your cue to wake up. The level of melatonin in your bloodstream is one of the ways your internal organs know what time it is. It functions as one hand on your circadian clock.[32]

Besides helping to regulate your sleep, melatonin is thought to play another role—suppressing cancer growth. Think of melatonin as helping to put cancer cells to sleep at night.[33] To see if this function applies to preventing breast cancer, researchers from Brigham and Women's Hospital in Boston and elsewhere came up with the clever idea of studying blind women. The thought was that because blind women can't see sunlight, their pineal glands never stop secreting melatonin into their bloodstreams. Sure enough, the researchers found that blind women may have just half the odds of breast cancer as sighted women.[34]

Conversely, women who interrupt their melatonin production by working night shifts appear to be at increased risk for breast cancer.[35] Even living on a particularly brightly lit street may affect the risk. Studies comparing night-time satellite photos against breast cancer rates have found that people living in brighter neighborhoods tend to have a higher breast cancer risk.[36,37,38] Therefore, it's probably best to sleep without any lights on and with the blinds down, though the evidence to support these strategies is limited.[39]

Melatonin production can be gauged by measuring the amount of melatonin excreted in our first pee in the morning. And, indeed, women with higher melatonin secretion have been found to have lower rates of breast cancer.[40] Other than minimizing nighttime light exposure, is there anything else you can do to keep up your production of melatonin? Apparently so. In 2005, Japanese researchers reported an association between higher vegetable intake and higher melatonin levels in the urine.[41] Is there anything in your diet that may lower melatonin production, thereby potentially increasing breast cancer risk? We didn't know until a comprehensive study of diet and melatonin was published in 2009. Researchers at Harvard University asked nearly a thousand women about their consumption of thirty-eight different foods or food groups and measured their morning melatonin levels. Meat consumption was the only food significantly associated with lower melatonin production, for reasons that are yet unknown.[42]

Minimizing melatonin disruption may therefore mean putting curtains on your windows, eating more vegetables, and lowering the curtain on eating too much meat.

Exercise and Breast Cancer

Physical activity is considered a promising preventive measure against breast cancer[43] not only because it helps with weight control but because exercise tends to lower circulating estrogen levels.[44] Five hours a week of vigorous aerobic exercise can lower estrogen and progesterone exposure by about 20 percent.[45] But do you need to work out that long for it to be protective?

Although even light exercise is associated with lowered risk of some other types of cancer, for breast cancer, leisurely strolls don't appear to cut it.[46] Even an hour a day of activities such as slow dancing or light

continued

housework may not help.[47] According to the largest study ever published on the subject, only women who worked up a sweat at least five or more times a week appeared to get significant protection.[48] Moderately intense activity may offer as much benefit as vigorous exercise, though.[49] Walking at a moderate pace for an hour a day is considered a moderately intense level of exercise, but it wasn't put to the test until a 2013 study reported that, indeed, walking an hour a day or more is associated with significantly lower breast cancer risk.[50]

Darwin was right: It's survival of the fittest—so get fit!

Heterocyclic Amines

In 1939, a curious finding was published in a paper titled "Presence of Cancer-Producing Substances in Roasted Food." A researcher described how he could induce breast cancers in mice by painting their heads with extracts of roasted horse muscle.[51] These "cancer-producing substances" have since been identified as heterocyclic amines (HCAs), described by the National Cancer Institute as "chemicals formed when muscle meat, including beef, pork, fish, and poultry, is cooked using high-temperature methods."[52] These cooking methods include roasting, pan frying, grilling, and baking. Eating boiled meat is probably the safest. People who eat meat that never goes above 212 degrees Fahrenheit produce urine and feces that are significantly less DNA-damaging compared to those eating meat dry-cooked at higher temperatures.[53] This means they have fewer mutagenic substances flowing through their bloodstreams and coming in contact with their colons. On the other hand, baking chicken for as few as fifteen minutes at about 350 degrees Fahrenheit leads to HCA production.[54]

These carcinogens are formed in a high-temperature chemical reaction between some of the components of muscle tissue. (The lack of some of these substances in plants may explain why even fried veggie burgers don't contain measurable HCAs.)[55] The longer meat is cooked, the more HCAs form. This process may explain why eating well-done meat is associated with increased risk of cancers of the breast, colon, esophagus, lung, pancreas, prostate, and stomach.[56] The situation creates what the *Harvard Health Letter* called a meat preparation "paradox"[57]: Cooking meat thoroughly reduces the risk of contracting foodborne infections (see chapter 5), but cooking meat *too* thoroughly may increase the risk of foodborne carcinogens.

Just because heterocyclic amines cause cancer in rodents doesn't mean they cause cancer in humans. In this case, though—it turns out people may be even *more* susceptible. The livers of rodents have shown an uncanny ability to detoxify 99 percent of the HCAs scientists stuffed down the animals' throats (a technique known as gavage).[58] But then, in 2008, researchers discovered that the livers of humans fed cooked chicken were only able to detoxify about half of these carcinogens, suggesting that the cancer risk is far higher than was previously thought based on experiments in rats.[59]

The carcinogens found in cooked meat are thought to explain why, as the Long Island Breast Cancer Study Project reported in 2007, women who eat more grilled, barbecued, or smoked meats over their lifetimes may have as much as 47 percent higher odds of breast cancer.[60] And the Iowa Women's Health Study found that women who ate their bacon, beefsteak, and burgers "very well done" had nearly five times the odds of getting breast cancer compared with women who preferred these meats served rare or medium.[61]

To see what was happening inside the breast, researchers asked women undergoing breast-reduction surgery about their meat-cooking methods. The scientists were able to link the consumption of fried meat with the amount of DNA damage found within the women's breast tissue,[62] the type of damage that can potentially cause a normal cell to mutate into a cancer cell.[63]

HCAs appear able both to initiate and to promote cancer growth. PhIP, one of the most abundant HCAs in cooked meat, was found to have potent estrogen-like effects, fueling human breast-cancer cell growth almost as powerfully as pure estrogen,[64] on which most human breast tumors thrive. But that result was based on research in a petri dish. How do we know that cooked-meat carcinogens find their way into human breast ducts, where most breast cancers arise? We didn't, until researchers measured the levels of PhIP in the breast milk of nonsmoking women. (HCAs are also found in cigarette smoke.)[65] In this study, PhIP was found in the breast milk of women who ate meat at the same concentration known to significantly boost breast cancer cell growth.[66] No trace of PhIP was found in the breast milk of the one vegetarian participant.[67]

A similar finding was reported in a study comparing the levels of PhIP in people's hair. The chemical was detected in hair samples of all six of the meat eaters tested, but in only one of the six vegetarians.[68] (HCAs can also be found in fried eggs.)[69]

Your body can rapidly rid itself of these toxins once exposure ceases. In fact, urine levels of PhIP can drop to zero within twenty-four hours of refraining from eating meat.[70] So if you practice Meatless Mondays, the level of PhIP passing through your body may become undetectable by Tuesday morning. But diet is not the only source of PhIP. HCA levels in vegetarians who smoke may approach those of nonsmoking meat eaters.[71]

The heterocyclic amine PhIP is not just a so-called complete carcinogen, able to both initiate cancers and then promote their growth. PhIP may also then facilitate cancer spread. Cancer develops in three major stages: 1) initiation, the irreversible DNA damage that starts the process; 2) promotion, the growth and division of the initiated cell into a tumor; and 3) progression, which can involve the invasion of the tumor into surrounding tissue and metastasis (spread) to other areas of the body.

Scientists can test how invasive, or aggressive, a certain cancer is by putting its cells into an instrument called an invasion chamber. They place cancer cells on one side of a porous membrane and then gauge their ability to penetrate and spread through the membrane. When researchers placed metastatic breast cancer cells from a fifty-four-year-old woman in an invasion chamber all by themselves, relatively few were able to breach the barrier. But within seventy-two hours of adding PhIP to the chamber, the cancer cells became more invasive, crawling through the membrane at an accelerated rate.[72]

PhIP in meat may therefore represent a three-strikes-you're-out type of carcinogen, potentially involved in every stage of breast cancer development. Staying away from the stuff isn't easy, though, eating the standard American diet. As the researchers note: "Exposure to PhIP is difficult to avoid because of its presence in many commonly consumed cooked meats, particularly chicken, beef and fish."[73]

Cholesterol

Remember earlier when we discussed the American Institute for Cancer Research? A study found that following its guidelines for cancer prevention appeared to reduce not just breast cancer risk but also heart disease risk.[74] What's more, not only may eating healthier to prevent cancer help to prevent heart disease but eating to prevent heart disease may also help to prevent cancer. One of the reasons? Cholesterol may play a role in the development and progression of breast cancer.[75]

Cancer appears to feed on cholesterol. LDL cholesterol stimulates the growth of breast cancer cells in a petri dish—they just gobble up the so-called bad cholesterol. Tumors may suck up so much cholesterol that cancer patients' cholesterol levels tend to plummet as their cancer grows.[76] This is not a good sign, as patient survival tends to be lowest when cholesterol uptake is highest.[77]

The cancer is thought to be using the cholesterol to make estrogen or to shore up tumor membranes to help the cancer migrate and invade more tissue.[78] In other words, breast tumors may take advantage of high circulating cholesterol levels to fuel and accelerate their own growth.[79] Cancer's hunger for cholesterol is such that pharmaceutical companies have considered using LDL cholesterol as a Trojan horse to deliver antitumor drugs to cancer cells.[80]

Though data have been mixed, the largest study on cholesterol and cancer to date—including more than a million participants—found a 17 percent increased risk in women who had total cholesterol levels over 240 compared with women whose cholesterol was under 160.[81] If lowering cholesterol may help lower breast cancer risk, what about taking cholesterol-lowering statin drugs?

Statins looked promising in petri-dish studies, but population studies comparing breast cancer rates among statin users and nonusers showed inconsistent results. Some suggested statins decreased breast cancer risk, while others showed increased risk. Nearly all these studies were relatively short term, however. Most considered five years to be long-term statin use, but breast cancer can take decades to develop.[82]

The first major study on the breast cancer risk of statin use for ten years or longer was published in 2013. It found that women who had been taking statins for a decade or more had twice the risk of both common types of infiltrating breast cancer: invasive ductal carcinoma and invasive lobular carcinoma.[83] The cholesterol drugs doubled the risk. If confirmed, the public health implications of these findings are immense: Approximately one in four women in the United States over the age of forty-five may be taking these drugs.[84]

The number-one killer of women is heart disease, not breast cancer, so women still need to bring down their cholesterol. You can likely achieve this without drugs by eating a healthy enough plant-based diet. And certain plant foods may be particularly protective.

PREVENTING (AND TREATING) BREAST CANCER BY EATING PLANTS

Not long ago, I received a very moving note from Bettina, a woman who had been following my work on NutritionFacts.org. Bettina had been diagnosed with stage two "triple-negative" breast cancer—the hardest type to treat. She underwent eight months of treatment, including surgery, chemotherapy, and radiation. A breast cancer diagnosis is stressful enough, but the anxiety and depression can be compounded by this type of rigorous cancer regimen.

Bettina, however, used the experience to make positive changes in her life. After watching a number of my videos, she started to eat healthier. She followed many of the recommendations you'll find in this chapter for helping to prevent a recurrence of cancer, such as eating more broccoli and flaxseeds. The good news: Bettina has been cancer-free for more than three years now.

Given all the studies I read through, it's easy for me to forget that the statistics refer to people's lives. Stories like Bettina's help me put faces to all the dry facts and figures. When real people make real changes, they can see real results.

Sadly, even after a breast cancer diagnosis, most women may not make the dietary changes that could help them most, such as consuming less meat and more fruits and vegetables.[85] Maybe they don't realize (or their doctors never told them) that a healthier lifestyle may improve their survival chances. For example, a study of nearly 1,500 women found that remarkably simple behavior changes—such as eating just five or more servings of fruits and veggies per day along with walking for thirty minutes six days a week—were associated with a significant survival advantage. Those who followed these recommendations appeared to have nearly half the risk of dying from their cancer in the two years following diagnosis.[86]

While stories like Bettina's can help make the statistics more inspiring, it all has to come back to the science. Over time, what to eat and feed our families are life-or-death decisions. How else can we decide but based on the best available balance of evidence?

Fiber

Inadequate fiber consumption may also be a risk factor for breast cancer. Researchers at Yale University and elsewhere found that premenopausal women who ate more than about six grams of soluble fiber a day (the equivalent of about a single cup of black beans) had 62 percent lower odds of breast cancer compared with women who consumed less than around four grams a day. Fiber's benefits appeared even more pronounced for estrogen-receptor-negative breast tumors, which are harder to treat: Premenopausal women on a higher fiber diet had 85 percent lower odds of that type of breast cancer.[87]

How did the researchers arrive at these figures? The Yale study was what's called a case-control study. Scientists compared the past diets of women who had breast cancer (the cases) to the past diets of similar women who did not have breast cancer (the controls) to try to tease out if there is something distinctive about the eating habits of women who developed the disease. The researchers found that certain women with breast cancer reported eating significantly less soluble fiber on average than the cancer-free women. Hence, soluble fiber may be protective.

The women in the study weren't getting their fiber from supplements, though; they were getting it from food. But this could mean that eating more fiber is merely evidence that the cancer-free women are eating more plant foods, the only place fiber is found naturally. Therefore, fiber itself might not be the active ingredient. Maybe there's something else protective in plant foods. "On the other hand," noted the researchers, "an increased consumption of fiber from foods of plant origin . . . may reflect a reduced consumption of foods of animal origin. . . ."[88] In other words, maybe it's not what they were eating *more* of but what they were eating *less* of. The reason high fiber intake is associated with less breast cancer may be because of more beans—or less bologna.

Either way, an analysis of a dozen other breast cancer case-control studies reported similar findings, with lower breast cancer risk associated with indicators of fruit and vegetable intake, such as vitamin C intake, and higher breast cancer risk associated with higher saturated-fat intake (an indicator of meat, dairy, and processed food intake). And according to these studies, the more whole plant foods you eat, the better it is for your health: Every twenty grams of fiber intake per day was associated with a 15 percent lower risk of breast cancer. [89]

One problem with case-control studies, though, is that they rely on people's memory of what they've been eating, potentially introducing what's known as "recall bias." For example, if people with cancer are more likely to selectively remember more of the unhealthy things they ate, this skewed recall could artificially inflate the correlation between eating certain foods and cancer. Prospective cohort studies avoid this problem by following a group (cohort) of healthy women and their diets forward (prospectively) in time to see who gets cancer and who doesn't. A compilation of ten such prospective cohort studies on breast cancer and fiber intake came up with similar results to the dozen case-control studies mentioned above, a 14 percent lower risk of breast cancer for every twenty grams of fiber intake per day.[90] The relationship between more fiber and less breast cancer may not be a straight line, though. Breast cancer risk may not significantly fall until at least twenty-five grams of fiber a day is reached.[91]

Unfortunately, the average American woman appears to eat less than fifteen grams of fiber per day—only about half the *minimum* daily recommendation.[92] Even the average vegetarian in the United States may only get about twenty grams daily.[93] Healthier vegetarians, though, may average thirty-seven grams a day, and vegans forty-six grams daily.[94] Meanwhile, the *whole*-food, plant-based diets used therapeutically to reverse chronic disease contain upward of sixty grams of fiber.[95]

Peeling Back Breast Cancer

"Does an Apple a Day Keep the Oncologist Away?" This was the title of a study published in the *Annals of Oncology* that set out to determine if eating an apple (or more) a day was associated with lower cancer risk. The results: Compared with people who average less than one apple a day, daily apple eaters had 24 percent lower odds of breast cancer, as well as significantly lower risks for ovarian cancer, laryngeal cancer, and colorectal cancer. The protective associations persisted even after considering these subjects' intake of vegetables and other fruits, suggesting daily apple consumption was more than just an indicator of eating a healthier diet.[96]

The cancer protection apples appear to offer is assumed to arise from their antioxidant properties. Apple antioxidants are concentrated in the peel, which makes sense: The skin is the fruit's first line of defense against the outside world. Expose the inner flesh, and it starts to brown (oxidize) within moments. The antioxidant power of the peel may be between two times (Golden Delicious) to six times (Idared) greater than the pulp.[97]

Beyond protecting against the initial free-radical hit to your DNA, apple extract has been shown to suppress the growth of both estrogen-receptor-positive and -negative breast cancer cells in a petri dish.[98] When researchers at my alma mater, Cornell University, separately dripped extracts of peel and flesh from the same apples on cancer cells, the peel stopped cancer growth ten times more effectively.[99]

Researchers found something in the peels of organic apples (presumably present in conventional ones as well) that appears to reactivate a tumor-suppressor gene called maspin (an acronym for mammary serine protease inhibitor). Maspin is one of the tools your body appears to use to keep breast cancer at bay. Breast cancer cells find a way to turn off this gene, but apple peels appear to be able to turn it back on. The researchers concluded that "apple peels should not be discarded from the diet."[100]

Preventing Breast Cancer by Any Greens Necessary

Earlier, I discussed the 2007 study of Long Island women that linked breast cancer risk to the heterocyclic amines formed in meat. Older women consuming the most grilled, barbecued, or smoked meat over their lifetimes were found to have 47 percent increased odds of breast cancer. Those with high meat intake who *also* had low fruit and vegetable intake had 74 percent higher odds.[101]

Low fruit and vegetable intake may just be a sign of unhealthy habits overall, but increasing evidence suggests that there may be something in produce that is actively protective against breast cancer. For example, cruciferous vegetables like broccoli boost the activity of detoxifying enzymes in your liver. Research has shown that if you feed people broccoli and brussels sprouts, they clear caffeine more quickly—meaning that if you eat a lot of cruciferous vegetables, you'd have to drink more coffee to get the same buzz because your liver (the body's purifier) has become so revved up.[102] Might this process work for those cooked meat carcinogens as well?

To find out, researchers fed a group of nonsmokers pan-fried meat. They then measured the levels of heterocyclic amines circulating in their bodies by sampling their urine. For two weeks, the study subjects added about three cups of broccoli and brussels sprouts to their daily diets and then ate the same meat meal. Though they consumed the same quantity of carcinogens, significantly less came out in their urine, consistent with the subjects' broccoli-boosted liver detox ability.[103]

What happened next was unexpected. The subjects stopped eating their veggies and, two weeks later, tried eating the meat meal again. Presumably, their ability to detox carcinogens would by then have reverted back down to baseline. But instead, the subjects' liver function remained enhanced even weeks later.[104] This finding suggests that not only might a heaping side of broccoli with your steak decrease carcinogen exposure but also that eating your veggies days or even weeks before the big barbecue may help shore up your defenses. Choosing the veggie burger may be the safest choice, though, as it may have no heterocyclic amines to detoxify.[105]

So are women who eat a lot of green vegetables less likely to get breast cancer? A study of fifty thousand African American women (a sadly neglected demographic in medical research, but a population group who tends to regularly eat more greens) found that those who ate two or more servings of vegetables a day had a significantly decreased risk of a kind of breast cancer that's hard to treat, estrogen- and progesterone-receptor-negative.[106] Broccoli appeared especially protective among premenopausal women, but collard green consumption was associated with less breast cancer risk at all ages.[107]

Breast Cancer Stem Cells

What if you're already fighting breast cancer or are in remission? Green vegetables may still be protective. Over the past decade, scientists have been developing a new theory of cancer biology based on the role of stem cells. Stem cells are essentially the body's raw materials—the "parents" from which all other cells with specialized functions are generated. As a result, stem cells are a critical component of the body's repair system, including regrowing skin, bone, and muscle. Breast tissue naturally has many stem cells in reserve, which are used during pregnancy to create new milk glands.[108] However, as miraculous as stem cells are, their immortality can also work against us. Instead of rebuilding organs, if they turn cancerous, they can build tumors.[109]

Cancerous stem cells may be why breast cancer can return, even up to twenty-five years after being fought off successfully the first time.[110] When people are told that they are cancer-free, it may mean their tumors are gone, but if their stem cells are cancerous, the tumors still might reappear many years later. Sadly, someone who has been cancer-free for ten years might consider herself cured but actually may just be in remission. Smoldering cancerous stem cells may be just waiting to reignite.

The current battery of sophisticated chemo drugs and radiation regimens is based on animal models. Success of a given treatment is often measured by its ability to shrink tumors in rodents—but rats in laboratories only live for about two or three years in any case. Doctors may be shrinking tumors, but mutated stem cells may still be lurking, able to slowly rebuild new tumors over the ensuing years.[111]

What we need to do is strike at the root of cancer. We need to devise treatments aimed not just at reducing tumor bulk but at targeting what has been called the "beating heart of the tumor":[112] cancer stem cells.

That's where broccoli may come in.

Sulforaphane, a dietary component of cruciferous vegetables like broccoli, has been shown to suppress the ability of breast cancer stem cells to form tumors.[113] This means that if you're currently in remission, eating lots of broccoli could theoretically help keep your cancer from returning. (I say theoretically because those results were from a petri dish.)

To be useful as a cancer fighter, sulforaphane would have to first be absorbed into your bloodstream when you eat broccoli. Then it would have to build up to the same concentration in breast tissue found to counter cancer stem cells in the lab. Is that possible? An innovative group at Johns Hopkins University sought to find out. The researchers asked women scheduled for breast reduction surgery to drink broccoli-sprout juice an hour before their procedure. Sure enough, after dissecting their breast tissue postsurgery, the researchers found evidence of significant sulforaphane buildup.[114] In other words, we now know that the cancer-fighting nutrients in broccoli do find their way to the right place when we swallow them.

To reach the concentration of sulforaphane in the breast found to suppress breast cancer stem cells, however, you would have to eat at least a quarter-cup of broccoli sprouts a day.[115] You can buy broccoli sprouts in the produce aisle, but they are cheap and easy to grow at home. They have a bit of a radishy bite to them, so I like to mix them into a salad to dilute their intensity.

There have yet to be randomized clinical trials to see if breast cancer survivors who eat broccoli live longer than those who don't, but with no downside and only positive side effects, eating broccoli and other cruciferous vegetables is something I would recommend for everyone.

Flaxseeds

Flaxseeds are one of the first items ever considered to be health foods, treasured for their purported healing properties since at least the times of ancient Greece, when the renowned physician Hippocrates wrote about using them to treat patients.[116]

Better known as one of the richest plant sources of essential omega-3 fatty acids, flaxseeds are really set apart by their lignan content. Though lignans are found throughout the plant kingdom, flaxseeds have around one hundred times more lignans than other foods.[117] What are lignans?

Lignans are phytoestrogens that can dampen the effects of the body's own estrogen. This is why flaxseeds are considered a first-line medical therapy for menstrual breast pain.[118] In terms of breast cancer risk, eating about a daily tablespoonful of ground flaxseeds can extend a woman's menstrual cycle by about a day.[119] This means she'll have fewer periods over the course of a lifetime and, therefore, presumably less estrogen exposure and reduced breast cancer risk.[120] Just as broccoli doesn't technically contain sulforaphane (only the precursors that turn into sulforaphane when chewed—see page 305), flaxseeds don't contain lignans, only lignan precursors, which need to be activated. This task is performed by the good bacteria in your gut.

The gut bacteria's role may help explain why women with frequent urinary tract infections may be at a higher risk of breast cancer: Every course of antibiotics you take can kill bacteria indiscriminately, meaning it may stymie the ability of the good bacteria in your gut to take full advantage of the lignans in your diet.[121] (Yet another reason you should take antibiotics only when necessary.)

Lignan intake is associated with significantly reduced breast cancer risk in postmenopausal women.[122] This effect is presumed to be due to lignans' further estrogen-dampening effects. But since lignans are found in healthy foods like berries, whole grains, and dark, leafy greens, could they just be an indicator of a healthy diet?

In a petri dish, lignans do directly suppress the proliferation of breast cancer cells.[123] But the strongest evidence to date that there really is something special about this class of phytonutrients comes from interventional trials, starting with a 2010 study funded by the National Cancer Institute. Researchers took about forty-five women at high risk of breast cancer—meaning they had suspicious breast biopsies or had previously suffered from breast cancer—and gave them the equivalent of about two teaspoons of ground flaxseeds every day. Needle biopsies of breast tissue were taken before and after the yearlong study. The results: On average, the women had fewer precancerous changes in their breasts after the year of flax lignans than before they started. Eighty percent (thirty-six of forty-five) had a drop in their levels of Ki-67, a biomarker (indicator) of increased cell proliferation. This finding suggests that sprinkling a few spoonfuls of ground flaxseeds on your oatmeal or whatever you're eating throughout the day may reduce the risk of breast cancer.[124]

What about women who already have breast cancer? Breast cancer survivors who have higher levels of lignans in their bloodstreams[125,126] and diets[127] appear to survive significantly longer. This outcome may be due to the fact that women who eat flaxseeds may also see a rise in the levels of endostatin in their breasts.[128] (Endostatin is a protein produced by your body to help starve tumors of their blood supply.)

The evidence from studies like these appeared so compelling that scientists performed a randomized, double-blind, placebo-controlled clinical trial of flaxseeds for breast cancer patients—one of the few times a food has ever been so rigorously put to the test. Researchers located women with breast cancer scheduled for surgery and divided them randomly into two groups: Every day, group one ate a muffin containing flaxseed, while group two ate a muffin that looked and tasted the same, but had no flaxseed in it. Biopsies of the tumors in the flax and no-flax groups were taken at the beginning of the study and then compared with the pathology of the tumor removed during surgery about five weeks later.

Was there any difference? Compared with the women who ate the placebo muffins, women consuming the muffins with flaxseed, on average, witnessed their tumor-cell proliferation decrease, cancer-cell death rates increase, and their c-erB2 scores go down. C-erB2 is a marker of cancer aggressiveness; the higher your score, the higher the potential for breast cancer to metastasize and spread throughout the body. In other words, the flaxseeds appeared to make the subjects' cancer less aggressive. The researchers concluded, "Dietary flaxseed has the potential to reduce tumor growth in patients with breast cancer. . . . [F]laxseed, which is inexpensive and readily available, may be a potential dietary alternative or adjunct to currently used breast cancer drugs."[129]

Soy and Breast Cancer

Soybeans naturally contain another class of phytoestrogens called isoflavones. People hear the word "estrogen" in the word "phytoestrogens" and assume that means soy has estrogen-like effects. Not necessarily. Phytoestrogens dock into the same receptors as your own estrogen but have a weaker effect, so they can act to block the effects of your more powerful animal estrogen.

There are two types of estrogen receptors in the body, alpha and beta. Your own estrogen prefers alpha receptors, while plant estrogens (phytoestrogens) have an affinity for the beta receptors.[130] The effects of soy phytoestrogens on different tissues therefore depend on the ratio of alpha to beta receptors.[131]

Estrogen has positive effects in some tissues and potentially negative effects in others. For example, high levels of estrogen can be good for the bones but can increase the likelihood of developing breast cancer. Ideally, you'd like what's called a "selective estrogen receptor modulator" in your body that would have proestrogenic effects in some tissues and antiestrogenic effects in others.

Well, that's what soy phytoestrogens appear to be.[132] Soy seems to lower breast cancer risk,[133] an antiestrogenic effect, but can also help reduce menopausal hot-flash symptoms,[134] a proestrogenic effect. So, by eating soy, you may be able to enjoy the best of both worlds.

What about soy for women *with* breast cancer? There have been five studies on breast cancer survivors and soy consumption. Overall, researchers have found that women diagnosed with breast cancer who ate the most soy lived significantly longer and had a significantly lower risk of breast cancer recurrence than those who ate less.[135] The quantity of phytoestrogens found in just a single cup of soy milk[136] may reduce the risk of breast cancer returning by 25 percent.[137] The improvement in survival for those eating more soy foods was found both in women whose tumors were responsive to estrogen (estrogen-receptor-positive breast cancer) and those whose tumors were not (estrogen-receptor-negative breast cancer). This also held true for both young women and older women.[138] In one study, for example, 90 percent of the breast cancer patients who ate the most soy phytoestrogens after diagnosis were still alive five years later, while half of those who ate little to no soy were dead.[139]

One way soy may decrease cancer risk and improve survival is by helping to reactivate BRCA genes.[140] BRCA1 and BRCA2 are so-called caretaker genes, cancer-suppressing genes responsible for DNA repair. Mutations in this gene can cause a rare form of hereditary breast cancer. As has been well publicized, Angelina Jolie decided to undergo a preventive double mastectomy. A National Breast Cancer Coalition survey found that the majority of women believe that most breast cancers occur among women with a family history or a genetic predisposition to the disease.[141] The reality is that as few as 2.5 percent of breast cancer cases are attributable to breast cancer running in the family.[142]

If the vast majority of breast cancer patients have fully functional BRCA genes, meaning that their DNA-repair mechanisms are intact, how did their breast cancer form, grow, and spread? Breast tumors appear able to suppress the expression of the gene through a process called methylation. While the gene itself is operational, the cancer has effectively turned it off or at least turned down its expression, potentially aiding the metastatic spread of a tumor.[143] That's where soy may come in.

The isoflavones in soy appear to help turn BRCA protection back on, removing the methyl straitjacket the tumor tried to place on it.[144] The dose breast cancer researchers used to achieve this result in vitro was pretty hefty, though—the equivalent to eating about a cup of soybeans.

Soy may also help women with variations of other breast cancer susceptibility genes known as MDM2 and CYP1B1. Women at increased genetic risk of breast cancer may therefore especially benefit from high soy intake.[145] The bottom line is that no matter which genes you inherit, changes in your diet may be able to affect DNA expression at a genetic level, potentially boosting your ability to fight disease.

Why Do Women in Asia Have Less Breast Cancer?

Though breast cancer is the most common cancer specific to women globally, Asian women are up to five times less likely to develop breast cancer than North American women.[146] Why?

One possibility is their intake of green tea, a common staple in many Asian diets. Green tea has been associated with about a 30 percent reduction in breast cancer risk.[147] Another strong possibility is a relatively high intake of soy, which, if consumed consistently during childhood, may cut the risk of breast cancer later in life by half. If women consume soy primarily as an adult, though, their risk reduction may only be closer to 25 percent.[148]

While intake of green tea and soy might account for a twofold reduction in Asian women's breast cancer risk, it doesn't fully account for the disparity between Eastern and Western breast cancer rates.

Asian populations also eat more mushrooms.[149] As noted in the box on red wine on page 181, white mushrooms have also been shown to block the estrogen synthase enzyme, at least in a petri dish. So researchers decided to investigate if there was a link between mushroom intake and breast cancer. They compared the mushroom consumption of one thousand breast cancer patients to one thousand healthy subjects of similar age, weight, and smoking and exercise status. The women whose mushroom consumption averaged just about one-half a mushroom or more per day had 64 percent lower odds of breast cancer compared with women who didn't eat mushrooms at all. Eating mushrooms *and* sipping at least half a tea bag's worth of green tea each day was associated with nearly *90 percent* lower breast cancer odds.[150]

Oncologists, doctors who treat cancer, can take pride in the strides they've made. Thanks to improvements in cancer treatment, cancer patients are living longer and healthier as has been celebrated in oncology journal editorials with such titles as "Cancer Survivors, 10 Million Strong and Growing!" Yes, more than 10 million cancer patients are still alive today, with "perhaps as many as 1 million new individuals in the United States joining those ranks each year."[151] That is an accomplishment, but wouldn't it be even better to prevent those million cases in the first place?

In medicine, a cancer diagnosis is considered a "teachable moment" when we can motivate a patient to improve his or her lifestyle.[152] By then, though, it may already be too late.

CHAPTER 12

How Not to Die from Suicidal Depression

Healthy food can have a powerful effect on mood. But don't take only my word for it. Take Margaret's too. After hearing me speak at her church, she sent me this e-mail:

Dear Dr. Greger,

I was diagnosed with clinical depression by a psychiatrist when I was ten years old. I spent all my teenage years and twenties on a cocktail of medications for depression. Even on medications, I was still haunted by intrusive thoughts of suicide on a daily basis. Worse yet, the medications gave me headaches, nausea, and vivid, often frightening, dreams. I was sleepy all the time, and despite the scary dreams, I had to nap every day. I slept a *lot*—a couple of hours midday and then close to ten hours every night. Even with these side effects, I was afraid not to take these medications because I really wanted to live, and I was scared that without meds I might get so depressed I would kill myself.

Eventually I got married . . . and divorced. Was hospitalized several times during my marriage for depression. To be honest, I just never had any sex drive, and my husband took it personally. I guess I'll never know if my missing libido was just a side effect of all the medications I was on or the depression itself.

About nine years ago, I heard you speak at my church. I realized I had just spent the last two decades in a medication-induced haze. And without ever really feeling good a single one of those days. I talked to my psychiatrist about how I wanted to completely overhaul my diet and try to back off the medications under her supervision. Much to my surprise, she was supportive. Well, I've been whole food and plant based for nine years and haven't had a further relapse. Not that I haven't been sad from time to time but I haven't had any more thoughts of suicide or any more hospitalizations. I sleep like a normal person now! Everyone tells me I am a different person since I changed my diet. I just wanted to thank you. My fiancé would like to thank you too! I owe you my life!

How can you prevent death by suicide? For those unfamiliar with the ravages of mental illness, the flippant answer is: Just don't do it. In fact, death from other leading killers, such as heart disease, type 2 diabetes, and hypertension, may be just as much a choice as death from suicide, since psychiatric disorders can cloud your judgment. Nearly forty thousand Americans take their own lives each year,[1] and depression appears to be a leading cause.[2] Thankfully, lifestyle interventions can help repair your mind as well as your body.

In 1946, the World Health Organization defined health as "a state of complete physical, mental and social well-being and not merely the absence of disease or infirmity."[3] In other words, you can be in excellent physical shape—enjoying low cholesterol, a healthy body weight, and good overall physical fitness—but that doesn't necessarily mean you're healthy. Mental health can be just as important as physical health.

Major depression is one of the most commonly diagnosed mental illnesses. An estimated 7 percent of American adults suffer from serious depression—that's about sixteen million people who have at least one depressive episode each year.[4] Now, everyone feels sad occasionally. A full range of emotions is part of what makes us human. Depression, however, is not just sadness. It is characterized by weeks of such symptoms as low or sad mood, diminished interest in activities that used to be pleasurable, weight gain or loss, fatigue, inappropriate guilt, difficulty concentrating, and recurrent thoughts of death.

Indeed, major depression can be a life-threatening ailment.

Good mental health isn't "merely the absence of disease," though. Just because you're not depressed doesn't necessarily mean you're happy. There are twenty times more studies published on health and depression than there are on health and happiness.[5] In recent years, however, the field of "positive psychology" has emerged, focusing on the relationship between optimal mental and physical health.

Growing evidence indicates that positive psychological well-being is associated with reduced risk of physical illness, but which came first? Are people healthier because they're happy, or are people just happier because they're healthy?

Prospective studies that follow individuals over time have found that people starting out happier do indeed end up healthier. An analysis of seventy such studies on mortality concluded that "positive psychological well-being has a favorable effect on survival in both healthy and diseased populations."[6] Those who are happier appear to live longer.

Not so fast, though. While positive mental states may be associated with less stress and more resilience to infection, positive well-being might also be accompanied by a healthy lifestyle. In general, people who feel satisfied appear to smoke less, exercise more, and eat healthier.[7] So is being happier just a marker of good health and not a cause of it? To find out, researchers set out to make people sick.

Scientists at Carnegie Mellon University took hundreds of individuals—some happy, some unhappy—and paid them $800 each to be allowed to drip the common cold virus into their noses. Even if someone with a cold sneezes right into your face and the virus gets into your nose, you won't get sick automatically, because your immune system may be able to fight it off. So the study question was: Whose immune system would be better at fighting off a common virus—those in the group initially rated as happy, peppy, and relaxed, or those in the group who were anxious, hostile, and depressed?

About one in three of the negative-emotion individuals failed to successfully fight off the virus and came down with a cold. But only one in five of the happy individuals became sick, even after the researchers took into account such factors as subjects' sleep patterns, exercise habits, and stress levels.[8] In a subsequent study, the researchers even exposed subjects (who had also been paid) to the influenza virus, a more serious infection. Once again, increased positive emotions were associated with decreased verified illness rates.[9] Happier people, it seems, are less likely to get sick.

So mental health does appear to play a part in physical health. That's why it's crucial that the food you eat support both your mind and your body. As you'll see, common foods from leafy green vegetables to your basic garden-variety tomato may positively affect your brain chemistry and help ward off depression. In fact, even simply *smelling* a common spice may improve your emotional state.

But avoiding the blues is not just about eating your greens. There are also components in certain foods that may increase the risk of depression, such as arachidonic acid, an inflammation-promoting compound found mostly in chicken and eggs in the diet that is blamed for potentially impairing mood by inflaming the brain.

Arachidonic Acid

Studies on the emotional health and mood states of those eating plant-based diets suggest that eating less meat isn't just good for us physically; it's good for us emotionally too. Researchers employed two psychological tests, the Profile of Mood States (POMS) and the Depression and Anxiety Stress Scale (DASS). POMS measures levels of depression, anger, hostility, fatigue, and confusion. The DASS gauges other negative mood states as well, including hopelessness, lack of interest, anhedonia (lack of pleasure), agitation, irritability, and impatience with other people. Subjects eating plant-based diets appeared to experience significantly fewer negative emotions than omnivores. Those eating better also reported feeling more "vigor."[10]

The researchers offered two explanations for their findings. First, people eating better diets may be happier because they're healthier.[11] Those eating plant-based diets don't just have lower rates of many of the leading killer diseases but also appear to have lower rates of such annoying ills as hemorrhoids, varicose veins, and ulcers; fewer surgeries; fewer hospitalizations; and only about half the odds of being on drugs, including tranquilizers, aspirin, insulin, blood pressure pills, pain medications, antacids, laxatives, or sleeping pills.[12] (Being able to avoid doctor visits and health insurance hassles would make anyone less irritable, stressed, and depressed!)

The researchers also suggested a more direct explanation for their results: Maybe the proinflammatory compound arachidonic acid found in animal products can "adversely impact mental health via a cascade of neuroinflammation."[13] The body metabolizes arachidonic acid into an array of inflammatory chemicals. In fact, that's how anti-inflammatory drugs like aspirin and ibuprofen work to relieve pain and swelling—by blocking the conversion of arachidonic acid into these inflammatory end products. Maybe the mental health of omnivores was being comparatively compromised by inflammation in their brains.

Inflammation isn't always bad, of course. When the area around a splinter gets all red, hot, and swollen, it's a sign that the body is using arachidonic acid to mount an inflammatory response to help fight off infection. But your body already makes all the arachidonic acid you need, so you don't need to take in any more via your diet.[14] In this way, arachidonic acid resembles cholesterol, another essential component that the body makes all on its own: When you add excess amounts through diet, it may upset your system's internal balance.[15] In this particular case, the researchers suspected arachidonic acid intake might impair the body's emotional state. There are data suggesting that people with higher levels of arachidonic acid in their blood may end up at significantly higher risk of suicide and episodes of major depression.[16]

The top-five sources of arachidonic acid in the American diet are chicken, eggs, beef, pork, and fish, although chicken and eggs alone contribute more than the other top sources combined.[17] Just a single egg's worth of arachidonic acid a day may significantly raise arachidonic acid levels in the blood.[18] Overall, omnivores appear to consume about nine times more arachidonic acid than those eating plant-based diets.[19]

The study showing improved moods and emotional states in those eating plant-based diets was a cross-sectional study, meaning it was a snapshot in time. What if people who start out mentally healthier go on to eat healthier, too, and not the other way around? To show cause and effect, researchers would have to perform an interventional study, the gold standard of nutritional science: Gather subjects, change their diets, and see what happens. The same research team did just that. They took men and women who ate meat at least once a day and took away their eggs and chicken, along with other meats, to see what would happen to their moods. Within just two weeks, the study subjects experienced a significant improvement in measures of their mood states.[20] The researchers concluded: "Perhaps eating less meat can help protect mood in omnivores, particularly important in those susceptible to affective disorders [such as depression]."[21]

Given these results, another research team decided to put a healthy diet to the test in a workplace setting, where healthy bodies and minds could potentially translate into improved productivity—and elevate the mood of shareholders as well. A group of overweight and diabetic employees at a major insurance company was encouraged to follow a whole-food, plant-based diet, cutting out all meat, eggs, dairy, oil, and junk foods. There was no portion-size restriction, no calorie counting, and no carb tracking, and participants were explicitly told not to change their exercise habits. Meals were not provided, but the company cafeteria did start offering such daily options as bean burritos and lentil and minestrone soups. A control group of employees received no dietary advice.[22]

Despite the dietary restrictions, over the course of about five months, the plant-eating group reported greater diet satisfaction than the control group. How well did they do? The plant-based group experienced improved digestion, increased energy, and better sleep, as well as significant improvement in their physical functioning, general health, vitality, and mental health. No surprise, then, that they showed measurable improvements in work productivity too.[23]

Based on this success, a much larger study of plant-based nutrition was conducted at ten corporate locations across the country from San Diego, California, to Macon, Georgia. The same resounding success was reported, showing improvements not only in subjects' body weight, blood sugar levels, and ability to control cholesterol[24] but also in their emotional states, including depression, anxiety, fatigue, sense of well-being, and daily functioning.[25]

Fighting the Blues with Greens

Here's a statistic you probably haven't heard: Higher consumption of vegetables may cut the odds of developing depression by as much as 62 percent.[26] A review in the journal *Nutritional Neuroscience* concluded that, in general, eating lots of fruits and veggies may present "a non-invasive, natural, and inexpensive therapeutic means to support a healthy brain."[27]

But how, exactly?

The traditional explanation of how depression works, known as the monoamine theory, proposes that the condition arises out of a chemical imbalance in the brain. The billions of nerves in your brain communicate with each other using chemicals called neurotransmitters. Your nerve cells don't physically touch one another. Instead, they manufacture and deploy neurotransmitters to bridge the gap between them. The levels of an important class of neurotransmitters called monoamines, which includes serotonin and dopamine, are controlled by an enzyme called monoamine oxidase (known as MAO) that breaks down any excess monoamines. People who are depressed appear to have elevated levels of this enzyme in their brains.[28] Thus, the theory goes, depression is caused by abnormally low levels of monoamine neurotransmitters due to elevated levels of the neurotransmitter-munching enzyme.

Antidepressant medications were developed to try to boost the levels of neurotransmitters to offset their accelerated breakdown. But if the excess MAO is responsible for depression, why not just develop a drug that blocks this enzyme? Such drugs do exist, but they have serious risks—not the least of which is the dreaded "cheese effect," in which eating certain foods (such as certain cheeses, cured meats, and fermented foods) while on the drug can potentially cause fatal brain hemorrhaging.[29]

If only there were a way to tamp down the monoamine oxidase enzyme safely. Well, it turns out that many plant foods, including apples, berries, grapes, onions, and green tea, contain phytonutrients that appear to naturally inhibit the MAO, as do such spices as cloves, oregano, cinnamon, and nutmeg.[30] This may help explain why those eating plant-rich diets have lower rates of depression.[31]

Even on a day-to-day basis, studies have shown that the more fruits and vegetables you eat, the happier, calmer, and more energetic you may feel that day—and this positivity can spill over into the next day. For your diet to have a meaningful psychological impact, though, you may need to consume approximately seven servings of fruits or eight servings of vegetables each day.[32]

Seeds and Serotonin

Although some plant foods contain significant amounts of serotonin,[33] the so-called happiness hormone, serotonin can't cross the blood-brain barrier. This means that dietary sources of serotonin can't make it into the brain, but the building block of serotonin, an amino acid called tryptophan, can get from your mouth to your blood to your brain. Tryptophan depletion experiments in the 1970s showed that people given specially concocted tryptophan-deficient diets suffered from irritability, anger, and depression.[34] So if you give people extra tryptophan, will they feel better?

That's the theory. However, in the 1980s, certain tryptophan supplements created a debacle, causing a rash of deaths.[35] But if tryptophan is an amino acid and if proteins are made out of amino acids, why can't you just give people high-protein meals to boost their serotonin levels by delivering extra tryptophan to the brain? It's been tried, and it's failed,[36] likely because other amino acids in protein-rich foods crowd out the tryptophan for access to the brain. However, carbohydrate ingestion does the opposite: It helps shunt many nontryptophan amino acids out from the bloodstream and into the muscles, allowing tryptophan greater access into the brain. For example, having a carb-rich breakfast like waffles and orange juice resulted in higher tryptophan levels in those studied than did a protein-rich breakfast of turkey, eggs, and cheese.[37]

This principle may explain why women suffering from premenstrual syndrome (PMS) sometimes crave carbohydrate-rich food. Consumption of even a single carb-rich, protein-poor meal has been shown to improve depression, tension, anger, confusion, sadness, fatigue, alertness, and calmness scores among women with PMS.[38] In a yearlong study, about one hundred men and women were randomly assigned to eat either a low-carb or high-carb diet. By the end of the year, the subjects eating the high-carb diets experienced significantly less depression, hostility, and mood disturbance than those in the low-carb group. This result is consistent with studies finding better moods and less anxiety among populations eating diets higher in carbohydrates and lower in fats and protein.[39]

Carbohydrates may facilitate tryptophan transport into the brain, but you would still need a dietary source. Ideally, it would have a high tryptophan-to-protein ratio to facilitate brain access.[40] Such seeds as sesame, sunflower, or pumpkin may fit the bill. Indeed, a double-blind, placebo-controlled trial of butternut squash seeds for social anxiety disorder reported a significant improvement in an objective measurement in anxiety within an hour of consumption.[41] All of these factors may contribute to the comprehensive improvement in mood one may achieve after just a few weeks on a plant-based diet.[42]

Saffron

The earliest recorded medical use of a spice appears to be more than 3,600 years ago, when saffron was evidently first used for healing.[43] A few thousand years later, scientists finally put saffron to the test in a head-to-head trial against the antidepressant drug Prozac for the treatment of clinical depression. Both the spice and the drug worked equally well in reducing depression symptoms.[44] As you can see in the box on pages 209–10, this may not be saying much, but at the very least, the saffron was safer in terms of side effects. For example, 20 percent of people in the Prozac group suffered sexual dysfunction, a common occurrence with many antidepressant medications, whereas no one in the saffron group did.

However, saffron may be one of those rare cases in which the natural remedy is more expensive than the drug. Saffron is the world's most expensive spice. It is harvested from crocus flowers, specifically the dried stigmas (the thread-like tips inside the flower), which are ground up to make the spice. You need more than fifty thousand crocuses—enough to cover a football field—to produce just a single pound of saffron.[45]

A Prozac-equivalent dose of saffron may cost more than twice as much as the drug, but a subsequent study found that even just smelling saffron appeared to have psychological benefits. Though researchers diluted the spice so much that the study subjects couldn't detect its odor, they still noted a significant drop in stress hormones measured in women who sniffed the saffron for twenty minutes compared with those who spent twenty minutes smelling a placebo, along with significant improvement in the women's symptoms of anxiety.[46]

So if you're feeling anxious, perhaps wake up and smell the saffron.

Coffee and Aspartame

Speaking of waking up to pleasant aromas, a cup of coffee may be doing more for the brain than making it feel less groggy in the morning. Researchers from Harvard University looked at data from three large-scale cohort studies of more than two hundred thousand American men and women. They found that people who drank two or more cups of coffee daily appeared to have about only half the suicide risk compared to non-coffee drinkers.[47] What about drinking more than four cups a day? A Kaiser Permanente study of more than one hundred thousand people found that suicide risk seemed to continue to drop with increases in coffee dose. People who drank more than six cups a day were 80 percent less likely to commit suicide,[48] though drinking *eight* or more cups a day has been associated with increased suicide risk.[49]

What you put in your coffee may also make a difference. The NIH-AARP study, which followed hundreds of thousands of Americans for a decade, found that frequent consumption of sweetened beverages may increase the risk of depression among older adults. Indeed, adding sugar to coffee may negate many of its positive effects on mood, and adding the artificial sweetener aspartame (found in Equal and NutraSweet) or saccharine (in Sweet'n Low) was associated with an increased risk of depression.[50]

The controversy surrounding the neurological effects of aspartame began in the 1980s.[51] At first, concern was limited to those with preexisting mental illness. An early study at Case Western Reserve University was halted prematurely for safety reasons because subjects with a history of depression appeared to be experiencing such severe reactions to the sweetener. The researchers concluded that "individuals with mood disorders are particularly sensitive to this artificial sweetener and its use in this population should be discouraged."[52]

Only recently were the neurobehavioral effects of aspartame investigated in a population free from mental illness. Healthy individuals were split into two groups—half were given a higher dose of aspartame (the equivalent of about three liters of Diet Coke's worth) and the other half received a lower dose (a single liter of Diet Coke's worth). Then the groups switched.[53] Bear in mind that the higher-aspartame diet contained just half the acceptable daily intake of the stuff, as determined by the U.S. Food and Drug Administration.[54] After only eight days on the higher-aspartame dose, participants exhibited more depression and irritability and performed worse on certain brain function tests.[55] So not only may aspartame cause adverse mental effects in sensitive populations but it may also harm the general public at sufficient doses.

Avoiding diet soda and those pastel paper packets seems easy enough, but artificial sweeteners are also present in more than six thousand products,[56] including breath mints, cereals, chewing gums, jams and jellies, juice drinks, puddings, and even nutritional bars and yogurts.[57] This prevalence has led researchers to assert that aspartame "is impossible to completely eradicate from daily encounters."[58] But, of course, that's only true for people who eat processed foods. This is yet another reason to spend most of your time at the grocery store in the produce aisle. Discriminating shoppers make it a priority to read ingredients lists, but the healthiest foods in the supermarket don't even have them.

Exercise versus Antidepressants

We've known for decades that even a single workout can elevate mood[59] and that physical activity is associated with decreased symptoms of depression. One study of nearly five thousand people across the country, for example, found that people who exercised regularly had 25 percent lower odds of a major depression diagnosis.[60]

Of course, studies like these may not mean that exercise reduces depression. Maybe it means that depression reduces exercise. In other words, if you're depressed, you might feel too lousy to get out of bed and go for a walk. What was needed to test this idea was an interventional study, one in which depressed subjects were split at random (randomized) into two groups, one that exercised and one that didn't.

That's what a team of researchers from Duke University attempted. They randomly assigned depressed men and women aged fifty or older to either begin an aerobic exercise program or take the antidepressant drug sertraline (Zoloft). Within four months, the mood of those in the drug group improved so much that they were, on average, no longer depressed. But the same powerful effect was found in the exercise group—that is, the group of people who weren't taking any drugs. Exercise, it seemed, works about as well as medication.[61]

Let's play devil's advocate for a moment: The drug-free group in the Duke study met three times each week for an exercise class. Could the social stimulation rather than the exercise have improved their mood?

continued

With this question in mind, the same researchers subsequently conducted the largest-ever exercise trial of patients with depression. This time, they added a group, so one group took antidepressants, one group took an exercise class, and a new group did exercises by themselves at home. The results? No matter the setting—whether subjects were alone or in a group—exercise appeared to work about as well as drugs at bringing depression into remission.[62]

So before your doctor writes you a prescription for an antidepressant, ask about prescribing a daily workout instead.

Antioxidants and Folate

Accumulating evidence suggests that free radicals—those highly unstable molecules that cause tissue damage and contribute to aging—may play an important role in the development of various psychiatric disorders, including depression.[63] Modern imaging techniques confirm autopsy studies showing a shrinkage of certain emotion centers in the brains of depressed patients that may be due to death of nerve cells in these areas caused by free radicals.[64]

This phenomenon may help explain why those who eat more fruits and vegetables, which are rich in the antioxidants that extinguish free radicals, appear protected against depression. A study of nearly three hundred thousand Canadians found that greater fruit and vegetable consumption was associated with lower risk of depression, psychological distress, mood and anxiety disorders, and poor perceived mental health. The researchers concluded that eating antioxidant-rich plant foods "may dampen the detrimental effects of oxidative stress on mental health."[65]

The Canadian study relied on questionnaires asking people to self-report fruit and vegetable intake, a method that's not always accurate. A nationwide American study took it one step further and measured the level of carotenoid phytonutrients in people's bloodstreams. These phytonutrients include some of the yellow, orange, and red antioxidant pigments found naturally in some of our healthiest foods, including sweet potatoes and green leafy vegetables. Not only did people with higher levels of these nutrients in their bloodstreams have a lower risk of depression symptoms but there was also an apparent "dose-response relationship," meaning that the higher the level of phytonutrients, the better people seemed to feel.[66]

Among the carotenoids, lycopene (the red pigment in tomatoes) has the highest antioxidant activity. Indeed, a study of nearly one thousand elderly men and women found that people who ate tomatoes or tomato products daily had just half the odds of depression compared with those who ate them once a week or less.[67]

If antioxidants are so helpful, why can't we just pop a few antioxidant pills? Well, only food sources of antioxidants appear to be protectively associated with depression. The same can't be said for dietary supplements.[68] This finding may indicate that the form and delivery of the antioxidants we consume are crucial to ensure their best effects. Alternatively, antioxidants may just be a marker for other components of plant-rich diets, such as folate.

Folate is a B vitamin concentrated in beans and greens. (Its name comes from the Latin word *folium*, meaning "leaf," because it was first isolated in spinach.) Early studies linking depression to low folate levels in the blood were cross-sectional in nature, meaning they were only snapshots in time. For this reason, we didn't know whether low folate intake led to depression or if depression itself led to low folate intake.[69] However, more recent studies following people over time suggest that low dietary folate intake may indeed increase the risk of severe depression by as much as threefold.[70] However, once again, folate *supplements* (folic acid) do not appear to help.[71]

Vegetables—including antioxidant-rich tomatoes and folate-packed greens—may be good for the body and the mind.

Do Antidepressant Drugs Really Work?

We've seen that saffron and exercise compare favorably to drugs in treating depression, but how much is that really saying? Thousands of published studies seem to have demonstrated that antidepressant drugs are effective.[72] The key word here, though, may be *published*. What if drug companies decided to publish only those studies that showed a positive effect but quietly shelved and concealed any studies showing the drugs didn't work? To find out if this was the case, researchers applied to the Food and Drug Administration under the U.S. Freedom of Information Act (FOIA) to get access to the published *and* unpublished studies submitted by pharmaceutical companies. What they found was shocking.

According to the published literature, the results of nearly all antide-

continued

pressant trials were positive. In contrast, FDA analysis of trial data—including the unpublished studies—demonstrated that roughly half of the trials showed the drugs didn't work after all. When all the data—published and unpublished—were combined, antidepressants failed to show a clinically significant advantage over placebo sugar pills.[73] This finding suggests that the placebo effect explains the apparent clinical effectiveness of antidepressants. In other words, improvements in mood may be a result of the patient's *belief* in the power of the drug—not the drug itself.[74]

Even worse, the FOIA documents revealed that the FDA knew that these drugs—such as Paxil and Prozac—didn't work much better than placebo yet made an explicit decision to shield drug companies by keeping this information from the public and prescribing physicians.[75] How could drug companies get away with this? The pharmaceutical industry is considered one of the most profitable and politically powerful industries in the United States, and mental illness is considered a golden goose: chronic, common, and often treated with multiple drugs.[76] Indeed, antidepressants are currently prescribed to more than 8 percent of the population.[77]

Just because antidepressant drugs may not work better than fake pills doesn't mean they don't work at all. Antidepressants offer substantial benefits to millions of people suffering from depression. And although the placebo effect is real and powerful, antidepressants do seem to beat out sugar pills in reducing symptoms in the most severely depressed—perhaps about 10 percent of patients (although admittedly, this statistic also means that about 90 percent of depressed patients may be prescribed medication with negligible benefit).[78]

If doctors are willing to give patients placebo-equivalent treatments, some argue that it would be better for them to just lie to patients and give them actual sugar pills.[79] Unlike the drugs, sugar pills do not cause side effects. For example, antidepressants cause sexual dysfunction in up to three-quarters of users. Other problems may include long-term weight gain and insomnia. And about one in five people have withdrawal symptoms when they try to quit.[80]

Perhaps most tragically, antidepressants may make people more likely to become depressed in the future. Studies show that patients are more likely to become depressed again after treatment with antidepressants than after treatment by other means, including placebos.[81] So even if the mood-boosting benefit of exercise is also a placebo effect, at least it's one with benefits rather than risks.

Just reading the dry statistics in all the studies, it's hard to appreciate the suffering. Seeing a graph in which depression scores drop for even hundreds of people doesn't hit me on the same gut level as seeing a single e-mail in my inbox of someone sharing his or her story of physical and emotional renewal.

Not long ago, a woman wrote to me about her battle with depression. Shay, in her forties, had always stuck to the standard American diet. In recent years, she had been suffering from severe migraines, unbearable constipation, and painful and irregular menstrual cycles. Meanwhile, her depression had become so bad that she was unable to go to work. Then Shay discovered my website and began educating herself about nutrition. Soon she came to understand how the Western diet was potentially contributing to her health problems, not to mention her unhappiness, and she became an ardent watcher of NutritionFacts.org videos.

Shay decided to switch to a whole-food, plant-based diet. She stopped eating animal products and junk and vastly increased her intake of fruits and vegetables. After four weeks, she had more energy and less-painful bowel movements. Within seven months, her bowel movements were effortless, her once-crippling migraines had stopped altogether, her periods were more regular, less painful, and shorter—and her depression was gone. Just months earlier, Shay had felt so bad that she couldn't get out of bed in the morning. But by improving her diet, she is now much healthier, both physically and mentally.

That is a great example of the power of a healthy diet.

CHAPTER 13

How Not to Die from Prostate Cancer

When Tony, a regular reader of NutritionFacts.org, heard that I was writing this book, he asked me to share his story with you in the hopes of helping other men avoid what happened to him. A happily married father, engineer, and self-described fitness nut, he always tried to make good choices out of respect for his body and was lucky to have descended from long-lived, healthy ancestors. Tony was a runner who had always been at a healthy weight. He stayed away from tobacco, alcohol, and drugs. In the 1980s, based on health recommendations from the USDA, he convinced his family to switch from whole milk to skim milk and from beef to fish and chicken—lots and lots of chicken.

Tony was the kind of patient doctors love to take care of—the type who says, "What else can I do to be at my very best?" So no one was more surprised than Tony when, in his early fifties, he was diagnosed with an aggressive prostate cancer. He sought care at a world-renowned medical center and underwent a radical prostatectomy, which successfully removed his cancer but left him with the daily challenge of dealing with the consequences of that surgery—namely, urinary leakage and erectile dysfunction.

He says he wishes he'd known about the conflicts of interest within the USDA (which I elaborated in chapter 5) that have affected the federal agency's ability to make recommendations in the best interests of the public independent of those of the food industry.

Eventually, Tony discovered the body of research you will be reading about in this chapter, and, being a scientist, he immediately understood the evidence that a healthy diet can improve male health. He has eaten a plant-based diet for the last several years, takes flaxseed every day, and has had no recurrence of cancer. As I will discuss, the same diet that may prevent prostate cancer has also been shown to potentially slow it down and even reverse its progression among those already diagnosed. So it is Tony's (and my) wish that this chapter will help you see the importance of healthy eating for a healthy prostate.

The prostate is a walnut-sized gland located between the bladder and base of the penis, just in front of the rectum. It surrounds the urethra, the outlet from the bladder, and secretes the fluid portion of semen. Just as glandular tissue in the breast can become cancerous, so can glandular tissue in the prostate.

Autopsy studies show that about half of men over the age of eighty have prostate cancer.[1] Most men die with prostate cancer without ever knowing they had it. That's the problem with the emphasis on screenings—many prostate cancers that are detected may never have led to harm even if they'd gone undiscovered.[2] Unfortunately, not all men are so lucky. Nearly twenty-eight thousand die each year from prostate cancer.[3]

Milk and Prostate Cancer

Since the U.S. National Dairy Board was first created by the Dairy and Tobacco Adjustment Act of 1983, it has spent more than $1 billion on advertising. By now, we're all familiar with its various slogans, such as "Milk is a natural." But is it? Think about it. Humans are the only species who drink milk after weaning. It also does seem a bit *un*natural to drink the milk of another species.

What about "Milk: It Does a Body Good"? All foods of animal origin contain sex steroid hormones, such as estrogen, but today's genetically "improved" dairy cows are milked throughout their pregnancies when their reproductive hormones are particularly high.[4] These hormones naturally found even in organic cow's milk may play a role in the various associations identified between milk and other dairy products and hormone-related conditions, including acne,[5] diminished male reproductive potential,[6] and premature puberty.[7] The hormone content in milk may explain why women who drink it appear to have five times the rate of twin births compared with women who do not drink milk.[8] When it comes to cancer, though, the greater concern may have to do with growth hormones.[9]

Mother Nature designed cow's milk to put a few hundred pounds on a baby calf within a few months. A lifetime of human exposure to these growth factors in milk may help explain the connections found between dairy consumption and certain cancers.[10] Leading Harvard University nutrition experts have expressed concern that the hormones in dairy products and other growth factors could stimulate the growth of hormone-sensitive tumors.[11] Experimental evidence suggests that dairy could also promote the conversion of precancerous lesions or mutated cells into invasive cancers.[12]

Concerns about milk and other dairy products first arose from population-scale data, such as the twenty-five-fold increase in prostate cancer in Japanese men since World War II, which coincided with a sevenfold increase in egg consumption, a ninefold increase in meat consumption, and a twentyfold increase in dairy consumption.[13] Though the rest of their diets remained comparatively stable and similar trends have been noted in other countries,[14] there were myriad changes in Japanese society beyond eating more animal products that could have contributed to these rising cancer rates. So scientists took a closer look.

To control for as many variables as possible, researchers devised an experiment in which they dripped milk on human prostate cancer cells in a petri dish. The researchers chose organic cow's milk to exclude any effect of added hormones, such as the bovine growth hormone, which is commonly injected into conventionally raised cows so they produce more milk.[15] The researchers found that cow's milk stimulated the growth of human prostate cancer cells in each of fourteen separate experiments, producing an average increase in cancer growth rate of more than 30 percent. In contrast, almond milk *suppressed* the growth of the cancer cells by more than 30 percent.[16]

What happens in a petri dish, though, doesn't necessarily happen in people. Nevertheless, a compilation of case-control studies did conclude that cow's milk consumption is a risk factor for prostate cancer,[17] and the same outcome was found for cohort studies.[18] A 2015 meta-analysis found that high intakes of dairy products—milk, low-fat milk, and cheese, but not nondairy sources of calcium—appear to increase total prostate cancer risk.[19]

But, you may be wondering, if you don't drink milk, what will happen to your bones? Doesn't milk help prevent osteoporosis? It turns out that the promised benefit may be just another empty marketing ploy. A meta-analysis of cow's milk intake and hip fracture studies shows no significant protection.[20] Even if you were to start drinking milk during adolescence in an attempt to bolster peak bone mass, it probably wouldn't reduce your chances of fracture later in life.[21] One recent set of studies involving one hundred thousand men and women followed for up to two decades even suggested milk may *increase* bone and hip fracture rates.[22]

Some babies are born with a rare birth defect called galactosemia, in which they lack the enzymes needed to detoxify galactose, a type of sugar found in milk. This means they end up with elevated levels of galactose in their blood, which can cause bone loss.[23] A group of Swedish researchers figured that even among normal people who can detoxify the stuff, it might not be good for their bones to be drinking all that galactose in milk every day.[24] And galactose may not just hurt bones. Scientists actually use galactose to induce premature aging in lab animals. When researchers slip lab animals some galactose, the "life-shortened animals showed neurodegeneration, mental retardation and cognitive dysfunction . . . diminished immune responses and reduction of reproductive ability."[25] And it doesn't take much, just the human equivalent of one to two glasses worth of milk a day.[26]

However, since humans aren't rodents, researchers investigated the connection between milk intake and mortality, as well as fracture risk in large populations of milk drinkers.[27] In addition to significantly *more* bone and hip fractures, researchers found higher rates of premature death, more heart disease, and significantly more cancer for each daily glass of milk women drank. Three glasses a day was associated with nearly twice the risk of dying early.[28] Men with higher milk consumption also had a higher rate of death, although they didn't have higher fracture rates.[29]

Overall, the study showed a dose-dependent higher rate of mortality (in both men and women) and fracture (in women), but the opposite was found for other dairy products, such as soured milk and yogurt, which would go along with the galactose theory, because the bacteria in these foods can ferment away some of the lactose.[30]

The medical journal editorial accompanying the published study emphasized that, given the rise in milk consumption around the world, the "role of milk in mortality needs to be established definitively now."[31]

Eggs, Choline, and Cancer

More than two million men are currently living with prostate cancer, but living with prostate cancer is better than dying from it. If the cancer is caught while still localized within the prostate, the chances of it killing you within the next five years are practically nil. However, if the cancer spreads far enough, your chances of surviving five years may be as low as one in three.[32] For this reason, scientists have been desperate to identify factors involved in the spread of prostate cancer once it has emerged.

Hoping to identify possible culprits, Harvard University researchers recruited more than one thousand men with early-stage prostate cancer and followed them for several years. Compared with men who rarely ate eggs, men who ate even less than a single egg a day appeared to have twice the risk of prostate cancer progression, such as metastasizing into the bones. The only thing potentially worse for prostate cancer than eggs was poultry: Men with more aggressive cancer who regularly ate chicken and turkey had up to four times the risk of prostate cancer progression.[33]

The researchers suggested that the link between consuming poultry and advancing cancer may be due to cooked-meat carcinogens (such as heterocyclic amines as discussed in chapter 11). For unknown reasons, these carcinogens build up more in the muscles of chickens and turkeys than in those of other animals.[34]

But what cancer-promoting substance is there in eggs? How could eating less than an egg a day double the risk of cancer invasion? The answer may be choline, a compound found concentrated in eggs.[35]

Higher levels of choline in the blood have been associated with increased risk of developing prostate cancer in the first place.[36] This may explain the link between eggs and cancer progression.[37] But what about cancer mortality? In a paper entitled "Choline Intake and Risk of Lethal Prostate Cancer," the same Harvard team found that men who consumed the most choline from food also had an increased risk of cancer death.[38] Men who consume two and a half or more eggs per week—basically an egg every three days—may have an 81 percent increased risk of dying from prostate cancer.[39] The choline in eggs, like the carnitine in red meat, is converted into a toxin called trimethylamine[40] by bacteria that exist in the guts of those who eat meat.[41] And trimethylamine, once oxidized in the liver, appears to increase the risk of heart attack, stroke, and premature death.[42]

Ironically, the presence of choline in eggs is something the egg industry boasts about even though most Americans get more than enough choline.[43] Mind you, the industry executives are aware of the cancer connection. Through the Freedom of Information Act, I was able to get my hands on an e-mail from the executive director of the Egg Nutrition Board directed to another egg industry executive that discussed the Harvard study suggesting that choline is a culprit in promoting cancer progression. "Certainly worth keeping in mind," he wrote, "as we continue to promote choline as another good reason to consume eggs."[44]

Diet Versus Exercise

Nathan Pritikin, the man who helped launch a lifestyle medicine revolution—and saved my grandma's life—wasn't a nutritionist or a dietitian. He wasn't even a doctor. He was an engineer. When he was diagnosed with heart disease in his forties, Pritikin reviewed all the available research himself and decided to try eating the type of diet followed by populations in places like rural Africa, where heart disease was rare. He figured that if he stopped eating a heart-disease-promoting diet, he could stop the advancement of the disease. What he found was even more remarkable. He didn't just stop the disease from getting worse, he reversed his condition.[45] He then went on to help thousands of others do the same.

After vanquishing our number-one killer, heart disease, Dr. Dean Ornish and Pritikin Research Foundation researchers moved on to killer number two: cancer. They developed an elegant series of experiments, placing people on different diets and then dripping their blood on human cancer cells growing in a petri dish. Whose bloodstream would be better at suppressing cancer growth?

The research showed that the blood of people randomized to a plant-based-diet group was dramatically less hospitable to cancer-cell growth than the blood of people in the control group who continued to eat their typical diet. The blood of those eating the standard American diet does fight cancer—if it didn't, many of us would be dead!—but the blood of people eating plant-based diets was shown to fight cancer about eight times better.[46]

The blood of men on the standard American diet slowed down the rate of prostate cancer cell growth by 9 percent. Place men on a plant-based diet for a year, though, and the blood circulating within their bodies can suppress cancer cell growth by 70 percent—that's nearly eight times the stopping power compared to a meat-centered menu.[47] Similar studies have shown that women eating plant-based diets appear to strengthen their bodies' defenses against breast cancer in just fourteen days (as detailed in chapter 11).[48] It's as if we're a totally different person inside after eating and living healthfully for just a couple of weeks.

It should be noted that the strengthening of cancer defenses in all these studies involved eating a plant-based diet *and* exercising. For example, in the breast cancer study, the women were asked to walk thirty to sixty minutes a day. How, then, do we know it was the diet that made their blood more effective at suppressing cancer growth? To tease out the effects of diet and exercise, a UCLA research team compared three groups of men: a plant-based diet-and-exercise group, an exercise-only group, and a control group of sedentary people eating standard fare.[49]

The diet-and-exercise group had been following a plant-based diet for fourteen years, along with participating in moderate exercise, such as a daily walk. The exercise-only group eating the standard American diet, on the other hand, had spent about fifteen years exercising strenuously for an hour a day at the gym at least five times a week. The researchers wanted to know if people who exercise hard enough for long enough develop cancer-fighting abilities that rival that of strolling plant eaters.[50]

To find out, blood from each of the three groups was dripped onto human prostate cancer cells growing in a petri dish to see whose blood kicked more cancer butt. The blood of the control group wasn't completely defenseless. Even if you're a french fry–eating couch potato, your blood may still be able to kill off 1–2 percent of cancer cells. But the blood of those who exercised strenuously every weekday for fifteen years killed 2,000 percent more cancer cells than the control groups'. Fantastic results, but the blood of those in the plant-based diet-and-exercise group wiped out an astounding 4,000 percent more cancer cells than that of the first group. Clearly exercise alone had a dramatic effect, but at the end of the day, thousands of hours in the gym appeared to be no match for a plant-based diet.[51]

Prostate Cancer Reversal Through Diet?

If a healthy diet can turn your bloodstream into a cancer-fighting machine, what about using it not just to prevent cancer but also to treat it? Other leading killers, including heart disease, type 2 diabetes, and hypertension, can be prevented, arrested, and even reversed, so why not cancer?

To test this question, Dr. Ornish and his colleagues recruited ninety-three men with prostate cancer who had chosen not to undergo any conventional treatment. Prostate cancer can be so slow growing and the side effects of treatment so onerous that men diagnosed with it often choose to be placed in a medical holding pattern called "watchful waiting" or "expectant management." Because the next step is often chemotherapy, radiation, and/or radical surgery that may leave men incontinent and impotent, doctors try to delay treatment as long as possible. And since these patients aren't actively doing anything to treat the disease, they represent an ideal population in whom to investigate the power of diet and lifestyle interventions.

The prostate cancer patients were randomized into two groups: a control group that wasn't given any diet or lifestyle advice beyond whatever their personal doctors told them to do, and a healthy-living group prescribed a strict plant-based diet centered around fruits, vegetables, whole grains, and beans, along with other healthy lifestyle changes, such as walking for thirty minutes, six days a week.[52]

Cancer progression was tracked using PSA levels, a marker of prostate cancer growth inside the body. After a year, the control group's PSA levels increased by 6 percent. That's what cancer tends to do: grow over time. But among the healthy-living group, PSA levels *decreased* by 4 percent, suggesting an average shrinkage of their tumors.[53] No surgery, no chemotherapy, no radiation—just eating and living healthfully.

Biopsies taken before and after the diet and lifestyle intervention showed that the expression of more than five hundred genes was affected. This was one of the first demonstrations that changing what you eat and how you live can affect you at a genetic level, in terms of which genes are switched on and off.[54] Within a year after the study ended, the cancers in the patients in the control group grew so much that 10 percent of them were forced to undergo a radical prostatectomy,[55] a surgery that involves the removal of the entire prostate gland and surrounding tissues. This treatment can lead not only to urinary incontinence (urine leakage) and impotence but to alterations in orgasmic function in approximately 80 percent of men undergoing the procedure.[56] In contrast, none in the plant-based diet and lifestyle group ended up on the operating table.

How were the researchers able to convince a group of older men to basically eat a vegan diet for a year? They evidently delivered prepared meals to their homes.[57] I guess the researchers figured men are so lazy they'll just eat whatever is put in front of them—and it worked!

Now, how about in the real world? Realizing that doctors apparently can't get most men with cancer to eat even a measly five servings of fruits and veggies daily,[58] a group of researchers at the University of Massachusetts settled on just trying to change their A:V ratio, or the ratio of animal to vegetable proteins in their diets.[59] Maybe just a reduction in meat and dairy and an increase in plant foods would be enough to put cancer into remission?

To test this, the researchers randomized prostate cancer patients into two groups, one group that attended classes on eating a more plant-based diet and a conventional-care group that received no dietary instruction. The healthy-eating advice group was able to drop their A:V ratio down to about 1:1, getting half their protein from plant sources. In contrast, the control group's ratio stayed up around 3:1 animal-to-plant protein.[60]

Those on the half-vegan diet did appear to slow down the growth of their cancer. Their average PSA doubling time—an estimate of how fast their tumors may have been doubling in size—slowed from twenty-one months to fifty-eight months.[61] In other words, the cancer kept growing, but even a part-time plant-based diet appeared to be able to significantly slow down their tumors' expansion. It is worth noting, though, that Dr. Ornish and colleagues were able to demonstrate that a full-time plant-based diet allowed for an apparent *reversal* in cancer growth: The subjects' PSA levels didn't just rise more slowly, but they trended downward. Thus, the ideal animal-to-plant protein ratio may be closer to zero to one.

The Worst A and the Best V

What if there's just no way Grandpa's going vegan, leaving you with only half measures? What would be on the short list of foods for him to avoid, or to include, in his diet?

Based on the Harvard University prostate cancer progression and mortality data detailed above, eggs and poultry may be the worst offenders: Patients may face twice the cancer progression risk from eating less than a single egg per day and up to quadruple the risk from eating less than a single serving of chicken or turkey daily.[62]

On the other hand, if you were to add only one thing to your diet, consider cruciferous vegetables. Less than a single serving a day of broccoli, brussels sprouts, cabbage, cauliflower, or kale may cut the risk of cancer progression by more than half.[63]

Watching your animal-to-plant protein ratio might be useful for cancer prevention in general. For example, the largest study ever performed on diet and bladder cancer—comprising nearly five hundred thousand people—found that an increase in animal protein consumption of just 3 percent was associated with a 15 percent increased risk of bladder cancer. On the other hand, an increase in plant protein intake of only 2 percent was associated with a 23 percent *decreased* cancer risk.[64]

Flaxseed

Prostate cancer rates vary tremendously around the world. African Americans, for example, may have an incidence of clinically apparent prostate cancer that is some 30 times greater than that of Japanese men and 120 times greater than that of Chinese men. This discrepancy has been attributed in part to the higher amounts of animal protein and fat in Western diets.[65] Another factor, though, may be the soy common in many Asian diets, which contains protective phytoestrogens called isoflavones.[66]

As detailed in chapter 11, the other major class of phytoestrogens is lignans, found throughout the plant kingdom but especially concentrated in flax-seeds. Higher levels of lignans tend to be found in the prostate fluids of populations of men with relatively low rates of prostate cancer,[67] and lignans have also been shown to slow the growth of prostate cancer cells in a petri dish.[68]

Researchers decided to put lignans to the test by asking men with prostate cancer scheduled for prostate-removal surgery the following month to consume three tablespoons a day of flaxseed. After surgery, their tumors were examined. Within just those few weeks, the flaxseed consumption appeared to have lowered their cancer-cell proliferation rates, while at the same time increasing their rate of cancer-cell clearance.[69]

Even better, flaxseeds may also be able to prevent prostate cancer from advancing to that stage in the first place. Prostatic intraepithelial neoplasia (PIN) is a precancerous prostate lesion found during a biopsy; it is analogous to ductal carcinoma in situ of the breast. Those with PIN have a high risk for cancer to appear during subsequent biopsies—25–79 percent.[70] Because men are repeatedly biopsied to monitor their condition, the procedures provide a perfect opportunity to see if a dietary intervention can keep these lesions from progressing to cancer.

After the first biopsies of their prostates came back PIN positive, fifteen men were asked to eat three tablespoons of flaxseed a day for the six months until their next biopsy. After that time, they showed a significant drop in PSA levels and biopsy cell-proliferation rates, suggesting that flaxseeds may indeed thwart the progression of prostate cancer. Two of the men saw their PSA levels drop to normal and didn't even need a second biopsy.[71]

Bottom line: The evidence suggests that flaxseed is a safe, low-cost source of nutrition and may reduce tumor-proliferation rates.[72] Why not give it a try? Just make sure to grind the flaxseeds first if you don't buy them preground—otherwise, the seeds may pass right through your body undigested.

Enlarged Prostate

If a healthy diet can slow down the abnormal growth of prostate cancer cells, can it also slow down the abnormal growth of normal prostate cells? Benign prostatic hyperplasia (BPH) is a condition characterized by enlargement of the prostate gland. In the United States, BPH affects millions of men[73]—as many as half of men by their fifties and 80 percent of men by their eighties.[74] Because the male prostate surrounds the outlet from the bladder, it can obstruct the normal flow of urine if it grows too large. This obstruction can cause a weak or hesitant stream and inadequate emptying of the bladder, requiring frequent trips to the bathroom. The stagnant urine retained in the bladder can also become a breeding ground for infection.

Unfortunately, the problem only seems to get worse as the gland continues to grow. Billions of dollars have been spent on drugs and supplements, and millions of American men have undergone surgery for BPH.[75] Surgical procedures involve a variety of Roto-Rooter techniques with innocent-sounding acronyms, such as TUMT, TUNA, and TURP. The *T*s stand for transurethral—meaning going up the penis with an instrument called a resectoscope. TUMT stands for transurethral microwave thermotherapy, in which doctors basically tunnel up the penis using an antenna-like tool and burn out a shaft with microwaves.[76] TUNA stands for transurethral needle ablation; here, a column is burned out with a pair of heated needles. And these are so-called minimally invasive techniques![77] The gold standard procedure is the TURP, wherein surgeons essentially use a loop of wire to core out the prostate. Side effects include "postoperative discomfort."[78] Ya think?!

There has to be a better way.

BPH is so common that most doctors may assume that it's just an inevitable consequence of aging. But it wasn't always so. In China in the 1920s and 1930s, for example, a medical college in Beijing reported that BPH affected not 80 percent of male patients but about eighty cases *total* over fifteen years. Both the historic rarity of BPH and prostate cancer in Japan and China have been attributed to the countries' traditional plant-based diets.[79]

This idea was studied by the same Pritikin Foundation researchers who pitted the blood of individuals before and after a plant-based diet against the growth of prostate cancer cells. This time, they performed the same experiment on the type of normal prostate cells that grow to obstruct urine flow. Within just two weeks, those eating plant-based diets saw their blood acquire the ability to suppress the abnormal growth of noncancerous prostate cells too—and the effect didn't seem to dissipate with time. The blood of those eating plant-based diets over the long term had the same beneficial effect for up to twenty-eight years straight. So it appears that as long as we continue to eat healthfully, prostate cell-growth rates will continue to go down and stay down.[80]

Some plants may be particularly prostate friendly. Research has found that flaxseeds can be used to treat BPH. Men given the equivalent of about three tablespoons of flaxseeds a day experienced relief comparable to that provided by commonly prescribed such drugs as Flomax or Proscar[81]—without the drugs' side effects, such as lightheadedness or sexual dysfunction.

Is it possible to prevent BPH in the first place? Eating garlic and onions has been associated with significantly lower risk of BPH.[82] In general, cooked vegetables may work better than raw ones, and legumes—beans, chickpeas, split peas, and lentils—have also been associated with lower risk.[83] TVP, short for textured vegetable protein, is a soybean product often used in pasta sauces and veggie chili. I would recommend that type of TVP over the one used in urology, which stands for transurethral vaporization of the prostate.[84]

IGF-1

Why do people who live to be one hundred or older seem to escape cancer? As you age, your risk of developing and dying from cancer grows every year—until you hit eighty-five or ninety, when, interestingly, your cancer risk begins to drop.[85] Indeed, if you don't get cancer by a certain age, you may never get it. What accounts for this relative resistance to cancer among centenarians? It may have to do with a cancer-promoting growth hormone called insulin-like growth factor 1 (IGF-1).[86]

Each year, you are reborn. You create and destroy nearly your entire body weight in new cells every year. Every day, about fifty billion of your cells die, and about fifty billion new cells are born to keep you in balance.[87] Of course, sometimes you need to grow, as when you're a baby or during puberty. Your cells don't become larger when you grow up; they simply become more numerous. An adult may have around forty trillion cells in his or her body, four times more than a child.

Once you've gotten through puberty, you no longer need to produce many more cells than you retire. You still need your cells to grow and divide, of course—out with the old, in with the new. You just don't want to make more cells than you're putting out to pasture. In adults, extra cell growth can mean the development of tumors.

How does your body keep itself in balance? By sending chemical signals called hormones to all the cells. A key signal is a growth hormone called IGF-1. It sounds like a droid from *Star Wars*, but IGF-1 is actually a crucial factor in regulating cell growth. Levels go up when you're a kid in order to power your development, but when you reach adulthood, IGF-1 levels diminish. It's your body's cue to stop producing more cells than it kills off.

Should your levels of IGF-1 remain too high when you reach adulthood, however, your cells will constantly receive a message to grow, divide, and keep going and growing. Not surprisingly, the more IGF-1 you have in your bloodstream, the higher your risk for developing cancers, such as prostate cancer.[88]

There is a rare form of dwarfism called Laron syndrome that is caused by the body's inability to produce IGF-1. Affected individuals grow to be only a few feet tall, but they also almost never get cancer.[89] Laron syndrome is a sort of cancer-proofing mutation, which led scientists to wonder: What if you could get all the IGF-1 you needed as a child to grow to a normal height but then down-regulate this hormone as adults and thereby turn off excess growth signals? It turns out you can do just that—not with surgery or medication but through simple dietary choices.

The release of IGF-1 appears to be triggered by the consumption of animal protein.[90] This may explain why you can so dramatically bolster the cancer-fighting power of your bloodstream within weeks of eating a plant-based diet. Remember the experiments in which dripping the blood from people eating healthy diets onto cancer cells wiped more of them out? Well, if you add back to the cancer cells the amount of IGF-1 that left the plant eaters' systems, guess what happens? The diet-and-exercise effect disappears. The cancer cell growth comes surging back. This is how we suspect plant-based eating boosts our blood defenses: By reducing animal protein intake, we reduce our levels of IGF-1.[91]

After just eleven days of cutting back on animal protein, your IGF-1 levels can drop by 20 percent, and your levels of IGF-1 *binding protein* can jump by 50 percent.[92] One of the ways your body tries to protect itself from cancer—that is, excessive growth—is by releasing a binding protein into your bloodstream to tie up any excess IGF-1. Think of it as the body's emergency brake. Even if you've managed to down-regulate production of new IGF-1 through diet, what about all that excess IGF-1 still circulating from the bacon and eggs you may have eaten two weeks before? No problem: The liver releases a snatch squad of binding proteins to help take it out of circulation.

How plant focused does a diet have to be to lower IGF-1 levels? Animal protein stimulates IGF-1 production whether it's the muscle proteins in meat, the egg-white protein in eggs, or the milk proteins in dairy. Vegetarians who include eggs and dairy in their diets don't seem to achieve a significant reduction in IGF-1. Only men[93] and women[94] who limit their intake of all animal proteins appear able to significantly drop their levels of the cancer-promoting hormone and raise their levels of the protective binding proteins.

Prostate cancer isn't inevitable. I once gave a speech in Bellport, New York, about preventing chronic disease through diet. Afterward, an audience member named John was inspired to e-mail me and recount his battle with prostate cancer. Diagnosed at age fifty-two, John had had six needle core biopsies performed, and each showed his cancer to be very aggressive. John's doctors immediately recommended surgery to remove his entire prostate.

Instead of going under the knife, John decided to switch to a plant-based diet. Eight months later, he had another biopsy. His doctors were astonished to see that only 10 percent of his cancer remained. What's more, his PSA tests have been completely normal ever since.

John was diagnosed in 1996. After changing his diet, his cancer went away and has stayed away.

John may have just gotten lucky, though. I do not recommend that people ignore their doctors' advice. Whatever you and your medical team decide together, healthy diet and lifestyle changes can presumably only help. That's the nice thing about lifestyle interventions—they can be implemented in addition to whatever other treatment options are chosen. In a research setting, that can complicate matters, as you don't know which action may be responsible for any improvement. But when facing a cancer diagnosis, you may want to opt for all the help you can get. Regardless of whether cancer patients elect for chemo, surgery, or radiation, they can always improve their diets. A prostate-healthy diet is a breast-healthy diet is a heart-healthy diet is a body-healthy diet.

CHAPTER 14

How Not to Die from Parkinson's Disease

Back in the 1960s at the height of the civil rights movement, my dad was dodging bullets during the Brooklyn riots and setting up shots at just the right angle to best capture images of my mother being arrested at protests and dragged away again and again. His most famous work—one of *Esquire*'s 1963 Photos of the Year—depicted family friend Mineral Bramletter suspended in a Christlike pose between two white police officers as another cop clutched his throat.

What a cruel twist of fate that a celebrated photojournalist got a disease that caused his hands to shake. For years, my dad suffered at the hands of Parkinson's. Slowly and all too painfully, he lost the ability to take care of himself, to live his life in any semblance of the way he had before. He became bedridden and compromised in every way imaginable.

After sixteen years of fighting, he went to the hospital one last time. As so often happens with chronic disease, one complication led to another. He got pneumonia and spent his last few weeks on a ventilator, suffering through a painful, prolonged death. The weeks he spent in that hospital bed before he passed were the worst weeks of both his and my life.

Hospitals are terrible places to be and terrible places to die. That is why each of us needs to take care of ourselves.

As my father's story shows, Parkinson's can end badly. It is the second most common neurodegenerative disease after Alzheimer's. Parkinson's is a disabling disorder affecting the speed, quality, and ease of movement. Its hallmark symptoms, which worsen as the disease progresses, include hand tremors, limb stiffness, impaired balance, and difficulty walking. It can also affect mood, thinking, and sleep. Parkinson's is not currently curable.

The disease is caused by the die-off of specialized nerve cells in a region of the brain that controls movement. It typically presents after age fifty. A history of head trauma can increase risk,[1] which may be why heavyweight boxers, including Muhammad Ali, and NFL players, including Hall of Famer Forrest Gregg, have fallen victim to the condition. However, most people may be more likely to develop the disease from toxic pollutants in our environment that can build up in the food supply and eventually affect the brain.

The National Cancer Institute's 2008/2009 U.S. Presidential Cancer Panel report discussed the degree to which we're being inundated with industrial chemicals. It concluded:

> The American people—even before they are born—are bombarded continually with myriad combinations of these dangerous exposures. The Panel urges you [Mr. President] most strongly to use the power of your office to remove the carcinogens and other toxins from our food, water, and air that needlessly increase health care costs, cripple our Nation's productivity, and devastate American lives.[2]

In addition to increasing your risk of developing many cancers, industrial pollutants may also play a role in the onset of such brain-deteriorating (neurodegenerative) diseases as Parkinson's.[3] And those toxins are residing in most peoples' bodies.

Every few years, the CDC measures the levels of chemical pollutants in the bodies of thousands of Americans from across the country. According to the agency's findings, the bodies of most women in the United States are contaminated with heavy metals, along with a number of toxic solvents, endocrine-disrupting chemicals, fire retardants, chemicals from plastics, polychlorinated biphenyls (PCBs), and banned pesticides such as DDT[4] (publicized by American biologist Rachel Carson in her 1962 bestseller *Silent Spring*).

In many cases, 99–100 percent of the hundreds of women tested were found to have detectable levels of these pollutants circulating in their bloodstreams. Pregnant women were found to harbor, on average, up to fifty different chemicals.[5] Could the presence of these potential toxicants in their bodies mean that they're also being passed on to their children? Researchers decided to put that question to the test by measuring pollutant levels right at delivery in the babies' umbilical cord blood. (As soon as the cord is cut, a little blood can be squirted into a vial.) After studying more than three hundred women who had recently given birth, researchers found that 95 percent of umbilical cord samples showed detectable DDT residues.[6] And this is now decades after the pesticide was banned.

What about men? Men tend to have even higher levels of certain pollutants than women. A clue to solving this mystery was found when breast-feeding history was taken into account. Women who never breast-fed had about the same level of certain toxicants in their bodies as men, but the longer they breast-fed their children, the lower their levels fell, suggesting that they were detoxing themselves by passing the pollution down to their children.[7]

It appears that blood levels of some pollutants in women may drop by nearly half during pregnancy,[8] in part because their bodies pass them off through the placenta.[9] That may be why breast milk concentrations of pollutants appear higher after the first pregnancy than in subsequent ones.[10] This could explain why birth order was found to be a significant predictor of pollutant levels in young people. Basically, firstborn kids may get first dibs on mom's store of toxic waste, leaving less for their baby brothers and sisters.[11]

Even mothers who were breast-fed as infants themselves tend to have higher levels of pollutants in their own breast milk when they grow up, suggesting a multigenerational passing down of these chemicals.[12] In other words, what you eat now may affect the levels of toxic chemicals in your grandchildren. When it comes to feeding babies, breast is still best—absolutely[13]—but rather than detoxing into our children, we should strive not to "tox" ourselves in the first place.

In 2012, researchers from the University of California–Davis, published an analysis of the diets of California kids aged two to seven. (Children are thought to be especially vulnerable to chemicals in the diet because they are still growing, and thus they have a comparatively greater intake of food and fluids relative to their weight.) Chemicals and heavy metals in children's bodies from the foods they ate were indeed found to exceed safety levels by a larger margin than in adults. Cancer risk ratios, for instance, were exceeded by a factor of up to one hundred or more. For every child studied, benchmark levels were surpassed for arsenic, the banned pesticide dieldrin, and potentially highly toxic industrial by-products called dioxins. They were also too high for DDE, a by-product of DDT.[14]

Which foods contributed the most heavy metals? The number-one food source of arsenic was poultry among preschoolers and, for their parents, tuna.[15] The top source for lead? Dairy. For mercury? Seafood.[16]

Those concerned about exposing their children to mercury-containing vaccines should know that eating just a single serving of fish each week during pregnancy can lead to more mercury in their infant's body than injecting them directly with about a dozen mercury-containing vaccines.[17] You should strive to minimize mercury exposure, but the benefits of vaccination far exceed the risks. The same cannot be said for tuna.[18]

Where in the food supply are these pollutants found? Today, most DDT comes from meat, particularly fish.[19] The oceans are essentially humanity's sewer; everything eventually flows into the sea. The same is true when it comes to dietary exposure to PCBs—another set of banned chemicals, once widely used as insulating fluid in electrical equipment. A study of more than twelve thousand food and feed samples across eighteen countries found that the highest PCB contamination was found in fish and fish oil, followed by eggs, dairy, and then other meats. The lowest contamination was found at the bottom of the food chain, in plants.[20]

Hexachlorobenzene, another pesticide banned nearly a half century ago, today may be found mainly in dairy and meat, including fish.[21] Perfluorochemicals, or PFCs? Overwhelmingly found in fish and other meats.[22] As for dioxins, in the United States, the most concentrated sources may be butter, followed by eggs, and then processed meat.[23] The levels in eggs may help explain why one study found that eating more than half an egg a day was associated with about two to three times higher odds for cancers of the mouth, colon, bladder, prostate, and breast compared to those who didn't eat eggs at all.[24]

If women want to clean up their diets before conception, how long does it take for these pollutants to leave their systems? To find out, researchers asked people to eat one large serving a week of tuna or other high-mercury fish for fourteen weeks to boost their levels of the heavy metal and then stop. By measuring how fast the subjects' mercury levels dropped, the scientists were able to calculate the half-life of mercury in the body.[25] The subjects appeared to be able to clear about half the mercury from their bodies within two months. This result suggests that within a year of stopping fish consumption, the body can detox nearly 99 percent of it. Unfortunately, other industrial pollutants in fish can take longer for our bodies to get rid of; the half-lives for certain dioxins, PCBs, and DDT by-products found in fish are as long as ten years.[26] So to get that same 99 percent drop, it could take more than a century—a long time to delay having your first child.

By now you are probably wondering how these chemicals get into your food in the first place. One reason is that we've so thoroughly polluted our planet that the chemicals can just come down in the rain. For example, scientists have reported eight different pesticides contaminating the snow-packed peaks of Rocky Mountain National Park in Colorado.[27] Once pollutants get into the soil, they can work their way up the food chain at increasing concentrations. Consider that before she's slaughtered for meat, a dairy cow may eat seventy-five thousand pounds' worth of plants. The chemicals in the plants can get stored in her fat and build up in her body. So when it comes to many of the fat-soluble pesticides and pollutants, every time you eat a burger, you are, in effect, eating everything that burger ate. The best way to minimize your exposure to industrial toxins may be to eat as low as possible on the food chain, a plant-based diet.

Reducing Dioxin Intake

Dioxins are highly toxic pollutants that accumulate in the fat of animal tissue, such that about 95 percent of human exposure comes from eating animal products.[28] Sometimes that's because of contaminated animal feed. In the 1990s, for example, a supermarket survey found that the highest concentration of dioxins was found in farm-raised catfish.[29] Apparently, the catfish were provided feed mixed with an anticaking agent laced with dioxins that may have originated from sewage sludge.[30]

That same feed was given to chickens, affecting approximately 5 percent of U.S. poultry production at the time.[31] That would mean that people ate hundreds of millions of contaminated chickens.[32] Of course, if it was in the chickens, then it was also in their eggs. Indeed, elevated dioxins levels were found in U.S. eggs too.[33] The U.S. Department of Agriculture estimated that less than 1 percent of feed was contaminated, but 1 percent of egg production would mean more than a million tainted eggs *per day*. But the catfish contamination was even more widespread: More than one-third of all U.S. farm-raised catfish tested were found to be contaminated with dioxins.[34]

In 1997, the Food and Drug Administration called on feed manufacturers to stop using these dioxin-tainted ingredients, stating that "[c]ontinued exposure to elevated dioxin levels in animal feed increases the risk of adverse health effects in animals and to humans consuming animal-derived food products."[35] So did the feed industry clean up their act? Up to a half billion pounds of catfish continued to be churned out of U.S. fish farms every year,[36] but it wasn't until more than a decade later that our government went back and checked for compliance. Researchers from the USDA tested samples of catfish from all over the country and in 2013 reported that *96 percent* of tested samples still contained dioxins or dioxin-like compounds. And when they checked the feed used to raise these fish? More than half the samples came back as contaminated.[37]

In other words, the feed industry has known for more than two decades that what they were feeding to animals (and, ultimately, to most of us[38]) may contain dioxins, but apparently, they continue this practice unabated.

The Institute of Medicine has made suggestions for reducing dioxin exposure, such as trimming fat from meat, including from poultry and fish, and avoiding the recycling of animal fat into gravy.[39] Wouldn't it be more prudent just to trim the amount of animal foods from your diet instead? Researchers have estimated that a plant based diet could wipe out about 98 percent of your dioxin intake.[40]

Smoking and Parkinson's Disease

The CDC recently celebrated the fifty-year anniversary of the landmark 1964 surgeon general's report on smoking, considered one of the great public health achievements of our time.[41] It's interesting to go back and read the reactions of the tobacco industry to such reports. For example, an industry insider argued that contrary to the surgeon general's argument that smoking costs our nation billions, "smoking *saves* the country money by increasing the number of people dying soon after retirement."[42] In other words, just think how much we're saving on Medicare and Social Security thanks to cigarettes.

The tobacco industry also criticized the surgeon general's "lack of balance regarding benefits of smoking."[43] As they testified before Congress, these "positive health benefits" include "the feeling of well-being, satisfaction, and happiness and everything else." Beyond all that happiness the surgeon general was trying to extinguish, the Tobacco Institute argued, "everything else" included protection against Parkinson's disease.[44]

As it happens, quite unexpectedly, more than five dozen studies over the past half century have collectively shown that smoking tobacco is indeed associated with significantly lower incidence of Parkinson's disease.[45] Valiant attempts have failed to explain away these findings. Maybe, public health scientists countered, it's because smokers are dying off before they get Parkinson's. No, smoking appears protective at all ages.[46] Maybe it's because smokers drink more coffee, which we know to be protective.[47] No, the protective effect remained even after researchers controlled studies for coffee intake.[48] Identical-twin studies helped rule out genetic factors in the link.[49] Even simply growing up in a home where your parents smoked appears protective when it comes to developing Parkinson's.[50] So was the tobacco industry right? Does it even matter?

Since the surgeon general's groundbreaking 1964 report, more than twenty million Americans have died as a result of smoking.[51] Even if you didn't care about dying from lung cancer or emphysema, even if you cared only about protecting your brain, you *still* shouldn't smoke, because smoking is a significant risk factor for stroke.[52] But what if you could get the benefits of smoking without the risks?

Maybe you can. The neuroprotective agent in tobacco appears to be nicotine.[53] Tobacco is part of the nightshade family, the group of plants that includes tomatoes, potatoes, eggplants, and peppers. It turns out they all contain nicotine, too, but in such trace amounts—hundreds of times less than what's found in a single cigarette—that the protective potential of vegetables was dismissed as inconsequential.[54] But then it was discovered that just one to two puffs of a cigarette can saturate half of your brain's nicotine receptors.[55] Then we learned that even exposure to secondhand smoke may lower the risk of Parkinson's[56] and that the amount of nicotine exposure sitting in a smoky restaurant is on the same order as what you might get from eating a healthy meal in a smoke-free restaurant.[57] So might eating lots of nightshade vegetables protect you from Parkinson's after all?

Researchers at the University of Washington decided to find out. When they tested for nicotine, they found none in eggplants, just a little in potatoes, some in tomatoes, and more significant amounts in bell peppers. These results were consistent with what researchers found when they studied nearly five hundred newly diagnosed Parkinson's patients compared to controls. Eating nicotine-rich vegetables, especially peppers, was associated with significantly lower risk of Parkinson's disease.[58] (This effect was found only in the nonsmokers, which makes sense because the flood of nicotine from cigarettes would likely overwhelm any dietary effect.) This study may help explain previous protective associations in terms of Parkinson's risk that had been tenuously found for tomato and potato consumption, as well as for the nightshade-rich Mediterranean diet.[59]

The University of Washington researchers concluded that more research is needed before individuals should consider dietary interventions to prevent Parkinson's disease, but when that intervention is simply enjoying more healthy dishes like stuffed peppers with tomato sauce, I don't see a reason why you should have to wait.

Dairy

Parkinson's patients have been found to have elevated levels of an organochlorine pesticide in their bloodstreams, the class of largely banned pesticides that includes DDT.[60] Autopsy studies have also found elevated levels of pesticides in the brain tissue of those with Parkinson's.[61] Elevated levels of other pollutants like PCBs were also found in their brains, and the higher certain PCB concentrations, the higher the degree of damage found specifically in the brain region thought to be responsible for the disease, called the substantia nigra.[62] As noted earlier, though many of these chemicals were banned decades ago, they may persist in the environment. You can continue to be exposed to them through the consumption of contaminated animal products in your diet, including dairy.[63] Indeed, people who eat dairy-free, plant-based diets were found to have significantly lower blood levels of the PCBs implicated in the development of Parkinson's disease.[64]

A meta-analysis of studies involving more than three hundred thousand participants found that overall dairy consumption was associated with significantly increased risk of Parkinson's disease. They estimated that Parkinson's risk may increase 17 percent for every daily cup of milk consumed.[65] "Contamination of milk with neurotoxins may be of critical importance," researchers offered by way of explanation.[66] For example, neurotoxic chemicals like tetrahydroisoquinoline, a compound used to induce parkinsonism in primates in laboratory studies,[67] appears to be found predominantly in cheese.[68] The concentrations found were low, but the concern is that they may accumulate over a lifetime of consumption,[69] resulting in the elevated levels found in the brains of Parkinson's patients.[70] There have been calls on the dairy industry to require screening of milk for such toxins,[71] but they have so far gone unanswered.

A recent nutrition journal editorial considered the case closed: "The only possible explanation for this effect is the evidence of the contamination of milk by neurotoxins."[72] But there are alternate explanations for the "clear-cut" link between dairy and Parkinson's.[73] For example, pollutant levels wouldn't explain why Parkinson's appears more closely tied to the consumption of the milk sugar lactose than to milk fat,[74] more closely tied to milk than to butter.[75] So maybe the culprit is galactose, the sugar in milk described in chapter 13, blamed for an increased risk of bone fractures, cancer, and death.[76] Those with an inability to detoxify the galactose in milk not only suffer damage to their bones but also to their brains.[77] This may help explain the link between milk intake and Parkinson's, as well as the link between milk and another neurodegenerative disease called Huntington's disease. Indeed, higher consumption of dairy products appears to double the risk of earlier-onset Huntington's.[78]

Another explanation is that milk consumption lowers blood levels of uric acid, an important brain antioxidant[79] shown to protect nerve cells against the oxidative stress caused by pesticides.[80] Uric acid may slow the progression of Huntington's[81] and Parkinson's,[82] and, most importantly, may lower the risk of getting Parkinson's in the first place.[83] Too much uric acid, however, can crystallize in your joints and cause a painful disease called gout, so uric acid can be thought of as a double-edged sword.[84] Too much uric acid is also associated with heart disease and kidney disease; too little, with Alzheimer's, Huntington's, Parkinson's, multiple sclerosis, and stroke.[85] Those on dairy-free, plant-based diets appear to hit the sweet spot[86] in terms of most optimal uric acid levels for longevity.[87]

Milk may *not* do a body good, at least when it comes to your bones and brain.

Plant-Based Diets and Pollutants

As we've discussed, organochlorines are a group of chemicals that includes dioxins, PCBs, and such insecticides as DDT. Although most were banned decades ago, they persist in the environment and creep up the food chain into the fat of the animals people eat.

What if you don't eat any animal products at all? Researchers have "found that vegans were significantly less polluted than omnivores" when measuring levels of organochlorines in their blood, including a variety of PCBs and one of Monsanto's long-banned Aroclor compounds.[88] This finding is consistent with studies showing higher levels of organochlorine pesticides in the body fat[89] and breast milk[90] of those who eat meat.

People eating completely plant-based diets have also been found to have markedly lower levels of dioxins in their bodies[91] as well as decreased contamination with PBDEs,[92] the flame-retardant chemical pollutants also linked to neurological problems.[93] No surprise: The highest levels of flame retardants in the U.S. food supply have been found in fish, though the primary source of intake for most Americans is poultry, followed by processed meat.[94] This discovery helps explain the significantly lower levels of PBDEs in the bodies of those eating meat-free diets.[95] It appears that the more plant-based foods you eat and the longer you go without eating animal products, the lower your levels fall.[96] No regulatory limits have been set for PBDEs in food, but as U.S. Department of Agriculture researchers noted in a survey of flame-retardant chemicals in domestic meat and poultry, "reducing the levels of unnecessary, persistent, toxic compounds in food and your diet is certainly desirable."[97]

Eating healthier can also reduce the concentrations of heavy metals in your body. The levels of mercury in the hair of those eating plant-based diets were found to be up to ten times lower than of those who ate fish.[98] Within three months of switching to a plant-based diet, the levels of mercury, lead, and cadmium growing out in your hair appear to drop significantly (but build back up when meat and eggs are added back into the diet).[99] Unlike heavy metals, though, some organochlorine pollutants can stick around for decades.[100] Any DDT in your KFC may stay with you for the rest of your life.

Berries

Dr. James Parkinson, in his original, centuries-old description of the disease that bears his name, described a characteristic feature: "torpid" bowels, or constipation that may precede the diagnosis by many years.[101] We've since learned that bowel-movement frequency may even be predictive of Parkinson's. Men with less than daily bowel movements, for instance, were found to be four times more likely to develop the disease years later.[102] Reverse causation has been suggested: Maybe constipation didn't lead to Parkinson's. Maybe Parkinson's— even decades before it was diagnosed—led to constipation. This idea was supported by anecdotal evidence suggesting that throughout their lives, many who would go on to develop Parkinson's reported never feeling very thirsty and, perhaps, decreased water intake contributed to their constipation.[103]

Alternatively, given the link between dietary pollutants and Parkinson's, constipation may be contributing directly to the disease: the longer feces stay in the bowel, the more neurotoxic chemicals in the diet may be absorbed.[104] There are now more than one hundred studies linking pesticides to an increased risk for Parkinson's disease,[105] but many of them are based on subjects' occupational or ambient exposure. Approximately one billion pounds of pesticides are applied annually in the United States,[106] and simply living or working in high-spray areas may increase your risk.[107] The use of common household pesticides like bug sprays is also associated with significantly increased risk.[108]

How exactly do pesticides increase your risk for Parkinson's? Scientists think they may cause DNA mutations that increase your susceptibility[109] or affect the way certain proteins fold in your brain. In order for proteins to function effectively, they have to be the right shape. As you make new proteins in your cells, if they come out folded incorrectly, they are simply recycled, and your body tries again. Certain misfolded proteins, however, can take a shape that your body has difficulty breaking down. Should this glitch happen continuously, the malformed proteins can accumulate and result in the death of the brain's nerve cells. Misfolded beta amyloid proteins, for example, are implicated in Alzheimer's disease (see chapter 3); misfolded prion proteins cause mad cow disease, a different malformed protein causes Huntington's; and misfolded alpha synuclein proteins can lead to Parkinson's disease.[110] In the most comprehensive study of this sort to date, eight out of twelve common pesticides tested were able to trigger the accumulation of alpha synuclein proteins in human nerve cells in a petri dish.[111]

As I've said, Parkinson's disease is caused by the die-off of specialized nerve cells in a region of the brain that controls movement. By the time the first symptoms arise, 70 percent of these critical cells may already be dead.[112] Pesticides are so good at killing these neurons that scientists often use pesticides in the laboratory to try to re-create Parkinson's in animals to test new treatments.[113]

If pesticides are killing off your brain cells, is there anything you can do to stop the process other than lowering your exposure to them? There are no known drugs that can prevent these misfolded proteins from accumulating, but certain phytonutrients called flavonoids—which are found in fruits and vegetables—may have protective effects. Researchers tested forty-eight different plant compounds able to cross the blood-brain barrier to see if any were able to stop alpha synuclein proteins from clumping together. To their surprise, not only did a variety of flavonoids inhibit these proteins from accumulating but they could also break up existing deposits.[114]

This study suggests that by eating healthfully, you can reduce your exposure to pollutants while countering their effects at the same time. And when it comes to countering the effects of pesticides, berries may be particularly useful. In a head-to-head battle between pesticides and berries, researchers found that preincubating nerve cells with a blueberry extract allowed them to better withstand the debilitating effects of a common pesticide.[115] But most such studies were performed on cells in a petri dish. Is there any evidence in people that eating berries could make a difference?

A small study published decades ago suggested that the consumption of blueberries and strawberries might protect against Parkinson's,[116] but the question remained largely unanswered until a Harvard University study of about 130,000 people found that people who eat more berries do indeed appear to have a significantly lower risk of developing the disease.[117]

The editorial that accompanied the study in the journal *Neurology* concluded that more research is necessary, but "until then, an apple a day might be a good idea."[118] Apples did appear protective against Parkinson's, but only for men. Everyone, however, appeared to benefit from the consumption of blueberries and strawberries, the only berries included in the study.[119]

If you do decide to follow my recommendation to eat berries every day, I would advise not serving them with cream. Not only has dairy been shown to block some of the beneficial effects of berries,[120] but, as we saw earlier, dairy products may contain compounds that cause the very damage the berries may be trying to undo.

Cannibalistic Feed Biomagnification

If people just eat from the bottom two levels of the food chain, only plants and plant eaters—that is, cows, pigs, and chickens fed grain and soybeans—why is the American populace so contaminated? Those of you who remember the mad cow disease story may know the answer. In modern agribusiness, there are essentially no more herbivores.

Millions of tons of slaughterhouse by-products continue to be fed to farm animals in the United States every year.[121] Not only have we turned these animals into meat eaters but virtual cannibals as well. When we feed farm animals millions of tons of meat and bonemeal, we're also feeding them any pollutants this feed may contain. Then, after those animals are slaughtered, their trimmings go to feed the next generation of farm animals, potentially concentrating the pollutant levels higher and higher.[122] So we can end up like polar bears or eagles at the top of the food chain and suffer the biomagnified pollutant consequences. When we eat these farmed animals, it's almost as if we're also eating every animal they ate.

The use of slaughterhouse by-products in animal feed can recycle both toxic heavy metals and industrial chemicals back into the food supply. Lead accumulates in animal bones and mercury in animal protein[123] (which is why egg whites contain up to twenty times more mercury than do yolks).[124] Persistent lipophilic organic pollutants (known as PLOPs[125]—really!) build up in animal fat. Reducing meat consumption can help reduce exposure, but these contaminants can come back to us in a variety of animal products. "Although a vegetarian lifestyle can lower the body burden of PLOP, MMHg [mercury], and lead," one toxicologist noted, "such benefits can be undermined by the consumption of contaminated milk and egg products. Farm animals that have been fed contaminated animal products produce contaminated milk and egg products."[126]

If you want to drop your PLOP, eat as low as possible on the food chain.

Coffee for Preventing and Treating Parkinson's Disease

Could your cup of morning joe help prevent and perhaps even help treat one of our most crippling neurodegenerative conditions? It appears so.

There have been at least nineteen studies performed on the role coffee may play in Parkinson's, and overall, coffee consumption is associated with about one-third lower risk.[127] The key ingredient appears to be the caffeine, since tea also seems protective[128] and decaf coffee does not.[129] Like the berry phytonutrients, caffeine has been shown to protect human nerve cells in a petri dish from being killed by a pesticide and other neurotoxins.[130]

What about coffee for *treating* Parkinson's? In a randomized controlled trial, giving Parkinson's patients the caffeine equivalent of two cups of coffee a day (or approximately four cups of black tea or eight cups of green tea) significantly improved movement symptoms within three weeks.[131]

Of course, there's only so much you can charge for a cup of coffee, so drug companies have tried to tweak caffeine into new experimental drugs, such as preladenant and istradefylline. But it turns out they don't appear to work any better than plain coffee, which is far cheaper and has a better safety record.[132]

There are a number of simple things you can do that may decrease your risk of dying from Parkinson's disease. You can wear seat belts and bicycle helmets to avoid getting hit in the head, you can exercise regularly,[133] avoid becoming overweight,[134] consume peppers, berries, and green tea, and minimize your exposure to pesticides, heavy metals, and dairy and other animal products. It's worth it. Trust me when I say that no family should have to endure the tragedy of Parkinson's.

CHAPTER 15

How Not to Die from Iatrogenic Causes (or, How Not to Die from Doctors)

As the saying goes, an ounce of prevention is worth a pound of cure. That's quaint, but a pound isn't all that heavy. Why change your diet and lifestyle when you can just let modern medicine do its job of fixing you back up?

Unfortunately, modern medicine isn't nearly as effective as most people think.[1] Doctors excel at treating acute conditions, such as mending broken bones and curing infections, but for chronic diseases, which are the leading causes of death and disability, conventional medicine doesn't have much to offer and, in fact, can sometimes do more harm than good.

For example, side effects from medications given in hospitals kill an estimated 106,000 Americans every year.[2] That statistic alone effectively makes medical care the sixth-leading cause of death in the United States. And this number reflects only the number of deaths from taking the drugs as prescribed. An additional 7,000 people die every year from receiving the wrong medication by mistake, and 20,000 others die from other hospital errors.[3] Hospitals are dangerous places, and that's not even counting the estimated 99,000 deaths each year due to hospital-acquired infections.[4] But can deaths from infections be blamed on doctors? They can if doctors won't even wash their hands.

We've known since the 1840s that hand washing is the best way to prevent hospital-acquired infections, yet compliance among health care workers rarely exceeds 50 percent. And doctors are the worst offenders.[5] One study found that even in a medical intensive care unit, slapping up a "contact precautions" sign (signaling particularly high risk of infection) leads less than a quarter of doctors to properly wash their hands or use a hand sanitizer when treating patients.[6] That's right. Not even one doctor out of four washed his or her hands before laying them on the ill. Many physicians are concerned that should it become widely known how many people doctors inadvertently kill every year, it could "undermine public trust."[7] But if doctors can't even be bothered to wash their hands, how much trust do we deserve?

This unfortunate (and gross!) situation means that you could go in for a simple operation and come out with a life-threatening infection—if you come out at all. Every year, 12,000 Americans die from complications due to surgeries that weren't even necessary in the first place. For those keeping score, that's more than 200,000 people dead from so-called iatrogenic causes (from the Ancient Greek *iatrós*, meaning "doctor"). And that figure is based only on the data on hospitalized patients. In outpatient settings—for instance, at your doctor's office—prescription drug side effects alone may result in 199,000 additional deaths.[8]

The Institute of Medicine estimates that medical errors may kill even more Americans, up to 98,000,[9] bringing the total annual death count closer to 300,000. That's more than the entire population of cities like Newark, Buffalo, or Orlando. Even using more conservative estimates of deaths due to medical errors, health care comes in as the *real* third-leading cause of death in America.[10]

How did the medical community respond to such damning conclusions? Deafening silence in both word and deed.[11] The first such report, which appeared in 1978, suggested that about 120,000 deaths occurring in hospitals could be prevented.[12] Then, sixteen years later, another scathing reminder was published in the *Journal of the American Medical Association*, suggesting the iatrogenic death toll may be "the equivalent of three jumbo-jet crashes every 2 days."[13] In the years between these two reports, as many as nearly two million Americans may have died due to medical errors, yet the medical community refused to comment on this tragedy and made no substantial effort to reduce the number of deaths.[14] Another estimated 600,000 deaths later, the prestigious Institute of Medicine released its own landmark report on the catastrophic consequences of medical error[15]—but again, little was done as a result.[16]

Eventually, a few changes were implemented. For instance, interns and residents could no longer be made to work for more than eighty hours a week (at least on paper), and shifts couldn't be more than thirty consecutive hours long. That may not sound like a big step, but when I started my internship after graduating from medical school, we worked thirty-six-hour shifts every three days—combined with our other days of work, that added up to a 117-hour work week.

When interns and residents are forced to pull all-nighters, studies suggest they may make 36 percent more serious medical errors, five times more diagnostic errors, and have twice as many "attentional failures" (such as nodding off during surgery).[17] The patient is supposed to be asleep during surgery, not the surgeon. It's no surprise, then, that overworked doctors may cause 300 percent more fatigue-related medical errors that lead to patient death.[18]

If every single day airliners crashed and killed hundreds of people, we would expect the Federal Aviation Administration to step in and do something. Why doesn't anyone confront the medical profession? Instead of just releasing reports, entities like the Institute of Medicine could have demanded that doctors and hospitals adopt at least a minimum set of preventive practices, such as bar-coding drugs to avoid mix-ups.[19] (You know, something they do even on a package of Twinkies at the grocery store.)

Only people on medications are killed by medication errors or the drugs' side effects, though. You have to actually be in the hospital to be killed by a hospital error or get an infection there. The good news is that most visits to doctors are for diseases that can be prevented with a healthy diet and lifestyle.[20]

The best way to avoid the adverse effects of medical tests and treatments is not to avoid doctors but to avoid getting sick in the first place.

Radiation

There are risks associated not only with medical treatment but also sometimes with diagnosis. A paper entitled "Estimated Risks of Radiation-Induced Fatal Cancer from Pediatric CT" out of Columbia University in 2001 reignited long-standing concerns about the risks associated with medical diagnostic radiation exposure. CT, or CAT, scans use multiple x-rays from different angles to create cross-sectional images, exposing the body to hundreds of times more radiation than a simple x-ray.[21] Based on the excess cancer risk of Hiroshima survivors exposed to similar doses of radiation,[22] it was estimated that out of all children who undergo abdominal or head CT scans every year, five hundred "might ultimately die from cancer attributable to the CT radiation."[23] In response to this revelation, the editor in chief of a leading radiology journal conceded, "We radiologists may be as guilty as others when it comes to not watching out for children."[24]

The risk of developing cancer after a single CT scan may be as high as 1 in 150 for a baby girl.[25] In general, the diagnostic medical radiation dealt out in one year is estimated to cause 2,800 breast cancers among American women, as well as 25,000 other cancers.[26] In other words, doctors may be causing tens of thousands of cancers every year.

Patients undergoing these scans are rarely informed of these risks. For example, did you know that getting a chest CT scan is estimated to inflict the same cancer risk as smoking seven hundred cigarettes?[27] One in every 270 middle-aged women may develop cancer due to a single angiogram.[28] CT scans and x-rays can be lifesaving, but good evidence suggests that one-fifth to one-half of all CT scans aren't necessary at all and could be replaced with a safer type of imaging or simply not performed at all.[29]

Many people expressed concern about the radiation exposure from the full-body scanners at airports using backscatter x-rays,[30] but those machines have since been phased out. The airplane itself, however, is a different story. Because you're exposed to more cosmic rays from outer space at higher altitudes, just one round-trip, cross-country flight may subject you to about the same level of radiation as a chest x-ray.[31] (Given my past speaking schedule, I should be glowing in the dark by now!)

Is there anything you can do to mediate the radiation risk? As with so many other health questions, the answer is that you can eat healthfully.

In an investigation funded by the National Cancer Institute, researchers studied the diets and chromosome integrity of airline pilots, who get zapped with radiation daily, to see which foods might be protective. They found that pilots who consumed the most dietary antioxidants suffered the least amount of DNA damage to their bodies. Note the word *dietary*. Antioxidant supplements, such as vitamins C and E, didn't seem to help. Pilots who consumed the most vitamin C through fruits and vegetables, though, appeared to be protected.[32] Taking antioxidant supplements may be more than just a waste of money. People given 500 mg of vitamin C a day were found to end up with *more* oxidative DNA damage.[33]

Remember that natural antioxidants in food work synergistically; it's the combination of many different compounds working together that tends to protect you, not high doses of single antioxidants found in supplements. Indeed, those pilots eating a mix of phytonutrients, concentrated in a variety of such plant foods as citrus, nuts, seeds, pumpkins, and peppers, had the lowest levels of DNA damage in response to the radiation they were bombarded with every day from the galaxy.[34]

The research team found that green, leafy vegetables like spinach and kale appear to have an edge over other vegetables and fruits when it comes to radiation protection.[35] All this time I've been packing kale chips on flights just because they're so lightweight, but it also turns out they may be protecting my DNA.

The same plant-based protection enjoyed by pilots was also found among atomic bomb survivors. For several decades, researchers have followed thirty-six thousand survivors of the nuclear attacks on Hiroshima and Nagasaki. Those who ate vegetable- or fruit-rich diets appeared to cut their cancer risk by about 36 percent.[36] We saw the same thing in the aftermath of the accident at the Chernobyl nuclear reactor in Ukraine, where consumption of fresh fruits and vegetables apparently protected children's immune systems, while egg and fish consumption was associated with a significantly increased risk of DNA damage. The researchers suggest this result could have been due to the possibility that the animal foods they ate were contaminated with radioactive elements or the role of animal fats in free-radical formation.[37]

Nuclear events offer a rare opportunity to study these effects on humans since, obviously, it is unethical to intentionally expose people to radiation. However, as we've learned from declassified documents about U.S. Cold War radiation experiments, this didn't stop our government from injecting "colored" people with plutonium[38] or feeding "retarded" children radioactive isotopes in their breakfast cereal.[39] Despite the Pentagon's insistence that these methods were the "only feasible means" of developing ways to protect people from radiation,[40] researchers have since come up with a few methods that don't violate the Nuremburg Code.

One is to study human cells in a test tube. Research has found, for example, that white blood cells blasted with gamma rays suffered less DNA damage when the cells had been pretreated with phytonutrients from ginger root. The ginger compounds protected DNA nearly as well as the leading radiation sickness drug[41] at 150 times lower the dose.[42] Those taking ginger in order to prevent motion sickness during air travel may be protecting themselves against more than just nausea.

Other common foods that may be protective against radiation damage include garlic, turmeric, goji berries, and mint leaves,[43] but none of these has been tested in clinical studies. How can we test the protective power of foods in people rather than petri dishes? To study how diet may protect against cosmic rays, airline pilots were studied. Guess who they studied to see if foods could be protective against x-rays? X-ray technicians.

Hospital workers who routinely operate x-ray machines have been found to suffer more chromosomal damage and to have higher levels of oxidative stress compared with other hospital workers.[44] For this reason, researchers recruited a group of x-ray techs and asked them to drink two cups of lemon balm tea each day for a month. (Lemon balm is an herb in the mint family.) Even in that short time frame, the lemon balm tea appeared able to boost the level of antioxidant enzymes in the subjects' bloodstreams while also reducing the amount of DNA damage they suffered.[45]

The Actual Benefit of Diet Versus Drugs

Based on a study of more than one hundred thousand Minnesotans, it appears that seven out of ten people may be prescribed at least one prescription drug in any given year. More than half are prescribed two or more drugs, and 20 percent are prescribed *five* or more medications.[46] All told, physicians dispense about four billion prescriptions for drugs every year in the United States.[47] That's about thirteen prescriptions a year for every man, woman, and child.

The two prescription drugs most often brought up in doctor visits are simvastatin, a cholesterol-lowering medication, and lisinopril, a blood-pressure pill.[48] So a lot of drugs are being doled out in an attempt to prevent disease. But how well are these billions of pills working?

An overconfidence in the power of pills and procedures for disease prevention may be one of the reasons doctors and patients alike may undervalue diet and lifestyle interventions. When surveyed, people tend to wildly overestimate the ability of mammograms and colonoscopies to prevent cancer deaths, or the power of drugs like Fosamax to prevent hip fractures, or drugs like Lipitor to prevent fatal heart attacks.[49] Patients believe cholesterol-lowering statin drugs are about twenty times more effective than they actually are in preventing heart attacks.[50] No wonder most people continue to rely on drugs to save them! But the dirty little secret is that most people surveyed said they wouldn't be willing to take many of these drugs if they knew how little benefit these products actually offered.[51]

How ineffectual are some of the most common drugs in America? When it comes to cholesterol, blood pressure, and blood-thinning drugs, the chance of even high-risk patients benefiting from them is typically less than 5 percent over a period of five years.[52] When asked, most patients say they want to be told the truth.[53] However, as doctors, we know that if we divulged this information, few of our patients would agree to take these drugs every day for the rest of their lives, which would be detrimental for the small percentage of people who do truly benefit from them. That's why doctors in the know and drug companies oversell the benefits by conveniently not mentioning how tiny these benefits actually are. When it comes to chronic disease management, practicing conventional medicine can be thought of as practicing deceptive medicine.

For the hundreds of millions of people on these drugs who don't benefit, it's not simply a matter of all the money spent and all the side effects endured. To me, the true tragedy is all the lost opportunities to address the root causes of patients' conditions. When people dramatically overestimate how much their prescription pills protect them, they may be less likely to make the dietary changes necessary to dramatically lower their risk.

Take cholesterol-lowering statin drugs, for example. The best they may be able to offer in terms of absolute risk reduction for a subsequent heart attack or death is about 3 percent over six years.[54] Meanwhile, a whole-food, plant-based diet may work twenty times better, potentially offering an absolute risk reduction of 60 percent after fewer than four years.[55] In 2014, Dr. Caldwell Esselstyn Jr. published a case series of about two hundred people with significant heart disease showing that a healthy enough plant-based diet may prevent further major cardiac episodes in 99.4 percent of patients who follow it.[56]

You don't really have the luxury of choosing between following a healthy diet or taking a pill to prevent a heart attack because pills may not work in the near term in 97 percent of the cases. Of course, diet and drugs are not mutually exclusive, and many under Dr. Esselstyn's care wisely continued to take their cardiac meds. You just need to have a realistic understanding of how limited a role the contents of your medicine cabinets play compared to the contents of your refrigerator. Heart disease may continue to be the number-one killer of men, women, and eventually our children if doctors continue to rely on drugs and stents. However, if you eat a healthy enough diet, you may be able to reverse the stranglehold it has on your heart. That is something doctors can be proud to divulge to our patients.

Aspirin

How well do over-the-counter drugs perform? For example, take aspirin. Perhaps the most commonly used medication in the world,[57] it's been around in pill form for over a century. Its active ingredient, salicylic acid, has been used in its natural form (as an extract of willow tree bark) to ease pain and fever for thousands of years.[58] One of the reasons it remains so popular—despite the fact that better anti-inflammatory painkillers exist now—is that it's used by millions of people on a daily basis as a blood thinner to reduce the risk of a heart attack. As we saw in chapter 1, heart attacks often occur when a blood clot forms in response to a ruptured atherosclerotic plaque in one of your coronary arteries. Taking aspirin may help stop this from happening.

Aspirin may also lower the risk of cancer.[59] It works by suppressing an enzyme within your body that creates pro-clotting factors, thereby thinning your blood. At the same time, aspirin suppresses proinflammatory compounds called prostaglandins, which in turn reduces pain, swelling, and fever.

Prostaglandins may also dilate the lymph vessels inside tumors, potentially allowing cancer cells to spread. One of the ways scientists think aspirin helps prevent cancer deaths is by counteracting a tumor's attempts to pry open the lymphatic bars on its cage and spread throughout the body.[60]

So should everyone take a "baby"-strength aspirin a day? (Note that aspirin should never actually be given to infants or children.)[61] No. The problem is that aspirin can cause side effects. The same blood-thinning benefit that can prevent a heart attack can also cause a hemorrhagic stroke, in which you bleed into your brain. Aspirin can also damage the lining of the digestive tract. For those who've already had a heart attack and continue to eat the same diet that led to the first one (and are therefore at exceedingly high risk of having another one), the risk-benefit analysis seems clear: Taking aspirin would probably prevent about six times more serious problems than it causes you. But among the general population who have yet to have their first heart attack, the risks and benefits are more closely matched.[62] Thus, taking an aspirin a day is generally not recommended.[63] Throw in even a 10 percent reduction in cancer mortality, though, and it could tip the risk-benefit balance in favor of aspirin.[64] Given that regular, low-dose aspirin use may reduce the risk of cancer mortality by one-third,[65] it is tempting to recommend it for nearly everyone. If only you could get the benefits without the risks.

Well, maybe you can.

The willow tree isn't the only plant that contains salicylic acid. It's widely found in many of the fruits and vegetables in the plant kingdom.[66] That's why you often find the active ingredient of aspirin in the bloodstreams of people who aren't taking it.[67] The more fruits and vegetables you eat, the higher your level of salicylic acid may rise.[68] In fact, the levels of people eating plant-based diets actually overlap with those of some people taking low-dose aspirin.[69]

With all that salicylic acid flowing through their systems, you might think plant eaters would have higher ulcer rates, because aspirin is known to chew away at the gut. But those following plant-based diets actually appear to have a significantly *lower* risk of ulcers.[70] How is that possible? Because in plants, the salicylic acid may come naturally prepackaged with gut-protective nutrients. For example, nitric oxide from dietary nitrates exerts stomach-protective effects by boosting blood flow and protective mucus production in the lining of the stomach, effects which demonstrably oppose the pro-ulcerative impact of aspirin.[71] So, for the general population, by eating plants instead of taking aspirin, individuals may not only get aspirin's benefits without its risks but also get the benefits—with benefits.

People who have had a heart attack should follow their physician's advice, which probably includes taking aspirin every day. But what about everyone else? I think everyone should take aspirin—but in the form of produce, not a pill.

The salicylic acid content in plants may help explain why traditional, plant-based diets were so protective. For instance, before their diets were Westernized, animal products made up only about 5 percent of the average Japanese diet.[72] During this period in the 1950s, age-adjusted death rates from colon, prostate, breast, and ovarian cancers were five to ten times lower in Japan than in the United States, while incidences of pancreatic cancer, leukemia, and lymphoma were three to four times lower. This phenomenon was not unique to the Japanese. As we've seen throughout this book, Western rates of cancers and heart disease have been found to be dramatically lower among populations whose diets are centered around plant foods.[73]

If part of this protection arises from the aspirin phytonutrients, which plants in particular are packed with the stuff? While salicylic acid is ubiquitously present in fruits and vegetables, herbs and spices contain the highest concentrations.[74] Chili powder, paprika, and turmeric are rich in the compound, but cumin has the most per serving. Indeed, just one teaspoon of ground cumin may be about the equivalent of a baby aspirin. This may help explain why India, with its spice-rich diets, has among the lowest worldwide rates of colorectal cancer[75]—the cancer that appears most sensitive to the effects of aspirin.[76]

And the spicier, the better! A spicy vegetable vindaloo has been calculated to contain four times the salicylic acid content of a milder madras-style veggie dish. Eat a single meal, and you can get the same spike in salicylic acid in your bloodstream as if you took an aspirin.[77]

The benefits of salicylic acid are another reason you should strive to choose organic produce. Because the plant uses the compound as a defense hormone, its concentration may be increased when that plant is bitten by bugs. Pesticide-laden plants aren't nibbled as much and, perhaps as a result, appear to produce less salicylic acid. For example, in one study, soup made from organic vegetables was found to contain nearly six times more salicylic acid than soup prepared from conventional, nonorganically grown ingredients.[78]

Another way to get more salicylic acid bang for your buck is by opting for whole foods. Whole-grain breads, for example, not only offer more salicylic acid but may contain one hundred times more phytochemicals in general than white bread—reportedly eight hundred compared with approximately eight.[79]

Attention has been focused on salicylic acid because of the voluminous data on aspirin, but hundreds of the other phytonutrients have been found to have anti-inflammatory and antioxidant activity as well. Still, given the strength of the aspirin evidence, there are those in the public health community who talk of a widespread "salicylic acid deficiency," proposing that the compound be classed as an essential vitamin: "Vitamin S."[80] Whether it's the salicylic acid or a combination of other phytonutrients that account for the benefits of whole plant foods, the solution is the same: Eat more of them.

Colonoscopies

The colonoscopy. You'll be hard pressed to find a more dreaded routine procedure. Every year, U.S. doctors may perform more than fourteen million colonoscopies,[81] an exam used to detect abnormal changes in the large intestine (colon) and rectum. During the procedure, doctors insert a five-foot-long flexible tube fitted with a tiny video camera and inflate the colon with air to visualize the colon lining. Any suspicious polyps or other abnormal tissue can be biopsied during the procedure. Colonoscopies can help doctors diagnose causes of rectal bleeding or chronic diarrhea, but routine colon cancer screenings may be the most common reason they are performed.

The reasons doctors often find it difficult to convince their patients to keep coming back for colonoscopies include the necessary bowel prep, during which you have to drink quarts of a powerful liquid laxative before the procedure to completely clean yourself out. There's also the pain and discomfort of the procedure itself[82] (though you're purposefully given drugs with amnesiac effects so you won't remember how it felt),[83] feelings of embarrassment and vulnerability, and the fear of complications.[84] These fears are not unfounded. Despite how routinely colonoscopies are performed, serious complications occur in about 1 out of every 350 cases, including such issues as perforations and fatal bleeding.[85] Perforations can occur when the tip of the colonoscope punctures the wall of the colon, when the colon is overinflated, or when a doctor cauterizes a bleeding biopsy site. In extremely rare cases, this cautery can ignite some residual gas and cause the colon to literally explode.[86]

Death from colonoscopy is rare, occurring in only about 1 in every 2,500 procedures.[87] Yet this means colonoscopies may be killing thousands of Americans every year, raising the question: Do the benefits outweigh the risks?

Colonoscopies are not the only screening technique for colon cancer. The U.S. Preventive Services Task Force (USPSTF), the official prevention guidelines body, considers colonoscopies just one of three acceptable colon-cancer screening strategies. Starting at age fifty, everyone should get either a colonoscopy once a decade, have their stool tested for hidden blood every year (which involves no scoping at all), or have a sigmoidoscopy every five years, along with stool testing every three. The evidence supporting "virtual" colonoscopies or DNA stool testing was judged insufficient.[88] Though routine screenings are no longer recommended at age seventy-five, this assumes you've been testing negative for twenty-five years. If you're now seventy-five and have never been screened, then it's probably a good idea to get screened at least into your eighties.[89]

Sigmoidoscopy uses a much smaller scope than in a colonoscopy and has ten times fewer complications.[90] However, because the scope may only go about two feet inside your body, it might miss tumors farther inside. So which is better overall? We won't know until randomized controlled colonoscopy trials are published in the mid-2020s.[91] Most other developed countries do not recommend either scoping procedure, though. For routine colon cancer screening, they still endorse the noninvasive stool blood testing.[92]

Which of the three options is best for you? The USPSTF recommends that the decision should be made on an individualized basis after weighing the benefits and risks with your doctor.

To what extent, though, do doctors inform patients of their options? Researchers audiotaped clinic visits to find out. They were looking for the nine essential elements of informed decision making, which include explaining the pros and cons of each option, describing the alternatives, and making sure the patient understands these options.[93]

Unfortunately, when it came to colon cancer screening, in most cases, the doctors and nurse practitioners studied communicated *none* of this vital information, zero out of nine elements.[94] As an editorial in the *Journal of the American Medical Association* put it: "There are too many probabilities and uncertainties for patients to consider and too little time for clinicians to discuss them with patients."[95] So doctors tend to just make up patients' minds for them. What do they choose? A National Cancer Institute–funded survey of more than one thousand physicians found that nearly all doctors (94.8 percent) recommended a colonoscopy.[96] Why do doctors push colonoscopies in the United States when most of the rest of the world appears to prefer noninvasive alternatives?[97] It may be because most doctors in the rest of the world don't get paid by procedure.[98] As one U.S. gastroenterologist put it, "Colonoscopy . . . is the goose that has laid the golden egg."[99]

An exposé in the *New York Times* on spiraling health care costs noted that in many other developed countries, colonoscopies cost just a few hundred dollars. In the United States? The procedure may cost thousands, which the journalists concluded has less to do with providing top-notch medical care and more with business plans aimed at maximizing revenue, marketing, and lobbying.[100]

Who's in charge of setting the prices? The American Medical Association. A *Washington Post* investigation exposed that each year, a secretive AMA committee determines billing standards for common procedures. The result is gross overestimates for the time it takes to perform common services like colonoscopies. As the *Post* pointed out, if AMA standards are to be believed, some doctors would have to work more than twenty-four hours a day to perform all the procedures they report to Medicare and private insurers. Is it any wonder that gastroenterologists bank nearly $500,000 per year?[101]

But why would your family doctor or internist push the procedure if they're not the ones doing it? Many doctors who refer their patients to gastroenterologists receive what are essentially financial kickbacks. The U.S. Government Accountability Office (GAO) reported on this practice of so-called self-referrals, a scheme where providers refer patients to entities in which they have a financial interest. The GAO estimated that doctors make nearly a million more referrals every year than they would have if they were not personally profiting.[102]

What to Take Before a Colonoscopy

Ever popped one of those breath mints after a big meal at a restaurant? Peppermint doesn't just make your breath smell better; it also helps to reduce the gastrocolic reflex—the urge to defecate following a meal. Nerves in your stomach stretch after eating, which triggers spasms in the colon to enable your body to make room for more food coming down the pike. Peppermint can reduce these spasms by relaxing the muscles that line your colon.[103]

What does this have to do with colonoscopies? If you take circular strips of human colons removed during surgery and lay them on a table, they spontaneously contract about three times per minute. Isn't that kind of creepy? But if you drip menthol (found in peppermint) onto the colon strips, the strength of the contractions diminishes significantly.[104] During a colonoscopy, such spasms can hinder the progress of the scope and cause the patient discomfort. By relaxing colon muscles, peppermint can make the procedure easier for both doctor and patient.

Doctors have experimented with spraying peppermint oil from the tip of the colonoscope,[105] as well as using a hand pump to flood the colon with a peppermint solution prior to the procedure.[106] The simplest solution might

be the best, though: asking the patient to swallow peppermint oil capsules. Premedicating with eight drops' worth of peppermint essential oil
four hours before a colonoscopy was found to significantly reduce colon
spasms, patient pain, and make the scope easier to insert and withdraw
compared with a placebo.[107]

If you do need a colonoscopy, ask your doctor about using this simple
plant remedy. It might make it easier on both of you.

Clearly, patients in America may be getting more medical care than they
really need. So said Dr. Barbara Starfield, who literally wrote the book on primary care.[108] One of our nation's most prestigious physicians, she composed
the scathing commentary in the *Journal of the American Medical Association* nam-
ing medical care as the third-leading cause of death in the United States.[109]

Her primary-care work has been widely embraced, but her findings on the
potentially ineffective and even harmful nature of U.S. health care received
almost no attention. "The American public appears to have been hoodwinked
into believing that more interventions lead to better health," she later said in
an interview.[110] As one health care quality advisor noted, the widespread dis-
regard of Dr. Starfield's evidence "recalls the dark dystopia of George Orwell's
1984, where awkward facts swallowed up by the 'memory hole' become as if
they had never existed at all."[111]

Sadly, Dr. Starfield is no longer with us. Ironically, she may have died from
one of the adverse drug reactions she so vociferously warned us about. After
she was placed on two blood thinners to prevent a stent in her heart from clogging up, she told her cardiologist she was bruising more and bleeding longer—
that's the drug risk you hope doesn't outweigh the benefits. Then Dr. Starfield
died after apparently hitting her head while swimming and bleeding into her
brain.[112]

The question I ask myself is not whether she should have been put on two
blood thinners for as long as she was—or whether she should have had the stent
inserted to begin with. Rather, I wonder if she could have avoided the medication and the surgery both by avoiding the heart disease in the first place. Heart
attacks are considered 96 percent avoidable in women who eat a wholesome
diet and engage in other healthy lifestyle behaviors.[113] The number-one killer
of women need almost never happen.

PART 2

Introduction

In part 1 of this book, I explored the science that demonstrates the role a plant-based diet rich in certain foods may play in helping to prevent, treat, and even reverse the fifteen leading causes of death. For those who may have already been diagnosed with one or more of these diseases, the information in part 1 can be lifesaving. But for everyone else—perhaps those worried about inheriting their family history of illness or those who simply want their diet to promote health and longevity—the primary question might concern food choices to make day in and day out. I have given more than a thousand presentations, and one of the most common questions I get is, "What do *you* eat every day, Dr. Greger?"

This, part 2 of *How Not to Die*, is my response to that question.

I've never had so much a sweet tooth as a grease tooth. Pepperoni pizza. Chicken wings by the basket. Sour cream–and-onion potato chips. A Hardee's bacon cheeseburger nearly every day during high school. Anything oily and fatty—and all washed down with an ice-cold Dr Pepper. Okay, so maybe a little sweet tooth. I also really liked strawberry-frosted doughnuts.

Even though my grandma's miraculous recovery from heart disease inspired me to pursue a career in medicine, I didn't clean up my own diet until the publication of Dr. Ornish's landmark Lifestyle Heart Trial in 1990. I was such a nerd in high school that I would spend my summer vacations hanging out in the science library at the local university. And there it was, published in the most prestigious medical journal in the world—proof that my family's story was not a fluke: Heart disease could be reversed. Dr. Ornish and his team had taken before-and-after x-rays of people's arteries and demonstrated how they could be opened up without angioplasty. No surgery. No miracle drug. Just a plant-based diet and other healthy lifestyle changes. That's what motivated me to change my own diet and ignited my twenty-five-year love affair with nutritional science. From that point forward, I have been determined to spread the word about food's power to make you healthy, keep you healthy, and, if necessary, return you to health.

For the purposes of this book, I've created two simple tools to help you integrate everything I've learned into your own daily life:

1. a Traffic Light system to quickly identify the healthiest options, and

2. a Daily Dozen checklist that will help you incorporate the foods that I consider essential to the optimal diet. (Check out the free app on iPhone and Android.)

So which foods are good for you, and which are bad?

This sounds like a simple enough question. In truth, I've found it difficult to answer. Whenever I'm asked at a lecture whether a certain food is healthy or not, I have to invariably reply, "Compared to what?" For example, are eggs healthy? Compared to oatmeal, definitely not. But compared to the sausage links next to them on the breakfast platter? Yes.

What about white potatoes? They're vegetables, so they must be healthy, right? Someone asked me this a few years ago after a group of Harvard University researchers raised concerns about baked and mashed potatoes.[1] So are they healthy? Compared to french fries, yes. Compared to a baked or mashed *sweet* potato? No, they're not.

I realize these may not be satisfying answers for people who just want to know whether or not to eat the darned potato, but the only way to answer the question meaningfully is to ask what your other options are. If you're in a fast-food joint, for example, a baked potato may very well be your healthiest option.

Compared to what? is not just a Socratic learning exercise I have practiced with my patients and students. Eating is essentially a zero-sum game: When you choose to eat one thing, you are generally choosing not to eat another. Sure, you could just go hungry, but eventually your body tends to balance things out by eating more later. So anything we choose to eat has an opportunity cost.

Every time you put something in your mouth, it's a lost opportunity to put something even healthier in there. Think of it as having $2,000 in your daily caloric bank. How do you want to spend it? For the same number of calories, you can eat one Big Mac, one hundred strawberries, or a five-gallon bucket of salad. Of course, these three options don't exactly fill the same culinary niche—if you want a burger, you want a burger, and I don't expect quarts of strawberries to make it on the Dollar Menu anytime soon—but this is an illustration of how mountainous a nutritional bang you can get for the same caloric buck.

The opportunity costs exacted are not only the nutrients you could otherwise be getting but the unhealthy components you could otherwise be avoiding. After all, when was the last time you had a friend diagnosed with kwashiorkor, scurvy, or pellagra? These are some of the traditional nutrient-deficiency diseases upon which the foundation of the field of nutrition was built. To this day, the nutrition and dietetic professions remain focused on what nutrients we may be lacking, but most of our chronic diseases may have more to do with what we're getting too much of. Know anyone suffering from obesity, heart disease, type 2 diabetes, or high blood pressure?

Isn't It Expensive to Eat Healthfully?

Researchers at Harvard University compared the cost and healthfulness of various foods across the country, hunting for the best bargains. They found that in terms of nutritional bang for your buck, people should buy more nuts, soy foods, beans, and whole grains, and less meat and dairy. They concluded: "The purchase of plant-based foods may offer the best investment for dietary health."[2]

Less healthy foods only beat out healthier foods on a cost-per-calorie basis, which is a way we measured food cost back in the nineteenth century. Back then, the emphasis was on cheap calories, no matter how you got them. So while beans and sugar both cost the same at that time (five cents a pound), the U.S. Department of Agriculture promoted sugar as more cost effective for pure "fuel value."[3]

The USDA can be excused for discounting the nutritional difference between beans and pure sugar. After all, vitamins hadn't even been discovered yet. Nowadays, we know better and can compare the cost of foods based on their nutritional content. An average serving of vegetables may

continued

cost roughly four times more than the average serving of junk food, but those veggies have been calculated to average twenty-four times more nutrition. So on a cost-per-nutrition basis, vegetables offer six times more nutrition per dollar compared to highly processed foods. Meat costs about three times more than vegetables yet yields sixteen times less nutrition based on an aggregate of nutrients.[4] Because meat is less nutritious *and* costs more, vegetables net you *forty-eight times* more nutrition per dollar than meat.

If your intent is to shovel as many calories as possible into your mouth for the least amount of money, then healthier foods lose out, but if you want to shovel the most *nutrition* into your mouth as cheaply as possible, look no further than the produce aisle. Spending just fifty cents more per day on fruits and vegetables may buy you a 10 percent drop in mortality.[5] Now that's a bargain! Imagine if there were a pill that could reduce your chance of dying by 10 percent over the next decade and only had good side effects. How much do you think the drug company would charge? Probably more than fifty cents.

Dining by Traffic Light

The U.S. government's official Dietary Guidelines for Americans has (as of this writing) a chapter "Food Components to Reduce," which specifically lists added sugars, calories, cholesterol, saturated fat, sodium, and trans fat.[6] At the same time, there are nine so-called shortfall nutrients, of which at least a quarter of the American population isn't reaching an adequate intake. These are fiber; the minerals calcium, magnesium, and potassium; and vitamins A, C, D, E, and K.[7] But you don't eat food "components." You eat food. There's no magnesium aisle in the grocery store. So which foods tend to have the most of the good stuff and the least of the bad? I've simplified it into a traffic light illustration (see figure 5).

Just as on the road, *green* means go, *yellow* means caution, and *red* means stop. (In this case, stop and think before you put it into your mouth.) Ideally, green-light foods should be maximized, yellow-light ones minimized, and red-light foods avoided.

Is *avoid* too strong a word? After all, the Dietary Guidelines for Americans merely encourage you to "moderate" your intake of unhealthy foods.[8] For example: "Eat less . . . candy."[9] From a health standpoint, though, shouldn't

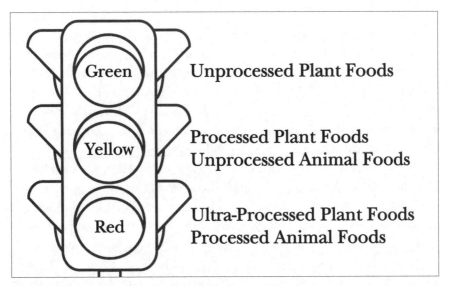

Figure 5

you generally try to avoid candy? Public health authorities don't just advise you to smoke *less* tobacco. They tell you to quit. They know only a small fraction of smokers will actually heed this advice, but it's the job of public health authorities to say what's best and let people make up their own minds.

That's why I appreciate the American Institute for Cancer Research (AICR) recommendations. Not beholden to the USDA, the AICR simply lays out the science. When it comes to the worst of the worst, the institute doesn't pull any punches. Instead of the Dietary Guidelines for Americans' advice to "Consume fewer . . . sodas,"[10] the AICR cancer prevention guidelines advise: "Avoid sugary drinks." Similarly, the AICR doesn't just say to cut back on bacon, ham, hot dogs, sausage, and lunch meats. The cancer guidelines tell you to "avoid processed meat." Period. Why? Because "data do not show any level of intake that can confidently be shown not to be associated with risk."[11]

The healthiest diet is one that maximizes the intake of whole plant foods and minimizes the intake of animal-based foods and processed junk. Simply put, eat more green-light foods. Eat fewer yellow-light foods. And, especially, eat even fewer red-light foods. Just like running red lights in the real world, you may be able to get away with it once in a while, but I wouldn't recommend making a habit out of it.

Given this, what we've seen in the previous chapters makes a lot of sense. Unprocessed plant foods tend to have more of the protective nutrients that Americans are lacking and fewer disease-promoting factors. No wonder the eating habit apparently best able to control our epidemics of dietary disease is a whole-food, plant-based diet. After all, food is a package deal.

This is one of the most important concepts in all of nutrition. Yes, there is calcium in cheese, protein in pork, and iron in beef, but what about all the baggage that comes along with these nutrients—the dose of dairy hormones, the lard, the saturated fat? As much as Burger King proclaims you can "Have It Your Way," you can't go up to the counter and ask for a burger, hold the saturated fat and cholesterol. Food is, indeed, a package deal.

Dairy is the number-one source of calcium in the United States, but it's also the number-one source of saturated fat. What kind of "baggage" do you get along with the calcium in green, leafy vegetables? Fiber, folate, iron, and antioxidants—some of the very nutrients lacking in milk. By getting most of your nutrition from whole plant foods, you get a bonus instead of baggage.

When the National Pork Board promotes ham as an "excellent source of protein,"[12] I can't help but think of the famous quote from a McDonald's senior vice president for marketing who, under oath in a court of law, described Coca-Cola as nutritious because it is "providing water."[13]

Why Don't the Dietary Guidelines Just Say No?

The green-light message shines brightly in pronouncements telling you to "eat more fruits and vegetables," but the yellow and red lights can be dim and cloudy thanks to politics. In other words, the guidelines are clear when there is eat-more messaging ("Eat more fresh produce"), but eat-less messaging is obscured into biochemical components ("Eat less saturated and trans fatty acids"). National health authorities rarely just say to "eat less meat and dairy." That's why my green-light message will sound familiar to you ("Oh, 'eat fruits and veggies'—I've heard that before") but the yellow- and red-light messages may sound controversial ("What? Minimize meat? Really?").

Part of the USDA's mission is "expanding markets for agricultural products."[14] At the same time, the federal agency is tasked with protecting public health by helping to develop the Dietary Guidelines for Americans. That's why, when those two directives are in sync, their eat-more language is clear: "Increase fruit intake." "Increase vegetable intake."[15] But when their dual mandates are in conflict—when "improving nutrition and health" is at odds with promoting "agriculture production"[16]—the eat-less messaging of the Dietary Guidelines gets repackaged and ends up referring to biochemical components: "Reduce intake of solid fats (major sources of saturated and trans fatty acids)."

What's the average consumer supposed to do with that obscure little nugget?

When the Guidelines tell you to eat less added sugar, calories, cholesterol, saturated fat, sodium, and trans fat, that's code for eat less junk food, less meat, less dairy, fewer eggs, and fewer processed foods. But they can't actually say that. When they did in the past, all heck broke loose. For example, when a USDA employee newsletter even suggested trying a meat-free lunch once a week as part of Johns Hopkins University's School of Public Health "Meatless Mondays" initiative,[17] the resulting political firestorm from the meat industry led the USDA to retract the advice just hours later.[18] "As a result of these conflicts [of interest]," concluded an analysis in the *Food and Drug Law Journal*, "the Guidelines sometimes favor the interests of the food and drug industries over the public's interest in accurate and impartial dietary advice."[19]

This reminds me of the landmark report on trans fat from the National Academy of Sciences' Institute of Medicine, one of our most prestigious institutions.[20] They concluded that no amount of trans fat is safe "because any incremental increase in trans fatty acid intake increases C[oronary] H[eart] D[isease] risk."[21] Since trans fats are found naturally in meat and dairy products,[22] this placed them in a quandary: "Because trans fats are unavoidable in ordinary, nonvegan diets, consuming 0 percent of energy would require significant changes in patterns of dietary intake."[23]

So if trans fats are found in meat and dairy and the only safe intake of trans fats is zero, that means the Institute of Medicine went on to encourage everyone to start eating a plant-based diet, right? No, they did not. The director of Harvard's Cardiovascular Epidemiology Program famously explained why: "We can't tell people to stop eating all meat and all dairy products," he said. "Well, we could tell people to become vegetarians," he added. "If we were truly basing this only on science, we would, but it is a bit extreme."[24]

We certainly wouldn't want scientists to base anything on science!

How SAD Is the Standard American Diet?

As cynical as I've become about diet and nutrition in this country, I was still surprised by a 2010 report from the National Cancer Institute on the status of the American diet. For example, three out of four Americans don't eat a single piece of fruit in a given day, and nearly nine out of ten don't reach the minimum recommended daily intake of vegetables. On a weekly

continued

basis, 96 percent of Americans don't reach the minimum for greens or beans (three servings a week for adults), 98 percent don't reach the minimum for orange vegetables (two servings a week), and 99 percent don't reach the minimum for whole grains (about three to four ounces a day).[25]

Then there was the junk food. The federal guidelines were so lax that up to 25 percent of your diet could be made up of "discretionary calories," meaning junk. A quarter of your calories could come from cotton candy washed down with Mountain Dew, and you'd still be within the guidelines. Yet we failed. Astoundingly, 95 percent of Americans exceeded their discretionary calorie allowance. Only *one in a thousand* American children between the ages of two and eight made the cutoff, consuming less than the equivalent of about a dozen spoonfuls of sugar a day.[26]

And we wonder why there is an obesity epidemic?

"In conclusion," the researchers wrote, "nearly the entire U.S. population consumes a diet that is not on par with recommendations. These findings add another piece to the rather disturbing picture that is emerging of a nation's diet in crisis."[27]

Producers of unhealthy commodities aren't out to make you sick. They're just trying to make a buck. Coca-Cola's profit margin, for example, is about one quarter of the soda's retail price, making soft-drink production, alongside tobacco, among the most profitable industries.[28] What's harder to understand is why the public health community isn't doing more about it.

"When the history of the world's attempt to address obesity is written," wrote the head of Yale University's Rudd Center for Food Policy & Obesity, "the greatest failure may be collaboration with and appeasement of the food industry."[29] For instance, Susan G. Komen, a leading U.S. breast cancer charity, linked up with fast-food giant KFC to sell pink buckets of fried chicken.[30]

Save the Children used to be a leader in the push for taxes on soda to offset some of the costs of childhood obesity. Then the organization did an abrupt 180-degree turn, withdrawing its support, saying that such campaigns no longer "fit with the way that Save the Children works." Perhaps it is only a coincidence that it was seeking a grant from Coca-Cola and had already accepted a $5 million grant from Pepsi.[31]

Even though our eating habits are now killing more Americans than our smoking habits,[32] I often hear the refrain in public health circles that we have to work with, rather than against, these companies, because unlike with tobacco, we don't have to smoke, but we do have to eat.[33] Well, yes, we need to breathe—but we don't need to breathe smoke. And yes, we need to eat, but we don't need to eat junk.

How I Define "Processed"

My Traffic Light model stresses two important general concepts: Plant foods, with their greater protective nutritional factors and fewer disease-promoting ones, are healthier than animal foods, and unprocessed foods are healthier than processed foods. Is that always true? No. Am I saying that all plant foods are better than all animal foods? No. In fact, one of the worst items on store shelves is partially hydrogenated vegetable shortening—a product that has *vegetable* right in its name! Even some unprocessed plants—such as blue-green algae—can be toxic.[34] Anyone who's had a bad case of poison ivy knows plants don't always like to be messed with. In general, though, choose plant foods over animal foods, and unprocessed over processed. Michael Pollan, bestselling author of *The Omnivore's Dilemma*, has said, "If it came from a plant, eat it. If it was made in a plant, don't."[35]

What do I mean by *processed*? The classic example is the milling of grains from whole wheat to white flour. Isn't it ironic that these are called "refined" grains, a word meaning improved or made more elegant? The elegance was not felt by the millions who died in the nineteenth century from beriberi, a vitamin B–deficiency disease that resulted from polishing rice from brown to white.[36] (White rice is now fortified with vitamins to compensate for the "refinement.") A Nobel Prize was awarded for the discovery of the cause of beriberi and its cure—rice bran, the brown part of rice that was removed. Beriberi can cause damage to the heart muscle, resulting in death from heart failure. Surely such a thing could never happen in modern times—an epidemic of heart disease that could be prevented and cured with a change in diet? Come on. (Please reread chapter 1.)

Sometimes, however, processing can make foods healthier. For example, tomato juice appears to be the one common juice that may actually be healthier than the whole fruit. The processing of tomato products boosts the availability of the antioxidant red pigment lycopene by as much as fivefold.[37] Similarly, the removal of fat from cacao beans to make cocoa powder improves the nutritional profile, because cocoa butter is one of the rare saturated plant fats (along with coconut and palm kernel oils) that can raise your cholesterol.[38]

So for the purposes of the Traffic Light model, I like to think of "unprocessed" as *nothing bad added, nothing good taken away*. In the above example, tomato juice could be thought of as relatively unprocessed because even much of the fiber is retained—unless salt is added, which would make it a processed food in my book and bump it right out of the green zone. Similarly, I would consider chocolate—but not cocoa powder—processed because sugar is added.

Using my definition of *nothing bad added, nothing good taken away*, steel-cut oats, rolled oats, and even (plain) instant oatmeal can all be considered unprocessed. Almonds are obviously a whole plant food. I would also consider no-salt-added almond butter to be a green-light food, but even unsweetened almond milk is a processed food, a food from which nutrition has been stolen. Am I saying almond milk is bad for you? Foods are not so much good or bad as they are better or worse. All I'm saying is that unprocessed foods tend to be healthier than processed ones. Think of it this way: Eating almonds is healthier than drinking almond milk.

The limited role I see for yellow-light foods in a healthy diet is to promote the consumption of green-light foods. For instance, if the only way I can get patients to eat oatmeal in the morning is if they make it creamy with almond milk, then I tell them to go right ahead. The same could be said for red-light foods. Without hot sauce, my intake of dark-green, leafy vegetables would plummet. Yes, I know there are all sorts of sodium-free, exotically flavored vinegars out there that I could use, and maybe one day I'll wean myself off Tabasco. But given my current tastes, the green ends justify the red means. If the *only* way you're going to eat a big salad is to sprinkle Bac-Os on top, then sprinkle away.

Bac-Os are what are referred to as *ultra*processed foods, bearing no redeeming nutritional qualities or resemblance to anything that grew out of the ground and often containing added garbage. Bac-Os, for example, have added trans fats, salt, sugar, and Red 40, a food dye banned in a number of European countries.[39] As a red-light food, it ideally should be avoided, but if the alternative to your big spinach salad with Bac-Os is KFC, then it's better to have the salad with the Bac-Os. They can be the spoonful of sugar that makes the medicine go down. The same goes for real bacon bits, for that matter.

I realize some people have religious or ethical objections to even trivial amounts of animal products. (Growing up Jewish near the largest pig factory west of the Mississippi, I can relate to both sentiments.) But from a human health standpoint, when it comes to animal products and processed foods, it's the overall diet that matters.

What Does "Whole-Food, Plant-Based" Mean, Exactly?

Sometimes people's diets take on a religiosity of their own. I remember a man once telling me that he could never "go plant based" because he could never give up his grandma's chicken soup. *Huh?* Then don't! After I asked him to say hello to his bubby for me, I told him that enjoying her soup shouldn't keep him from making healthier choices the rest of the time. The problem with all-or-nothing thinking is that it keeps people from even taking the first steps. The thought of *never* having pepperoni pizza again somehow turns into an excuse to keep ordering it every week. Why not scale down to once a month or reserve it for special occasions? We cannot let the "perfect" be the enemy of the good.

It's really the day-to-day stuff that matters most. What you eat on special occasions is insignificant compared to what you eat day in and day out. So don't beat yourself up if you really want to put edible bacon-flavored candles on your birthday cake. (I'm not making those up![40]) Your body has a remarkable ability to recover from sporadic insults as long as you're not habitually poking it with a fork.

This book is not about vegetarianism, veganism, or any other "-ism." There are people who completely eliminate any and all animal products as part of a religious or moral stance and may indeed end up better off as a side benefit.[41] But strictly from a human health standpoint, you would be hard pressed to argue, for example, that the traditional Okinawan diet, which is 96 percent plant based,[42] is inferior to a typical Western, 100 percent vegan diet. In Kaiser Permanente's guide "The Plant-Based Diet: A Healthier Way to Eat," the authors define a plant-based diet as one that excludes animal products completely, but they make sure to note: "If you find you cannot do a plant-based diet 100 percent of the time, then aim for 80 percent. Any movement toward more plants and fewer animal products can improve your health!"[43]

From a nutrition standpoint, the reason I don't like the terms *vegetarian* and *vegan* is that they are only defined by what you *don't* eat. When I used to speak on college campuses, I would meet vegans who appeared to be living off french fries and beer. Vegan, technically, but not exactly health promoting. That's why I prefer the term *whole-food, plant-based nutrition*. As far as I can discern, the best available balance of evidence suggests that the healthiest diet is one centered on unprocessed plant foods. On a day-to-day basis, the more whole plant foods and the fewer processed and animal products, the better.[44]

Preparing Yourself for Healthier Habits

First, you need to know your own psychology. There are certain personality types that do better when they go all in. If you tend to have an "addictive" personality, or if you are the kind of person who takes things to extremes—for instance, you either don't drink at all or you drink in excess—it's probably best for you to try to stick with the program. But some individuals can get away with "social smoking," for example; they can light up a few times a year and escape nicotine dependence.[45] The reason we as physicians advocate for smokers to quit completely is not because we think that one cigarette every once in a while is going to do irreversible damage but because we're afraid that one cigarette may lead to two, and, before long, the unhealthy habit has taken hold. Similarly, one (well-cooked) hamburger is not going to kill anyone. It's what you eat day to day that adds up. You have to take stock of your disposition to know if you can overcome the risk of sliding down the slippery slope.

There's a concept in psychology called "decision fatigue" that marketers use to exploit consumers. It appears humans have a limited capacity to make many decisions in one short stretch of time, and the quality of our decisions will deteriorate to the extent that we eventually begin making downright irrational choices. Ever wonder why supermarkets stack the junk food at the checkout counter? After wading through the forty thousand items in the average supermarket,[46] we end up with less willpower to resist impulse purchases.[47] So making rules for yourself and sticking to them may help you make more sensible choices over the long run. For instance, making a strict decision to never cook with oil, to avoid meat entirely, or to eat only whole grains may paradoxically make for sturdier life changes. By not having junk food in the house, you remove the temptation by removing the choice. I know if I get hungry enough I'll eat an apple.

There may also be a *physiological* argument for not wildly deviating from a well-planned diet. After a vacation cruise during which you indulged in all manner of rich foods, your palate may get dulled to the point where the natural foods you enjoyed just the week before no longer deliver the same taste satisfaction. For some, this may simply require a period of readjustment. But for others, this departure from an otherwise healthy diet may lead back to a dietary glut involving added salt, sugar, and fat.

For those of us who grew up eating SAD (the Standard American Diet), starting to eat healthfully can be a big shift. I know it was for me. Though my mom tried to keep us eating good-for-us foods at home, when I was hanging out with friends, we'd go through boxes of Little Debbie snack cakes and indulge in greasy meals at the local Chinese restaurant, where I'd order spareribs or any other dish with chunks of deep-fried meat. One of my favorite snacks was nacho cheese–flavored Slim Jims.

Thankfully, I was able to escape SAD's clutches before any overt health problems arose. That was twenty-five years ago. Looking back, I view that as one of the best decisions of my life.

Some go cold turkey, if you will, while others transition more slowly using a variety of approaches. One I've used personally in my medical practice is Kaiser Permanente's three-step method. Realizing that most American families tend to rotate through the same eight or nine meals, step one suggests that you think of three meals you already enjoy that are plant based, like pasta and marinara sauce that could be easily tweaked to whole-grain pasta with some added veggies. Step two asks you to think of three meals you already eat that could be *adapted* to become a green-light meal, like switching from beef chili to five-bean chili. Step three is my favorite: Discover new healthy options.[48]

Ironically, many people following healthy diets report eating an even greater variety of foods than when they ate their former "unrestricted" diet. Before widespread use of the Internet, I used to tell people to go to their public libraries and borrow cookbooks. Today, Google whole-food, plant-based recipes, and a million hits pop up. If you're feeling overwhelmed, good places to start include:

- **ForksOverKnives.com:** This site of the wildly popular documentary and book of the same name offers hundreds of recipes.
- **StraightUpFood.com:** Cooking instructor Cathy Fisher shares more than one hundred recipes on this site.
- **HappyHealthyLongLife.com:** This site's tagline reads: "A [Cleveland Clinic] medical librarian's adventures in evidence-based living." She used the *e* word—I think I'm in love!

Once you've found three new meals you enjoy and can prepare with ease, step three is complete. You now have a nine-meal rotation, and you're off! After that, moving on to breakfast and lunch is easy.

If you hate to cook and just want the cheapest, easiest way to make healthy meals, I highly recommend dietitian Jeff Novick's *Fast Food* DVD series. Using common staples like canned beans, frozen vegetables, quick-cook whole grains, and spice mixes, Jeff shows you how you can feed your family healthfully in no time for about four dollars a day per person. The DVDs also include grocery store walk-throughs, shopping tips, and information on how to decipher nutrition labels. Check out his cooking series at JeffNovick.com/RD/DVDs.

If you crave more structure and social support, the Physicians Committee for Responsible Medicine (PCRM), a nonprofit nutrition research and policy advocacy organization in Washington, D.C., has a fantastic three-week kickstart program for plant-based eating. Check it out at 21DayKickstart.org. This free online nutrition program starts the first of every month and offers a full meal plan, recipes, tips, resources, a restaurant guide, and a community forum. As of this writing, it's offered in four languages. Hundreds of thousands of people have already benefited from it, so feel free to give it a try.

I've always tried to get my patients to think of healthy eating as an experiment. It can be overwhelming to think of such a sweeping change as permanent. That's why I ask them to give me just three weeks. I find that if my patients think of it simply as an experiment, they're more likely to go whole hog (whole grain?) and realize the maximum benefits. But that's just me being sneaky. I know that once those three weeks are up, if they really gave it their all, they will be feeling so much better, their lab values will be looking so much better, and their palates will have started to change. Healthy eating tastes better and better the longer you stick with it.

I remember talking about this with Dr. Neal Barnard, founding president of PCRM, which publishes a great deal of research pitting a healthy diet against a variety of common ailments—everything from acne and arthritis to menstrual cramps and migraines. He often uses what's called an "A-B-A" study design. Participants' health is assessed at baseline on their regular diets, and then they're switched to a therapeutic diet. In an effort to make sure any health changes participants experience on the new diet aren't merely a coincidence, they are then switched back to their regular diet to see if the changes disappear.

This kind of rigorous study design improves the validity of the results, but the problem, Dr. Barnard related, is that sometimes people improve *too* much. After a few weeks on a plant-based diet, sometimes people feel so much better that they refuse to go back on their baseline diet[49]—even though it's required by the study protocol. Since they didn't complete the study as planned, their data have to be effectively thrown out and may never make it into the final paper. Ironically, healthy eating can be so effective that it undermines its own studies of effectiveness!

WWDGE: What Would Dr. Greger Eat?

I'm regularly asked what I eat every day. I've always been hesitant to answer for a number of reasons. First, it shouldn't matter what I or anyone else eats, says, or does. The science is the science. Too much of the nutrition world is split into camps, each following their respective guru. What other field of serious scientific inquiry is like that? After all, $2 + 2 = 4$ regardless of what your favorite mathematician thinks. This is because there isn't a trillion-dollar industry that profits from confusing people about arithmetic. If you were getting conflicting messages from all sides about basic math, in desperation, you might have to choose one authority to stick with, hoping that person will accurately represent the available research. Who has time to read and decipher all the original source material?

Early on in my practice, I decided that I didn't want to rely on anyone else's interpretation for what could ultimately be life-or-death decisions for my patients. I had the access, the resources, and the background to interpret the science on my own. When I initially began my annual reviews of the nutrition literature, it was really just to make myself a better doctor. But when I discovered such a treasure trove of information, I knew I couldn't keep it to myself. My hope is to disseminate it in a way that removes me as much as possible from the equation. I don't want to present the trademarked Dr. Greger Diet; I want to present the best-available-evidence diet. That's why I show the original papers, charts, graphs, and quotes with links to all the primary sources in my Nutrition Facts.org videos. I try to keep my own interpretation to a minimum—though admittedly, I sometimes can't help myself!

What a person chooses to do with information is highly personalized and often depends on such factors as his or her current life situation and how risk averse he or she is. Given the same information, two people can make two entirely different but legitimate decisions. For this reason, I've been hesitant to share my own personal choices, because I'm afraid they'll unduly sway people to make decisions that might not be right for them. I'd rather just present the science and let others decide for themselves.

In addition, everyone's taste buds are different. I can imagine someone thinking, *He puts hot sauce on what?* When people hear me talk about the wonders of hummus (a Middle Eastern chickpea spread) but not baba ganoush (a Middle

Eastern roasted-eggplant spread), they might come away with the impression that I think one is healthier than the other. This may be (and probably is, actually), but my real reason is simple: I don't like the taste of eggplant.

Conversely, just because I eat something doesn't mean it's healthy. For example, people are surprised to hear I use dutched (alkali-processed) cocoa. In that process, more than half of the antioxidants and flavanol phytonutrients are wiped out.[50] Why would I use it, then? Because it tastes so much better to me than unprocessed cocoa. While I encourage people to use natural cocoa, I don't take my own advice in that regard. In some cases, it would be better if people would do as I say, not as I do.

And what if I shared a recipe that someone found utterly repulsive? I would hate for him or her to think, *If this is healthy eating, count me out!* As you eat healthier, your palate actually changes. It's an amazing phenomenon. Your taste buds are constantly adapting—minute to minute, in fact. If you drank some orange juice right now, it would taste sweet. But if you first ate some candy and then drank the same OJ, it could taste unpleasantly bitter. Over the long term, the more you eat healthfully, the better healthy foods taste.

I remember the first time I sipped a green smoothie. I was speaking somewhere in Michigan, hosted by a darling physician couple. They told me that they drank "blended salads" for breakfast. Intellectually, I loved the idea. Greens, the healthiest food on the planet, in convenient liquid form? I envisioned myself drinking a salad on my way to work every day. But then I tasted it. It felt like I was drinking someone's lawn. I gagged and almost threw up over my hosts' kitchen table.

Green smoothies are something you have to build up to. Everyone loves fruit smoothies. A frozen banana, strawberries—yum! And surprisingly, you can throw a handful of baby spinach in there and you may hardly even taste it. Give it a try! You'll be surprised. Okay, so if one handful is good, how about two? Slowly, your taste buds can adapt to increasing quantities of greens. This happens with all your senses. Walk into a dark room, and your eyes will slowly adapt. Stick your foot into a hot bath, and though at first it may be too hot, your body equilibrates to a new normal. Likewise, in just a couple of weeks, you can be drinking—and enjoying—concoctions you'd now consider absolutely wretched.

Having said all that, I will now proceed to tell you what I eat, what I drink, what I do, and how I do it. In each subsequent chapter, I will dive deeper into each of the entries on my Daily Dozen checklist to describe which types of these green-light foods are my favorites, as well as the tricks and techniques I use to prepare them. I will not be detailing every type of bean, fruit, vegetable, nut, or spice that I eat. Rather, my goal here is to explore some of the interesting science behind a few of my favorite options in each category.

Please understand that my strategy is *a* way to do it rather than *the* way to do it. If it happens to work for you too, great. If not, I hope you'll explore the myriad other ways you could use this same body of evidence to help improve and prolong your life.

Dr. Greger's Daily Dozen

Whole-food, plant-based nutrition—pretty self-explanatory, right? But aren't some green-light foods better than others? For example, you can apparently live extended periods eating practically nothing but potatoes.[1] That would, by definition, be a whole-food, plant-based diet—but not a very healthy one. All plant foods are not created equal.

The more I've researched over the years, the more I've come to realize that healthy foods are not necessary interchangeable. Some foods and food groups have special nutrients not found in abundance elsewhere. For example, sulforaphane, the amazing liver-enzyme detox-boosting compound I profiled in chapters 9 and 11, is derived nearly exclusively from cruciferous vegetables. You could eat tons of other kinds of greens and vegetables on a given day and get no appreciable sulforaphane if you didn't eat something cruciferous. It's the same with flaxseeds and the anticancer lignan compounds. As I mentioned in chapters 11 and 13, flax may average one hundred times more lignans than other foods. And mushrooms aren't even plants at all; they belong to an entirely different biological classification and may contain nutrients (like ergothioneine) not made anywhere in the plant kingdom.[2] (So technically, maybe I should be referring to a whole-food, plant- and fungus-based diet, but that just sounds kind of gross.)

It seems like every time I come home from the medical library buzzing with some exciting new data, my family rolls their eyes, sighs, and asks, "What can't we eat now?" Or they'll say, "Wait a second. Why does everything seem to have parsley in it all of a sudden?" My poor family. They've been very tolerant.

As the list of foods I tried to fit into my daily diet grew, I made a checklist

Daily Dozen

No. of servings

☑☑☑   Beans

☑   Berries

☑☑☑   Other Fruits

☑   Cruciferous Vegetables

☑☑   Greens

☑☑   Other Vegetables

☑   Flaxseeds

☑   Nuts

☑   Spices

☑☑☑   Whole Grains

☑☑☑☑☑   Beverages

☑   Exercise

Figure 6

and had it on a little dry-erase board on the fridge. We would make a game out of ticking off the boxes. This evolved into the Daily Dozen (see figure 6).

By *beans*, I mean legumes, which comprise all the different kinds of beans, including soybeans, split peas, chickpeas, and lentils. While eating a bowl of pea soup or dipping carrots into hummus may not seem like eating beans, it is. You should try to get three servings a day. A serving is defined as a quarter cup of hummus or bean dip; a half cup of cooked beans, split peas, lentils, tofu, or tempeh; or a full cup of fresh peas or sprouted lentils. Though peanuts are technically legumes, nutritionally, I've grouped them in the Nuts category, just as I would consider green (snap or string) beans to be better placed in the Other Vegetables category.

A serving of berries is a half cup of fresh or frozen, or a quarter cup of dried.

While biologically speaking, avocados, bananas, and even watermelons are technically berries, I'm using the colloquial term for any small edible fruit, which is why I include kumquats and grapes (and raisins) in this category, as well as fruits that are typically thought of as berries but aren't technically, such as blackberries, cherries, mulberries, raspberries, and strawberries.

For other fruits, a serving is a medium-sized fruit, a cup of cut-up fruit, or a quarter cup of dried fruit. Again, I'm using the colloquial rather than the botanical definition, so I place tomatoes in the Other Vegetables group. (Interestingly, this is something the U.S. Supreme Court actually ruled on in 1893.[3] Arkansas decided to have it both ways, declaring tomatoes both the official state fruit *and* the official state vegetable.[4])

Common cruciferous vegetables include broccoli, cabbage, collards, and kale. I recommend at least one serving a day (typically a half cup) and at least two additional servings of greens a day, cruciferous or otherwise. Serving sizes for other greens and vegetables are a cup for raw leafy vegetables, a half cup for other raw or cooked vegetables, and a quarter cup for dried mushrooms.

Everyone should try to incorporate one tablespoon of ground flaxseeds into his or her daily diet, in addition to a serving of nuts or other seeds. A quarter cup of nuts is considered a serving, or two tablespoons of nut or seed butters, including peanut butter. (Chestnuts and coconuts don't nutritionally count as nuts.)

I also recommend one-quarter teaspoon a day of the spice turmeric, along with any other (salt-free) herbs and spices you may enjoy.

A serving of whole grains can be considered a half cup of hot cereal such as oatmeal, cooked grain such as rice (including the "pseudograins" amaranth, buckwheat, and quinoa), cooked pasta, or corn kernels; a cup of ready-to-eat (cold) cereal; one tortilla or slice of bread; half a bagel or english muffin; or three cups of popped popcorn.

The serving size in the beverage category is one glass (twelve ounces), and the recommended five glasses a day is in addition to the water you get naturally from the foods in your diet.

Finally, I advise one daily "serving" of exercise, which can be split up over the day. I recommend ninety minutes of moderate-intensity activity, such as brisk (four miles per hour) walking or forty minutes of vigorous activity (such as jogging or active sports) each day. Why so much? I'll explain my reasoning in the Exercise chapter.

This may all sound like a lot of boxes to check, but it's not difficult to knock off a bunch at one time. One simple peanut butter and banana sandwich and you just checked off four boxes. Or imagine sitting down to a big salad. Two cups of spinach, a handful of arugula, a handful of toasted walnuts, a half cup of chickpeas, a half cup of red bell pepper, and a small tomato. You just knocked out *seven* boxes in one dish. Sprinkle on your flax, add a handful of goji berries, and enjoy it with a glass of water and fruit for dessert, and you could wipe out nearly half your daily check boxes in a single meal. And then if you ate it on a treadmill . . . just kidding!

Do I check off each glass of water I drink? No. In fact, I don't even use the checklist anymore; I just used it initially as a tool to get me into a routine. Whenever I was sitting down to a meal, I would ask myself, *Could I add greens to this? Could I add beans to that?* (I always have an open can of beans in the fridge.) *Can I sprinkle on some flax or pumpkin seeds, or maybe some dried fruit?* The checklist just got me into the habit of thinking, *How can I make this meal even healthier?*

I also found the checklist helped with grocery shopping. Although I always keep bags of frozen berries and greens in the freezer, if I'm at the store and want to buy fresh produce for the week, it helps me figure out how much kale or blueberries I need.

The checklist also helps me picture what a meal might look like. Looking over the checklist, you'll see there are three servings each of beans, fruits, and whole grains, and about twice as many veggies in total than any other food component. Glancing at my plate, I can imagine one quarter of it filled with grains, one quarter with legumes, and a half plate filled with vegetables, along with maybe a side salad and fruit for dessert. I prefer one-bowl meals where everything's mixed together, but the checklist still helps me to visualize. Instead of a big bowl of spaghetti with some veggies and lentils on top, I think of a big bowl of vegetables with some pasta and lentils mixed in. Instead of a big plate of brown rice with some stir-fried vegetables on top, I picture a meal that's mostly veggies—and oh look! There's some rice and beans in there too.

But there is no need to be obsessive about the Daily Dozen. On hectic travel days when I've burned through my snacks and I'm trying to piece together some semblance of a healthy meal at the airport food court, sometimes I'm lucky if I even hit a quarter of my goals. If you eat poorly on one day, just try to eat better the next. My hope is that the checklist will serve you as a helpful reminder to try to eat a variety of the healthiest foods every day.

But should you eat your veggies raw or cooked? Do you need to choose organic or is conventional okay? What about GMOs? Gluten? All these questions and more will be answered as I go through each of the Daily Dozen in detail in the following chapters.

Beans

The federal government's MyPlate campaign was developed to prompt Americans to think about building healthy meals. Most of your plate should be covered with vegetables and grains, preferably whole grains, with the rest of the plate split between fruits and the protein group. Legumes were given special treatment, straddling both the protein and the vegetable groups. They're loaded with protein, iron, and zinc, as you might expect from other protein sources like meat, but legumes also contain nutrients that are concentrated in the vegetable kingdom, including fiber, folate, and potassium. You get the best of both worlds with beans, all the while enjoying foods that are naturally low in saturated fat and sodium and free of cholesterol.

The most comprehensive analysis of diet and cancer ever performed was published in 2007 by the American Institute for Cancer Research. Sifting through some half a million studies, nine independent research teams from around the globe created a landmark scientific consensus report reviewed by twenty-one of the top cancer researchers in the world. One of their summary cancer-prevention recommendations is to eat whole grains and/or legumes (beans, split peas, chickpeas, or lentils) with every meal.[1] Not every week or every day. *Every meal!*

Having some oatmeal in the morning makes it easy enough to fulfill the whole grains recommendation, but legumes? Who eats beans for breakfast? Well, lots of people around the world do. A traditional English breakfast includes savory combinations of baked beans on toast, mushrooms, and grilled tomatoes. Japanese breakfasts traditionally include miso soup, and many children in India start their days with idli, a type of steamed lentil cake. More familiar ways for American palates to meet the cancer prevention guidelines might be a whole-grain bagel schmeared with hummus. My friend Paul mashes cannellini beans into his oatmeal and swears you can't even see or taste them. Why not?

Soy

Soybeans are probably the beans Americans are most comfortable incorporating into their breakfasts. Soy milk, for instance, has grown into a billion-dollar business. But soy milk and even tofu are processed foods. When it comes to the nutrients you tend to associate with legumes—fiber, iron, magnesium, potassium, protein, and zinc—about half are lost when soybeans are converted into tofu. However, beans are so healthy that you can throw away half the nutrition and *still* have a really healthy food. If you do eat tofu, choose varieties made with calcium (you'll see it in the ingredients list), which can weigh in at a whopping 550 mg of calcium per (3 oz) slice.[2]

Even better than tofu, though, would be a *whole* soy food like tempeh, which is a type of fermented soybean patty. If you look closely at tempeh, you can actually see all the little soybeans. I don't usually eat tempeh for breakfast, but I do like to slice it thin, dip it into a thick flax "egg" mixture (see page 341 for my recipe), dredge it through some rosemary-seasoned whole-grain bread crumbs or coarse blue cornmeal, and bake it in my toaster oven at about 400°F until golden brown. Then I dip it in buffalo hot sauce for a healthier approximation of the chicken wings I enjoyed in my youth.

What About GMO Soy?

A prominent scientific journal recently editorialized that although we are now swimming in information about genetically modified crops, much of what we're being told is wrong—from both sides of the debate. "But a lot of this incorrect information is sophisticated, backed by legitimate-sounding research and written with certitude," the editorial read, quipping that when it comes to GMOs, a good gauge of a statement's fallacy may be "the conviction with which it is delivered."[3]

Monsanto's Roundup Ready soybeans are the number-one genetically modified crop, engineered to be resistant to the herbicide Roundup (also sold by Monsanto), which allows farmers to spray the crops to kill weeds while leaving the soy standing.[4]

Though much debate continues to swarm around the hypothetical risks of GMO crops, the greater concern for human health may be the potential for GMO crops to contain elevated pesticide residues.[5] This fear was realized in 2014 when high levels of Roundup pesticides were reported on GMO soybeans (but not on non-GMO or organic soybeans).[6] The pesticide levels were considered high compared to maximum allowable residue levels at the time, but were they high enough to have adverse effects on consumers?

Anti-GMO activists point to studies showing Roundup may interfere with embryonic development and disrupt hormones. These studies were, respectively, on sea urchin embryos[7] and cells from mouse testicles.[8] Blogs scream headlines like "Men! Save Your Testicles," citing articles with concerning names like "Prepubertal Exposure to Commercial Formulation of the Herbicide Glyphosate Alters Testosterone Levels and Testicular Morphology."[9] But that study was about puberty in rats. I doubt the blog would have gotten as many hits if it had been titled "Men! Save Prepubescent Rats' Testicles!"[10]

Am I being too harsh? After all, where could scientists find live human tissue to experiment on? A research team came up with a brilliant solution—study placentas! Millions of women in the United States give birth each year, and the placenta, the temporary organ formed in the uterus to nourish the fetus during pregnancy, is typically incinerated after delivery. Why not test Roundup on human placental tissue? The researchers did so and found that at the concentration that's sprayed on crops in the fields, the pesticides did indeed have toxic effects on human tissue.[11]

That finding may help explain the few tentative studies suggesting adverse effects on pesticide workers[12,13] and their children,[14] but by the time the pesticides enter the food supply, they are highly diluted. Concentrations of Roundup pesticides may only reach a few parts per million in food and a few parts per billion in your body. Researchers, however, discovered the pesticide may still have effects at a few parts per *trillion*. Even at that minuscule dose, Roundup pesticides were found to have estrogenic effects in vitro, stimulating the growth of estrogen-receptor-positive human breast cancer cells.[15]

As we saw in chapter 11, though, soy consumption is associated with *lower* breast cancer risk and improved breast cancer survival. That may be because most GMO soy in the United States is used as feed for chickens, pigs, and cattle, whereas most of the major soy *food* manufacturers use non-GMO soy. It could also be because the benefits of eating any kind of soy far outweigh the risks. Regardless, why accept any risk at all when you can choose organic soy products, which by law exclude GMOs?

The bottom line is that there is no direct human data suggesting any harm from eating GMO crops, though such studies haven't been done (which critics say is exactly the point).[16] That's why mandatory labeling on GMO products would be helpful, so that public health researchers can track whether or not GMOs are having any adverse effects.

But I believe it is important to put the GMO issue in perspective. As I've tried to show, there are dietary and lifestyle changes we can make that could eliminate most heart disease, strokes, diabetes, and cancer. *Millions* of lives could be saved. For this reason, I'm sympathetic to the biotech industry's exasperation about GMO concerns when we still have people dropping dead from everything else they're eating.[17] As one review concluded: "Consumption of genetically modified food entails risk of undesirable effects similar to the consumption of traditional food."[18] In other words, buying the non-GMO Twinkie isn't doing your body much good.

Miso is another fermented whole soy food. This thick paste is commonly mixed with hot water to make a delicious soup that's a staple in Japanese cuisine. If you want to give it a try, I suggest white miso, which has a mellower flavor than red miso. Making miso soup can be as easy as mixing one tablespoon of miso with two cups of hot water and whatever vegetables you prefer. That's it!

Because miso may contain probiotic bacteria,[19] it's probably best not to actually cook the miso, lest the good bugs be wiped out. When I prepare it, I boil dried mushrooms, a pinch of arame seaweed, a few sun-dried tomatoes, and greens in a pot and ladle off about a quarter cup of hot broth into a large bowl, add the miso, and mash it with a fork until only a thin paste remains. I then pour the rest of the soup into the bowl and stir to combine it with the miso. And, because I'm a bit of a hot-sauce freak, I add some Sriracha for a little kick. My new favorite addition is freshly toasted sesame seeds. I pour out a layer of raw, hulled sesame seeds, put them in the toaster oven until they just start to turn golden, and then throw them sizzling into the soup. Makes the whole kitchen smell heavenly.

Miso Soup: Soy Versus Sodium

The process of producing miso involves adding salt—lots of salt. A single bowl of miso soup could contain half the American Heart Association's recommended daily limit, which is why I always reflexively avoided it when I'd see it on a menu. But when I actually looked into it, I was surprised by what I found.

There are two principal reasons to avoid salt: stomach cancer and high blood pressure. Considered a "probable cause" of stomach cancer,[20] excess salt intake may cause thousands of cases every year in the United States.[21] The elevated stomach cancer risk associated with salt intake appears on par with that of smoking or heavy alcohol use but may only be half as bad as opium use[22] or a daily serving of meat. A study of nearly a half-million people found that a daily portion of meat (about the size of a deck of cards) was associated with up to five times the odds of stomach cancer.[23]

This may explain why people eating plant-based diets appear to be at significantly lower risk.[24] But it's not just sodium-rich animal products like processed meats and salted fish that are associated with higher stomach cancer risk—pickled plant foods are as well.[25] Kimchi, a spicy pickled vegetable side dish, is a staple in Korean cuisine and could help explain why that country may have the highest stomach cancer rates in the world.[26]

Miso, however, was *not* associated with increased cancer risk.[27] The carcinogenic effects of the salt may be counteracted by the anticarcinogenic effects of the soy. For example, tofu intake has been associated with about 50 percent less stomach cancer risk[28] and salt with about 50 percent more risk,[29] which explains how they may effectively cancel each other out. Further protection apparently offered by allium (onion) family vegetables[30] may tip the cancer-fighting scale in favor of miso soup that's garlicky or has some scallions thrown in.

Cancer isn't the primary reason people are told to avoid salt, though. What about miso soup and high blood pressure? There may be a similar relationship. The salt in miso may push up your blood pressure while the soy protein in miso may lower it back down.[31] For example, if you compare the effects of soy milk to skim milk (to make a fairer comparison by removing the saturated butterfat factor), soy milk lowers blood pressure about nine times more effectively than skim dairy milk.[32] Would the benefits of soy be enough to counter the effects of the salt in miso, though? Japanese researchers decided to find out.

Over a four-year period, they tracked men and women in their sixties who started out with normal blood pressures to see who was more likely to be diagnosed with high blood pressure: those who had two or more bowls of miso soup a day or those who had one or less. Two bowls a day would be like adding half a teaspoon of salt to your daily diet, yet those who consumed at least that much miso were found to have five times *lower* risk of becoming hypertensive. The researchers concluded: "Our results on miso-soup have shown that [the] anti-hypertensive effect of miso is possibly above [the] hypertensive effect of salt."[33] So miso soup may actually be protective overall.

Edamame is about as whole a soy food as you can get. After all, these are soybeans still in their pods. You can buy them frozen and just throw a handful into some boiling water anytime you want a healthy snack. They cook in about five minutes. All you need to do is strain them and, if you're like me, crack lots of fresh pepper onto the pods and nibble the beans right out. (You can also buy them pre-shelled, but then they're not as fun to eat.)

On the opposite end of the processing spectrum are plant-based meat alternatives like veggie burgers, which are healthy only insofar as they replace the real thing. Beyond Chicken, for example, has fiber, zero saturated fat, zero cholesterol, and equal protein to and fewer calories than an actual chicken breast (plus presumably less food-poisoning risk). But Beyond Chicken pales in comparison to the nutrition found in the soybeans, yellow peas, and amaranth grain from which it was made. Of course, people choosing these meat alternatives are not standing in the grocery store agonizing between Beyond Chicken Grilled Strips and a bowl of legumes and whole grains. So if fajitas are the foregone conclusion, then it would certainly be healthier to choose the plant-based mock meat to the meat itself. I see the value of these meat-alternative products as healthier transition foods to wean people off the standard American diet. Even if you just stopped there, you'd be better off, but the more you can move toward whole-food nutrition, the better. You don't want to get stuck at the yellow light.

Peas

Like edamame, raw english peas (also known as shell or garden peas) can be a great au naturel snack. I fell in love with peas in the pod when I first picked them off the vine at a farm my brother and I spent time on one summer as kids. They were like candy. Every year, I look forward to the few weeks I can find them fresh.

Lentils

Lentils are little lens-shaped legumes. (Lenses were actually named after lentils; *lens* is lentil in Latin.) They gained fame in 1982 upon the discovery of the "lentil effect," or the ability of lentil consumption to blunt the sugar spike of foods consumed hours later at a subsequent meal.[34] Lentils are so rich in prebiotics that they create a feast for your friendly flora, which in turn feed you right back with beneficial compounds, such as propionate, that relax your stomach and slow the rate at which sugars are absorbed into your system.[35] Chickpeas and other legumes were found to have a similar influence, and so this phenomenon was later renamed the "second-meal effect."[36]

Lentils are already one of the most nutrient-dense legumes. But when sprouted, their antioxidant power doubles (and even quintuples for chickpeas).[37] Lentils can be easily sprouted into one of the healthiest possible snacks. I was amazed when I first tried making them. What start out looking like hard little pebbles transform into tender morsels in just a couple of days. Why add protein powder to your smoothies when you can add sprouted lentils? In a sprouting jar, or simply a mason jar covered with cheesecloth secured with a rubber band, soak lentils overnight in water, drain, and then rinse and drain twice daily for another couple of days. Sprouting to me is like gardening on steroids—I can create fresh produce in three days right on my kitchen counter. (Of course, if you open a can of lentils, you can enjoy them in about three seconds.)

Are Canned Beans as Healthy as Home Cooked?

Canned beans are convenient, but are they as nutritious as home cooked? A recent study discovered that indeed canned beans are as healthy as boiled beans—with one exception: sodium. Salt is often added to canned beans, resulting in sodium levels up to one hundred times more than if you cooked them without any salt.[38] Draining and rinsing your canned beans can remove about half the added salt, but then you'd also be rinsing away some of the nutrition. I recommend purchasing the no-salt-added varieties and cooking with the bean liquid in whatever dish you're whipping up.

Home-cooked beans may come out tastier, particularly texture-wise. Canned beans can sometimes be a bit mushy, whereas when properly soaked and cooked, beans can come out nice and firm yet tender. Using dried beans is also cheaper. Some bean-counting researchers found that canned beans can be about three times as expensive as home cooked, but the difference only came out to about twenty cents per serving.[39] My family chooses to spend that extra twenty cents to save the hours beans can take to cook.

The only legumes I have the patience to cook from scratch are lentils. They cook quickly and don't need to be presoaked. You can just simmer them as you would pasta, in a pot with an abundance of water, for about half an hour. In fact, if you're making pasta and have the time, why not let some lentils boil in the water for twenty minutes before adding in the pasta? Lentils are great in spaghetti sauce. That's what I do when I make rice or quinoa: I throw a handful of dried lentils into the rice cooker, and they're done when the grain is cooked. Mashed and seasoned cooked lentils also make a great veggie dip. Double check marks!

Dipping veggies in hummus is a double-check-box snack. And don't forget other bean blending, from garlicky white bean spreads and pinto pâtés to spicy black bean dip. Another fantastic snack (can you tell I love snacking?) is roasted chickpeas. Google it. My favorite, not surprisingly, is the buffalo ranch flavor (from the *Kid Tested Firefighter Approved* blog[40]), using a silicone baking mat.

Mealtime options can include dishes like bean burritos; chili; pasta e fagioli; red beans and rice; minestrone; Tuscan white bean stew; and black bean, lentil, or split pea soup. My mom turned me on to dehydrated precooked pea soup mixes. (The lowest sodium brand I've been able to find is from Dr. John McDougall's food line.) You simply add the mix to boiling water with some frozen greens and stir. (Whole Foods Market sells inexpensive one-pound frozen bags of a prechopped blend of kale, collard, and mustard greens. Couldn't be easier!) I pack pea soup mix when I travel. It's lightweight, and I can prepare it in the hotel room coffeemaker.

Big Bucks on Beans' Benefits

For more than a decade, soy foods have enjoyed the rare privilege of an "FDA-approved" food-label health claim about soy's ability to protect against heart disease. A billion-dollar industry, Big Soy has a lot of money to fund research touting the benefits of their bean. But is soy really the top bean, or are other legumes just as powerful? It turns out that *non*-soy beans, including lentils, lima beans, navy beans, and pinto beans, drop bad cholesterol levels[41] as effectively as soy protein.[42] One study, for example, found that eating a half a cup a day of cooked pinto beans for two months may drop your cholesterol by nineteen points.[43]

One of my favorite go-to quickie meals starts with toasting some corn tortillas. (Food for Life, the same company that makes Ezekiel bread, makes a sprouted yellow corn tortilla usually sold in the frozen section.) Then I mash some canned beans on them with a fork and add a spoonful or two of jarred salsa. All the better if I have fresh cilantro, salad greens, or avocado to top it all off. If I'm lucky enough to have fresh collard greens, I'll steam a few leaves and use them as burrito wraps to replace the tortillas. We call them collardritos in our house. Greens and beans—can't get healthier than that!

Any leguminous dessert options? Three words: black-bean brownies. I don't have a recipe of my own, but if you poke around online, you'll find many good ones, including the one Dr. Joel Fuhrman shared on *The Dr. Oz Show*, which uses almond butter as the green-light source of fat and dates as the green-light source of sugar.[44]

Mostly, I just add beans to whatever I happen to be making. I try to always keep an open can front and center in the fridge as a reminder. We buy black beans by the case. (Black beans appear to have more phenolic phytonutrients than other common legumes,[45] but the best bean is probably whichever one you'll eat the most of!)

Clearing the Air About Beans and Gas

Beans, beans. Good for your heart. The more you eat 'em, the . . . longer you live? Legumes have been found to be "the most important predictor of survival in older people"[46] around the globe. Whether it was the Japanese eating soy products, the Swedes eating brown beans and peas, or those in the Mediterranean region eating lentils, chickpeas, and white beans, legume intake was consistently associated with a longer life span. Researchers found an 8 percent reduction in risk of premature death for every twenty-gram increase in daily legume intake— that's barely two tablespoons' worth![47]

So why aren't more people taking advantage of this dietary "fountain of youth"? Fear of flatulence.[48] Is that really the choice you're left with, then? Breaking wind or breaking down? Passing gas or passing on?

Are the concerns about the gassiness of beans just a bunch of hot air?

When researchers tried adding a half cup of beans to people's diets, the majority experienced no symptoms at all. Even among people who did get gassy, 70 percent or more reported that it diminished by the second or third week of the study. The researchers concluded: "People's concerns about excessive flatulence from eating beans may be exaggerated."[49]

Flatulence may be more common than you think. Americans report passing gas an average of fourteen times a day,[50] with the normal range extending up to twenty-three times daily.[51] Flatulence comes from two places: swallowed air and fermentation in the bowel. Factors that might cause you to swallow extra air include chewing gum, wearing ill-fitting dentures, sucking on hard candies, drinking through a straw, eating too fast, talking while you eat, and smoking cigarettes. So, if the fear of lung cancer doesn't get you to quit smoking, maybe fear of flatulence will.

The main source of gas, though, is the normal bacterial fermentation in the colon of undigested sugars. Dairy products are a leading cause of excessive flatulence,[52] which is due to poor digestion of the milk sugar lactose.[53] One of the most flatulent patients ever reported in the medical literature was effectively cured once all dairy products were removed from his diet. The case, reported in the *New England Journal of Medicine* and submitted to the *Guinness Book of World Records*, involved a man who, after consuming dairy, experienced "70 passages in one four-hour period."[54] Cutting the cheese, indeed.

Long term, most people bulking up on high-fiber plant foods do not appear to have significantly increased problems with gas.[55] The buoyancy of floating stools from trapped gases can in fact be seen as a sign of adequate fiber intake.[56] The indigestible sugars in beans that make it down to your colon may even function as prebiotics to feed your good bacteria and make for a healthier colon.

Even if at first they make you gassy, beans are so health promoting that you should experiment with ways to keep them in your diet at all costs. Lentils, split peas, and canned beans tend to produce less gas, and tofu isn't usually an offender. Repeated soakings of dried beans in water containing a quarter teaspoon of baking soda per gallon[57] and tossing out the cooking water may help if you boil your own beans. Of the spices that have been tested, cloves, cinnamon, and garlic seem to be the most gas reducing, followed by turmeric (but only if uncooked), pepper, and ginger.[58] If worse comes to worst, there are cheap supplements that contain alpha-galactosidase, an enzyme shown to break up the bean sugars and take the sail out of your wind.[59]

Odor is a separate issue. The smell appears to come primarily from the digestion of sulfur-rich foods. So to cut down on the stench, experts have recommended cutting back on such foods as meat and eggs.[60] (Hydrogen sulfide is called "rotten egg gas" for a reason.) This may be why people who eat meat regularly were found to generate as much as fifteen times the sulfides as those eating plant-based diets.[61]

There *are* healthy sulfur-rich foods, such as garlic and cauliflower. If you're about to embark on a long trip in a confined space after a big meal of aloo gobi, Pepto-Bismol and generic equivalents can act as a windbreaker by binding up the sulfur in your gut to eliminate odors. But this should be used only as a short-term solution due to the potential for bismuth toxicity with chronic use.[62]

Then there are the high-tech solutions, such as carbon-fiber, odor-eating underwear (cost: $65), which were put to the test in a series of studies that included such gems as "Utilizing gas-tight Mylar pantaloons, the ability of a charcoal-lined cushion to absorb sulfur-containing gases instilled at the anus of eight subjects was assessed."[63] The name of the charcoal-lined cushion? The "Toot Trapper."

The bottom line: Intestinal gas is normal and healthy. No less an expert than

Hippocrates himself was attributed as saying, "Passing gas is necessary to well-being."[64] In a review of degassing drugs and devices, Dr. John Fardy, a chair of gastroenterology, wrote: "Perhaps increased tolerance of flatus would be a better solution, for we tamper with harmless natural phenomena at our peril."[65] And, yes, Dr. Fardy is his real name.

Legume consumption is associated with a slimmer waist and lower blood pressure, and randomized trials have shown it can match or beat out calorie cutting for slimming tummy fat as well as improving the regulation of blood sugar, insulin levels, and cholesterol. Beans are packed with fiber, folate, and phytates, which may help reduce the risk of stroke, depression, and colon cancer. The phytoestrogens in soy in particular appear to both help prevent breast cancer and improve breast cancer survival. No wonder the cancer guidelines suggest you should try to fit beans into your meals—and it's so easy! They can be added to nearly any meal, easily incorporated into snack times, or served as the star attraction. The possibilities are endless.

Berries

Dr. Greger's Favorite Berries

Açai berries, barberries, blackberries, blueberries, cherries (sweet or tart), concord grapes, cranberries, goji berries, kumquats, mulberries, raspberries (black or red), and strawberries

Serving Sizes:

½ cup fresh or frozen
¼ cup dried

Daily Recommendation:

1 serving per day

The case for berries has been made throughout this book. Berries offer potential protection against cancer (chapters 4 and 11), a boost to the immune system (chapter 5), and a guard for the liver (chapter 8) and brain (chapters 3 and 14). An American Cancer Society study of nearly one hundred thousand men and women found that those who ate the most berries appeared significantly less likely to die of cardiovascular disease.[1]

Wait a second—tastes great *and* may help you live longer? Yes. That's what plant-based eating is all about.

Greens are the healthiest vegetables, and berries are the healthiest fruits—in part due to their respective plant pigments. Leaves contain the green pigment chlorophyll, which sets off the firestorm of photosynthesis, so greens have to be packed with antioxidants to deal with the charged high-energy electrons that are formed. (Remember superoxide from chapter 3?) Meanwhile, berries evolved to have bright, contrasting colors to attract fruit-eating critters to help disperse their seeds. And the same molecular characteristics that give berries such vibrant colors may account for some of their antioxidant abilities.[2]

Americans eat a lot of pale and beige foods: white bread, white pasta, white potatoes, white rice. Colorful foods are often healthier because they contain antioxidant pigments, whether it's the beta-carotene that makes carrots and sweet potatoes orange, the lycopene antioxidant pigment that makes tomatoes red, or the anthocyanin pigments that make blueberries blue. The colors *are* the antioxidants. That knowledge alone should revolutionize your stroll down the produce aisle.

Guess which have more antioxidants—red onions or white onions? You don't need to look up the answer. You can see the difference with your own eyes. (Indeed, red onions have 76 percent more antioxidant capacity than white, with yellow onions in between.[3]) So, given the choice, why buy another white onion ever again?

Red cabbage may contain eight times more antioxidants than green cabbage,[4] which is why you'll never find a green cabbage in my house.

Pop quiz: Which wipes out more free radicals—pink grapefruit or regular grapefruit? Granny Smith or Red Delicious? Iceberg lettuce or romaine? Red grapes or green? Yellow corn or white corn? See, you don't need me to go to the grocery store with you. You can make all these calls yourself.

What about a purple-skinned eggplant or a white-skinned eggplant? Trick question! Remember, the pigment is the antioxidant, so the color of the skin doesn't matter if you peel it off. As we learned in chapter 11, that's why you never want to peel apples. It's for this same reason kumquats may be the healthiest citrus fruit, since you can eat them rind and all.

Shop for the reddest of strawberries, the blackest of blackberries, the most scarlet tomato, the darkest green broccoli you can find. The colors *are* the antiaging, anticancer antioxidants.

Antioxidant content is one of the reasons I've singled out berries for special treatment. They are second only to herbs and spices as the most antioxidant-packed food category. As a group, they average nearly ten times more antioxidants than other fruits and vegetables (and exceed fifty times more than animal-based foods).[5]

290 | HOW NOT TO DIE

The Antioxidant Power of Berries

As with other green-light foods, the healthiest variety is the one you'll eat most often, but if you have no particular preference, why not put the berry with the most antioxidants in your morning oatmeal? Thanks to a study that compared more than a hundred different berries and berry products, we now know which one that is.[6]

America's favorite fruits are apples and bananas, with antioxidant power of about 60 units and 40 units, respectively. Mangos, the preferred fruit around the world outside of the United States, have even more antioxidant punch at around 110 units. (It makes sense when you consider how much more colorful they are on the inside.) But none of these fruits are a match for berries. Strawberries weigh in at about 310 units per cup, cranberries at 330, raspberries at 350, blueberries at 380 (though wild blueberries may have twice as much[7]), and blackberries at a whopping 650 units. Above even those are exotic types you can pick wild in the Arctic tundra, like red whortleberries. (They sound like something from a Dr. Seuss book!) But in terms of what you can find readily in the store, it's blackberries for the win. (I share my whole-fruit cocktail recipe for using one of the runners-up, cranberries, on page 151.) I'm happy as long as you're eating a serving of any type of berry every day, but in terms of antioxidant content, choosing blackberries over strawberries appears to give you twice the bang for your berry.[8]

What About All the Sugar in Fruit?

There are a few popular diets out there that urge people to stop eating fruits because their natural sugars (fructose) are thought to contribute to weight gain. The truth is, only fructose from added sugars appears to be associated with declining liver function,[9] high blood pressure, and weight gain.[10] How could the fructose in sugar be bad but the same fructose in fruit be harmless? Think about the difference between a sugar cube and a sugar beet. (Beets are the primary source of sugar in the United States.[11]) In nature, fructose comes prepackaged with the fiber, antioxidants, and phytonutrients that appear to nullify adverse fructose effects.[12]

Studies show that if you drink a glass of water with three tablespoons of sugar (similar to what would be in a can of soda), you'll have a big spike in your blood sugar levels within the first hour. That causes your body to release so much insulin to mop up the excess sugar that you actually overshoot and become hypoglycemic by the second hour, meaning that your blood sugar drops even lower than it would if you were fasting. Your body detects this low blood sugar, thinks you might be in some sort of famine situation, and responds by dumping fat into your bloodstream as an energy source to keep you alive.[13] This excess fat in the blood can then go on to cause further problems. (See chapter 6.)

But what if you eat a cup of blended berries in *addition* to the sugar? The berries, of course, have sugars of their own—an additional tablespoon's worth—so the blood sugar spike should be even worse, right? Actually, no. Study participants who ate berries with their cup of sugar water showed no additional blood sugar spike and no hypoglycemic dip afterward; their blood sugar levels merely went up and down, and there was no surge of fat into the blood.[14]

Consuming sugar in fruit form is not only harmless but actually helpful. Eating berries can blunt the insulin spike from high-glycemic foods like white bread, for example.[15] This may be because the fiber in fruit has a gelling effect in your stomach and small intestine that slows the release of sugars[16] or because of certain phytonutrients in fruit that appear to block the absorption of sugar through the gut wall and into your bloodstream.[17] So eating fructose the way nature intended carries benefits rather than risks.

Low-dose fructose may actually benefit blood sugar control. Eating a piece of fruit with each meal could be expected to lower, rather than raise, the blood sugar response.[18] What about people with type 2 diabetes? Diabetics randomized into a group restricted to no more than two daily pieces of fruit had no better blood sugar control than those randomized into a group told to eat a *minimum* of two pieces of fruit per day. The researchers concluded that "the intake of fruit should not be restricted in patients with type 2 diabetes."[19]

Surely there must be *some* level of fructose consumption that's harmful even when served in Mother Nature's green-light form, right? Apparently not.

Seventeen people were asked to eat *twenty* servings of fruit per day for months. Despite the extraordinarily high fructose content of this fruit-based diet—the sugar equivalent of about eight cans of soda a day—the

continued

investigators reported beneficial outcomes with no overall adverse effects for body weight, blood pressure,[20] insulin, cholesterol, and triglyceride levels.[21] More recently, the research group who invented the glycemic index found that feeding subjects a fruit-, vegetable-, and nut-based diet that included about twenty servings of fruit per day for a couple of weeks had no adverse effects on weight, blood pressure, or triglycerides—all while lowering LDL ("bad") cholesterol by an astounding thirty-eight points.[22]

Cholesterol lowering was not the only record broken: Participants were asked to eat forty-three servings of vegetables a day in addition to the fruit, the result of which was that the researchers recorded the largest-ever bowel movements documented in a dietary intervention.[23]

Are frozen berries as nutritious as fresh ones? Studies on cherries,[24] raspberries,[25] and strawberries[26] suggest that most of their nutrition is retained even when frozen. I usually opt for frozen berries since they last longer, are available year round, and tend to be cheaper. If you looked in our freezer right now, you'd see it's about half frozen greens and half frozen berries. What do I do with those berries? Make ice cream, of course.

The favored dessert in our home is soft-serve "ice cream" made by blending frozen fruit. You whip up frozen fruit in a blender, food processor, or juicer, and voilà! Instant all-fruit ice cream. You have to taste it to believe it. The simplest recipe has one ingredient: frozen bananas. Peel and freeze some ripe bananas (the riper, the better—I'm talking brown). Once frozen, throw them in a food processor and blend. They transform into a smooth, light, fluffy dessert cheaper, healthier, and tastier than anything you might get in a trendy frozen yogurt shop.

Of course making *berry* ice cream or at least a berry-banana mix is even healthier. My favorite is chocolate. To make it, blend dark, sweet cherries or strawberries mixed with a tablespoon of cocoa power, a splash of a milk of your choice (more if you want a milkshake), a capful of vanilla extract, and some pitted dates. If you didn't yet get your nuts for the day, you can add some almond butter. Either way, you get an instant, decadent, chocolate dessert so nutritious that the more you eat, the healthier you are. Let me repeat that: The more you eat, the healthier you are. That's my kind of ice cream!

Tart Cherries

Research dating back half a century suggests tart cherries are so anti-inflammatory that they can be used to successfully treat a painful type of arthritis called gout.[27] Delicious dietary treatments are much welcomed, as some gout drugs can cost $2,000 a dose,[28] carry no clear-cut distinction between nontoxic, toxic, and lethal doses,[29] or can cause a rare side effect in which your skin detaches from your body.[30] Of course, the best way to deal with gout is to try to prevent it in the first place with a more plant-based diet.[31]

Cherries can reduce the level of inflammation among healthy people too (as measured by a drop in C-reactive protein levels),[32] so I was excited to find a green-light source available year-round—a canned product with only two ingredients: cherries and water. I drain off the liquid (which then goes into my hibiscus punch recipe on page 390) and mix the cherries in a bowl of cooked oatmeal along with cocoa powder and pumpkin seeds. If you sweeten it with date sugar or erythritol (see page 389), it's like eating chocolate-covered cherries for breakfast.

A note of caution: For the same reason that high doses of anti-inflammatory drugs such as aspirin should be avoided during the third trimester of pregnancy, cocoa, berries, and other foods high in anti-inflammatory polyphenols should only be eaten in moderation in late pregnancy.[33]

Goji Berries

Tart cherries naturally contain melatonin and have been used to improve sleep without any side effects.[34] Goji berries, however, have the highest concentrations of melatonin.[35] Gojis have the third-highest antioxidant capacity of any common dried fruit—five times more than raisins and second only to dried pomegranate seeds and barberries (a fruit commonly found in Middle Eastern markets and spice stores).[36] Gojis also have a specific antioxidant pigment that makes corn yellow—zeaxanthin. When eaten, zeaxanthin is shuttled into your retinas (the back of your eyes) and appears to protect against macular degeneration, a leading cause of vision loss.[37]

The egg industry boasts about the zeaxanthin content in yolks, but goji berries have about fifty times more than eggs.[38] A double-blind, randomized, placebo-controlled trial found that gojis may even help people already suffering from macular degeneration.[39] The researchers used milk to improve the absorption of zeaxanthin (which, like all carotenoids, is fat soluble), but a healthier way would be to use green-light sources of fat, such as nuts and seeds—in other words, goji trail mix!

Aren't goji berries expensive, though? In natural foods stores, they can go for twenty dollars a pound, but in Asian supermarkets, you can buy them as "Lycium" berries, and they're even cheaper than raisins. So, however you used to eat raisins—as a snack, in baked goods, in your breakfast cereal or oatmeal, whatever—I recommend you make the switch to gojis.

Black Currants and Bilberries

Speaking of berries and eyesight, a double-blind, placebo-controlled, crossover trial of black currants found they can improve the symptoms of computer eye strain (known in doctor-speak as "video display terminal work-induced transient refractive alteration").[40] What passes for currants in the United States are usually champagne grape raisins, not actual black currants, which were banned in the country a century ago at the behest of the lumber industry. (The industry feared they might spread a plant disease that affects white pines, a tree we hardly harvest anymore, so the ban has since been lifted in some states.) Real black currants are currently making a comeback, but if—as the researchers suspected—the benefits have to do with the anthocyanin pigments, other berries like bilberries, blueberries, or blackberries may help as well. Anthocyanin pigments are responsible for many of the intense blue, black, purple, and red colors of berries and other fruits and vegetables. The highest concentrations are found in aronia berries and elderberries, followed by black raspberries, blueberries (especially the smaller "wild" varieties), and blackberries. The cheapest source, though, is probably red cabbage.[41]

Bilberries gained notoriety during World War II when it was said that pilots in the British Royal Air Force "were eating bilberry jam to improve their night vision."[42] It turns out this may have been a story concocted to fool the Germans. The more likely reason the Brits were able to suddenly target Nazi bombers in the middle of the night wasn't because of bilberries but thanks to a top-secret new invention: radar.

Unfortunately, these anthocyanin pigments take a hit when berries are processed into jam. As much as 97 percent of anthocyanins are lost when strawberries are turned into strawberry jam.[43] Freeze-drying, however, appears to be remarkably nutrient preserving.[44] I remember trying "astronaut ice cream" as a kid when I visited the Smithsonian's Air and Space Museum. That's what freeze-dried strawberries taste like to me. They just melt in your mouth. Delicious, nutritious, but expensive.

Fresh berries, of course, are divine. My family enjoys pick-your-own out-ings and then freezes the abundance. I've also been known to lay a sheet under branches of mulberry trees that grow in a park by our house and gently knock down a ripe bounty with a broom handle. Evidently, nearly all wild "aggregate" berries (meaning berries that look like clusters of little balls, like blackberries, raspberries, and mulberries) in North America are edible,[45] but please be sure you make an ironclad identification before foraging.

Berries in all their colorful, sweet, and flavorful glory are protective little anti-oxidant powerhouses. The issue shouldn't be how you are going to get your one minimum daily serving but rather how you are going to pry yourself away from them. In your smoothie, as a dessert, on your salad, or just popped right into your mouth—they are nature's candy.

Other Fruits

It took years for nearly five hundred researchers from more than three hundred institutions in fifty countries to develop the 2010 Global Burden of Disease Study. Funded by the Bill & Melinda Gates Foundation, it is the largest analysis of risk factors for death and disease in history.[1] In the United States, the massive study determined that the leading cause of both death and disability was the American diet, followed by smoking.[2] What did they determine to be the worst aspect about our diet? Not eating enough fruit.[3]

Don't limit yourself to eating fruit just the way it comes plucked off the tree.

Although fruit makes for a perfect, quick snack, don't forget that it can be cooked as well. Think baked apples, poached pears, and grilled pineapple.

If you like drinking your fruit, blending is better than juicing to preserve nutrition. Juicing removes more than just fiber. Most of the polyphenol phytonutrients (see chapter 3) in fruits and vegetables appear to be bound to the fiber and are only liberated for absorption by the friendly flora in your gut. When you merely drink the juice, you lose out on the fiber and all the nutrition that was attached to it.[4] Even just cloudy apple juice, which retains a bit of the fruit fiber, appears to have nearly triple the phenolics compared to clear apple juice.[5]

Whereas greater consumption of whole fruits has been associated with a lower likelihood of developing type 2 diabetes, Harvard University researchers found that greater juice consumption was associated with higher diabetes risk. So, by choosing yellow-light sources of fruit, like juice or jelly, you may not only be missing out on nutrients but actively working against your health.[6]

An Apple a Day

Anyone who says they don't have time to eat healthfully has never met an apple. Talk about a convenience food! For those who grew up in a world dominated by Red Delicious and Granny Smith, I'm happy to report there are thousands of varieties. Health-wise, crab apples (gross!) probably top the charts,[7] but taste-wise, my personal favorite is Honeycrisp—or any pick-your-own variety I can find locally. If you've never tried an apple you picked right off a tree, you don't know what you're missing. Failing that, farmers' markets can offer good deals on great produce. My family buys apples by the half bushel.

Dates

My favorite fruit snack in the fall and winter is apple slices with dates, for the perfect mix of tart and sweet. Growing up, I never liked dates. They tasted dry and kind of waxy. But then I discovered there were soft, plump, moist varieties that didn't taste like the chalky ones that haunted my childhood. Barhi dates, for example, are wet and sticky, but when frozen, they acquire the taste and chew of caramel candy. Seriously. Paired with my Honeycrisp, it's like eating a butterscotch-flavored caramel apple.

Locally, you should be able to find decent Medjool dates in Middle Eastern grocery stores and many natural foods markets, but for the too-moist-to-be-sold-commercially varieties, you'll probably have to shop online. I have tried dates from most of the major online retailers and always go back to ordering from the Date People, a small farm in California. I am averse to commercial endorsements, but I've never tasted consistently better dates from any other source (although Black Sphinx dates from Phoenix come close!). Date People's annual harvest comes in around my birthday in October, and I always splurge as a present to myself and get a big box to put in our freezer.

Olives and Olive Oil

Olives and extra-virgin olive oil are yellow-light foods. Olive consumption should be minimized because they're soaked in brine—a dozen large olives could take up nearly half your recommended sodium limit for an entire day. Olive oil is sodium-free, but most of its nutrition has been removed. You can think of extra-virgin olive oil a little like fruit juice: It has nutrients, but the calories you get are relatively empty compared to those from the whole fruit. (Olives are, after all, fruits.)

Freshly squeezed olive juice already has less nutrition than the whole fruit, but then olive-oil producers also throw away the olive wastewater, which contains the water-soluble nutrients. As a result, you end up getting just a small fraction of the nutrition of the whole fruit by the time extra-virgin olive oil is bottled. Refined olive oil (nonvirgin) is even worse. I would classify it, along with other vegetable oils, as red-light foods, as they offer such scant nutrition for their heavy caloric loads. One tablespoon of oil can contain more than one hundred calories without filling you up. (Compare that single tablespoon to the one-hundred-calorie serving sizes of other foods on page 110.)

I think of oil as the table sugar of the fat kingdom. Similar to the way manufacturers take healthy foods like beets and throw out all their nutrition to make sugar, they take wholesome corn and scorch-earth it down to corn oil. Like sugar, corn oil calories may be worse than just empty. In chapter 1, I touched on the impairment of artery function that can occur within hours of eating red-light fare like fast food and cheesecake. The same detrimental effect happens after the consumption of olive oil[8] and other oils[9] (but not after eating green-light sources of fat like nuts).[10] Even extra-virgin olive oil may impair your arteries' ability to relax and dilate normally.[11] So, like any yellow-light food, its use should be curtailed.

Cooking without oil is surprisingly easy. To keep foods from sticking, you can sauté in wine, sherry, broth, vinegar, or just plain water. For baking, I've successfully used green-light ingredients such as mashed bananas or avocado, soaked prunes, and even canned pumpkin to substitute for oil to provide a similar moistness.

The reduction of yellow-light foods is all about frequency and quantity. If you are going to trek outside the green zone, my advice is simple: Make it count. Don't waste precious indulgences on crappy food. I don't want to sound like a food snob, but if you're going to eat something less than maximally healthy, I say pamper yourself and truly relish it. When I eat olives, there's no way I'm going to eat those waxy black abominations in a can. I'm going to slice up some purple kalamatas that actually have some flavor. If you're going to spoil yourself once in a while, I say do it right!

Mangos

Mangos are my favorite fruit treat during spring and summer, but you have to know where to look to get good ones. Check out Hispanic markets and Indian grocery stores. The difference between a mango from Walmart and one from an Indian spice store is like the difference between a hard, pale, tasteless, pink tomato and a ripe, flavorful, farm-stand heirloom. You should be able to smell the mango at arm's length.

My favorite way to eat a mango is like sipping a Capri Sun drink pouch. When the fruit gets soft and ripe, I roll it between my palms, kneading it with my fingers until it becomes essentially liquid pulp in a pouch. Then I nip off the tip with my teeth, gently squeeze, and suck the mango right out of its peel.

Watermelon

Are some whole fruits better than others? Berries contain the most antioxidants, whereas melons wallow down around iceberg lettuce levels. Watermelon *seeds*, on the other hand, have pretty respectable antioxidant levels, so I try to avoid seedless varieties. A spoonful of watermelon seeds may have as many antioxidants as a whole cup of melon balls.[12] Seedless or not, watermelon contains a compound called citrulline that can boost the activity of the enzyme responsible for dilating the blood vessels in the penis that result in erections. A group of Italian researchers found that citrulline supplementation at the level of five servings of red watermelon a day improved erection hardness in men with mild erectile dysfunction, allowing for a 68 percent increase in monthly intercourse frequency.[13] Yellow watermelon has four times more citrulline,[14] though, so just about one wedge a day (one-sixteenth of a modest melon) may have the same effect. If this information is new to you, perhaps it's because the advertising budgets of drug companies like Pfizer, which rake in billions of dollars each year from the sale of erectile dysfunction drugs, are about a thousand times[15] that of the entire budget of the National Watermelon Promotion Board.[16]

Dried Fruit

I love dried mangos, but they are hard to find without added sugar. I remember naïvely asking a friend in the food business why the industry felt the need to sugar-up an already sweet fruit. "Added weight," he explained. Just as poultry processors inject salt water into chickens to add water weight, processed food companies often use sugar as a cheap way to bulk up products sold by the pound.

This made me determined to make my own. I bought an inexpensive dehydrator from eBay, and I'm so glad I did. Fruit is about 90 percent water, so imagine intensifying the flavor of a fresh, ripe mango tenfold. Mind-blowing! Mangos can be a messy pain to peel, but once that's done, I slice them about a centimeter thick and sprinkle them with chia seeds before putting them in the dehydrator. If I'm taking them on a plane or a hike, I'll dry them completely. Otherwise, I only wait until just the outside is dry. The outer layer, encrusted with chia, gets a crispy texture while the core remains moist and ready to burst. It's the kind of thing I can't eat while watching a movie or reading a book. It tastes so good I just have to stop, close my eyes, and savor it.

I also like drying thin apple slices. I either sprinkle them with cinnamon or rub them with freshly grated ginger. They can be just dried until chewy or completely dehydrated into crunchy apple chips. Eating a dozen dried apple rings a day may drop LDL cholesterol levels 16 percent within three months and 24 percent within six months.[17]

If you buy dried fruit, I recommend choosing unsulfured varieties. Sulfur-containing preservatives, such as sulfur dioxide in dried fruit and sulfites in wine, can form hydrogen sulfide in your gut—this is the rotten egg gas implicated in the development of the inflammatory bowel disease ulcerative colitis. The main source of hydrogen sulfide is the metabolism of animal protein,[18] but you can further lower your exposure by avoiding sulfur additives (either by reading labels or choosing organic, in which such preservatives are forbidden). The sulfur naturally contained in cruciferous vegetables does not appear to elevate colitis risk,[19] so feel free to add kale chips to your healthy snacking menu.

Prescribing Kiwifruit

There appear to be a disproportionate number of articles in the medical literature about the clinical benefits of kiwifruit. Is that because they're better than other fruits? Or is it because the kiwi industry has more research dollars? One country, New Zealand, holds a substantial share of the global kiwi market, so it's in its best interest to underwrite research on the fruit. As a result, there is no shortage of papers touting the benefits of kiwifruit.

Kiwi is one of the fruits I've prescribed to my patients with insomnia (two an hour before bedtime appears to significantly improve sleep onset, duration, and efficiency)[20] and also to help with constipation-type irritable bowel syndrome (two kiwifruit a day seem to significantly improve bowel function). Kiwi certainly seems like a better option than the leading IBS drug, which was pulled from the market for apparently killing too many people.[21]

Kiwifruit also appear to benefit immune function. Preschoolers randomized to eat gold kiwifruits every day appeared to cut their risk of contracting a cold or flu-like illness nearly in half compared to those randomly selected to eat bananas instead.[22] A similar experiment was tried on elderly individuals, another high-risk group. Those in the banana control group who got an upper-respiratory-tract infection suffered for about five days with a sore throat and congestion, compared to the kiwifruit eaters, who felt better after just a day or two.[23] About 1 in 130 children may be allergic to kiwifruit, though,[24] which may rank kiwis as the third-most-common food allergen (second only to milk and eggs),[25] so they are not for everyone.

Citrus

Adding citrus zest to your meals not only adds color, flavor, aroma, and a bit of culinary flair but also nutrition. Citrus zest lives up to its name in terms of enlivening dishes, and it may do the same to your DNA-repair capabilities. On average, humans appear to suffer eight hundred hits to their DNA per hour.

If not fixed, this can cause mutations that give rise to cancer.[26] Comparing identical and fraternal twins, researchers have determined that only part of your DNA-repair function is determined genetically. The rest may be under your control.[27]

The dietary factor found best able to boost DNA repair was citrus fruit.[28] Within two hours of consuming citrus, your DNA becomes significantly more resistant to damage,[29] which may help explain why citrus consumption is associated with lower risk of breast cancer.[30] Some of the citrus compounds thought responsible—which concentrate in the breast[31] and enhance DNA repair[32]—are found in the peel, though. This may be why people who eat at least some citrus peel appear to have lower skin cancer rates than those who don't.[33]

Stick with the whole fruit, because supplements don't appear to boost DNA repair,[34] and citrus juice doesn't appear to help, either. In fact, drinking orange juice every morning may even increase skin cancer risk.[35] Green-light forms of foods always seem to be the best, and you can eat citrus in an even *less* processed way by slipping some of the rind into your diet through zesting. I like to freeze lemons, limes, and oranges whole so we always have them on hand to grate onto meals that could use a little zing.

My only whole-citrus caveat: Inform your physician if you eat grapefruit. This fruit can suppress the enzymes that help clear more than half of commonly prescribed drugs, and less drug clearance means higher drug levels in the body.[36] This may actually be good if you want a better caffeine buzz from your morning coffee[37] or if your doctor wants to help you save money by boosting the effects of expensive drugs instead of just peeing them away.[38] But higher drug levels may also mean higher risk of side effects, so if you regularly eat grapefruits, your physician may want to change your prescription or alter the dosing.

Exotic Fruits

The medical school I attended sits in the middle of Boston's Chinatown. I remember the first time I perused the produce aisle at a large Asian supermarket. With options from bizarre-looking dragon fruit to tribble-like rambutans, I felt like I was on another planet. Every week I tried something new. Some stuck with me—I still sneak lychees into the movies—but others were one-time affairs. Let me share with you the Durian Incident.

Durians are the most badass of all fruits. Imagine a five-pound football covered in sharp spikes like some medieval mace. What other fruit could be described in the medical literature as causing "severe body injury" in papers with titles like "Penetrating Ocular Injury by Durian Fruit"?[39] And I haven't even gotten to its most distinctive quality: its smell. With an odor perhaps best described as "pig-shit, turpentine and onions, garnished with a gym sock,"[40] durian fruits are banned from many public spaces, like subways and airports, in Southeast Asia, where they are grown.

I had to try eating one of these crazy things!

Durian fruits are sold frozen. (I would soon come to understand why.) I took one back to campus and managed to hack off a piece without impaling myself on a spike. The fruit tasted like a caramelized onion popsicle. I left the rest in my locker. Big mistake! I arrived the next day to find an entire floor of the medical center—including the dean's office—cordoned off. They were going locker to locker, cutting off all the locks, searching in vain for the cause of a stench so overpowering you couldn't even locate it. It was like a fog of stink. Hospital staff seriously thought someone had stolen body parts from the gross anatomy cadaver lab. And then it struck me. *Uh-oh.* The durian had thawed. When I realized it was all my fault, I crawled to the dean to beg forgiveness. I already had a history of run-ins with the administration over issues I had raised about the curriculum, and now this. I'll never forget what he said to me that day: "Why am I not surprised you had something to do with this?"

When adding as much fruit as possible to your diet, you certainly don't have to seek out weapons-grade stinky fruit, but you also don't have to stick with the same old, same old. Treat yourself! Have fun sampling the many varieties of the many different fruits around. How lovely it can be to stroll through your farmers' market on a weekend and pick up locally grown fruits that you can zest onto your meals, blend into smoothies, chew when dried, incorporate into your favorite dishes, or best of all, bite right into. The opportunities are ripe for the picking!

Cruciferous Vegetables

When I used to teach medical students at Tufts, I gave a lecture about this amazing new therapeutic called "iloccorB." I'd talk about all the evidence supporting it, the great things it could do, and its excellent safety profile. Just as the students would start scrambling to buy stock in the company and prescribe it to their future patients, I'd do the big reveal. Apologizing for my "dyslexia", I would admit that I'd gotten it backward. All this time, I had been talking about broccoli.

I've mentioned broccoli more than any other food in this book, and for good reason. We've seen how cruciferous vegetables like broccoli can potentially prevent DNA damage and metastatic cancer spread in chapter 2, activate defenses against pathogens and pollutants in chapter 5, help to prevent lymphoma in chapter 9, boost your liver detox enzymes and target breast cancer stem cells in chapter 11, and reduce the risk of prostate cancer progression in chapter 13. The component responsible for these benefits is thought to be sulforaphane, which is formed almost exclusively in cruciferous vegetables. This is why they get their own spot on the Daily Dozen.

Beyond being a promising anticancer agent,[1] sulforaphane may also help protect your brain[2] and your eyesight,[3] reduce nasal allergy inflammation,[4] manage type 2 diabetes,[5] and was recently found to successfully help treat autism. A placebo-controlled, double-blind, randomized trial of boys with autism found that about two to three cruciferous vegetable servings' worth[6] of sulforaphane a day improves social interaction, abnormal behavior, and verbal communication within a matter of weeks. The researchers, primarily from Harvard University and Johns Hopkins University, suggest that the effect might be due to sulforaphane's role as a "detoxicant."[7]

Strategies to Enhance Sulforaphane Formation

The formation of sulforaphane in cruciferous vegetables is like a chemical flare reaction. It requires the mixing of a precursor compound with an enzyme called myrosinase, which is inactivated by cooking[8] (though microwaved broccoli appears to retain some cancer-fighting capacity). This may explain why we see dramatic suppression of test-tube cancer-cell growth by raw broccoli, cauliflower, and brussels sprouts, but hardly any reaction when they're cooked.[9] But who wants to eat raw brussels sprouts? Not me. Thankfully, there are ways to get the benefits of raw vegetables in cooked form.

Biting into broccoli is like snapping that chemical flare. When raw broccoli (or any other cruciferous vegetable) is chopped or chewed, the sulforaphane precursor mixes with the myrosinase enzyme and sulforaphane is created as the vegetable sits on the cutting board or lies in your upper stomach waiting to be digested.[10] Though the enzyme is destroyed by cooking, both the precursor and the final product are resistant to heat. So here's the trick: Use what I call the "Hack and Hold" technique (maybe I should call it Whack and Wait?).

continued

If you chop the broccoli (or brussels sprouts, kale, collards, cauliflower, or any other cruciferous vegetable) and then wait forty minutes, you can cook it as much as you want. At that point, the sulforaphane has already been made, so the enzyme is no longer needed to achieve maximum benefit. It's already done its job. (You can also buy bags of fresh greens and other crucifers that are prechopped or shredded, which can presumably be cooked immediately.)

Given this understanding, can you see how most people prepare broccoli soup incorrectly? Typically, they first cook the broccoli and then blend it. But, when you blend it, you're merely mixing the precursor with an enzyme that's been inactivated by cooking. Do it in the opposite order: First blend your veggies and then wait forty minutes before cooking them. This way, you can maximize sulforaphane production.

What about *frozen* broccoli and other crucifers? Commercially produced frozen broccoli lacks the ability to form sulforaphane because the vegetables are blanched (flash-cooked) before they're frozen for the very purpose of deactivating enzymes.[11] This process prolongs shelf life, but when you take the veggies out of your freezer, the enzyme is inert. At that point, it doesn't matter how much you chop or how long you wait—no sulforaphane is going to be made. This may be why fresh kale has been shown to suppress cancer cell growth in vitro up to ten times better than frozen kale.[12]

The frozen crucifer is still packed with the precursor, though—remember, it's heat resistant. You could make lots of sulforaphane from it by adding back some enzyme.[13] But where can you get myrosinase? Scientists buy theirs from chemical companies, but you can just walk into any grocery store.

Mustard greens are also cruciferous vegetables. They grow from mustard seeds, which you can buy ground up in the spice aisle as mustard powder. If you sprinkled some mustard powder on frozen broccoli that's been cooked, would it start churning out sulforaphane? Yes!

Boiling broccoli prevents the formation of any significant levels of sulforaphane due to inactivation of the enzyme. However, the addition of powdered mustard seeds to cooked broccoli significantly increases sulforaphane formation.[14] Then it's almost as good as eating it raw! So, if you don't have forty minutes to spare between chopping and cooking, or if you're using frozen greens, just sprinkle the crucifers with some mustard powder before you eat them, and you'll be all set. Daikon radishes, regular radishes, horseradish, and wasabi are all cruciferous vegetables and may have the same effect. All it appears to take is a pinch to revitalize sulforaphane production.[15] You can also add a small amount of fresh greens to your cooked greens. So when I add shreds of purple cabbage to my finished dishes, it not only adds a beautiful garnish with a delightful crunch, it's filled with the sulforaphane-producing enzyme.

One of my first tasks every morning used to be chopping greens for the day, using my Hack and Hold technique. But now, with the Mustard Powder Plan, I have one less to-do on my list.

Horseradish

The serving sizes I offer on page 304 correspond roughly to the daily intake required to achieve cancer-preventive levels according to the innovative breast-surgery study I detailed in chapter 11. As you can see, horseradish has the smallest serving size, which means it's the most concentrated of the cruciferous vegetables. One tablespoon and your Daily Dozen is down to an Everyday Eleven. Horseradish can be made into a sauce, relish, or dressing to score an extra check mark with a kick. It's great in mashed potatoes or, for a healthier option still, mashed cauliflower. Just boil cauliflower for about ten minutes until tender and then mash with a fork or potato masher or purée in a food processor with some of the reserved cooking liquid until smooth. I season it with pepper, roasted garlic, and a dollop of horseradish and then pour mushroom gravy on it. Delicious!

Roasting Cruciferous Vegetables

As much as I love mashed cauliflower, roasted cauliflower (or broccoli, for that matter) is my favorite. Roasting brings out a nutty, caramelized flavor. I slice raw cauliflower into "steaks," roast at 400°F for about a half hour, and then smother it in a lemon-tahini sauce. Sometimes I go minimalist and just sprinkle on lemon juice, zest, capers, and garlic. (This chapter is making me hungry!)

Kale Chips

I'll talk about some of the more traditional ways I prepare greens in the next section, but kale chips deserve a special mention. You can use a dehydrator if you have one, but I often don't have the patience. When I'm in the mood for kale chips, I want them *now*. They can be as simple as one ingredient: kale. Pull the leaves off the stems and tear into large pieces. Make sure that they are dry, or they'll steam rather than crisp. Lay out the torn leaves in a single layer on a cookie tray lined with parchment paper or a silicone mat to prevent sticking, and bake at a low temperature (about 250°F) and check often to make sure they don't burn. Within about twenty minutes, they transform into light, crispy snacks. Preseason the leaves before you roast them, or add your spices after they're done. There are thousands of recipes online. I recommend starting with Ann Esselstyn's recipe on her son Rip's website, Engine2Diet.com.[16] With kale chips, the more you snack, the healthier you are.

Cruciferous Garnishes

Similar to the way I use an open can of beans in the fridge as a reminder to try to bean-up any dish, we always have a purple (or red) cabbage in the crisper to help us cruciferize our meals. I slice off shreds and garnish nearly anything with them. Red cabbage averages about one dollar per pound,[17] is found at pretty much any grocery store or market, can last weeks in the fridge (though if it does, that means you're not using it enough!), and has more antioxidants per dollar than anything else you'll find in the produce aisle. There are healthier foods you can buy, but not for the same amount of money. For example, purple cabbage may have nearly three times the antioxidant power per dollar that blueberries do.[18] In terms of eating healthfully on a budget, purple cabbage can't be beat. Or can it?

After chopping and discarding the waste, red cabbage averages 45 cents a cup.[19] But broccoli sprouts—if you make them yourself—may be even cheaper. Broccoli sprout seeds can be purchased online or at natural foods stores for about twenty dollars a pound, but that makes about seventy-five cups of sprouts. In terms of sulforaphane content, that may be around three hundred cups of mature broccoli. So DIY broccoli sprouts provide a green-light sulforaphane source for about a nickel a day.

Sprouting broccoli sprouts is as easy as sprouting lentils. Start with a mason jar with a sprouting (screen) lid. Add a tablespoon of seeds, let them soak overnight in water, drain in the morning, and then after that, just quickly rinse and drain twice a day. Most people wait for about five days, until the seeds fully sprout (taking on the look of alfalfa sprouts), but new science suggests sulforaphane content peaks at forty-eight hours after the seeds are initially drained.[20] This makes them even quicker and easier to grow and eat. When I'm not traveling, I usually have a few jars in rotation. It can be the middle of winter, and

I'm growing my own salad on my kitchen counter! Every day, you can get cups of fresh produce for your family without ever having to go to the store.

Cruciferous Supplements?

If you don't like the taste of cruciferous vegetables but still want the benefits of the sulforaphane, what about the broccoli supplements currently on the market? Researchers recently put a leading commercial supplement to the test. Broc coMax boasts the equivalent of a half pound of broccoli in every capsule. Study subjects were given either six capsules a day or a single cup of broccoli sprouts. The supplement hardly worked at all, whereas the sprouts boosted blood levels about eight times higher for eight times less cost. The researchers concluded that "our data provide further evidence that bioavailability of [sulforaphane] is dramatically lower when subjects consume broccoli supplements compared to fresh broccoli sprouts."[21]

Too Much of a Good Thing?

If broccoli sprouts are so cheap and effective, why not eat bowls of them? A formal safety analysis found no significant adverse effects to about one and a half cups a day,[22] but we didn't have data on a potential upper limit until a team of Italian researchers tried to push the envelope. They were attempting to come up with an intravenous infusion dose to use as chemotherapy, and so they wanted to know how high they could go. The researchers discovered that blood levels achieved by four or more cups of broccoli sprouts may indeed be detrimental.[23] They concluded, however, that no harm was found at "nutritionally attainable concentrations." But that's not really true. Broccoli sprouts do have a radishy bite, but someone *could* theoretically eat four cups of sprouts a day. (They don't know health nuts like I know some health nuts.)

Let me tell you a story. A few years ago, someone came up to me after a lecture in Miami and told me he had heard that wheatgrass juice was good for you. "It cleans you out," he had read. So he thought, *Why not?* and decided to stuff himself with it. He told me how he calculated the volume of the human digestive tract (all ten yards or so) and proceeded to

continued

drink that amount continuously, quart after quart, until it started coming out the other end. Intrigued, I asked him what happened. He looked up at me with an expression that I can only describe as rapturous and said, "It was *volcanic*."

It would be hard for me to say too many good things about crucifers. These vegetables do wonders for your health, from fighting cancer progression and boosting defenses against pathogens and pollutants to helping protect your brain and vision and more. And you can use this family of veggies as your excuse to play Mad Scientist in the kitchen, manipulating enzyme chemistry to maximize the health benefits.

Greens

Popeye was right when he bragged that he was strong to the finish because he ate his spinach. Dark-green, leafy vegetables are the healthiest foods on the planet. As whole foods go, they offer the most nutrition per calorie. Just to emphasize the point, there was a study published in the journal *Nutrition and Cancer* entitled "Antioxidant, Antimutagenic, and Antitumor Effects of Pine Needles."[1] Edible leaves, in all their shapes and sizes, it seems, can be healthy foods.

In 1777, General George Washington issued a general order that American troops should forage for wild greens growing around their camps "as these vegetables are very conducive to health, and tend to prevent . . . all putrid disorders."[2] Since then, however, Americans have declared their independence from greens. Today, only about one in twenty-five even reach a dozen servings throughout the course of an entire month.[3] I advise getting more than a dozen servings per week.

IMPORTANT CAVEAT: Greens and Warfarin

In 1984, the tragic case of a thirty-five-year-old woman unfolded when she failed to inform her physician about her change in diet. Because of her mechanical heart valve, the woman was on a blood-thinning drug called warfarin. But because she wanted to lose weight, she started eating a diet composed almost entirely of salad, broccoli, turnip greens, and mustard greens. Five weeks later, she suffered a blood clot and died.[4]

If you are on the drug warfarin (also known as Coumadin), talk with your physician before you increase your greens intake. The drug works (both as a rat poison and a human blood-thinner) by crippling the enzyme that recycles vitamin K, which is involved in clotting your blood. If your system gets an influx of fresh vitamin K, which is concentrated in greens, you can thereby undermine the effectiveness of the drug. You should still be able to eat your greens, but your physician will have to titrate the dose of the drug to match your regular greens intake.

Eating greens nearly every day may be one of the most powerful steps you can take to prolong your life.[5] Of all the food groups analyzed by a team of Harvard University researchers, greens turned out to be associated with the strongest protection against major chronic diseases,[6] including up to about a 20 percent reduction in risk for both heart attacks[7] and strokes[8] for every additional daily serving.

Imagine if there were a pill that could prolong your life and only had good side effects. Everyone would be taking it! It would be making billions of dollars for the lucky drug company that created it. All health plans by law would have to cover it. People from every walk of life and every corner of the globe would be clamoring for it. But when that "pill" is just eat-your-greens, people lose interest.

Drug companies have yet to patent broccoli (though Monsanto is trying![9]). Doctors, however, don't have to wait for perky pharmaceutical sales reps to wine, dine, and cajole them into prescribing Pfizer-brand spinach or GlaxoSmithKline-brand collards. Here's my prescription for you:

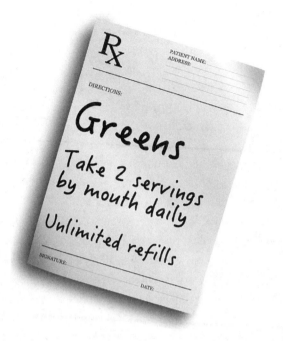

If the full spectrum of colorful plant pigments are good for you, why are greens the healthiest? When autumn in New England becomes aflame with brilliant hues, where do those oranges and yellows come from? They were there all along, actually—just masked by the green pigment chlorophyll that starts to break down in the fall.[10] Similarly, the dark-green leaves of vegetables contain many of the other plant pigments all wrapped up in one package. As I mentioned, these colorful compounds are often the very same antioxidants implicated in many of the benefits of fruit and vegetable consumption. So, in essence, when you eat your greens, you are eating the rainbow.

How to Regenerate Coenzyme Q10 Naturally

One of the reasons greens are some of the healthiest green-light foods may be due to their green color. Decades ago, a search began for "interceptor" molecules that could serve as the body's first line of defense against cancer. The theory was that if we could find something that could tightly bind to carcinogens and prevent them from slipping into our DNA, we might be able

continued

to prevent some of the mutations that lead to cancer. After years of combing for the existence of such carcinogen-binding molecules, an interceptor was found: chlorophyll, the most ubiquitous plant pigment in the world. It was right under our noses all along (provided we were eating healthfully!).[11]

In a petri dish, certain DNA damage in human cells exposed to a carcinogen could be "totally abolished" by chlorophyll.[12] But what about in people? In the name of science, volunteers drank a solution of radioactive aflatoxin (a carcinogen) with or without spinach chlorophyll. Six cups of spinach worth of chlorophyll appeared to block about 40 percent of the carcinogen.[13] Amazing! But that's not all chlorophyll can do.

In college, you learn that pretty much everything you were taught in high school biology wasn't true. Then in graduate school, you unlearn all the oversimplifications you learned in college. Just when you think you understand something in biology, it always seems a little more complicated than you thought. For example, until recently, we assumed plants and plantlike organisms were the only ones that could directly capture and utilize the energy from the sun. Plants photosynthesize. Animals don't. That's because plants have chlorophyll and animals do not. Well, technically, you *do* have chlorophyll in your body—temporarily, at least—after you eat greens. But it would seem there's no way the chlorophyll that enters your bloodstream after that salad could react with sunlight. After all, light can't penetrate through your skin, right?

Wrong. Any kid who's ever shined a flashlight through her or his fingers could have told you that.

The red wavelengths of sunlight do penetrate into your body.[14] In fact, if you step outside on a sunny day, there's enough light reaching your brain that you could actually read this page inside your skull.[15] Your internal organs are bathed in sunlight, along with any chlorophyll circulating in your bloodstream. Although any energy produced by the chlorophyll would be negligible,[16] it turns out that light-activated chlorophyll in your body may help regenerate a critical molecule called coenzyme Q10.[17]

CoQ10, also known as ubiquin*ol*, is an antioxidant. When ubiquin*ol* extinguishes a free radical, it is oxidized to ubiquin*one*. To act as an effective antioxidant again, the body must regenerate ubiquinol from ubiquinone. Think of it like an electrical fuse: Ubiquinol can only be used once before having to be reset. That's where sunlight and chlorophyll may come in.

Researchers exposed some ubiquinone and dietary chlorophyll metabolites to the kind of light that reaches your bloodstream . . . and poof! CoQ10 was reborn. However, without the chlorophyll, or without the light, nothing happened. All along, we've been thinking that the main benefit of sunlight was only the formation of vitamin D and that the main benefit of greens was the antioxidants they contain. But now we suspect the combination of the two may actually help the body create and maintain its own internal stock of antioxidants.

Eating a plant-based, chlorophyll-rich diet may be especially important for those on cholesterol-lowering statin drugs, as these medications can interfere with CoQ10 production.

Green Can Taste Great

I hope I've been able to convince you to eat greens as often as possible. The problem for many people is getting them to *taste* good. I'm afraid too many of us still suffer flashbacks from overcooked, slimy green lumps on school cafeteria trays.

Take kale, for example. Fibrous and grassy tasting, right? Kind of bitter too? Some varieties are more palatable than others. In a good supermarket produce section, you may be able to find three types: green, black, and red. Nutritionally, the differences among them appear to be insignificant compared to how much of each you may be willing to eat.[18,19] The healthiest kale is the one you'll eat the most of.

I would suggest using black kale (also called lacinato, dinosaur, or Tuscan kale), red kale (also found as red Russian kale), or baby kale, since these varieties are all milder and more tender than the more common mature green (curly) kale.

Start by rinsing the leaves thoroughly under running water. Then rip off the stems and tear the leaves into bite-sized pieces. Alternatively, after the leaves are removed from their stems, roll them up and slice into thin ribbons. If you want to make it even easier on yourself, just use whatever type you can find frozen. Frozen greens are cheaper, last longer, and come prewashed and prechopped.

There's a phenomenon called flavor-flavor conditioning in which you can change your palate by linking a less pleasant flavor (for instance, sour or bitter) with a more pleasant one (say, sweet). For example, when researchers tried adding sugar to sour grapefruit juice, people liked it better. No surprise. But within a few days, the study subjects began to like even *unsweetened* grapefruit juice more than they did before the experiment started. In fact, this reconditioning of the palate lasted for at least weeks after the sugar was removed.[20]

The same happens when researchers dip or spritz broccoli with sugar water or aspartame.[21] I know that sounds gross, but they're not actually making the broccoli taste sweet. The added sweetness merely masks the bitterness by fooling your taste buds.[22] This is why the so-called secret ingredient in many collard greens recipes is a spoonful of sugar. Certainly, if there were ever a food to justify the use of a yellow- or red-light condiment to boost consumption, it would be the single healthiest of all foods: greens. I use a balsamic glaze even though it has some added sugar in it. It would be healthier, though, to add green-light sweetness in the form of something like figs or grated apples.

The sweetness trick is why green smoothies can be so delicious (if not a little odd looking). Smoothies can be a great way to introduce greens into children's diets. The basic triad is a liquid, ripe fruit, and fresh greens. I'd start with a two-to-one ratio of fruits to greens to start with before tipping heavier toward greens on the scale. So, for example, one cup of water, a frozen banana, a cup of frozen berries, and a cup of packed baby spinach would be a classic green smoothie 101.

I like to add fresh mint leaves as well for a boost of flavor (and even more greens). Fresh herbs can be expensive at the store, but mint can grow like a weed in your yard or in a pot on your windowsill. Eating greens for breakfast can be as delicious as mint chocolate oatmeal—cooked oatmeal, chopped mint leaves, cocoa powder, and a healthy sweetener (see page 388).

When you're thinking about ways to pair your greens with something you already love to make the greens more palatable, consider mixing them with a green-light source of fat: nuts, seeds, nut or seed butters, or avocados. Many of the nutrients greens are famous for are fat soluble, including beta-carotene, lutein, vitamin K, and zeaxanthin. So pairing your greens with a green-light source of fat may not only make them taste better but will maximize nutrient absorption. This can mean enjoying a creamy tahini-based dressing on your salad, putting walnuts in your pesto, or sprinkling some toasted sesame seeds on your sautéed kale.

The jump in nutrient absorption is no small effect. When researchers tried feeding people a healthy salad of spinach, romaine, carrots, and tomatoes along with a source of fat, there was an impressive spike in carotenoid phytonutrients in their bloodstream over the next eight hours. With a fat-free dressing, carotenoid absorption flatlined down to negligible amounts; it was as if they'd never eaten the salad at all.[23] Similarly, adding some avocado to your salsa may triple the amount of fat-soluble nutrients that make it into your bloodstream (in this case, the lycopene in the tomatoes).[24] It doesn't take much. Just three grams of fat in an entire hot meal may be sufficient to boost absorption.[25] That's just a single walnut or a spoonful of avocado or shredded coconut. Snack on a few pistachios after a meal, and you're all set. The greens and the source of fat just have to end up in your stomach at the same time.

Another way to remove bitterness from greens is to blanch or boil them, but unfortunately this works by leaching some of the healthy compounds into the cooking water.[26] If you're making soup, that's not a problem, because the nutrients aren't destroyed as much as they are displaced. If the cooking liquid is poured off, however, you could be losing some nutrition. But even if 50 percent of these healthy compounds go down the drain, if the decreased bitterness motivates you to eat twice as many greens, problem solved! Whenever I'm boiling pasta, for example, I'll add a bunch of fresh greens to the pot a few minutes before I'm ready to drain the pasta. I know I'll be losing some nutrients when I pour off the cooking water, but it's worth it to me for the convenience of throwing everything into one pot and getting my family to eat even more greens.

Try to incorporate greens into as many meals as possible. I put just about everything I eat on a bed of greens. That way, the greens take on the flavor of the rest of the dish. However, if you want to eat cooked greens "straight," you can try adding lemon juice, flavored vinegars, red pepper flakes, garlic, ginger, low-sodium soy sauce, or caramelized onions. I personally like mine hot, sweet, smoky, and salty. I use hot sauce for heat, balsamic glaze for sweetness, and both smoked paprika and liquid smoke. For saltiness, I used to be fond of a soy sauce substitute called Bragg Liquid Aminos until I got more serious about cutting down my sodium intake. The best sodium-free salt substitute I've been able to find is something called Table Tasty. (What's with these names?)

There are whole grocery aisles full of prepared sauces with which you can experiment. Most have added salt, oil, or sugar, so I try to reserve them for exceptionally healthy foods. Mixing yellow- and red-light foods together (like dipping your fries and McNuggets in barbecue sauce) may just add insult to injury, but I wouldn't eat half as many baked rosemary sweet-potato fries if I weren't dipping them in hot-sauce-spiked ketchup. And if there were ever an excuse to dip out of the green-light zone, it would be for green, leafy vegetables.

During my bachelor days, I would regularly order Chinese food for delivery—usually broccoli and garlic sauce (hold the white rice). Then I'd throw brown rice or quinoa along with dried lentils into my rice cooker and steam or microwave a pound of greens. By the time the delivery arrived, everything was ready and I would just mix it all together and have more than enough for leftovers.

You can also find prepackaged pouches of Indian food online or at Indian or natural foods markets. Again, I'd use them as sauces rather than eat them as a meal in themselves. My favorite is spinach dal—that way, I'm eating greens in a greens sauce! That's like the kale-pesto principle: Use one green (basil) to make the other green (kale) taste better.

The Health Benefits of Vinegar

Vinegar may be one condiment that's good for you. Randomized, controlled trials involving both diabetic and nondiabetic individuals suggest that adding two teaspoons of vinegar to a meal may improve blood sugar control, effectively blunting the blood sugar spike after a meal by about 20 percent.[27] So adding vinegar to potato salad or to rice (like the Japanese do to make sushi rice) or dipping bread in balsamic vinegar may blunt the effects of these high-glycemic foods.

We've known about the antiglycemic effect of vinegar for more than twenty-five years, but we're still not sure of the mechanism.[28] Originally, it was thought that vinegar slowed stomach emptying, but even consuming vinegar outside of meals appears to help. Type 2 diabetics consuming two tablespoons of apple cider vinegar at bedtime, for example, were found to wake up with better blood sugars in the morning.[29] Consuming pickles or vinegar *pills* does not seem to have the same effect.[30] Do not, however, drink vinegar straight, as it can burn your esophagus,[31] or in excess—a cup a day for six years (that's two thousand cups!) was discovered to be a bad idea.[32]

Vinegar may also help with polycystic ovary syndrome (PCOS), improve arterial function, and help reduce body fat. A daily tablespoon of apple cider vinegar restored ovarian function within a few months in four out of seven women with PCOS.[33] A tablespoon of rice vinegar was found to acutely improve artery function in postmenopausal women. We're not sure why, but the acetate from the acetic acid in vinegar may lead to improved nitric-oxide production (see page 136).[34] Such an effect would be expected to help with hypertension, and indeed there is a study purporting to show blood pressure benefits from a tablespoon of vinegar a day.[35]

Despite folk wisdom to the contrary, vinegar does not appear to be an effective treatment for head lice,[36] but it may help with weight loss. A double-blind, placebo-controlled (but vinegar company–funded) study was performed, in which obese subjects consumed daily vinegar drinks with either one or two tablespoons of apple cider vinegar, or a placebo drink that tasted like vinegar but contained no acetic acid. Both vinegar groups lost significantly more weight than the control group. Though the effect was modest—about four pounds over a three-month period—CT scans showed the vinegar groups' subjects lost a significant amount of their "visceral" fat, the abdominal fat that is particularly associated with chronic disease risk.[37]

There are all sorts of flavorful, exotic vinegars to explore these days, including fig, peach, and pomegranate. I encourage you to experiment and find ways to incorporate some into your diet.

Salad Days

Having a big salad every day is a great way to burn through the Daily Dozen. To a base of mesclun greens and arugula, I add tomato, red bell pepper, beans, and barberries, along with toasted nuts if I'm using a fat-free dressing. My current favorite dressing recipe is a Caesar spin-off shared by Dr. Michael Klaper from the TrueNorth Health Center:

2 tablespoons almond meal
3 cloves crushed garlic
3 tablespoons dijon mustard
3 tablespoons nutritional yeast flakes
2 tablespoons white miso
3 tablespoons lemon juice
⅓ cup water

Blend and enjoy! (If you have a high-speed blender, you could probably use whole almonds instead of meal.)

Baby spinach may have higher levels of phytonutrients than mature spinach leaves,[38] but what about *real* baby spinach—so-called microgreens, the seedlings of vegetables and herbs? A nutritional analysis of twenty-five commercially available microgreens found they did have significantly higher nutrient densities. For example, red cabbage microgreens have a sixfold higher vitamin C concentration than mature red cabbage and nearly seventy times the vitamin K.[39] But they're eaten in such microquantities that even the healthiest upscale restaurant garnish probably isn't going to do much for you.

If, however, you want to grow your own, you could have rotating trays of microgreens that you snip off with scissors for probably the healthiest salad out there. (On a lecture tour, I once stayed with someone who did just that, and

I've been jealous ever since.) Microgreens are the perfect plants for the impatient gardener—fully grown in just one to two weeks.

The One Green to Avoid

Although greens are the healthiest of foods, there's one green I caution against eating: alfalfa sprouts. Over a dozen years, twenty-eight outbreaks of *Salmonella* food poisoning linked to sprouts have been documented in the United States, affecting 1,275 people.[40] Of course, *Salmonella*-tainted eggs sicken an estimated 142,000 Americans every year,[41] but that doesn't make it any less tragic for those hospitalized and killed in "sproutbreaks." Alfalfa sprout seeds have all sorts of microscopic nooks and crannies where bacteria from manure-contaminated irrigation water can hide. So even home-sprouted alfalfa seeds should not be considered safe.

I will never forget a presentation I gave in Boston. It was in a game show—style format in which contestants from the audience tried to rank, from healthiest to unhealthiest, the foods I'd brought with me. There was a lively cacophony of conflicting advice shouted from the crowd. You can imagine the groans when I revealed that alfalfa sprouts—a quintessential health food—belonged way at the top on the foods-to-avoid list.

Later that night, I was stuck with the sprouts after all the healthier and yummier items had been given away as prizes. I had just told my audience not to eat them—but I hate wasting food. In a do-as-I-say-not-as-I-do moment, I added them to my salad that night. Yes, they had been sitting in the car all day and on stage for hours. Yes, they were at the top of my game show's list of foods you should not eat. But, what were the odds that that one particular package was contaminated? I went back to work the next day at the New England Medical Center emergency room—not as a physician but as a patient with *Salmonella* food poisoning.

So other than the dreaded alfalfa sprout, greens truly are the healthiest foods on the planet. You simply can't do better in terms of nutrition per calorie. Explore, innovate, taste test, play, and teach your palate to enjoy them. Whether you sneak them into a refreshing smoothie, incorporate them into sauces and dressings, use them as a base for main dishes, or eat them straight in a big, vibrant salad—just do it. Your body will thank you with every bite of greens you take.

Other Vegetables

Dr. Greger's Other Favorite Vegetables

Artichokes, asparagus, beets, bell peppers, carrots, corn, garlic, mushrooms (button, oyster, portobello, and shiitake), okra, onions, purple potatoes, pumpkin, sea vegetables (arame, dulse, and nori), snap peas, squash (delicata, summer, and spaghetti squash varieties), sweet potatoes/yams, tomatoes, and zucchini

Serving Sizes:

1 cup raw leafy vegetables
½ cup raw or cooked nonleafy vegetables
½ cup vegetable juice
¼ cup dried mushrooms

Daily Recommendation:

2 servings per day

The mammoth Global Burden of Disease Study identified the typical American diet as the primary cause of Americans' death and disability[1] and inadequate vegetable intake as our fifth-leading dietary risk factor, nearly as bad as our consumption of processed meat.[2] The Union of Concerned Scientists estimates that if the nation increased its consumption of fruits and veggies to meet the dietary guidelines, we might save the lives of more than one hundred thousand people a year.[3]

You should eat more fruits and vegetables as if your life depended on it, because maybe it does.

Garden Variety: Diversifying Your Vegetable Portfolio

Perhaps the least controversial advice in all of nutrition is to eat more fruits and vegetables, which is to say eat more plants, since the term *vegetable* basically just means all parts of the plant that aren't fruit. There are root vegetables like sweet potatoes, stem vegetables like rhubarb, pod vegetables like peas, and even flower vegetables like broccoli. (It isn't called cauli*flower* for nothing.) We've already talked about the leaf vegetables in the greens section. If dark-green, leafy vegetables are the healthiest foods around, then why branch out to other parts of the plant? (Pun intended!) Yes, you're supposed to eat the rainbow, but didn't we just learn that green leaves have an entire spectrum of colors hidden inside?

Unlike more generic compounds like vitamin C, which is broadly available in various fruits and vegetables, other nutrients are not so evenly distributed. Just as certain fruits like citrus offer unique nonpigment phytonutrients not found in other fruits, different vegetables contribute different compounds. White cauliflower, lacking antioxidant pigments, doesn't appear to have much to offer at first glance, but because it belongs to the cruciferous family, it's one of your healthiest options. Similarly, white mushrooms may look pretty drab, but they can provide *myco*nutrients not found in the entire plant kingdom.

We now know that certain phytonutrients bind to specific receptors and other proteins in the body. I talked about the Ah "broccoli receptors" in chapter 5. There are also effectively green-tea receptors in your body—that is, receptors for EGCG, a key component of green tea. There are binding proteins for the phytonutrients in grapes, onions, and capers. Recently, a cell surface receptor was even identified for a nutrient concentrated in apple peels. These specific proteins may not be activated, though, unless you eat specific foods.[4]

The different phytonutrient profiles may then result in different clinical effects. For example, drinking tomato juice can rescue the immune function of study subjects crippled by two weeks of fruit and vegetable deficiency, but carrot juice apparently cannot.[5] Even different parts of the same vegetable can have different effects. One of the reasons certain tomato products appear to be protective against heart attacks[6] is because the yellow fluid surrounding the seeds concentrates a compound that suppresses platelet activation.[7] (Platelets are what help trigger the blood clots that cause heart attacks and most strokes.) Aspirin has a similar effect, but it doesn't work in everyone and can increase bleeding risk—two limitations that the tomato compound may be able to overcome.[8,9] But if you only consume tomato sauce, juice, or ketchup, you may be missing out[10] since the seeds are removed during processing. So when picking out canned tomato products, choose whole, crushed, or diced tomatoes instead of tomato sauce, purée, or paste.

Different plants may also affect the same part of the body in different ways. Consider mental function, for instance. In a study of dozens of fruits and vegetables, from raspberries to rutabagas, certain plants appear to shore up specific cognitive domains. For example, the consumption of some plant foods was associated with better executive function, perceptual speed, and semantic (fact-based) memory, while the consumption of others was more consistently associated with visual-spatial skills and autobiographical memory.[11] In other words, you may need to build up a portfolio of many fruits and vegetables to cover all your bases.

One of the reasons studies may underestimate the protective effects of plant foods is that they tend to measure *quantity* of fruit and vegetable consumption rather than *quality* of fruit and vegetable consumption. People are more likely to eat bananas and cucumbers than blueberries and kale. But variety is important too. Half the fruit servings in the United States are taken up by just five fruits—apples and apple juice, bananas, grapes, orange juice, and watermelon—and most vegetable servings are from canned tomatoes, potatoes, and iceberg lettuce.[12]

In one of the few studies that looked specifically at the diversity of fruit and vegetable consumption, the variety of intake was an even better predictor of decreased inflammation in the bodies of middle-aged adults than the absolute quantity of consumption.[13] Even after removing the effects of quantity, the addition of two different types of fruits and vegetables per week has been associated with an 8 percent reduction in the incidence of type 2 diabetes.[14] These kinds of data led the American Heart Association to add a recommendation in their latest dietary guidelines to also eat a *variety* of fruits and vegetables.[15] It's an important addition; otherwise, a big bag of potato chips or one head of iceberg lettuce could technically fulfill or exceed your recommended nine servings a day.

It's better to eat a whole orange rather than take a vitamin C pill, since the pill deprives you of all the other wonderful nutrients in the oranges themselves. The same principle applies when you don't diversify your fruit and vegetable consumption. By only eating apples, you also miss out on oranges' nutrients. You don't get the limonoids in citrus, like limonin, limonol, or tangeretin, though you may get more malic acid (from the Latin *malum*, meaning apple). When it comes to the unique phytonutrient profile of each fruit and vegetable, it's like comparing apples to oranges! That's why you should mix it up.

In a sense, though, all fruits are just fruits, whereas vegetables can be any other part of the plant. Roots may harbor different nutrients than shoots. For this reason, it may be even more important to get in a variety of vegetables, so you can benefit from all parts of the plant, as one large cancer study of nearly a half-million people did indeed find.[16] "Because each vegetable contains a unique combination," a recent review concluded, "a great diversity of vegetables should be eaten . . . to get all the health benefits."[17] Variety is not only the spice of life; it may prolong it as well.

Eating Better to Look Better

We've all heard of the proverbial golden glow that's often equated with health, vitality, and youth. But instead of using a tanning bed to achieve a more golden hue, you can do it with a bed of greens.

There are certain animals who use diet to increase their sexual attractiveness. Great tits, distinctive olive-and-black songbirds ubiquitous throughout Europe and Asia, tend to prefer carotenoid-rich caterpillars, which make their breast plumage brighter yellow, to become more attractive to potential mates.[18] Can a similar phenomenon be found in humans?

Researchers took digital photographs of African, Asian, and Caucasian men and women and asked others to manipulate the skin tone of their faces with a dial until they reached what they perceived to be the healthiest-looking color.[19] Sure enough, both men and women preferred the yellow "golden glow" that can be achieved through "dietary carotenoid deposition in the skin."[20] In other words, by eating the yellow and red pigments in fruits and vegetables, like beta-carotene in sweet potatoes and lycopene in tomatoes, men and women may be able to naturally acquire more of a golden and rosy glow. Researchers decided to put it to the test.

Based on a six-week study of college students, the complexion achieved by eating my Daily Dozen recommendation of nine servings of fruits and vegetables a day was found to be significantly healthier and more attractive looking than that achieved by eating three daily servings.[21] The healthier you eat, the healthier you look. Indeed, studies find that "individuals with the lowest fruit and vegetable intake may enjoy the most improvement in appearance."[22]

What about wrinkles? A study out of Japan used the six-point Daniell scale to rate the extent of crow's-feet wrinkles around the eyes of more than seven hundred women, with a score of one being the least severe and a score of six being the most severe. The researchers found that "a higher intake of green and yellow vegetables was associated with decreased facial wrinkling." Women who ate less than one daily serving of green and yellow veggies averaged about a three on the Daniell scale, while women who ate more than two servings a day averaged closer to a two. The researchers celebrated "the potential for these studies to promote a healthy diet . . ."[23]

I am certainly not above appealing to vanity, especially for my younger patients who have seemed more interested in which dietary changes will clear their acne than which will clear their future risk of chronic disease. So I'm happy to see articles embrace these types of studies with headlines like "Greens to Be Gorgeous."[24] Still, although looking great on the outside is fine, looking great on the inside is even better.

Mushrooming Benefits

Ergothioneine is an unusual amino acid. Although it was discovered more than a century ago, it was ignored until recently when researchers found that humans have a transporter protein in their bodies specifically designed to pull ergothioneine out of food and into body tissue. This suggests that this amino acid plays some important physiological role. But what? Our first clue was the tissue distribution. Ergothioneine concentrates in parts of your body where there is a lot of oxidative stress—your liver and the lenses of your eyes, for example, as well as such sensitive tissues as bone marrow and semen. Researchers guessed, then, that it might act as a so-called cytoprotectant, a cell protector, and that's indeed what was subsequently found.[25]

Ergothioneine appears to function as a potent intramitochondrial antioxidant, meaning it can get inside the mitochondria—the microscopic power plants within your cells. The DNA inside the mitochondria is especially vulnerable to free-radical damage, since many other antioxidants are unable to penetrate the mitochondrial membrane. This is one reason ergothioneine may be so important. Depriving human cells of this amino acid leads to accelerated DNA damage and cell death. Unfortunately, the human body cannot make ergothioneine; you can only get it through food. "Because of its dietary origin and the toxicity associated with its depletion," Johns Hopkins University researchers concluded, "ET [ergothioneine] may represent a new vitamin . . ."[26] If it were classified as such, that would make it the first new vitamin since vitamin B12 was isolated back in 1948.[27]

What are the best dietary sources of ergothioneine? The highest levels by far have been reported in mushrooms. For example, oyster mushrooms, which you can grow yourself in only two weeks from a just-add-water kit, have more than one thousand units (µg/dag) of ergothioneine, about nine times more than their closest competitor, black beans. And a serving of black beans has about eight times more than a serving of the third-leading source, chicken liver. Chicken meat, along with beef and pork, only has about ten units, one hundred times less than oyster mushrooms. Kidney beans have about four times more than meat, but even at forty-five units, they pale in comparison to some of the mushrooms.[28]

Ergothioneine is heat stable, which means it's not destroyed when mushrooms are cooked.[29] This is good news, because it's best not to eat mushrooms raw; there's a toxin in edible mushrooms called agaritine to which you should minimize your exposure. Thankfully, the toxin is destroyed by cooking. Just thirty seconds in the microwave wipes out most agaritine in mushrooms. Freezing also gets rid of most of it, but drying does not. If you put dried mushrooms in your soup, it's best to boil them for at least five minutes.[30] Morel mushrooms are a special case. The toxin levels appear higher and may react with alcohol even after cooking.[31] I consider all other cooked edible mushrooms to be green-light foods and all other edible raw mushrooms yellow-light foods. However, raw morel mushrooms, cooked morels served with alcohol, and all wild-foraged mushrooms should be on the red-light list in my opinion.

Do you have to eat mushrooms to be healthy? No. (Otherwise, it would be the Daily Baker's Dozen.) Famously in our family, my mom has never eaten a mushroom in her life and never will, because they "look funny." But given the potential immune and anticancer benefits documented in chapters 5 and 11, I would encourage you to try to find ways to incorporate them into your diet.

My favorite way to enjoy mushrooms is to grill portobellos. I picked up a George Foreman Grill from my local thrift store, and my family has officially renamed it the Portobello Mushroom Grill. I know people tend to marinate portobellos first, but I just drizzle them with balsamic vinegar, grill until the juice starts dripping, and then add cracked pepper. They're so good we eat them just like that.

Pop quiz: Which is healthier? Plain white mushrooms or portobellos? Trick question! They're the same mushroom. The little white button mushrooms grow up to be portobellos. White mushrooms are just baby 'bellos.

Mushrooms can be stuffed, enjoyed in soups like mushroom barley, act as the star of a creamy risotto or pâté, serve as the base of a great gravy or as a flavorful addition to any pasta sauce, or simply be braised with crushed garlic in red wine.

Even More Vegetables!

My favorite way to eat raw veggies is to dip bell pepper strips, carrots, or snap peas in a hummus or bean dip, and my favorite way to eat them cooked is by roasting them. Roasting can transform vegetables into otherworldly creations. If you don't believe me, try roasting red bell peppers, brussels sprouts, beets, or squash. Never thought you liked okra because it's too slimy? Try it roasted.

One of my favorite springtime dishes is roasted asparagus dipped in guacamole. (Here's an interesting asparagus fact: Did you know there are four types of people in the world? Those whose pee turns stinky after eating asparagus, and those whose doesn't, *and* those who are apparently genetically incapable of smelling the asparagus pee odor, and, finally, those who can. So some people may not think they get stinky pee from asparagus, but they actually do and just can't smell it![32])

Sweet potatoes are one of my favorite snacks. During harsh Boston winters while I was in medical school, I would take two freshly microwaved sweet potatoes and pop them in my coat pockets as natural hand warmers. When they cooled down, my hand warmers became instant healthy snacks! It's actually better to boil them, though, to best preserve their nutritional content.[33] Regardless of your cooking method, be sure to keep on the skin. The peel of the sweet potato has nearly ten times the antioxidant power as the inner flesh (on a per-weight basis), giving them an antioxidant capacity approaching that of blueberries.[34]

Sweet potatoes themselves can be considered a superfood.[35] They are ranked as one of the healthiest foods on the planet[36] and one day, perhaps, even off the planet—NASA has chosen them for future space missions.[37] In fact, they're among the healthiest *and* cheapest, with one of the highest nutrient-rich food scores per dollar.[38] When picking out varieties at the supermarket, remember that a sweet potato's nutritional content is tied directly to the intensity of its color. The more yellow or orange its flesh, the healthier it may be.[39]

Sweet potatoes are healthier than plain potatoes, but if you're going to choose the latter, seek out those with blue or purple flesh. The consumption of one boiled purple potato a day for six weeks was found to significantly decrease inflammation, something neither white nor yellow potatoes were able to accomplish.[40] The same was found for oxidation, but much faster. Within hours of consumption, purple potatoes increased the antioxidant capacity of study subjects' bloodstream, whereas white potato starch appeared to actually have a pro-oxidant effect.[41] Blue potatoes may have ten times more antioxidant power than regular white ones.[42] The most exciting purple potato study to date had people with hypertension eat six to eight microwaved small purple potatoes a day, and they were able to significantly bring down their blood pressure levels within a month.[43]

Purple *sweet* potatoes may offer the best of both worlds.[44] I was so excited to discover them that I bought them as holiday gifts for my family one year—stocking stuffers they could stuff themselves with!

Getting Kids (and Parents) to Eat Their Veggies

Published strategies for getting kids (of all ages) to eat their vegetables include cutting them into slices, sticks, or stars—the most popular shape.[45] Supposedly, putting an Elmo sticker on veggies swayed 50 percent of children to choose broccoli over a chocolate bar.[46] If they're still not biting, though, you can apply the same trick I use to get our dog to take her pills: Dip the veggies in peanut butter. A study found that pairing vegetables with peanut butter successfully increases intake "even in vegetable-resistant children."[47] Offering a salad dressing dip has also been found to help.[48]

Simply having healthy foods out and available can boost intake. Guess what happened when researchers put out bowls of cut-up fresh fruit in addition to the regular party fare brought by parents for kindergarten or preschool celebrations? No special effort was made to encourage students to choose the fruit—the researchers just put it out on the table with all the other food. Would kids actually eat fruit when such foods as birthday cake, ice cream, and cheese puffs were available? Yes! On average, each kid ate a full fruit serving.[49] Take that, cheese puffs!

Even just calling vegetables by different names can help. Elementary schools were able to double vegetable consumption simply by coming up with names that better appealed to the kids. Students ate twice the number of carrots if they were called "X-Ray Vision Carrots," compared to when they were just carrots or generically called the "Food of the Day."[50] Are adults as gullible? Apparently so. For example, grown-ups reported "Traditional Cajun Red Beans and Rice" tasted better than just "Red Beans with Rice" . . . even though they were the exact same dish.[51]

When school cafeterias put out signs like Power Punch Broccoli and Silly Dilly Green Beans, or called broccoli Tiny Tasty Tree Tops, selection of broccoli increased by about 110 percent, and selection of green beans jumped by nearly 180 percent.[52] The researchers concluded that "these studies demonstrate that using an attractive name to describe a healthy food in a cafeteria is robustly effective, persistent, and scalable with little or no money or experience. These names were *not* carefully crafted, discussed in focus groups, and then pretested." They were just invented out of thin air. And kids were suckered into eating healthier for weeks simply by adults' putting out silly little signs. Indeed, in the school displaying these playful new names in the cafeteria line, vegetable purchasing went up nearly 100 percent, while in the control school without signs, vegetable purchases started low and actually got worse.[53] So why isn't every single school in the country doing this right now? Bring it up at your next PTA meeting.

Let's not forget the hide-the-veggies strategy. Studies have shown that broccoli, cauliflower, tomatoes, squash, and zucchini can be added covertly to familiar entrées such that the appearance, flavor, and texture of the original recipes are maintained (like puréeing vegetables into a pasta sauce).[54] Studies found the trick works for adults too. Researchers were able to slip in up to a pound of clandestine vegetables a day (resulting in 350 fewer calories eaten).[55] Surreptitiously incorporating vegetables into foods shouldn't be the only way that vegetables are served to children, though. Since the appetite for an initially unappetizing vegetable can be increased through repeated exposure, it is important to use several strategies to ensure that kids experience whole vegetables. After all, they're not always going to be eating at home. One of the most important predictors of children's fruit and vegetable consumption has been found to be parents' consumption,[56] so if you want your kids to eat healthfully, it helps to be a healthy role model.

The Top Cancer-Fighting Vegetables

According to a landmark American Institute for Cancer Research report, any effect of plant-based diets is "likely to be due not only to the exclusion of meat, but also to the inclusion of a larger number and of wider range of plant foods, containing an extensive variety of potential cancer-preventive substances."[57] In other words, it may not be enough to cut down on meat; you need to eat as many whole, healthy plant foods as possible. Meatless Mondays are great, but even more so when followed by Tomato Tuesdays, Watercress Wednesdays, and so on.

Different vegetables may target different cancers—sometimes even in the same organ. For example, cabbage, cauliflower, broccoli, and brussels sprouts are associated with lower risk of colon cancer in the middle and right side of your body, whereas risk of colon cancer farther down on the left side appears to be lowered more by carrots, pumpkins, and apples.[58]

An extraordinary study published in the journal *Food Chemistry* pitted thirty-four common vegetables in vitro against eight different types of human cancer cells: breast cancer, brain tumors, kidney cancer, lung cancer, childhood brain tumors, pancreatic cancer, prostate cancer, and stomach cancer. Take breast cancer, for example. Seven vegetables (eggplant, bok choy, carrot, tomato, endive, fennel bulb, and romaine lettuce) appeared useless, suppressing breast cancer cell growth no more than the control. Six vegetables (orange bell pepper, english cucumber, radicchio, jalapeño, potato, and beetroot) nearly halved cancer growth, but five veggies (cauliflower, brussels sprouts, green onion, leek, and garlic) "abolished" cancer growth completely, stopping breast tumor cells dead in their tracks.[59]

There were two take-home messages to come out of this remarkable study. The first is that you should eat a portfolio of vegetables. Radishes, for example, are completely unable to stop pancreatic cancer cell growth. However, radishes were 100 percent effective at halting the growth of stomach cancer cells. Orange bell peppers were useless against stomach cancer, but they were able to suppress prostate cancer cell growth by more than 75 percent. In the words of the researchers, "a diversified diet, containing several distinct classes of vegetables (and hence of phytochemicals) is essential for effective prevention of cancer."[60]

How to Make a Cancer-Fighting Salad

Imagine you're standing in line at one of those made-to-order salad places where you get to choose your lettuce, your toppings, and your dressing. You start with the greens. For the sake of this example, let's say you are offered a choice between the five covered in the *Food Chemistry* study: Boston lettuce, endive, radicchio, romaine lettuce, and spinach. Which should you choose? Based on the study findings: spinach. Out of the five options, spinach beat out the others against breast cancer, brain tumors, kidney cancer, lung cancer, pediatric brain tumors, pancreatic cancer, prostate cancer, and stomach cancer. The runner up? Radicchio.[61]

Which toppings should you add to your spinach salad? You only get five to choose from and, after consulting the Daily Dozen cheat sheet in your wallet, you can tick three check boxes immediately: beans, berries, and nuts. Now you only have two toppings left. Out of the thirty-two remaining vegetables included in the study, which two of the following should you pick? Choose carefully:

Acorn squash	Curly cabbage	Leek
Asparagus	Eggplant	Orange bell pepper
Beetroot	Endive	Potato
Bok choy	English cucumber	Radicchio
Boston lettuce	Fennel bulb	Radish
Broccoli	Fiddleheads	Red cabbage
Brussels sprouts	Garlic	Romaine lettuce
Cabbage	Green beans	Rutabaga
Carrot	Green onions	Tomato
Cauliflower	Jalapeño	Yellow onion
Celery	Kale	

Which two did you choose? If one of your choices was brussels sprouts, cabbage, curly cabbage, or kale, *and* the other choice was garlic, green onions, or leek, you get a gold star! Of all the vegetables tested, those had the most cancer-preventing potential. Notice anything they have in common? All the top choices belong to one of only two superfood families: cruciferous vegetables and the allium veggie family, which includes garlic and onions. As the researchers put it, "the inclusion of cruciferous and Allium vegetables in the diet is essential for effective dietary-based chemopreventive [cancer-preventing] strategies."[62]

Note that the most common vegetables didn't make the cut. "The majority of the vegetable extracts tested in this study, including vegetables that are commonly consumed in Western countries such as potato, carrot, lettuce and tomato," the researchers concluded, "had little effect on the proliferation of the tumour cell lines."[63]

The single most effective vegetable was garlic, which came in first against breast cancer, both child and adult brain cancer, lung cancer, pancreatic cancer, prostate cancer, and stomach cancer, and second after leeks against kidney cancer. So might I suggest a garlicky salad dressing like the one on page 319?

Garlic and Onions

As the above salad example illustrates, garlic, onions, leeks, and other vegetables in the allium family appear to have special properties. Wait a second, though. Like chemotherapy, maybe garlic isn't just toxic to cancer cells but toxic to *all* cells? That wouldn't be good. Researchers also wondered about this, so they decided to compare the effects of garlic and other vegetables on the growth of both cancer cells and normal cells. The same garlic dose that blocked nearly 80 percent of cancer cell proliferation appeared to have no effect whatsoever against normal cells, and similar results were found for the other allium and cruciferous vegetables. In other words, vegetables are selective; they destroy cancer cells but leave normal cells alone.

These results were seen in a petri dish, though, and while such studies may have direct relevance for digestive-tract cancers that come in close contact with these foods, for these foods to be protective against other cancers, the anti-cancer compounds would have to be absorbed into the bloodstream. And in the case of brain tumors, the anticancer compounds would additionally have to cross the blood-brain barrier. The findings do seem to sync with other studies, though, both among human populations and in other laboratories, that corroborate the cancer-fighting benefits of cruciferous vegetables,[64] garlic, and onions.[65] Regardless, this study illustrates the dramatic differences between the biological capacities of individual vegetables and families of veggies and underscores the importance of including a variety of vegetables in your diet.

Which Is the Best Cooking Method?

Is it better to eat your vegetables raw or cooked? If you're thinking raw, you're right. But if you guessed cooked, you're also right.[66] Confused? Well, a number of nutrients, like vitamin C, are partially destroyed by cooking. For example, steamed broccoli may have about 10 percent less vitamin C than raw broccoli.[67] If, however, you prefer cooked broccoli enough to eat seven florets of steamed rather than six florets of raw, then you just more than made up the difference.

Other nutrients, however, actually become *more* absorbable after cooking. For example, you end up with more than six times the vitamin A in your bloodstream from cooked carrots compared to raw ones.[68] A study of long-term raw foodists found surprisingly low blood levels of the red antioxidant pigment lycopene.[69] It's not what you eat but what you absorb, and cooked to-matoes appear able to better boost your lycopene levels.[70] Steaming may also improve the bile acid–binding capacity of vegetables,[71] which may help lower breast cancer risk.[72]

Raw-food diets automatically eliminate most red- and yellow-light foods, which is not only an improvement over the standard American diet but also over many plant-based diets. There is no evidence to suggest, however, that eating raw foods largely or exclusively is healthier than eating a combination of cooked and raw whole plant foods.

Some cooking methods, though, are preferable to others. Deep-fried foods, whether of plant origin (like french fries) or from animals (like fried chicken), have been associated with higher cancer risk.[73] Deep-frying leads to the pro-duction of dangerous heterocyclic amines in meat (as detailed in chapter 11) and to acrylamide in deep-fried plant foods. The excess lifetime cancer risk attributable to the consumption of french fries in young children, for example, may be as high as one or two in ten thousand—meaning about one in ten thousand boys and girls eating french fries may develop cancer that would have otherwise not occurred had they *not* eaten french fries. The researchers urge deep-fryer cooking times and temperatures be set as low as possible "while still maintaining a tasty quality."[74] (They wouldn't want to reduce can-cer so much that the deep-fried foods wouldn't be as tasty!) Blanching potatoes first can reduce acrylamide formation, but potato chip companies argue that this might have a negative impact on the "nutritional properties of the fried product," because it would leach away some of the vitamin C.[75] But if you're relying on potato chips to get your vitamin C, acrylamide is probably the least of your worries.

What is the best way to cook vegetables to preserve nutrition? I am often asked that question, and it's difficult to answer, as it varies for different vegeta-bles. What we would need is a study that measures a variety of different cook-ing methods with a variety of different vegetables. Thankfully, we got exactly that in 2009. A Spanish research team pulled out all the stops, performing more than three hundred separate experiments with twenty vegetables and six cooking methods, all while considering three different measures of antioxidant activity. They tested baking, boiling, frying, griddling (cooking in a thick fry-ing pan with no oil), microwaving, and pressure-cooking.[76]

Let's start with the worst methods in terms of antioxidant loss: boiling and pressure-cooking. When you use these wet-cooking methods, some of the nutrition is lost into the cooking water, but less than I would have thought. For instance, the researchers found that boiling removes an average of 14 percent of the vegetables' antioxidant capacity. So, if you like your corn on the cob boiled, you could just add an extra quarter ear to the pot. (Six quarters boiled may have all the antioxidant power of five quarters raw, baked, or microwaved.[77]) Of the six cooking methods studied, griddling and microwaving were actually the gentlest. Nuking your veggies appears to preserve, on average, more than 95 percent of antioxidant capacity.[78]

Those are averages across twenty vegetables, however. Some vegetables are more resistant, and antioxidant power actually *increases* with cooking in some veggies. Which do you think was the most vulnerable vegetable—that is, the one probably best eaten raw? If you guessed bell peppers, you're right. They've been shown to lose up to 70 percent of their antioxidant capacity when baked in an oven. I'm going to continue to roast my peppers because of how much I love the taste, but I realize I'm getting less nutritional bang for my buck. (No biggie, though, because I can just add an extra sprinkle of oregano to my roasted red pepper pasta sauce.)

On the other hand, three vegetables hardly seem to be affected at all by cooking: artichokes, beets, and onions. You can even boil them, and they'll still retain 97.5 percent of their antioxidant power.

Finally, there are two vegetables that may actually become *healthier* through cooking: the humble carrot and the celery stalk. No matter how you prepare them—even by boiling—carrots and celery appear to gain in antioxidant power. Green beans get an honorable mention, because they increase in antioxidant power when cooked by all methods except boiling or pressure-cooking. Microwaved green beans, for example, have more antioxidants than raw. So go ahead and make a nice vegetable soup and boost the ingredients' antioxidant content at the same time.

How to Make Your Own Fruit and Vegetable Wash

Buying organic foods reduces your exposure to pesticides, but it doesn't eliminate them entirely. Pesticide residues have been detected in 11 percent of organic crop samples due to accidental or fraudulent use, cross-contamination from neighboring nonorganic fields, or the lingering presence of persistent pollutants like DDT in the soil.[79]

There are many commercial fruit and vegetable wash products that purport to improve the removal of pesticides, but a variety have been tested and appear to be a complete waste of money.[80] For example, Procter & Gamble had a product that claimed it was "proven to be 98% more effective than water in removing pesticides." When it was put to the test, though, it did no better than plain tap water.[81] Rinsing produce under running water generally removes less than half of the pesticide residue.[82] A fingernail-polish-remover acetone bath has been found to be more effective at removing pesticides,[83] but of course I'm not advocating dunking your fruits and veggies in that! The goal is to make your tomato *less* toxic.

One effective method is to use a 5 percent acetic-acid bath—in other words, plain white vinegar, which has been found to remove the bulk of certain pesticide residues.[84] But 5 percent is full strength, and it would get expensive buying gallons of white vinegar just to wash your fruits and veggies. Unfortunately, a diluted white-vinegar bath only seems marginally more effective than tap water.[85]

Thankfully, there is a solution that is both cheap and effective: salt water. A 10 percent saltwater rinse has been found to work as well as full-strength vinegar.[86] To make your own pesticide-reducing bath, add one part salt to nine parts water. Just make sure to rinse off all the salt before eating.

Is Buying Organic Worth It?

Stroll down the produce aisle of your grocery store. You'll see lots of foods labeled "organic," but what does that really mean?

According to the USDA, organic farming practices preserve the environment and avoid most synthetic materials, including pesticides and antibiotics. Among other requirements, organic farmers must receive annual on-site inspections, use only USDA-approved materials, and not use genetically modified crops. In order to be counted in the $35 billion U.S. organic retail market, products receive a USDA organic stamp.[87]

The fact is that being organic doesn't mean a food is healthy. The organic food industry didn't become so lucrative by selling carrots. For instance, you can now buy pesticide-free potato chips and organic jelly beans.[88] There are even organic Oreo cookies. Junk food is still junk food, even if it was produced organically. The organic label cannot turn red lights green.

Many are surprised to learn (I know I was!) that a review of hundreds of studies found that organic produce does not seem to have significantly more vitamins and minerals. Organic fruits and vegetables do, however, appear to have more nontraditional nutrients like polyphenol antioxidants,[89] thought to be because conventionally grown plants given high-dose synthetic nitrogen fertilizers may divert more resources to growth rather than defense.[90] This may be why, as we learned in chapter 4, organic berries appear to suppress cancer growth better than conventional berries in vitro.

Based on its elevated antioxidant levels, organic produce may be considered 20–40 percent healthier, the equivalent of adding one or two servings' worth to a five-a-day regimen. But organic produce may be 40 percent more expensive, so for the same money, you could just buy the extra servings' worth of conventional produce. From a purely nutrients-per-dollar standpoint, it's not clear that organic foods are any better.[91] But people don't just buy organic foods because they're healthier—what about safety?

Conventional produce appears to have twice the levels of cadmium, one of the three toxic heavy metals in the food supply, along with mercury and lead.[92] The cadmium is thought to come from the phosphate fertilizers that are added to conventional crops.[93] The greatest concern most people have about conventionally grown produce, though, is the pesticide residues.

People not only tend to overestimate the nutritional benefit of organic food, they also overestimate the risks of pesticides.[94] For example, surveys have found that many consumers erroneously believe that just as many people die from pesticide residues on conventional food as they do from automobile accidents,[95] or that eating nonorganic produce is almost as bad as smoking a daily pack of cigarettes.[96] This kind of thinking is dangerous, as it could lead to a decrease in overall fruit and vegetable consumption.

If just half of the U.S. population were to increase fruit and vegetable consumption by a single serving per day, an estimated twenty thousand cancer cases might be avoided each year. This estimate was calculated using conventional produce, so the additional pesticide burden from all that extra produce might be expected to cause ten new cancer cases. On balance, the study suggested, if half of Americans ate one more serving of produce per day, we'd prevent 19,990 people from becoming cancer patients every year. Sounds good to me!

Unfortunately, this paper was written by scientists-for-hire paid by conventional produce growers, so they had an incentive to exaggerate the benefits and downplay the risks.[97] Nevertheless, I think the bottom line is sound. You receive tremendous benefit from eating conventional fruits and vegetables that far outweighs whatever little bump in risk you may get from the pesticides.[98] But why accept any risk at all when you can choose organic? My own family buys organic whenever we can, but we never let concern about pesticides stop us from stuffing our faces with as many fruits and vegetables as possible.

At least half your plate should be filled with vegetables. Here's a simple rule: Include vegetables in everything, and the more the better. Bean burritos are better than carnitas, but better still is a bean burrito with lots of veggies wrapped inside. Instead of spaghetti with marinara sauce, make it spaghetti with marinara sauce . . . and loads of veggies. Marinara is certainly better than Alfredo, but it's even better still to go the extra veggie mile and heap on your favorite vegetables.

Flaxseeds

I have talked about the wonders of flaxseeds in a few of this book's earlier chapters, including those on high blood pressure (chapter 7), breast cancer (chapter 11), and prostate cancer (chapter 13). Remember how flaxseeds apparently offer "miraculous defense against some critical maladies"?

Okay, you're convinced. But just where do you get flaxseeds, and how do you best use them?

You can buy flaxseeds in bulk at natural foods stores for just a few dollars per pound. They come in nature's finest packaging: a hard natural hull that keeps them fresh. However, Mother Nature packs them a little too well. If you eat flaxseeds whole, they're likely to pass right through you without releasing any of their nutrients. So, for best results, first grind up the seeds with a blender or coffee or spice grinder, or buy them preground or "milled." (The other option is to chew them really well.) Thanks to their antioxidant content, ground flaxseeds should last at least four months at room temperature.[1]

Ground flax is a light, nutty powder that can be sprinkled on oatmeal, salads, soups—frankly, just about anything you're eating. You can even bake with flax without damaging the lignans[2] or omega-3 fatty acids[3] (unlike flaxseed *oil*). During medical school, I used to make a few dozen flaxseed muffins at a time and put them in the freezer. Then I'd pop one in the microwave every morning before I ran out the door and get my daily flax fix while eating breakfast surreptitiously on the subway.

Are Fruit-and-Nut Bars Fattening?

There are a number of energy bars on the market containing only green-light ingredients, such as dried fruits, seeds, and nuts. People love them because they're so easy to throw into a briefcase, backpack, or purse and eat as a convenient snack on the go.

Dried fruits, seeds, and nuts are all nutrient-dense foods, but they're also calorie dense. Might concentrating so many calories into such a small energy bar contribute to weight gain? To find out, Yale University researchers split about one hundred overweight men and women into two groups. All the participants ate their normal diet, but half were told to add two fruit-and-nut bars daily. After two months, despite the extra 340 calories a day from the bars, the fruit-and-nut bar group did not gain any weight.[4]

Dried fruits and nuts appear to be so satiating that people feel full and unintentionally offset the calories elsewhere throughout the day. Studies on apple rings,[5] figs,[6] prunes,[7] and raisins[8] have found similar results. In the apple study, postmenopausal women who added two apples' worth of apple rings to their daily diet for six months not only didn't gain weight but experienced a whopping 24 percent drop in their LDL ("bad") cholesterol.[9] (That's nearly the effect you can get with some statin drugs!) In general, the 7 percent of Americans who average a tablespoon or more of dried fruit per day tend to be less overweight and less obese, and they have slimmer waistlines and less abdominal obesity than Americans who don't eat as much dried fruit.[10]

Of course, when shopping for energy bars, it's imperative that you read their labels, as many brands have added sugars. Or you can just save yourself some money and choose good old-fashioned trail mix. Better yet, how

continued

about eating a piece of fresh fruit? Still, if the choice is between an energy
bar and a candy bar as an afternoon snack, the choice is clear.

Other Ways to Eat Flaxseeds

When you're not sprinkling ground flax on your cereal, salads, or soups or baking it into your muffins, there are plenty of other ways to get your daily serving
of flaxseeds. There are a lot of convenient flax bars, crackers, and snacks on the
market these days, a few of which even have all green-light ingredients.

Honestly, it's pretty easy to make your own flax crackers. Mix two cups of
ground flaxseeds with a cup of water, add whatever herbs and spices you want,
and then spread the dough thinly on a parchment- or silicone-lined baking sheet.
Score the dough into thirty-two crackers and bake at 400°F for about twenty
minutes. To flavor mine, I use a half teaspoon each of smoked paprika, garlic
powder, and onion powder, but you should play around until you find a (salt-
free) spice profile you prefer. When cut into thirty-two pieces, each cracker
meets your Daily Dozen serving requirement.

I also use my trusty discount dehydrator to make raw flax crackers. All you
do is mix a cup of whole flaxseeds with a cup of water along with flavorful ingredients like sun-dried tomatoes and basil. After it firms for about an hour
and gets a jelly-like consistency, I spread it out thinly and dehydrate away. Give
it a try! Dip your flax crackers in hummus or another bean dip for double
check marks. Since you're using whole flaxseeds, though, make sure to chew
thoroughly for maximum benefit.

Flaxseeds have a wonderful binding quality that makes them a great ingredient for thick, milkshake-like smoothies. Toss a tablespoon of ground flax into
a blender with some frozen berries, unsweetened soy milk, and half a ripe banana or mango or a few dates for sweetness, and you have a delicious drink
containing both classes of protective phytoestrogens—lignans in flax and isoflavones in soy. (See chapter 11.) Blend in some cocoa powder for a chocolate
milkshake that could help improve your chances of both preventing and surviving breast and prostate cancers.

This same binding quality makes flaxseeds a green-light thickener to replace cornstarch. I use flax to make my favorite quickie stir-fry sauce. I start
with some bok choy and fresh mushrooms. The water clinging to the bok choy
after it's rinsed, along with the liquid that gets released from the mushrooms
while cooking, is enough to flash-steam the veggies in a hot pan without any

added oil. Once the bok choy is tender-crisp, I add a cup of water mixed with a tablespoon each of tahini, ground flaxseeds, and Asian black-bean garlic sauce, a fermented yellow-light condiment you can find in a jar at most large grocery stores. Once the sauce thickens, it's ready for some fresh ground pepper (and hot sauce, if you've got that spicy tooth like I do) and . . . voilà!

You can even use ground flaxseeds to replace eggs in baking. For each egg in the recipe, whisk one tablespoon of ground flaxseeds with three tablespoons of water until the mixture becomes gooey. Unlike chicken eggs, "flax eggs" are not only cholesterol-free but they're also packed with soluble fiber to bring your cholesterol down[11] instead of up.

It never ceases to amaze me how these tiny little seeds can pack such a health-promoting punch. With just a measly tablespoon a day and so many delicious, easy ways to incorporate ground flax into your sips and bites, there's no reason you shouldn't be able to tick this Daily Dozen check box every day.

Nuts and Seeds

Sometimes it feels like there just aren't enough hours in a day to get everything done. So instead of trying to make your day longer, why not make your life longer by an extra two years? That's about how long your life span may be increased by eating nuts regularly—one handful (or about a quarter of a cup) five or more days a week.[1] Just that one simple and delicious act alone may extend your life.

The Global Burden of Disease Study calculated that not eating enough nuts and seeds was the third-leading dietary risk factor for death and disability in the world, killing more people than processed meat consumption. Insufficient nut and seed intake is thought to lead to the deaths of millions of people every year, fifteen times more than all those who die from overdoses of heroin, crack cocaine, and all other illicit drugs combined.[2]

The Uses of Blended Nuts

Nuts make for quick and delicious snacks on their own, but my personal favorite use for them is as green-light sources of fat to make rich, creamy sauces. Whether in a cashew Alfredo, a ginger-peanut sauce, or a tahini-based green goddess dressing, nuts and seeds can maximize nutrient acquisition by both improving absorption and increasing your total intake of vegetables by adding some creamy cachet.

An often overlooked use for nuts is as a key ingredient in soups, such as African peanut stew. When blended and heated, cashews thicken to make an amazingly creamy soup base. Nut and seed butters also pair well with veggies and fruits. Most everyone loves the classic childhood pairings of peanut butter with celery or apples. One of my favorite treats is dipping fresh strawberries into a decadent chocolate sauce. All you need is a half cup of an unsweetened milk, one tablespoon of chia seeds, one tablespoon of cocoa, one teaspoon of almond butter, and sweetener to taste. (I use one tablespoon of erythritol, discussed on page 389.) Mix all the ingredients, and heat until the almond butter melts and the sweetener dissolves. Pour into a bowl, whisk until smooth, and put it in the fridge to cool. The chia and fiber from the cocoa powder help it thicken into an indulgent delight. (You can grind up the chia seeds first, but I like the tapioca-like texture the little chia balls form.)

Walnuts for the Win

Which nut is healthiest? Normally, my answer is whichever you're most willing and able to eat regularly, but walnuts really do seem to take the lead. They have among the highest antioxidant[3] and omega-3[4] levels, and they beat out other nuts in vitro in suppressing cancer cell growth.[5] But how do walnuts fare outside the laboratory in real life?

PREDIMED is one of the largest interventional dietary trials ever performed. Interventional studies, if you remember, are those in which participants are randomized to different diets to see who fares better. This helps researchers avoid the problem of confounding variables when trying to determine cause and effect in cohort studies. For example, in major study[6] after study[7] after study,[8] people who eat nuts tend to live longer and suffer fewer deaths from cancer, heart disease, and respiratory disease. There was a lingering question, though:

Did these findings show causation or merely correlation? It could be possible, after all, that nut eaters also tend to have other healthy lifestyle behaviors. Maybe those who eat nuts are more likely to be, well, health nuts. On the other hand, if scientists randomly assign thousands of people to various levels of nut consumption and the nuttier group ends up the healthiest, we could have more confidence that nuts aren't just *associated* with better health but actually *cause* better health. This is what PREDIMED ended up doing.[9]

More than seven thousand men and women at high cardiovascular risk were randomized into different diet groups and followed for years. One of the groups received a free half pound of nuts every week. In addition to eating more nuts, they were told to improve their diets in other ways, such as eating more fruits and vegetables and less meat and dairy, but weren't as successful at any of those other goals compared to the control group. Nevertheless, having a free half pound of nuts sent to them every week for four consecutive years did indeed persuade them to start eating more nuts.[10] (It's too bad the researchers couldn't have slipped in a little free broccoli too!)

At baseline, before the study even started, the thousands assigned to the nut group were already eating about half an ounce of nuts a day. Thanks to the ensuing freebies, they ended up bumping up their consumption to a whole ounce (about a handful). As a result, the study was able to determine what happens when people at high risk for heart disease following a particular diet eat an extra half ounce of nuts every day.

With no significant differences in meat and dairy intake, there were no significant differences in saturated fat or cholesterol intake. So, unsurprisingly, there were no significant differences in their blood cholesterol levels or the subsequent number of heart attacks. However, the added-nuts group did end up having significantly fewer strokes. In a sense, all the dietary groups were eating stroke-promoting diets. People in all the groups had strokes after eating each of the diets for years—so, ideally, they'd instead choose diets that can stop or reverse the disease process rather than encourage it. But for those not willing to make major shifts in their diet, just the minor tweak of adding nuts appeared to cut stroke risk in half.[11] Those in the extra-nut-eating group still had strokes, but only about half as many. If this works as well in the general population, eighty-nine thousand strokes a year would be prevented in the United States alone. That would be like ten strokes an hour, around the clock, prevented simply by adding about four walnuts, almonds, and hazelnuts to the nation's daily diet.

Regardless of which group participants were assigned to, those eating more nuts each day had a significantly lower risk of dying prematurely overall.[12] Those who consumed more red- and yellow-light sources of fat—olive oil or extra virgin olive oil—failed to have any survival benefit.[13] This is consistent with the way Ancel Keys, the so-called father of the Mediterranean diet, viewed olive oil. He thought of its benefit more as a means of replacing animal fats—that is, anything to get people to eat less lard and butter.[14]

Of all the nuts studied in PREDIMED, the researchers found the greatest benefits associated with walnuts, particularly for preventing cancer deaths.[15] People who ate more than three servings of walnuts per week appeared to cut their risk of dying from cancer in half. A review of the scientific literature concluded that "the far-reaching positive effects of a plant-based diet that includes walnuts may be the most critical message for the public."[16]

The Power of a Pea-"Nut"

Did you know that peanuts actually aren't nuts? Technically, they're legumes, but they're often lumped together with true nuts in dietary surveys and studies, so it's been hard to tease out their effects. Harvard University researchers worked to change that in the Nurses' Health Study by specifically asking people about their peanut butter intake. They found that women at high risk for heart disease who ate nuts *or* a tablespoon of peanut butter five or more days a week appeared to nearly halve their risk of suffering a heart attack compared to women who ate a serving or less per week.[17] This cross-protection between true nuts and peanuts also appears to extend to fibrocystic breast disease. Adolescent girls in high school who consumed just one or more servings of peanuts a week appeared to have significantly lower risk of developing lumpy breasts, which can be a marker for increased breast cancer risk.[18] PB&J to the rescue!

Nuts and Obesity: Weighing the Evidence

Nuts and nut butters are packed with nutrition—and calories. For example, just two tablespoons of a nut or seed butter might contain nearly two hundred calories. Nevertheless, it's probably better to eat two hundred calories of nut butter than two hundred calories of what most Americans would eat otherwise. Given how concentrated nut calories are—you'd have to eat nearly an entire head of cabbage to get the same amount—if you add a serving of nuts to your daily diet, won't you gain weight?

To date, there have been about twenty clinical trials on nuts and weight, and not a single one showed the weight gain you might expect. All the studies showed less weight gain than predicted, no weight gain at all, or weight *loss*—even after study subjects added a handful or two of nuts to their daily diets.[19] However, these studies lasted just a few weeks or months. Perhaps prolonged nut consumption leads to weight gain? That question has been examined six different ways in studies lasting up to eight years. One found no significant change, and the other five measures found significantly *less* weight gain and reduced risk of abdominal obesity in those who ate more nuts.[20]

The first law of thermodynamics states that energy can neither be created nor destroyed. If calories, which are units of energy, can't just disappear, then where are they all going? In one trial, for instance, participants who ate up to 120 pistachios as an afternoon snack every day for three months didn't appear to gain a pound.[21] How could thirty thousand calories vanish into thin air?

One theory offered was dubbed the Pistachio Principle: Maybe nuts just take a lot of work to eat. Pistachios are typically bought in their shells, which slows consumption time, allowing your brain to better regulate your appetite.[22] Sounds plausible, but what about shelled nuts like almonds and cashews? A study out of Japan did suggest that increasing "dietary hardness" (meaning chewing difficulty) is associated with a slimmer waist.[23] Perhaps all that chewing simply tires you out?

Then there's the fecal-excretion theory. Many of the cell walls of chewed almonds, for example, remain intact in the gastrointestinal tract. In other words, it's possible a lot of the calories in nuts just never get digested and wind up in your waste because you didn't chew well enough. Both of these theories were put to the test by an international group of researchers who gave participants either a half cup of unshelled peanuts or a half cup of peanuts ground into peanut butter. If either the Pistachio Principle or the fecal-extraction theory were correct, the peanut-butter group would gain weight, since no calories would be left in undigested nuts, and no calories would be burned chewing. But in the end, neither group gained weight, so there must be another answer.[24]

What about the dietary-compensation theory? The idea here is that nuts are so satiating and good at suppressing appetite that you end up eating less food overall. This could explain why some studies found that people lost weight after eating nuts. To test this idea, Harvard Medical School researchers gave two groups smoothies with the same number of calories, but one contained walnuts, and the other didn't. Despite drinking the same amount of calories, the placebo (nut-free) smoothie group reported feeling significantly less full than the walnut group.[25] So, yes—it does seem that nuts can make you feel fuller faster than some other foods.

At this point, it looks as if 70 percent of nut calories are lost through dietary compensation and 10 percent are flushed as fat in your feces.[26] But what about the last 20 percent? Unless all the calories are accounted for, you would still expect some weight gain. The answer appears to lie in the ability of nuts to boost metabolism. When you eat nuts, you burn more of your own fat. Researchers have found that while control-diet subjects were burning about twenty grams of fat within an eight-hour period, a group eating the same number of calories and fat, but with walnuts included in their diet, burned off more—about thirty-one grams of fat.[27] If a pill could do that, drug companies would be raking it in!

The bottom line? Yes, nuts are high in calories, but through a combination of dietary compensation mechanisms, your body's failure to absorb some of the fat, and increased fat-burning metabolism, nuts can be a lifeline without expanding your waistline.

Pistachio Nuts for Sexual Dysfunction

Erectile dysfunction (ED) is the recurrent or persistent inability to attain or maintain an erection for satisfactory sexual performance. It is present in up to thirty million men in the United States and approximately one hundred million men worldwide.[28] Wait a second. The United States has less than 5 percent of the world's population yet up to 30 percent of the impotence? We're number one!

The reason may be due to our artery-clogging diet. Erectile dysfunction and our number-one killer, coronary artery disease, are actually two manifestations of the same disease—inflamed, clogged, and crippled arteries— regardless of which organs are affected.[29] Not to worry, though, because Americans have red, white, and blue pills like Viagra . . . right? The problem is that these pills just cover up the symptoms of vascular disease and don't do anything for the underlying pathology.

Atherosclerosis is considered a systemic disorder that uniformly affects all major blood vessels in the body. Hardening of the arteries can lead to softening of the penis, since stiffened arteries can't relax open and let the blood flow. Thus, erectile dysfunction may just be the flaccid tip of the iceberg in terms of a systemic disorder.[30] For two-thirds of men showing up at emergency rooms with crushing chest pain, their penises had been trying to warn them for years that something was wrong with their circulation.[31]

Why does atherosclerosis tend to hit the penis first? The arteries in the penis are half the size of the "widow-maker" coronary artery in the heart. Therefore, the amount of plaque you wouldn't even feel in the heart could clog half the penile artery, causing symptomatic restriction in blood flow.[32] This is why erectile dysfunction has been called "penile angina."[33] In fact, by measuring blood flow in a man's penis with ultrasound, doctors can predict the results of his cardiac stress test with an accuracy of 80 percent.[34] Male sexual function is like a penile stress test, a "window into the hearts of men."[35]

In medical school, we were taught the forty-over-forty rule: 40 percent of men over age forty have erectile dysfunction. Men with erection difficulties in their forties have a fiftyfold increased risk of having a cardiac event (like sudden death).[36]

We used to think of erectile dysfunction in younger men (those under age forty) as "psychogenic"—meaning it's all in their heads. But now we're realizing that ED is more likely an early sign of vascular disease. Some experts believe that a man with erectile dysfunction—even if he doesn't have cardiac symptoms—"should be considered a cardiac . . . patient until proved otherwise."[37]

The reason even young men should care about their cholesterol levels is because they predict erectile dysfunction later in life,[38] which in turn predicts heart attacks, strokes, and a shortened life span.[39] As one medical journal put it, the take-home message is that "ED = Early Death."[40]

What does this have to do with nuts? A clinical study found that men who ate three to four handfuls of pistachios a day for three weeks experienced a significant improvement in blood flow through the penis, accompanied by significantly firmer erections. The researchers concluded that three weeks of pistachios "resulted in a significant improvement in erectile function . . . without any side effects."[41]

This is not just a male issue. Women with higher cholesterol levels report significantly lower arousal, orgasm, lubrication, and sexual satisfaction. Atherosclerosis of the pelvic arteries can lead to decreased vaginal engorgement and "clitoral erectile insufficiency syndrome," defined as "failure to achieve clitoral tumescence [engorgement]." This is thought to be an important factor in female sexual dysfunction.[42] We learned from the Harvard Nurses' Health Study that eating just two handfuls of nuts weekly may extend a woman's life as much as jogging four hours a week.[43] So eating healthier may not only extend your love life but also your entire life.

Why are beans, nuts, and whole grains so health promoting? Maybe it's because they are all seeds. Think about it: All it takes for an acorn to explode into an oak tree is water, air, and sunlight. Everything else is contained within the seed, which possesses the entire complex of protective nutrients required to mature into a plant or tree. Whether you're eating a black bean, a walnut, a grain of brown rice, or a sesame seed, in essence you're getting the whole plant in a tiny little package. As two noted nutrition experts concluded, "[D]ietary recommendations should embrace a wide array of seeds as part of a plant-based dietary pattern . . ."[44]

Nuts may be the easiest and tastiest Daily Dozen check box to check off. For those with peanut or tree nut allergies, seeds and seed butters can often be used as safe alternatives. But what about nut consumption if you have diverticulosis? For fifty years, doctors have told patients with this common intestinal condition to avoid nuts, seeds, and popcorn, but when the issue was finally put to the test, it turns out these healthy foods actually appear to be protective.[45] So diverticulosis shouldn't stop you from meeting this Daily Dozen mark, either. This one simple and delicious act could add years to your life without adding on pounds.

Herbs and Spices

Here's a simple tip: Use your senses to pick out healthy foods. There is a good biological reason you should be so attracted to the vibrant colors found in the produce aisle: In many cases, the colors *are* the antioxidants. You can figure out which of two tomatoes has more antioxidants just by looking at which has a deeper red color. Of course, the food industry tries to hijack this natural instinct for colorful foods with abominations like Froot Loops, but if you stick to green-light foods, you can let color guide you. The same is true, we're now realizing, with flavor.

Just as many of the plant pigments are beneficial, scientists are discovering that many of the flavor compounds in herbs and spices are powerful antioxidants as well.[1] Guess where the antioxidant rosmarinic acid is found? What about cuminal, thymol, and gingerols? The flavors *are* the antioxidants. You can use this knowledge to help you make decisions at the grocery store. You can see that red onions have more antioxidants than white, and you can taste that regular onions have more antioxidants than mellower, milder Vidalia-type onions.[2]

The bitter and pungent compounds in the cruciferous and allium families are thought to be responsible for their health benefits. Intense colors and intense flavors can be signs of intense benefit. For optimum health, you should try to eat both colorful and flavorful foods. Indeed, the dietary guidelines for a number of countries now specifically encourage the consumption of herbs and spices, not only as a substitute for salt but for the healthy properties they have in their own right.[3] And on the top of my list of healthful herbs and spices is turmeric—a spice that is both colorful *and* flavorful.

Why You Should Include Turmeric in Your Daily Diet

In recent years, more than five thousand articles have been published in the medical literature about curcumin, the pigment in turmeric that gives it that bright yellow color. Many of these papers sport impressive-looking diagrams suggesting that curcumin can benefit a multitude of conditions with a dizzying array of mechanisms.[4] Curcumin was first isolated more than a century ago, yet out of the thousands of experiments, only a few in the twentieth century were clinical studies involving actual human participants. But since the turn of the century, more than fifty clinical trials have tested curcumin against a variety of diseases, and dozens more studies are on the way.[5]

We have seen how curcumin may play a role in preventing or treating lung disease, brain disease, and a variety of cancers, including multiple myeloma, colon cancer, and pancreatic cancer. But curcumin has also been shown to help speed recovery after surgery[6] and effectively treat rheumatoid arthritis better than the leading drug of choice.[7] It also may be effective in treating osteoarthritis[8] and other inflammatory conditions, such as lupus[9] and inflammatory bowel disease.[10] In the latest trial for ulcerative colitis, a multicenter, randomized, placebo-controlled, double-blind study found that more than 50 percent of patients achieved remission within just one month on curcumin compared to *none* of the patients who received the placebo.[11] If you are as convinced as I am that you should include turmeric in your diet to benefit from its pigment curcumin, the next questions, then, are: how much do you eat, how do you eat it, and what are the risks?

A Quarter Teaspoon of Turmeric Every Day

Turmeric is potent stuff. If I took a sample of your blood and exposed it to an oxidizing chemical, researchers could quantify the damage it caused to the DNA in your blood cells with sophisticated technology that allows them to count the number of breaks in DNA strands. If I then gave you a single pinch of turmeric to eat once a day for a week, redrew your blood, and again exposed your blood cells to the same free radicals, you would see that with the tiny bit of turmeric on board, the number of cells with DNA damage could be cut in half.[12] That's not mixing turmeric with cells in a petri dish—that's having you ingest the spice and then measuring the effects in your blood. And this was not some fancy curcumin supplement, not some turmeric *extract*. It was just the plain spice you can buy at any grocery store. And, the dose was tiny, about one-eighth of a teaspoon.

Now that's powerful!

The doses of turmeric that have been used in human studies range from less than one-sixteenth of a teaspoon up to nearly two tablespoons a day.[13] Few adverse effects have been reported even at high doses, but the studies typically have lasted only a month or so. We don't know what long-term effects of high doses there may be. Because turmeric can have such powerful drug-like effects, until we have better safety data, I would not advise anyone to take more than the culinary doses that have a long-standing record of apparent safety. How much is that? Though traditional Indian diets can include up to about a teaspoon of turmeric daily, the average intake in India is closer to a quarter teaspoon a day.[14] So that's how much I recommend you get as part of your Daily Dozen.

How to Eat Turmeric

Primitive peoples often used spices in sophisticated ways. For instance, quinine from cinchona bark was used to treat the symptoms of malaria long before the disease was even identified, and the raw ingredients of aspirin have been used as a popular painkiller long before Mr. Friedrich Bayer came along.[15] Over the last twenty-five years, about half of new drug discoveries have come from natural products.[16]

There's a plant in South Asia called adhatoda (*adu*, meaning "goat," and *thoda*, meaning "not touch"—it's so bitter even the goats won't eat it). Its leaves are steeped with pepper to make a folk remedy effective for treating asthma. Somehow it was figured out what scientists didn't discover until 1928: Adding pepper vastly boosted the plant's antiasthmatic properties. And now we know why. About 5 percent of black pepper by weight is composed of a compound called piperine, which accounts for pepper's pungent flavor and aroma. But piperine is also a potent inhibitor of drug metabolism.[17] One of the ways your liver gets rid of foreign substances is by making them water soluble so you can pee them out. This black pepper molecule, however, inhibits that process, thereby boosting blood levels of the medicinal compounds in adhatoda—and it can do the same for curcumin in turmeric root.

Within an hour of eating turmeric, curcumin appears in your blood-stream, but only in small traces. Why only scant amounts? Presumably, your liver is actively working to get rid of it. But what if you suppress that elimination process by eating some black pepper? If you consume the same amount of curcumin but add a quarter teaspoon of black pepper, the level of curcumin in your blood shoots up by 2,000 percent.[18] Even just the littlest pinch of pepper, just one-twentieth of a teaspoon, can significantly boost curcumin blood levels.[19] And guess what is a common ingredient in many curry powders besides turmeric? Black pepper. Curry powder in India is also often served with a source of fat, which alone can enhance the bioavailability of curcumin seven- to eightfold.[20] (Unfortunately, traditional knowledge appeared to fail here as to the best source of that fat. Indian cuisine employs a great deal of clarified butter, or ghee, which may explain the country's relatively high rates of heart disease despite its otherwise relatively healthy diet.[21])

My favorite way to incorporate turmeric is to use fresh turmeric root. Any large Asian market should carry it in the produce aisle. It looks like skinny fingers of gingerroot, but when you snap it open, you are greeted by the most unreal, Day-Glo, fluorescent-orange color. My quarter teaspoon of dried turmeric recommendation translates into about a quarter inch of fresh turmeric root. The roots are about two inches long, cost about ten cents each, and can last for weeks in the fridge or basically forever in the freezer. Every year you can go to the store and buy a twelve-month supply of fresh turmeric for about five dollars.

There's evidence to suggest that the cooked and raw forms may have different properties. Cooked turmeric appears to offer better DNA protection, while raw turmeric may have greater anti-inflammatory effects.[22] I enjoy it both ways. I use a grater to add my daily quarter inch into whatever I may be cooking (or right onto a cooked sweet potato), or I throw a raw slice into a smoothie. You probably won't even taste it. Fresh turmeric has a much more subtle flavor than dried, so it may be an especially good option for those who don't like turmeric's taste. You will see it, though. Be careful—it can stain clothing and surfaces. Turmeric may not just make your health golden but your fingertips, as well.

Consuming turmeric with soy may offer a double benefit for osteoarthritis sufferers.[23] Scrambled tofu is the classic turmeric-soy combination, but let me share two of my favorites: one raw and one cooked. You can whip up a pumpkin pie smoothie in less than three minutes. Simply blend a can of pumpkin purée, a handful of frozen cranberries and pitted dates, pumpkin pie spice to taste, a quarter-inch turmeric slice (or quarter-teaspoon of powder), and unsweetened soy milk to reach your preferred consistency.

Another favorite is my pumpkin custard (aka crustless pie). All you need to do is blend one can of pumpkin purée with about ten ounces of silken tofu (the Mori-Nu brand is convenient because it stays fresh without refrigeration), as much pumpkin pie spice as you like, and one to two dozen pitted dates (depending on how much of a sweet tooth you have). Pour into a dish and bake at 350°F until cracks appear on the surface. By skipping the piecrust and sticking with a custard, you're left with vegetables, tofu, spices, and fruit. The more you eat, the healthier you are.

Fresh or powdered, turmeric is a natural flavor fit for Indian and Moroccan cuisines, but I add it to most anything. I find it pairs particularly well with brown rice dishes, lentil soup, and roasted cauliflower. Prepared yellow mustard typically already has turmeric in it for color, but try to find a salt-free variety—one that's essentially just vinegar, a cruciferous vegetable (mustard seeds), and turmeric. I can't think of a healthier condiment.

What About Turmeric Supplements?

Wouldn't it be more convenient to just take a curcumin supplement every day? Added expense aside, I see three potential downsides. First, curcumin is not equivalent to turmeric. Supplement manufacturers often fall into the same reductionist trap as the drug companies do. Herbs are assumed to have only one main active ingredient, so the thinking goes that if you can isolate and purify it into a pill, you should be able to boost the effects. Well, curcumin is described as the active ingredient in turmeric,[24] but is it *the* active ingredient or just *an* active ingredient? In fact, it's just one of many different components of the whole-food spice.[25]

Few studies have compared turmeric with curcumin, but some that have suggest that turmeric may work even better. For example, researchers at the MD Anderson Cancer Center in Texas pitted both turmeric and curcumin against seven different types of human cancer cells in vitro. Against breast cancer, for instance, curcumin kicked butt, but turmeric kicked even more butt. The same was true against pancreatic cancer, colon cancer, multiple myeloma, myelogenous leukemia, and others—turmeric came out on top, above just its yellow pigment curcumin. These findings suggest that components other than curcumin can also contribute to anticancer activities.[26]

Although curcumin is believed to account for most of turmeric's health-promoting activities, research published over the past decade has indicated that curcumin-*free* turmeric—turmeric with the so-called active ingredient removed—may be as effective as or even more effective than turmeric with curcumin. There are turmerones, for example, in turmeric (but processed out of curcumin supplements) that may exhibit both anticancer and anti-inflammatory activities. I naïvely assumed that the researchers who discovered this would advocate that people consume turmeric rather than take curcumin supplements, but instead, they suggested the production of all sorts of different turmeric-derived supplements.[27] After all, who can make any money on a whole food that costs pennies a day?

My second concern involves dosing. While the turmeric trials have used modest amounts that could conceivably be achieved through diet, curcumin-only trials have tested the amount of curcumin found in entire cupfuls of turmeric spice—one hundred times more than what curry lovers have been eating for centuries.[28] Some supplements add black pepper as well, potentially boosting levels to the equivalent of twenty-nine cups a day of turmeric, which might result in enough curcumin in the blood to potentially *cause* DNA damage based on in vitro data.[29]

Finally, there is a concern about contamination with toxic metals, such as arsenic, cadmium, and lead. None of the tested samples of powdered turmeric on the U.S. market has been found to be contaminated with heavy metals, but the same cannot be said of curcumin supplements.[30]

None of these concerns (except cost) applies to supplements containing only whole ground turmeric powder. Nearly all turmeric supplements are extracts, however. How else could they get away with selling a small bottle of pills for twenty dollars when the bulk spice may be less than twenty dollars a pound? A bottle might last two or three months. For the same price, bulk turmeric could offer two or three years' worth at Daily Dozen dosing.

One compromise between convenience and cost may be to make your own turmeric capsules. There are capsule-stuffing gadgets that allow you to fill your own. Given the cost discrepancy between bulk turmeric and supplements, such a gadget would probably pay for itself after your first batch. A "00"-sized capsule would fit a day's quarter-teaspoon dose. Making your own capsules might be a little time consuming, but if you won't otherwise consume turmeric in your daily diet, it might be time well spent. If there were ever such thing as a magic pill, single-ingredient, ground turmeric root would probably come closest.

Who Should Not Take Turmeric

If you suffer from gallstones, turmeric may trigger pain. Turmeric is a chole-cystokinetic agent, meaning it facilitates the pumping action of the gallbladder to keep bile from stagnating.[31] Ultrasound studies show that a quarter tea-spoon of turmeric causes the gallbladder to contract, squeezing out half of its contents.[32] In this way, it may help *prevent* gallstones from forming in the first place. But what if you already have a stone obstructing your bile duct? That turmeric-induced squeeze could be painful.[33] For everyone else, though, the effect of turmeric would be expected to reduce the risk of gallstone formation and ultimately even reduce the risk of gallbladder cancer.[34]

Too much turmeric, however, may increase the risk of certain kidney stones. Turmeric is high in soluble oxalates, which can bind to calcium and de-velop into the most common form of kidney stone—insoluble calcium oxalate, which is responsible for about 75 percent of all cases. Those who have a tendency to form those stones should probably restrict consumption of total dietary oxalate to no more than 50 mg per day. This would mean no more than a teaspoon of turmeric daily at most.[35] (Turmeric, by the way, is consid-ered safe during pregnancy, but curcumin supplements may not be.[36])

My recommended daily quarter teaspoon of turmeric is in addition to what-ever other (salt-free) herbs and spices you enjoy. The reason the Daily Dozen encourages herb and spice consumption in general and not just turmeric is not because they're all interchangeable—turmeric appears to have unique benefits—but because there's evidence other herbs and spices have health ben-efits as well. I've talked about the role of saffron, for example, in the treat-ment of Alzheimer's (chapter 3) and depression (chapter 12). Spices don't just make food taste better; they make food better for you. I encourage you to keep a well-stocked spice cabinet and make it a habit to add whatever herbs and spices you find appealing to any dish you might be eating.

What follows here is a more in-depth examination of some of the herbs and spices for which we have the most scientific data. I will describe some of the fascinating studies that illustrate the benefits of these flavor boosters and ex-plain some of the easiest ways to add them to your meals.

Fenugreek

Powdered fenugreek seed is a spice found commonly in Indian and Middle East-ern cuisines. Fenugreek appears to significantly improve muscle strength and weight-lifting power output, allowing men in training, for example, to leg press an extra eighty pounds compared to those ingesting a placebo.[37] Fenugreek may also possess "potent anticancer properties" in vitro.[38] I don't like the taste of the powder, so I just throw in fenugreek seeds with my broccoli seeds when I'm sprouting.

There is a side effect of fenugreek seed consumption, however: It can make your armpits smell like maple syrup.[39] I kid you not. It's a harmless phe-nomenon, but what isn't harmless, however, is maple syrup urine disease, a serious congenital disorder. Breast-feeding infants with mothers who use fenu-greek to boost their milk production may be misdiagnosed with this com-pletely unrelated disorder.[40] If you're pregnant or breast-feeding and eating fenugreek, make sure to tell your obstetrician just so she or he doesn't think your baby has maple syrup urine disease.

Cilantro

One sign of changing U.S. demographics is that salsa has replaced ketchup as America's top table condiment.[41] One popular salsa ingredient is cilantro, one of the most polarizing and divisive food ingredients known to humankind. Some people absolutely love it, and some people absolutely hate it. What's interesting is that the lovers and the haters appear to experience the taste differently. In-dividuals who like cilantro may describe it as fresh, fragrant, or citrusy, whereas people who dislike the herb report that it tastes like soap, mold, dirt, or bugs.[42] I'm not sure how people know what bugs taste like, but rarely are polarizing opinions about flavors so extreme.

Different ethnic groups do seem to have different rates of cilantro dislike, with Ashkenazi Jews scoring among the highest on the cilantro hate-o-meter.[43] Another clue came from twin studies that show that identical twins tend to share cilantro preferences, whereas fraternal twins do not have such a strong correlation.[44] The human genetic code contains about three billion letters, so we'd have to analyze the DNA of roughly ten thousand people to find a cilan-tro gene. Obviously, genetic researchers have better things to do than under-take that challenge . . . right?

Maybe not. Genetic studies of more than twenty-five thousand participants who reported their cilantro preferences discovered an area on chromosome 11 that seemed to be a match. What's there? A gene called OR6A2 that enables you to smell certain chemicals like E-(2)-decenal, which is both a primary constituent of cilantro and a defensive secretion of stink bugs. So maybe cilantro does taste like bugs! Cilantro lovers may just be genetic mutants who have an inability to smell the unpleasant compound.[45]

This may actually be an advantage, though, because cilantro is healthy stuff. Mother Nature has been described as the most comprehensive pharmacy of all time, and cilantro is one of her oldest herbal prescriptions.[46] About twenty sprigs of cilantro daily for two months reduced inflammation levels in arthritis sufferers and cut uric-acid levels in half, suggesting that lots of cilantro may be useful for people suffering from gout.[47]

Cayenne Pepper

In a study published as "Secretion, Pain and Sneezing Induced by the Application of Capsaicin to the Nasal Mucosa in Man," researchers found that if you cut a hot pepper and rub it inside your nostrils, your nose will start running and hurting, and you'll start sneezing. (Capsaicin is the burning component of hot peppers.) Why would they perform such an experiment? People who have handled hot peppers know that if they get some up their nose, they can experience an intense burning sensation. (And it doesn't even have to get up your nose, which I was chagrined to learn after I once failed to wash my hands before using the restroom!) However, the researchers noted that "these phenomena have not been investigated." So they decided it "appeared worthwhile to study the effects produced by topical application of capsaicin in the human [nose] . . ."[48]

The researchers enlisted a group of medical students and dripped some capsaicin in their noses. The students started sneezing, burning, and snotting, describing the pain at about eight or nine on a scale of one to ten. No surprise. But it gets a little more interesting. What happened when they repeated the experiment day after day? You'd think the students might be more sensitive to capsaicin, with their nose still irritated from the day before, causing even greater pain and discomfort, right? Actually, the capsaicin hurt less. By day five, in fact, it hardly hurt at all—they didn't even get a runny nose anymore.

Were the poor med students permanently numbed? No. After a month or so, the desensitization wore off, and they were back in agony whenever the researchers tried dripping capsaicin back in their noses. What was likely happening is that the pain fibers—the nerves that carry pain sensation—used up so much of the pain neurotransmitter (called substance P) that they ran out. Exposed day after day, the nerves exhausted their stores and could no longer transmit pain messages until they made more neurotransmitter from scratch, which takes a couple of weeks.

How could this be exploited for medical purposes? There's a rare headache syndrome called cluster headache, which has been described as one of the worst pains humans can experience. Few, if any, medical disorders are more painful. It's nicknamed the "suicide headache" because patients have taken their lives because of it.[49]

Cluster headaches are thought to be caused by pressure on the trigeminal nerve in the face. Treatments involve everything from nerve blocks to Botox to surgery. But that same nerve goes down to the nose. What if you cause the whole nerve to dump all its substance P? Researchers tried the daily capsaicin experiment with cluster headache sufferers. Unlike the wimpy medical students who rated the nose burning as an eight or nine on the ten-point pain scale, those used to the violence of cluster headache attacks rated the pain caused by capsaicin at only a three or four. By day five, they too became desensitized to the pain of the capsaicin. What happened to their headaches? Those who rubbed capsaicin in the nostril on the side of the head where the headaches occurred cut the average number of attacks in half. In fact, half the patients were apparently cured—their cluster headaches were gone completely. All in all, 80 percent responded, which is at least equal to, if not better than, all the current available therapies.[50]

What about other pain syndromes? Irritable bowel syndrome is thought to be caused by a hypersensitivity of the lining of the colon. How do you determine if someone's gut is hypersensitive? Innovative Japanese researchers developed a device to deliver "repetitive painful rectal distention," which is basically a half-quart balloon hooked up to a fancy bicycle pump that is inserted and inflated until you can't stand the pain anymore. Those with IBS had a significantly lower pain threshold, significantly less "rectal compliance."[51]

So how about trying to desensitize the gut by depleting substance P stores? It's bad enough to have to rub hot peppers up your nose, but where would you have to stick them for irritable bowel? Thankfully, researchers chose the oral route. They found that the enteric-coated capsules of red pepper powder were able to significantly decrease the intensity of abdominal pain and bloating, suggesting "a way of dealing with this frequent and distressing functional disease . . ."[52]

What about red pepper powder for the pain of chronic indigestion (dyspepsia)? Within a month of taking about one and a half teaspoons' worth of cayenne pepper a day, stomach pain and nausea improved.[53] The frequently prescribed drug Propulsid (cisapride) worked almost as well as the red pepper powder and was considered generally well tolerated—until, that is, it started killing people. Propulsid was pulled from the market after causing fatal heart rhythms.[54]

Ginger

Many successful natural treatments start like this: Some doctor learns that a plant has been used in some ancient medical tradition and figures, "Why not try it in my practice?" Ginger has been used for centuries for headaches, and so a group of Danish physicians advised one of their migraine patients to give it a go. At the first sign of a migraine coming on, the patient mixed a quarter teaspoon of powdered ginger in some water and drank it. Within thirty minutes, the migraine disappeared. And it worked every time for her, with no apparent side effects.[55]

This is what's called a case report. Though they're really just glorified anecdotes, case reports have played an important role in the history of medicine, from the discovery of AIDS[56] to a failed chest-pain drug with a billion-dollar side effect—Viagra.[57] Case reports are considered the weakest form of evidence, but that's often where investigations begin.[58] So the case report of successfully treating one migraine patient with ginger isn't so much helpful in itself, but it can inspire researchers to put it to the test.

Eventually, a double-blind, randomized, controlled clinical trial was performed comparing the efficacy of ginger for the treatment of migraine headaches to sumatriptan (Imitrex), one of the top-selling, billion-dollar drugs in the world. Just one-eighth of a teaspoon of powdered ginger worked just as well and just as fast as the drug (and costs less than a penny). Most migraine sufferers started with moderate or severe pain, but after taking the drug or the ginger, ended up in mild pain or were entirely pain-free. The same proportion of migraine sufferers reported satisfaction with the results either way.

As far as I'm concerned, ginger won. Not only is ginger a few billion dollars cheaper, but it caused significantly fewer side effects. While on the drug, people reported dizziness, a sedative effect, vertigo, and heartburn, but the only side effect reported for ginger was an upset stomach in about one out of twenty-five people.[59] (A whole tablespoon of ginger powder at one time on an empty stomach could irritate anyone, though,[60] so don't overdo it.) Sticking to one-eighth of a teaspoon is not only up to three thousand times cheaper than taking the drug, you're probably less likely to end up as a case report yourself, like the people who have had a heart attack after taking sumatriptan for a migraine,[61] or have died.[62]

Migraines are described as "one of the most common" pain syndromes, affecting as much as 12 percent of the population.[63] That's common? How about menstrual cramps, which plague up to 90 percent of younger women?[64] Can ginger help? Even just one-eighth of a teaspoon of ginger powder three times a day dropped pain from an eight to a six on a scale of one to ten, and down further to a three in the second month.[65] And these women hadn't been taking ginger all month; they started the day before their periods began, suggesting that even if it doesn't seem to help much the first month, women should try sticking with it.

What about the duration of pain? A quarter teaspoon of ginger powder three times a day was found to not only drop the severity of menstrual pain from about seven down to five but decrease the duration from a total of nineteen hours in pain down to about fifteen hours,[66] significantly better than the placebo, which were capsules filled with powdered toast. But women don't take bread crumbs for their cramps. How does ginger compare to ibuprofen? Researchers pitted one-eighth of a teaspoon of powdered ginger head-to-head against 400 mg of ibuprofen, and the ginger worked just as effectively as this leading drug.[67] Unlike the drug, ginger can also reduce the amount of menstrual bleeding, from around a half cup per period down to a quarter cup.[68] What's more, ginger intake of one-eighth of a teaspoon twice daily started a week before your period can yield a significant drop in premenstrual mood, physical, and behavioral symptoms.[69]

I like sprinkling powdered ginger on sweet potatoes or using it fresh to make lemon-ginger apple chews as an antinausea remedy. (Ever since I was a little kid, I've suffered from motion sickness.) There is an array of powerful antinausea drugs, but they come with a nausea-inducing list of side effects, so I've always striven to find natural remedies whenever possible for myself and for my patients.

Ginger has been used for thousands of years in traditional healing systems. In India, it's known as *maha-aushadhi*, meaning "the great medicine." However, it wasn't proven to reduce nausea until 1982, when it beat out Dramamine in a head-to-head test in blindfolded volunteers who were spun around in a tilted, rotating chair.[70] Ginger is now considered a nontoxic, broad-spectrum antiemetic (antivomiting agent) effective in countering nausea during motion sickness, pregnancy, chemotherapy, and radiation, and after surgery.[71]

Try making my lemon-ginger apple chews: In a blender, liquefy one peeled lemon with a palm-sized "hand" of fresh gingerroot. Use the mixture to coat thin slices of four apples, and then place them in a dehydrator until they reach desired chewiness. I like them a little moist, but you can dehydrate them further to make lemon-ginger apple chips, which store longer than the chews. For me, a few pieces eaten about twenty minutes before travel works wonders.

Note: Ginger is generally considered safe during pregnancy, but the maximum recommended daily dose of fresh ginger while pregnant is 20 grams (about four teaspoons of freshly grated gingerroot).[72] Any more may have uterus-stimulating effects. Women using my apple chews recipe to combat morning sickness should spread out the four apples' worth of chews or chips over several days.

Peppermint

Which herbs have the most antioxidants? The most antioxidant-packed herb is dried Norwegian bearberry leaf. (Good luck finding that!) The most antioxidant-packed *common* herb is peppermint.[73] That's why I add mint to my favorite hibiscus cocktail recipe (see page 390) and why I try to add it to food whenever possible. Mint is a traditional ingredient in Middle Eastern salads like tabbouleh, Indian chutneys, and Vietnamese soups and fresh summer rolls. I like to put it into anything chocolaty as well.

Oregano and Marjoram

Oregano is such an antioxidant-rich herb that researchers decided to test if it could reduce the DNA-damaging effects of radiation. Radioactive iodine is sometimes given to people with overactive thyroid glands or thyroid cancer to destroy part of the gland or mop up any remaining tumor cells after surgery. For days after the isotope injection, patients are so radioactive that they are advised not to kiss anyone or to sleep close to anyone (including their pets), and to maximize the distance between themselves and children or pregnant women.[74] The treatment can be very effective, but all that radiation exposure appears to increase the risk of developing new cancers later on.[75] Hoping to prevent the DNA damage associated with this treatment, researchers tested the ability of oregano to protect chromosomes of human blood cells in vitro from exposure to radioactive iodine. At the highest dose, chromosome damage was reduced 70 percent. The researchers concluded that oregano may "act as a potent radioprotective agent."[76]

Other petri-dish studies with oregano suggest anticancer and anti-inflammatory properties. In a comparison of the effects of various spice extracts—bay leaves, fennel, lavender, oregano, paprika, parsley, rosemary, and thyme—oregano beat out all but bay leaves in its ability to suppress cervical cancer cell growth in vitro while leaving normal cells alone.[77] Of 115 different foods tested for anti-inflammatory properties in vitro, oregano made it into the top five, along with oyster mushrooms, onions, cinnamon, and tea leaves.[78]

Marjoram is a closely related herb and also shows promise in laboratory studies. It appears to significantly inhibit the migration and invasion of breast cancer cells in vitro.[79] None of these studies on oregano family herbs was done on people, though, so we have no idea how, if at all, these effects will translate to a clinical setting. One of the only randomized, controlled trials I'm aware of is a study of marjoram tea for polycystic ovary syndrome (PCOS). The tea was purportedly used in traditional herbal medicine to "restore hormonal balance," so researchers decided to put it to the test. They instructed women with PCOS to drink two cups of marjoram tea on an empty stomach every day for a month. Beneficial effects on hormone levels were observed, which, the researchers concluded, "may justify the improvement claimed by traditional medicine practitioners and patients."[80]

Cloves

The most antioxidant-packed common *spice* is the clove.[81] It has an exceptionally strong flavor, so try adding just a teensy pinch to anything you'd normally put cinnamon or ginger on. Ground cloves are great on stewed pears and baked apples, giving them a pleasant, mulled cider taste, and a mug of chai tea is a fantastic way to pack in a bunch of high-impact common spices at once.

Amla

The most antioxidant-packed *uncommon* spice is amla,[82] which is powdered dried Indian gooseberry fruit. As a Western-trained physician, I had never heard of amla despite its common use in Ayurvedic herbal preparations. I was surprised to find four hundred articles on this lesser-known spice in the medical literature, and even more surprised to find papers with titles like "Amla . . . a Wonder Berry in the Treatment and Prevention of Cancer." Amla is arguably the most important plant in Ayurvedic medicine, used traditionally as everything from a neutralizer of snake venom to a hair tonic.[83] I eat it because it's apparently the single most antioxidant-packed green-light food on Earth.[84]

Using an argon laser, researchers can measure and track human carotenoid antioxidant levels in real time. The most important finding from this body of work is that antioxidant levels can plummet within two hours of an oxidatively stressful event. When you're stuck in traffic breathing diesel fumes, deprived of sleep, or suffering from a cold, for example, your body starts using up some of its antioxidant stores. What may only take two hours to lose can take up to three days to build back up.[85]

Even ordinary body processes, such as turning food into energy, can produce free radicals. This is okay as long as the food you eat comes prepackaged with antioxidants. But if it doesn't—if you chug straight sugar water, for example—the level of free radicals and oxidized fat in your bloodstream rises over the next few hours, while vitamin E levels drop as your body's antioxidant stores are expended.[86] If you were to eat the same amount of sugar in the form of an orange, though, you wouldn't get a spike in oxidation.[87] Researchers concluded: "This argues strongly for the need to include high antioxidant foods in each and every meal in order to prevent this redox [free-radical versus antioxidant] imbalance."[88]

The standard American diet (SAD) isn't exactly antioxidant packed. Here is the antioxidant content (in modified FRAP assay daμmol antioxidant units) of some typical American breakfast foods: bacon (7) and eggs (8), a bowl of corn flakes (25) with milk (10), an Egg McMuffin (11), pancakes (21) with maple syrup (9), and a bagel (20) with cream cheese (4). A typical breakfast may average about 25 antioxidant units.[89]

Compare those to the smoothie I had for breakfast this morning. I started with a cup of water (0), a half cup of frozen blueberries (323), and the pulp of a ripe mango (108). I added a tablespoon of ground flaxseeds (8), along with a half cup of fresh mint leaves (33) and a palmful of bulk white tea leaves (103). (For more about tea leaves, see page 385.) While the typical SAD breakfast may give you only about 25 antioxidant units, my breakfast smoothie offered more than 500. And, when I add the final ingredient, a single teaspoon of amla, I get an additional 753 antioxidant units. That's about four cents' worth of amla, and it just doubled the antioxidant content of my entire smoothie. Before I've even fully woken up, I've already consumed more than 1,000 antioxidant units. That's more than the average person may get in an entire week. I could drink my smoothie and eat nothing but doughnuts for the rest of the week, and most people *still* wouldn't catch up. Notice that even though I packed the blender with amazing foods like blueberries and tea leaves, fully half the antioxidant power came from that single, four-cent teaspoon of powdered gooseberries.

You can buy amla online or at any Indian spice store. Ayurvedic herbal supplements are typically something you'd want to stay away from, as they have been found to be heavily contaminated with heavy metals,[90] some of which are actually added intentionally.[91] But none of the samples of powdered amla tested so far has been found to be contaminated. You can find whole Indian gooseberries in the frozen section of Indian grocery stores, but frankly, I find them inedible—astringent, sour, bitter, and fibrous all at the same time. The powder isn't much tastier, but it can be disguised in something with a strong flavor, like a smoothie. Alternatively, you could pack amla into capsules like the turmeric. Whenever I'm out on the road on a speaking tour, I try to take daily capsules of turmeric and amla until I can get back home and wrest back control over my diet.

Spice Mixes

While there have been a considerable number of studies done with individual spices, few have looked at increasing spice consumption in general. One group at Pennsylvania State University did compare the effects of a high-fat chicken meal with and without a mixture of nine herbs and spices. Herbs and spices were chosen because, ounce for ounce, they have more antioxidants than any other food group (and because the study was funded by the McCormick spice company).[92]

Unsurprisingly, the people in the spice group experienced a doubling of the antioxidant power in their bloodstreams compared to participants in the spice-free group. Remarkably, though, the spice group ended up with 30 percent less fat (triglycerides) in their blood after the meal and improved insulin sensitivity. The researchers concluded that "the incorporation of spices into the daily diet may help normalize postprandial [after-meal] disturbances in glucose [sugar] and lipid [fat] homeostasis [control] while enhancing antioxidant defense."

But why experience such disturbances in the first place? The study reminds me of those that show eating greens is particularly protective against cancer among smokers.[93] That is, the take-home message shouldn't be telling smokers to eat greens—it should be telling smokers to quit smoking. Of course, they could do both, which in the context of the spice study would mean adopting an antioxidant-rich, green-light diet, offering the best of both worlds.

Some of my favorite spice mixes are pumpkin pie spice, curry powder, chili powder, Chinese five-spice powder, a savory Indian spice blend called garam masala, an Ethiopian blend called berbere, Italian seasoning, poultry seasoning, and a Middle Eastern blend called za'atar. Spice mixes are a convenient way to provide a balance of flavors while boosting the variety of your spice intake, but make sure to check that the mixes are salt-free.

Is Liquid Smoke Safe?

I don't know how I lived so long without smoked paprika. I swear it tastes like barbecue potato chips. After I first discovered it, I became a smoked-paprika zealot and put it on almost everything, but now I reserve it mostly for greens and when toasting fresh squash and pumpkin seeds. (I'll bet you aren't surprised to learn that's my favorite part of Halloween!) I was concerned there might be carcinogenic combustion products in smoked seasonings (similar to the benzo[a]pyrene found in cigarette smoke and diesel exhaust), but these compounds tend to be fat soluble. So when you smoke a spice or make a water-based solution like liquid smoke, the smoke flavor compounds are captured without capturing most of the smoke *cancer* compounds. The same can't be said for smoked fatty foods. While you'd have to chug three bottles of hickory smoke flavoring to exceed the safety limit, a smoked ham or smoked turkey sandwich could take you halfway there, and a single barbecued chicken leg would take you over the top. Smoked fish, such as herring or salmon, appears to be the worst. One bagel with lox could take you ten times over the safety limit.[94]

Some Risks to Spicing Up Your Life

There are a few spices, however, of which you can have too much of a good thing. Take poppy seeds, for example.

The opium poppy used to make heroin is the same opium poppy that produces the poppy seeds in muffins and bagels. The idea that poppy seeds could serve as the source of appreciable amounts of narcotics was not given much credence despite the existence of an old European custom recommending a poppy seed–filled pacifier to quiet a noisy baby.[95] It wasn't given much credence, that is, until a mother tried giving her six-month-old some strained milk in which she had boiled some poppy seeds with the very best intentions of helping the child sleep better. The baby stopped breathing—but luckily survived.[96]

The cases of poppy seed overdose aren't limited to children. There's another case in the literature of an adult who felt "dim feelings in the head" after eating spaghetti with a half cup of poppy seeds on top.[97] So what's the upper limit of poppy seed consumption that's probably safe? Based on median morphine levels,[98] about one teaspoon for every ten pounds of body weight. This means that someone weighing about 150 pounds should probably eat no more than five tablespoons of raw poppy seeds at a time.[99]

Cooking may wipe out half of the morphine and codeine contained naturally in poppy seeds, which gives you some more leeway when baking.[100] Soaking the poppy seeds for five minutes and then discarding the water before adding the seeds to your recipe can eliminate half of that remaining, if you're making some poppy seed–filled pastry or other baked goods for children. Otherwise, there shouldn't be any risk at usual levels of intake—unless you're going in for a drug test, in which case you may want to avoid poppy seeds altogether.[101]

Too much nutmeg can also be a problem. A paper entitled "Christmas Gingerbread . . . and Christmas Cheer: Review of the Potential Role of Mood Elevating Amphetamine-like Compounds . . ." suggested that certain natural constituents of spices like nutmeg may form amphetamine compounds within the body sufficient "to elevate the mood and to help provide some added Christmas cheer" during the holiday season.[102]

This hypothetical risk was raised as far back as the 1960s in the *New England Journal of Medicine* in an article called "Nutmeg Intoxication."[103] The paper pondered whether the age-old custom of adding nutmeg to eggnog arose from the "psychopharmacological effect" described in cases of nutmeg intoxication. Such cases evidently go back to the 1500s, when nutmeg was used as an abortifacient to induce a miscarriage.[104] In the 1960s, the spice was used as a psychotropic drug.[105] During that decade, mental health professionals concluded that while nutmeg "is much cheaper for use and probably less dangerous than the habit-forming heroin, it must be stated that it is not free from danger and may cause death."[106]

The toxic dose of nutmeg is two to three teaspoons. I had assumed no one would ever come close to that amount unintentionally until I saw a report in which a married couple ate some pasta, collapsed, and were subsequently hospitalized. What had happened was a big mystery until the husband revealed that he had accidentally added one-third of a jar of nutmeg to the meal while cooking.[107] That's about four teaspoons of the spice. I don't know how they could have eaten it! I imagine the poor wife was just trying to be polite.

Another popular and powerful spice is cinnamon, which has been prized for its ability to lower blood sugar levels.[108] It works so well that you can even "cheat" on a diabetes test by consuming two teaspoons of cinnamon the night before. Twelve hours later, your blood sugar spike in response to meals will still be significantly dampened.[109] Even just a teaspoon a day appears to make a significant difference.[110] Unfortunately, cinnamon can no longer be considered a safe and effective treatment for diabetes.

There are two main types of cinnamon: Ceylon cinnamon and cassia cinnamon (also known as Chinese cinnamon). In the United States, anything simply labeled "cinnamon" is probably cassia, since it's cheaper. This is unfortunate, because cassia contains a compound called coumarin, which may be toxic to the liver at high doses. Unless it's specifically labeled Ceylon cinnamon, a quarter teaspoon of cinnamon even a few times a week may be too much for small children, and a daily teaspoon would exceed the tolerable upper safety limit for adults.[111] Can't you just switch to Ceylon cinnamon and get the benefits without the risks? Without the risks, yes, but we're no longer so sure about the benefits.

Nearly all the studies showing blood sugar benefits of cinnamon have been performed with cassia. We've just assumed that the same would apply for the safer Ceylon cinnamon, but it was only recently put to the test. The nice blunting of blood sugars you see in response to cassia cinnamon disappeared when the researchers tried using Ceylon cinnamon instead.[112] In fact, all along it may actually have been the toxic coumarin itself that was the active blood-sugar-lowering ingredient in the cassia cinnamon. Thus, sidestepping the toxin by switching to Ceylon cinnamon may sidestep the benefit. So, in a nutshell, when it comes to lowering blood sugars, cinnamon may not be safe (cassia), or it may be safe, but apparently not effective in reducing blood sugar (Ceylon).

I still encourage Ceylon cinnamon consumption, given that it is one of the cheapest common food sources of antioxidants, second only to purple cabbage. But what's a type 2 diabetic to do? Even the cassia cinnamon only brought down blood sugars modestly—in other words, it was only as good as the leading diabetes drug in the world, metformin, sold as Glucophage.[113] Yes, cassia cinnamon may work as effectively as the leading drug, but that's not saying much. The best way to treat diabetes is to attempt to cure it entirely with a healthy diet. (See chapter 6.)

Who knew that the herbs and spices you've been tossing into sauces and sprinkling onto dishes could have such impacts on your health? Work your creativity in the kitchen and spice up your meals and drinks to make them more flavorful and more healthful—but don't forget the quarter teaspoon of daily turmeric. I am sufficiently convinced by the available body of evidence to single turmeric out as something everyone should add to his or her daily diet.

Whole Grains

Consistent with recommendations from leading cancer[1] and heart disease[2] authorities, I recommend at least three servings of whole grains a day. Harvard University's preeminent twin nutrition studies—the Nurses' Health Study and the Health Professionals Follow-Up Study—have so far accumulated nearly three million person-years of data. A 2015 analysis found that people who eat more whole grains tend to live significantly longer lives independent of other dietary and lifestyle factors.[3] No surprise, given that whole grains appear to reduce the risk of heart disease,[4] type 2 diabetes,[5] obesity, and stroke.[6] Eating more whole grains could save the lives of more than a million people around the world every year.[7]

There are so many nutrition claims floating around the Internet that lack scientific backing, but a few especially persistent memes directly contradict the available evidence. When I see books, websites, articles, and blogs parroting claims like "grains are inflammatory—even whole grains," I can't help but wonder what alternate dimension the authors call home.

Pick your indicator of inflammation. Take C-reactive protein (CRP), for instance. CRP levels rise within the body in response to inflammatory insults and are therefore used as a screening test for systemic inflammation. Each daily serving of whole grains is estimated to *reduce* CRP concentrations by approximately 7 percent.[8] Furthermore, there's a whole alphabet soup of inflammation markers that appear to be improved by whole grains: ALT, GGT,[9] IL-6,[10] IL-8,[11] IL-10,[12] IL-18,[13] PAI-1,[14] TNF-α,[15] TNF-R2,[16] whole blood viscosity, and erythrocyte filtration.[17] Or, as presented in less technical terms in the *American Journal of Clinical Nutrition*, "Whole-grain intake cools down inflammation."[18] Even excluding heart disease and cancer, habitual whole-grain intake is linked to a significantly lower risk of dying from inflammatory diseases.[19]

What About Gluten?

You've probably heard about an autoimmune disorder called celiac disease, in which the consumption of gluten causes adverse reactions, including gastrointestinal problems. Gluten is a group of proteins found in certain grains, including wheat, barley, and rye. Celiac disease is relatively rare, though, affecting less than 1 percent of the population.[20] For the more than 99 percent of the rest of us who don't have the disorder, is gluten okay or, indeed, health-promoting like other plant proteins?

In 1980, researchers in England reported a series of women suffering from chronic diarrhea who were cured by a gluten-free diet, yet none of the women had evidence of celiac disease.[21] They appeared to have some sort of *non*-celiac gluten sensitivity. At the time, the medical profession expressed skepticism that there was such a thing,[22] and even now there are experts who question its existence.[23] In fact, doctors commonly referred their patients claiming non-celiac gluten sensitivity to psychiatrists because they were believed to have an underlying mental illness.[24]

The medical profession has a history of dismissing diseases as existing "just in your head." Examples of these include post-traumatic stress disorder

(PTSD), ulcerative colitis, migraines, ulcers, asthma, Parkinson's, Lyme disease, and multiple sclerosis. Despite resistance from the prevailing medical community, each one of these conditions has subsequently been confirmed as a legitimate disorder.[25] On the flip side, the Internet is rife with unsubstantiated claims about gluten-free diets that have spilled over into the popular press, making gluten the diet villain du jour.[26] And, of course, the gluten-free processed food industry, today worth billions, has a financial interest in the public's confusion.[27] Whenever that much money is at stake, it's hard to trust anyone, so as always, stick to the science. And what sort of evidence is there for the existence of a condition presumed to be so widespread?

The first double-blind, randomized, placebo-controlled gluten challenge was published in 2011. Patients complaining of irritable bowel–type symptoms who claimed they felt better on a gluten-free diet—despite not having celiac disease—were tested to see if they could tell if bread and muffins they were given contained gluten or were gluten-free. All the subjects started out gluten-free and symptom-free for two weeks, and then were challenged with one of the two types of bread and muffins. Even those who ate the gluten-free placebo products felt worse, meaning they started out on a gluten-free diet and continued on a gluten-free diet, yet they reported feeling crampy and bloated. This is what's called the nocebo effect. The placebo effect takes place when you give patients something useless and they feel better; the nocebo effect occurs when you give someone something harmless and they feel worse. Nevertheless, the subjects who received actual gluten felt even worse. So the researchers concluded that non-celiac gluten intolerance may indeed exist.[28]

However, this was a small study, and even though the researchers claimed the gluten-free products were indistinguishable from those containing gluten, it's possible that the patients were able to tell which foods were which. So, in 2012, Italian researchers created a double-blinded test with 920 patients diagnosed with non-celiac gluten sensitivity. Each was given capsules filled with either wheat flour or a placebo powder. More than two-thirds failed the test: Those on the placebo got worse, or those on the wheat felt better. But for those who passed, there was a clear benefit to staying on the wheat-free diet, confirming the "existence of non-celiac WS [wheat sensitivity]."[29] Note that they said *wheat* sensitivity, though, not *gluten* sensitivity. In other words, gluten itself may not be causing gut symptoms at all.

Most people who are sensitive to wheat are sensitive to a variety of other foods too. For example, two-thirds of people with wheat sensitivity have also been found to be sensitive to cow's milk protein. Eggs appear to be the next leading culprit.[30] If you put people on a diet low in common triggers of irritable bowel symptoms and *then* challenge them with gluten, there's no effect, calling into question the existence of non-celiac gluten sensitivity.[31]

Interestingly, despite being informed that avoiding gluten was apparently not helping their gut symptoms, many participants opted to continue following a gluten-free diet as they subjectively described "feeling better." This led the researchers to wonder if avoiding gluten might improve the mood of those with wheat sensitivity and, indeed, short-term exposure to gluten appeared to induce feelings of depression in these patients.[32] Regardless of whether non-celiac gluten sensitivity is a disease of the mind or the gut, it is no longer considered a condition that can be dismissed.[33]

The next question, then, is what percentage of the population should avoid wheat and other gluten-containing grains? About one in one thousand may have an allergy to wheat,[34] and nearly one in one hundred have celiac disease,[35] which appears to be on the rise. Still, there's less than a one-in-ten-thousand chance that an American will be diagnosed with celiac disease in a given year.[36] Our best estimate for the prevalence of wheat sensitivity is in the same general range of celiac disease: slightly higher than 1 percent.[37] So only about 2 percent of the population appears to have a problem with wheat, but that's potentially millions of people who may have been suffering for years and could have been cured by simple dietary means, yet were unrecognized and not helped by the medical profession until recently.[38]

For the 98 percent of people who don't have wheat issues, there is no evidence to suggest that following a gluten-free diet has any benefits.[39] In fact, there is some evidence suggesting that a gluten-free diet may adversely affect gut health in people without celiac disease, wheat sensitivity, or wheat allergy. A month on a gluten-free diet was found to adversely affect gut flora and immune function, potentially setting up those on gluten-free diets for an overgrowth of harmful bacteria in their intestines.[40] This is due, ironically, to the beneficial effects of the very components wheat-sensitive individuals have problems with—such as the "FODMAP" fructans that act as prebiotics and feed your good bacteria, or the gluten itself, which may boost immune function.[41] Less than a week of added gluten protein may significantly increase natural killer cell activity,[42] which could be expected to improve the body's ability to fight cancer and viral infections.

The greatest threat gluten-free diets may pose, though, is that they may undermine our ability to diagnose celiac disease, the much more serious form of wheat intolerance. Doctors diagnose celiac by looking for the inflammation caused by gluten in celiac sufferers. But if patients complaining of digestive problems come to the doctor having already eliminated much of the gluten in their diets, physicians might miss the disease.[43] Why would getting a formal diagnosis matter if you're already on a gluten-free diet? First of all, it's a genetic disease, so you'll know to test your family. More significantly, though, many people on so-called gluten-free diets are not actually on truly gluten-free diets. Even twenty parts per million can be toxic to someone with celiac. Sometimes, even foods labeled "gluten-free" may not be safe for celiac sufferers.[44]

What's the best course of action to take if you suspect you might be sensitive to gluten? First off, do *not* go on a gluten-free diet. If you suffer from chronic irritable bowel–type symptoms, such as bloating, abdominal pain, and irregular bowel habits, ask your doctor about getting a formal evaluation for celiac disease. If you have celiac, *then* go on a strict gluten-free diet. If you don't have the disease, the current recommendation is that you first try a healthier diet that includes more fruits, vegetables, whole grains, and beans, all the while avoiding processed foods.[45] The reason people may feel better on a gluten-free diet—and therefore conclude they have a problem with gluten—is because they've suddenly stopped eating so much fast food and other processed junk. In other words, if you eat a deep-fried Twinkie and your stomach aches, it may not be the gluten.

If a healthy diet doesn't help, I suggest you try to rule out other causes of chronic gastrointestinal distress. When researchers have studied PWAWGs— that's what they're called in the medical literature: People Who Avoid Wheat and/or Gluten—they've found that about one-third of them didn't appear to have gluten sensitivity but instead had other conditions like an overgrowth of bacteria in their small intestines, were fructose or lactose intolerant, or had a neuromuscular disorder like gastroparesis or pelvic floor dysfunction.[46] After each of these is ruled out as well, *then* I'd suggest people suffering from chronic, suspicious symptoms try a gluten-free diet.

No current data suggest that the general population should try to avoid gluten, but for those with celiac disease, a wheat allergy, or a wheat sensitivity *diagnosis*, gluten-free diets can be a lifesaver.[47]

Eat Whole . . . Within Minutes

Eating whole grains should be more than just swapping out white bread for whole wheat and white rice for brown. There is a wonderful universe of whole grains out there. You may have tried quinoa, but what about kañiwa or fonio? Even wild rice (which is not actually even rice) may not sound as wild as

374 | HOW NOT TO DIE

the grain called freekeh. Have fun and try some amaranth, millet, sorghum, or teff to expand the amber waves of your horizon. Buckwheat is my mom's favorite.

As with vegetables, use color to make decisions at the grocery store. If you have a choice, pick red quinoa over white quinoa, blue corn over yellow, and yellow corn over white. Beyond just comparing antioxidant content, there's experimental evidence to suggest that pigmented rice—red, purple, or black—has benefits over brown. For example, in addition to having about five times more antioxidants,[48] colored rice varieties have shown greater antiallergy activity in vitro,[49] as well as superior anticancer effects against breast cancer[50] and leukemia cells.[51]

For convenience's sake, there are a number of quick-cooking grains: amaranth, millet, regular oats, quinoa, and teff can all be prepared in less than twenty minutes. For grains that take longer, such as barley, farro, or steel-cut oats, consider cooking a big pot in advance on the weekend so you can simply reheat for your meals throughout the week. Or get a rice cooker—you can buy one for less than twenty dollars.

Whole-wheat pasta cooks in about ten minutes. Improved production technologies have created a new generation of whole-grain pastas that no longer have the rough and mealy texture of yesteryear. My favorite brand is Bionaturae because of its deliciously nutty taste—try it with my Eight Check-Mark Pesto.

Dr. Greger's Eight Check-Mark Pesto

2 cups fresh basil leaves
¼ cup freshly toasted walnuts
2 cloves fresh garlic
¼ of a peeled lemon
¼ teaspoon lemon zest
¼ inch of fresh turmeric root (or ¼ teaspoon turmeric powder)
¼ cup pinto beans
¼ cup water or liquid from bean can
1 tablespoon white miso
Pepper to taste

Combine all ingredients in a food processor. Blend until smooth.
Scoop onto a cup and a half of cooked whole-grain pasta.

Popcorn is a whole grain that takes less than five minutes to prepare. A hot-air popper is another inexpensive, useful appliance. There's an endless variety of savory, sweet, and spicy toppings you can use. I like the combination of chlorella and nutritional yeast. (In my family, the green color earned it the name "zombie corn.") By lightly misting air-popped popcorn with a spray bottle, you can get dry seasonings to stick. I like to spritz with balsamic vinegar. Be sure to stay away from artificial butter flavorings. Originally, we thought the artificial butter flavor chemical diacetyl was just an occupational health hazard, resulting in the deaths of workers who handled the chemical from a condition that became known as "popcorn lung."[52] Now we know consumers are also at risk, given a case series of serious lung disease thought to be caused by butter-flavored microwave popcorn consumption.[53]

There are even one-minute whole-grain options: fully precooked bowls and pouches of brown rice and quinoa that can be microwaved and don't even need to be refrigerated—just heat and eat.

The Five-to-One Rule

If you buy packaged grain products, anything labeled on the front with words like "multigrain," "stone-ground," "100% wheat," "cracked wheat," "seven-grain," or "bran" is usually *not* a whole-grain product. They're trying to distract you from the fact that they're using refined grains. Here, color may not help. Ingredients like "raisin juice concentrate" are used to darken white bread to make it look healthier. Even if the first word in the ingredients list is "whole," the rest of the ingredients could be junk.

I suggest using the Five-to-One Rule. When buying healthier, whole-grain products, look at the Nutrition Facts label on the package and see if the ratio of grams of carbohydrates to grams of dietary fiber is five or less (see figure 7). For example, let's see if 100 percent whole-wheat Wonder Bread passes the test: Per serving, the package lists 30 grams of carbohydrates and 3 grams of fiber. Thirty divided by 3 is 10. Well, 10 is more than 5, so the 100 percent whole-wheat Wonder Bread goes back on the shelf even though, technically, it's a whole-grain product. Compare that to Ezekiel bread, a sprouted-grain bread based on a biblical verse. It has 15 grams of carbohydrates and 3 grams of fiber, and, just like that, passes the test. So do Ezekiel english muffins, which taste great with fruit-only jam and nut butter. Though the science on the potential benefits of sprouted grains is still in its infancy, available data look promising.[54]

Apply the same Five-to-One Rule to breakfast cereals, another grocery

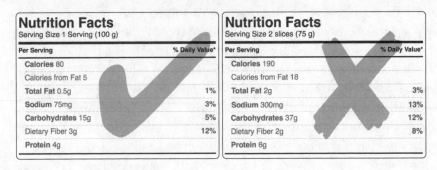

Figure 7

category that can lull you into believing nearly everything is healthy. Multi-Grain Cheerios, for example, sounds good, but it has a ratio over 7. And then it just goes downhill from there with Frosted Cheerios and Fruity Cheerios, which have carbohydrate-to-fiber ratios that exceed 10. Compare that with Uncle Sam cereal, sliding in with a ratio under 4. Others that make the cut include some no-added-sugar puffed-grain cereals like puffed barley, but the healthiest whole grains are the least processed, the so-called intact grains.

Even though wheat berries, shredded wheat, whole-wheat flour, and puffed-wheat cereal may all be 100 percent whole wheat, they are handled by the body very differently. When grains are ground into flour or puffed, they are digested more rapidly and more completely. This increases their glycemic index and leaves fewer leftovers for the friendly flora down in your colon.

Researchers have experimented with this by splitting people into two groups. One group ate nuts, seeds, and beans more or less intact. The other group ate the same exact foods, but ground into flours and pastes. The first group ate nuts instead of nut butters, whole chickpeas instead of hummus, and muesli instead of muesli ground into a cream-of-wheat texture. Note that both groups were eating whole foods, just in different forms.

What happened? The intact-whole-grain diet group doubled their stool size, which was significantly greater than that of the ground-whole-grain group, even though they were eating the same foods in the same quantities.[55] How is that possible? There is so much more left over for your gut flora to eat when you eat your grains intact. Few people realize that the bulk of stool is not undigested food but pure bacteria—trillions and trillions of bacteria.[56] That may be why you get an increase of nearly two ounces of stool for every one ounce of fiber you eat. That's not just water weight—you're feeding your good bacteria so they can be fruitful and multiply.[57]

As the study demonstrated, when you eat grains intact, even if you chew your food thoroughly, pieces of whole seeds and grains transport starch and other goodies all the way down to your colon for your flora to feast on.[58] But when grains are unnaturally processed into flour, almost all of the starch is digested in the small intestine, and you end up starving your microbial self. When that happens regularly, it can result in dysbiosis, an imbalance in which bad bacteria can take over and increase your susceptibility to inflammatory diseases or colon cancer.[59] The moral of the story: Whole grains are great, but intact whole grains may be even better.

Instead of a puffed brown-rice cereal, how about just brown rice? Brown rice for breakfast may sound weird, but warm bowls of grains are traditional breakfast foods in many parts of the world. There are savory versions, or you can sweeten it up with fresh, frozen, dried, or freeze-dried berries. There are online sites where you can buy freeze-dried strawberries in bulk for less than a dollar per cup.

Oats

Oatmeal, of course, is the classic whole-grain breakfast. Just as cruciferous vegetables and flaxseeds harbor beneficial compounds found in abundance nowhere else, oats contain a unique class of anti-inflammatory compounds called avenanthramides. They're thought to be responsible in part for the fresh odor and flavor of oats[60] as well as the ability of oatmeal lotion to relieve skin itching and irritation.[61] Studies on human skin fragments from plastic surgery that were subjected to inflammatory chemicals reveal that oatmeal extract can suppress inflammation[62]—so much that oatmeal now appears to be the treatment of choice for certain serious chemotherapy-induced skin rashes.[63] Ironically, two of the cancer cell lines found to be resistant to that type of chemotherapy[64] were found to be sensitive to avenanthramides in vitro, suggesting that people should be applying oatmeal to their insides as well.[65] Oatmeal is more than just a whole grain.[66]

Oatmeal is my go-to breakfast when I travel. If there isn't a nearby Starbucks where I can pick up some oatmeal, I prepare instant oatmeal with dried fruit in the coffeemaker in my hotel room. At home, if you want to spice up your oatmeal routine, Google "savory oatmeal" for all sorts of interesting dishes involving sautéed mushrooms, herbs, spinach, curry, roasted vegetables—you name it!

The Daily Dozen calls on you to eat three servings of whole grains a day. This might seem like a lot, but when you look at the actual size of those recommended servings, it'll be a snap for you to succeed. Just one pasta dish at an Italian restaurant may average the equivalent of six servings![67] A morning oatmeal habit is a great way to kick-start your day, and then there are a variety of quick-cooking whole grains that serve as convenient, filling ways to fight chronic disease risk all day long.

Beverages

There are plenty of dietary guidelines for eating, but what about for drinking? The Beverage Guidance Panel was assembled to provide "recommendations on the relative health and nutritional benefits and risks of various beverage categories." The panel included such heavyweights as Dr. Walter Willett, chair of the nutrition department at Harvard University School of Public Health and professor of medicine at Harvard Medical School.

The panel's nutrition experts ranked beverage categories on a six-tier scale from best to worst. Unsurprisingly, soda ranked last. Whole milk, meanwhile, was grouped with beer, with a recommendation for zero ounces a day. Their justification included concerns about links between milk and prostate cancer, as well as aggressive ovarian cancer, perhaps "related to its well-documented effect on circulating concentrations of insulin-like growth factor 1." (See chapter 13.) Tea and coffee—preferably without creamer or sweetener—tied as the number-two healthiest beverages, second only to water, the top-ranked drink.[1]

Water

More than two thousand years ago, Hippocrates said, "If we could give every individual the right amount of nourishment and exercise, not too little and not too much, we would have found the safest way to health."[2] Water is the healthiest beverage to drink—but how much is too little, and how much is too much? Water has been described as a "neglected, unappreciated and under researched" subject,[3] but many of the studies extolling the need for proper hydration have been funded by the bottled water industry.[4] It turns out the oft-quoted "drink at least eight glasses of water a day" recommendation actually has little underpinning scientific evidence.[5]

The eight-a-day recommendation can be traced back to a 1921 paper in which the author measured his own urine and sweat output and determined he lost about 3 percent of his body weight in water a day, which comes out to about eight cups.[6] Consequently, for the longest time, water requirement guidelines for humanity were based on just one person's urine and sweat measurements.

But now there's actually extensive evidence suggesting that not drinking enough water may be associated with a variety of problems, including falls and fractures, heat stroke, heart disease, lung disorders, kidney disease, kidney stones, bladder and colon cancer, urinary tract infections, constipation, dry-eye disease, cavities, decreased immune function, and cataract formation.[7] The problem with many of these studies, though, is that low water intake is also associated with several unhealthy behaviors, including low fruit and vegetable intake, more fast-food consumption, and even less "shopping at farmers markets."[8] And think about it—who drinks lots of water? People who exercise a lot. So perhaps it's no wonder that heavy water drinkers have lower disease rates.

Only large and expensive randomized trials could definitively settle these questions. But given that water cannot be patented, such trials seem unlikely.[9] As a result, we're left with studies that just link disease with low water intake. But are people sick because they don't drink enough water, or are they not drinking enough because they're sick? There have been a few large prospective studies in which fluid intake was measured before disease developed. For example, a Harvard University study of nearly forty-eight thousand men found that the risk of bladder cancer decreased by 7 percent for every extra daily cup of fluid consumed. A high intake of water—say, eight cups a day—may reduce the risk of bladder cancer by about 50 percent, potentially saving thousands of lives.[10]

Probably the best evidence we have for a specific recommendation for how much water you should be drinking comes from the Adventist Health Study. Twenty thousand men and women were studied. Those who drank five or more glasses of water a day had about half the risk of dying from heart disease compared to those who drank two glasses or less daily. About half of the cohort consisted of vegetarians, so they were also getting extra water by eating more fruits and vegetables. As in the Harvard study, this protection remained even after controlling for other factors, such as diet and exercise, suggesting that water indeed was the cause, perhaps by lowering blood "viscosity" (that is, by improving blood flow).[11]

If protection against cancer and heart disease isn't enough motivation, perhaps the prospect of being a better kisser will be. Brushing artificial skin against the lips of young women, researchers found that hydrated lips showed greater sensitivity to light touch.[12]

Based on the best evidence to date, authorities from Europe, the U.S. Institute of Medicine, and the World Health Organization recommend about eight to eleven cups of water a day for women and ten to fifteen cups a day for men.[13] These recommendations include water from all sources, though, not solely beverages. You get about four cups from the food you eat and the water your body actually produces on its own,[14] so these guidelines roughly translate into a daily recommendation for drinking four to seven cups of water for women and six to eleven cups for men (assuming only moderate physical activity at moderate ambient temperatures).[15]

You can also get water from all the other drinks you consume, including caffeinated beverages, with the exception of stronger alcoholic drinks like wines and spirits. Coffee,[16] tea,[17] and beer can leave you with more water than you started with, but wine actively dehydrates you.[18] Note, though, in the cancer and heart disease studies mentioned earlier, the health benefits were almost exclusively associated with increased consumption of water, not other beverages. I address the problems with alcoholic drinks in chapters 8 and 11.

Bottom line: Unless you have a condition like heart or kidney failure or your physician otherwise advises you to restrict your fluid intake, I recommend you drink five glasses of tap water a day. I prefer tap not only because it's less economically and environmentally costly but because it may have less chemical and microbial contamination than bottled water.[19]

Can Drinking Water Make You Smarter?

Your brain is 75 percent water.[20] When you become dehydrated, your brain actually shrinks.[21] How might this affect brain function?

Based on urine samples obtained from groups of nine- to eleven-year-old kids in Los Angeles and Manhattan, nearly two-thirds of children may arrive at school in a state of mild dehydration,[22] which may in turn negatively affect scholastic performance. If you take a group of schoolkids and randomly assign them to drink either one or zero cups of water before taking a test, guess which group does significantly better? The group given the water. These results, the researchers concluded, suggest that "even children in a state of mild dehydration, not induced by intentional water deprivation or by heat stress and living in a cold climate, can benefit from drinking more water and improve their cognitive performance."[23]

Your hydration status may also affect your mood. Restriction of fluid intake has been shown to increase sleepiness and fatigue, lower levels of vigor and alertness, and increase feelings of confusion. But as soon as study subjects are allowed to drink again, the deleterious effects on alertness, happiness, and clarity of thought are almost immediately reversed.[24] Water absorption begins very rapidly, within five minutes from mouth to bloodstream, peaking around minute twenty.[25] Interestingly enough, cold water gets sucked in about 20 percent faster than body-temperature water.[26]

How can you tell if you're dehydrated? Just ask your body. If you chug some water and pee most of it out soon after, this would be your body's way of saying it was all topped off. But if you drink a bunch of water and your body keeps most of it, then your tank was running low. Researchers used this concept to develop a formal dehydration assessment tool: Empty your bladder, chug three cups of water, and then see how much you pee an hour later. They determined that if you drink three cups and urinate less than one cup within that hour, there's a good chance you were dehydrated.[27]

But you know, water can be so *boring*. So try adding fresh fruit or veggies as they do in fancy spas and upscale hotels. I like adding frozen strawberries in place of ice cubes. Sometimes I add a few drops of a potent juice concentrate, like tart cherry or pomegranate. Cucumber slices, ginger shavings, a cinnamon stick, lavender, and a mint leaf or two are also common refreshing additions. My latest favorite flavor fusions involve mixing tangerine slices and fresh basil or frozen blackberries and fresh sage.

Bubbles! One of my colleagues at work has a SodaStream on his desk, and he makes his own sparkling water for about twenty-five cents a cup. In addition to making water more interesting, carbonation may also help relieve gastrointestinal symptoms. A randomized trial of the effects of sparkling versus still water found that drinking carbonated water may improve symptoms of constipation and dyspepsia, including bloating and nausea.[28]

What if you took water and added beans or greens—that is, coffee beans or tea leaves? Wouldn't you get all the water you need plus a bonus of additional nutrients? A cup of black coffee, tea, or herbal tea only has two calories, potentially offering nutrition at little caloric cost. Think of healthy beverages as the opposite of junk food: Junk food offers calories with scarce nutrition, whereas healthy beverages offer nutrition with scarce calories. But just how healthy are coffee and tea?

Coffee

I have already discussed the benefits of coffee for the liver (chapter 8), mind (chapter 12), and brain (chapter 14). What about overall longevity? Do people who drink coffee live longer lives than people who don't?

The National Institutes of Health–AARP Diet and Health Study, the largest-ever prospective study conducted on diet and health, put that question to the test. Yes, drinking lots of coffee *is* associated with a longer life, but the effect is relatively modest. People who drank six or more cups per day had a 10–15 percent lower mortality rate due to fewer deaths from heart disease, respiratory disease, stroke, injuries and accidents, diabetes, and infections.[29] However, when a study looked at people under the age of fifty-five, the opposite effect was found: Drinking more than six cups of coffee daily was found to *increase* the risk of death. "Hence," the researchers concluded, "it may be appropriate to recommend that younger people, in particular, avoid heavy coffee consumption (less than 28 cups per week or less than 4 cups in a typical day)."[30]

The bottom line, based on all the best studies to date, is that coffee consumption may indeed be associated with a small reduction in mortality,[31] on the order of a 3 percent lower risk of premature death for each cup of coffee consumed daily.[32] Don't worry, it's not "wake up and smell the coffee or don't wake up at all"—the findings are less prescriptive than they are reassuring for those concerned about their coffee addiction.

Coffee is not for everyone. For example, be careful if you have gastro-esophageal reflux disease (GERD). While a population study found no link between coffee consumption and subjective symptoms of GERD, such as heartburn and regurgitation,[33] scientists who actually stuck tubes down people's throats to measure their pH found that coffee does seem to induce significant acid reflux, whereas tea does not. Caffeine does not appear to be the culprit, since caffeinated water doesn't cause a problem. However, the coffee decaffeination process seems to reduce the level of whichever compounds are responsible, since decaf coffee appeared to cause less reflux. The researchers advised that people who suffer from GERD should consider switching to decaf or—even better—drink tea instead.[34]

Daily coffee consumption is also associated with a slightly increased risk of bone fractures among women, but, interestingly, a decreased fracture risk among men.[35] However, no association was found between coffee and *hip* fracture risk. Conversely, tea may reduce hip fracture risk[36] but appears to have no significant effect on fracture risk in general.[37] This is an important distinction, because hip fractures are associated with a shortened life span more than other types of bone fractures.[38]

People with glaucoma,[39] or perhaps even with merely a family history of glaucoma,[40] may also want to stay away from caffeinated coffee. Coffee intake is associated with urinary incontinence in both women[41] and men.[42] And there are case reports of individuals with epilepsy having fewer seizures after laying off coffee, so avoiding it is certainly worth a try for people with seizure disorders.[43] Finally, it almost goes without saying that people who have trouble sleeping might not want to drink too much coffee. Just a single cup at night can cause a significant deterioration in sleep quality.[44]

The mystery as to why some studies showed that coffee consumption increased cholesterol and others did not was solved when it was discovered that the cholesterol-raising compound thought to be responsible was fat soluble. The culprit compound, cafestol, is found in the oils of coffee beans that become trapped in the paper filter, so drip coffee doesn't raise cholesterol as much as french press, boiled, or Turkish ("mud"-style) coffee. Neither the degree of roasting nor decaffeination appears to make a difference, though Robusta beans have less cafestol than Arabica beans. If you don't have optimal cholesterol levels, you should consider sticking to filtered coffee or using instant coffee, which also lacks these compounds.[45] If these tweaks don't help, consider eliminating coffee completely, as even paper-filtered coffee may raise cholesterol levels a small amount.[46]

We used to think caffeine might increase the risk of an irregular heart rhythm called atrial fibrillation, but this was based on anecdotal case reports involving the acute ingestion of very large quantities of caffeine[47] (including a case blamed in part on a woman's "chocolate intake abuse").[48] As a result, the erroneous notion that caffeine ingestion may trigger abnormal heart rhythms became "common knowledge," an assumption that led to changes in medical practice. More recently, however, actual studies were performed that revealed caffeine intake does *not* appear to increase the risk of atrial fibrillation after all.[49] Moreover, "low-dose" caffeine, which was defined as drinking fewer than about six cups of coffee a day, may even have a protective effect on heart rhythm.[50]

Moderate caffeine consumption in healthy, nonpregnant adults is not only safe but has been found to increase energy and alertness and enhance physical, motor, and cognitive performance.[51] Despite these benefits, one medical journal editorialized that doctors should "temper any message that suggests that caffeine is beneficial . . . given the proliferation of energy drinks that contain massive quantities of caffeine . . ."[52] Indeed, drinking a dozen highly caffeinated energy drinks within a few hours could cause a lethal caffeine overdose.[53] That said, drinking a few cups of coffee a day may actually extend your life a bit[54] and even has the potential to slightly lower your overall cancer risk.[55]

I cannot recommend drinking coffee, though. Why? Because every cup of coffee is a lost opportunity to drink a potentially even healthier beverage—a cup of green tea.

Tea

Black, green, and white teas are all made from the leaves of the same evergreen shrub. Herbal tea, on the other hand, involves pouring hot water over any plant in the world *other* than the tea plant.

What's so special about the tea bush? Phytonutrients exclusive to the tea plant appear so powerful that they can reverse disease even when merely applied to the skin. For example, the topical application of green tea in ointment form on genital warts results in an astounding 100 percent clearance in more than half the patients tested.[56] It's no wonder that this wonder treatment is now officially incorporated into the Centers for Disease Control STD Treatment Guidelines.[57] There was even a remarkable case report of a woman whose skin cancers were apparently stopped with topical green tea application.[58] If green tea can do that on the outside of your body, what might it be able to do internally?

I already discussed the role green tea may play in breast cancer prevention in chapter 11. Drinking tea may protect against gynecological malignancies, such as ovarian cancer[59] and endometrial cancer,[60] as well as lower your cholesterol,[61] blood pressure,[62] blood sugar,[63] and body fat.[64] It may protect the brain from both cognitive decline[65] and stroke.[66] Tea consumption is also associated with decreased risk of diabetes,[67] tooth loss,[68] and up to half the risk of dying from pneumonia.[69] Those who suffer from seasonal allergies may also benefit from drinking tea. Randomized trials have shown that drinking about three cups of Japanese Benifuuki green tea per day starting six[70] to ten[71] weeks before pollen season significantly reduces allergy symptoms. That's nothing to sneeze at!

Riding the Waves

The invention of the electroencephalogram (EEG) to measure brain-wave activity has been described as "one of the most surprising, remarkable, and momentous developments in the history of clinical neurology."[72] Scientists discovered that humans have four main mental states—two while sleeping and two while awake. Delta waves, in which your brain is electrically pulsing slowly at about one wave per second, are typically only seen in deep sleep. Then there's theta-wave sleep. At about five cycles per second, this mental state occurs when you're dreaming. The two waking states are alpha and beta. The alpha state is relaxed, aware, and attentive, such as when you close your eyes and meditate. Beta, meanwhile, is the stimulated, hustle-and-bustle state in which most of us live our lives.

Alpha, however, is where you want to be—fully alert and focused, yet calm. How do you get there? If you relax in a pleasant, peaceful place, after about ninety minutes, you can start to generate some significant alpha activity (though such practicing meditators as Buddhist monks can achieve this state much earlier and maintain it even with their eyes open). To acquire this talent, you could meditate every day for a few years—or you could just drink some tea. Within minutes of tea consumption, anyone may be able to attain that same relaxed but alert brain-wave pattern.[73] That dramatic alteration in brain activity may explain why tea is the world's single most popular beverage after water.

Both white and green teas are less processed than black tea and are probably preferable.[74] White tea is made from young leaves and is named after the silvery-white hairs on the immature buds; green tea is made from more mature leaves. Which tea is healthier? The answer seems to depend on whether or not you add lemon. If you drink your tea without lemon, green tea appears preferable to white tea. But if you add lemon, white tea jumps ahead.[75] The reason is that while there are more phytonutrients in white tea, they may only be released at a certain pH level.[76]

In terms of cancer prevention potential, both green and white teas have been shown to protect against DNA damage in vitro against PhIP, the cooked-meat carcinogen I described in chapter 11. White tea won out, though, blocking upward of 100 percent of DNA damage compared to green tea, which at the same concentration only blocked about half. The "potent antimutagenic activity of white tea in comparison with green tea" was achieved at a brewing time of one minute. For most of the teas tested, steeping longer than a minute had no additional effect. In terms of antioxidant activity, though, it may be better not to brew at all.[77]

Cold-steeping is a popular way to prepare tea in Taiwan, especially during the summer months. Cold-steeped tea is not like conventional iced tea, in which you brew your tea hot and then cool it down. Rather, cold-steeping involves tossing the tea in cold water and letting it sit at room temperature or in the fridge for at least two hours. This method has been found to reduce the caffeine content and is said to reduce bitterness and improve the aroma.[78] But what does cold-steeping do to the nutrient content? You would think that cold water wouldn't draw out as many antioxidants. After all, nutrient extraction is presumably the whole point of brewing tea with hot water, right? A group of scientists took it upon themselves to compare the antioxidant activity of hot- versus cold-steeped tea. Essentially, they mixed LDL ("bad") cholesterol with free radicals and timed how long it took the cholesterol to oxidize in the presence of both hot- and cold-steeped tea.

In a surprise upset, cold-steeped white tea was significantly better at slowing down oxidation.[79] (No significant effect of brewing temperature on the antioxidant activity of green tea was found.) The researchers surmised that traditional tea water is so hot that it manages to destroy some of the more sensitive antioxidants in white tea. I no longer brew my tea; I just let it sit overnight in the fridge. Cold-steeping saves prep time and energy, and may even be healthier.

You don't have to care how much nutrition is extracted from tea leaves, though, if you simply eat them. Matcha is powdered green tea, produced by milling whole tea leaves into a fine powder that can be added straight to water. Why waste nutrition by dumping a tea bag when you're done, when you can drink the leaves instead? Think of it this way: Drinking steeped tea is akin to boiling a pot of collard greens and then throwing away the veggies and just drinking the cooking water. Sure, some of the nutrition leached into the water, but wouldn't it be better to eat the leaves themselves? That's why I now just throw whole tea leaves straight into my smoothies (see page 364). This is also a great way to incorporate tea in your diet if drinking tea on an empty stomach causes discomfort. If you develop a taste for matcha (I find it a bit grassy), you can carry around little packets of it wherever you go and just put some in your water bottle and shake. For essentially zero calories, you can drink dark-green leafies all day.

If green tea is so good, why not just take green-tea extract pills? Because of dozens of reported cases of liver toxicity linked to their use[80]—yet another demonstration that it's better to eat the whole food than some glorified "active ingredient" concentrate. There is one tea beverage I'd stay away from, though. Based on a few cases of serious, life-threatening outcomes linked to kombucha tea, a type of fermented tea, the consumption of kombucha "should be discouraged," according to one case report of a person who ended up in a coma after drinking the stuff.[81]

Are there any caveats to regular tea consumption? The fluoride content of tea appears to be the limiting factor. The tea plant naturally concentrates fluoride from the soil, which is one of the reasons tea consumption may help fight cavities,[82] but too much fluoride can be toxic. A recent case reported in the *New England Journal of Medicine* described a woman who started experiencing bone pain after seventeen years of habitually consuming a pitcher of tea made from 100 to 150 tea bags daily.[83] That's too much.

To prevent skeletal fluorosis, adults should probably not drink more than about twenty tea bags' worth of black tea a day for twenty years straight, or thirty bags of green daily, or eighty bags of white tea a day.[84] To prevent dental fluorosis, a harmless but unsightly mottled tooth discoloration, children should probably refrain from drinking more than about three bags of black tea a day (or around four bags of green or twelve of white)[85] while their teeth are still developing, up until around age nine.[86]

The Best Sweetener

In chapter 12, I shared research suggesting that adding sugar may negate some of the benefits of beverages, while adding artificial sweeteners like aspartame or saccharine may even make things worse. Are there any health-promoting sweeteners? The only two concentrated, green-light sweeteners may be blackstrap molasses and date sugar. Other natural caloric sweeteners, such as honey, less processed cane sugars, and maple, agave, and brown rice syrups don't appear to have much to offer nutritionally.[87] Date sugar is a whole food—just dried dates ground up into a powder—as are date and prune pastes, which can be homemade or purchased. These are all good options for baking, but for sweetening drinks, the taste of molasses may be too strong, and the whole-food sweeteners don't fully dissolve.

How about stevia? During the 1990s, research out of Japan found that steviosides, the "active" ingredient in stevia, appeared harmless. But in the guts of rats, intestinal bacteria transformed steviosides into a toxic substance called steviol, which can cause a big spike in mutagenic DNA damage in vitro.[88] Unfortunately, it turns out that humans have the same bacterial activity in their guts.[89] It's the dose that makes the poison, though. The World Health Organization considers up to 1.8 mg of stevia compounds per pound of body weight to be a safe amount. Given the American sweet tooth, though, if we sweetened everything with stevia, you could exceed that safety limit. But just drinking up to two stevia-sweetened beverages a day should be considered harmless.[90]

The sugar alcohols sorbitol and xylitol are harmless in themselves, but they aren't absorbed by the body and end up in the colon, where they can draw in fluid and cause diarrhea. This is why they're only used commercially in small quantities, such as in mints or chewing gum, as opposed to beverages. A related compound, however, erythritol, is absorbed and may have the harmlessness of xylitol without the laxative effect.

Erythritol is found naturally in pears and grapes, but industrially, yeast is used to produce it. Erythritol doesn't cause cavities,[91] and it hasn't been implicated in fibromyalgia,[92] preterm birth,[93] headaches,[94] hypertension,[95] brain disorders,[96] or platelet disorders[97] like other low-calorie sweeteners. Moreover, erythritol may actually have some antioxidant properties.[98] As with any highly processed product, though, its utility should be confined to increasing your consumption of green-light foods. So, for example, if the only way for you to eat half a grapefruit is to sprinkle some sugar on it, then it's probably better to eat a sugared grapefruit than no grapefruit at all—though sprinkling it with erythritol would be even better. With this logic in mind, I use erythritol to increase my consumption of cranberries (remember my Pink Juice recipe in chapter 8?), cocoa powder (see page 264), and hibiscus tea.

My Hibiscus Punch

In 2010, an antioxidant analysis of three hundred different beverages was published, examining everything from Red Bull to red wine.[99] And the winner is . . . hibiscus tea! I documented its potent antihypertensive effects in chapter 7. I've always had "normal" blood pressure by U.S. standards, but I wanted to shoot for optimal, so hibiscus became a daily staple for me. Give this recipe a try:

To eight cups of water, add a handful of bulk dried hibiscus or four bags of tea in which hibiscus is the first ingredient. Then add the juice of one lemon and three tablespoons of erythritol, and leave it in your fridge to cold-brew overnight. In the morning, strain out the hibiscus or take out the tea bags, shake well, and drink throughout the day. That's something I try to do every day I'm home.

For extra credit, add green foam: Pour a cup of the tea into a blender with a bunch of fresh mint leaves, blend on high, and enjoy. You end up with dark-green leafies blended into what may be the highest antioxidant beverage in the world, and it tastes like fruit punch. Your kids will love it!

As with any sour food or beverage, make sure to rinse your mouth with water after consumption to prevent the natural acids from dissolving your enamel.[100] Do *not* brush your teeth within an hour after eating or drinking something sour, as your enamel may be in a softened state and be further damaged by brushing.[101] If you sip continuously throughout the day, I suggest using a straw to bypass your teeth.[102]

Be careful, though. There are three ways that even harmless sweeteners could theoretically be harmful. Over the years, numerous large-scale studies have found a correlation between artificial-sweetener use and weight gain.[103] The most common explanation for this counterintuitive finding is reverse causation: People aren't fat because they drink diet soda; they drink diet soda because they're fat.

But there are at least three other less benign alternative explanations. The first is called "overcompensation for expected caloric reduction." If you covertly switch people's soda for diet soda without their knowing it, their caloric intake drops.[104] This makes sense, since they're not drinking all that sugar anymore. But what if you fess up to what you did? People who knowingly consume artificial sweeteners may actually end up eating *more* calories; they may figure after their zero-calorie drink, they can indulge in that second piece of pie. Indeed that's what studies have shown. For example, if you give subjects an aspartame-sweetened cereal for breakfast, but only inform half the participants that the sweetener was artificial, when lunchtime comes, the aspartame-informed group ends up eating significantly more than the aspartame-naïve group.[105] I think of this concept anytime I see someone at a fast-food restaurant ordering a diet soda with their meal.

A second explanation for gaining weight while using artificial sweeteners is based on how humankind evolved: When your brain registers the sensation of sweetness on your tongue, millions of years of evolution remind your brain to boost your appetite to eat as much as possible—after all, naturally sweet plant foods like fruits or sweet potatoes are among the healthiest. When you drink a can of diet soda, your brain thinks you just stumbled across a wild blueberry bush, and it sends urgent signals to eat large and eat fast before someone else gets wind of your bounty. At the same time, your body knows that if you eat too many calories, you might get too fat and not be able to outrun that saber-toothed tiger, so when your gut senses that you've absorbed enough calories, it sends signals up to your brain to urge you to stop eating. When you ingest low-calorie sweeteners, however, you experience the familiar hunger-boosting effect due to the sensation of sweetness on your tongue, yet you may lack the hunger-suppressing effect of calories entering your gut. The result can be a revved-up appetite that can lead to eating more food than you otherwise would have.[106] That's the second way diet soda could counterintuitively lead to weight gain.

The third way involves maintaining cravings for, and dependency on, all things sweet. By continuing to consume any sweeteners—with or without calories—you are unable to train your flavor preferences away from intensely sweet foods.[107] Let's say that you use erythritol at home. That's great, but what happens when you go on vacation and don't have ready access to it? Your preference for intensely sweet food travels with you, and that may end up translating into the increased consumption of less-than-healthy foods.

The bottom line? Erythritol seems safe, but only if you don't use it as an excuse to eat more junk food. With great sweetness comes great responsibility.

Drink five glasses of water a day, be they plain tap water or flavored with fruit, tea leaves, or herbs. Keeping hydrated may elevate your mood (and vigor!), improve your thinking, and even help cut your risk for heart disease, bladder cancer, and other diseases. Bottoms up!

Exercise

Moderate-Intensity Activities

Bicycling, canoeing, dancing, dodgeball, downhill skiing, fencing, hiking, housework, ice-skating, in-line skating, juggling, jumping on a trampoline, paddle boating, playing Frisbee, roller-skating, shooting baskets, shoveling light snow, skateboarding, snorkeling, surfing, swimming recreationally, tennis (doubles), treading water, walking briskly (4 mph), water aerobics, waterskiing, yard work, and yoga

Vigorous Activities

Backpacking, basketball, bicycling uphill, circuit weight training, cross-country skiing, football, hockey, jogging, jumping jacks, jumping rope, lacrosse, push-ups and pull-ups, racquetball, rock climbing, rugby, running, scuba diving, tennis (singles), soccer, speed skating, squash, step aerobics, swimming laps, walking briskly uphill, and water jogging

Serving Sizes:

90 minutes of moderate-intensity activity
40 minutes of vigorous activity

Daily Recommendation:

1 serving per day

More than two-thirds of American adults are overweight.[1] Think about that. Fewer than one in three people maintain a healthy weight. What's more, by 2030, more than *half* the country's population may be clinically obese. Over the last three decades, childhood obesity has tripled, and most overweight kids will continue to be overweight into adulthood.[2] As mentioned earlier, we may be in the process of raising the first generation of children in America with a shorter predicted life span than their parents.[3]

The food industries like to blame inactivity as the prime cause of obesity, not the promotion and consumption of their calorie-rich products.[4] On the contrary, however, research suggests that the level of physical activity may have actually *increased* in the United States over the past few decades.[5] We know that obesity is rising even in areas where people are exercising more.[6] This is likely explained by the fact that eating activity levels are outstripping physical activity levels.[7]

Compared to eating habits in the 1970s, every day, children are consuming the caloric equivalent of an extra can of soda and small fries, and adults are eating an extra Big Mac's worth of calories. Just to make up for the extra calories Americans are taking in compared to a few decades ago, as a nation, we'd need to walk an extra two hours a day, every day of the week.[8]

Surveys suggest that most people believe controlling diet and getting enough exercise are equally important for weight control.[9] It's a lot easier to eat, however, than to move. To walk off the calories found in a single pat of butter or margarine, you'd have to add about an extra half mile to your evening stroll. For every additional sardine on your Caesar salad, that's another quarter-mile jog. If you eat two chicken legs, you'll need to get up on your own two legs and run three miles just to make up for it—and that's stewed chicken, skin removed.[10]

Researchers who accept grants from the Coca-Cola Company[11] call physical inactivity "the biggest public health problem of the 21st century."[12] Actually, physical inactivity ranks down at number five in terms of risk factors for death in the United States and number six in terms of risk factors for disability.[13] And inactivity barely makes the top ten globally.[14] As we've learned, diet is by far our greatest killer, followed by smoking.[15]

Of course, that doesn't mean you should sit on the couch all day. As we've seen in this book, in addition to helping you enjoy a healthy body weight, exercise can also ward off and possibly reverse mild cognitive decline, boost your immune system, prevent and treat high blood pressure, and improve your mood and quality of sleep, among many other benefits. If the U.S. population collectively exercised enough to shave just 1 percent off the national body mass index

(BMI), 2 million cases of diabetes, 1.5 million cases of heart disease, and up to 127,000 cases of cancer might be prevented.[16]

Stand Up for Your Health

It turns out your mom and dad were right about the hazards of watching too much television—although it may not rot the brain so much as the body. Based on a study of about nine thousand adults followed for seven years, researchers calculated that every additional hour spent watching TV per day may be associated with an 11 percent increased risk of death.[17] Screen time in general—including playing video games—appears to be a risk factor for premature death.[18] So does that mean you have to kill your TV and PlayStation before they kill you?

It's not the electronics themselves but the sedentary behavior associated with enjoying them. Of course, not all sedentary behaviors are bad.[19] Consider sleeping—you can't be more sedentary than that! The problem appears to be sedentary *sitting*. After tracking the health of more than one hundred thousand Americans for fourteen years, an American Cancer Society study found that men who sit for six hours or more per day have a 20 percent higher overall death rate compared to men who sit for three hours or less, while women who sit for more than six hours have a 40 percent higher death rate.[20] A meta-analysis of forty-three such studies found that excess sitting was associated with a shorter life span,[21] and this may be "regardless of physical activity level." In other words, people who religiously hit the gym after work may still have shortened life spans if they are otherwise sitting throughout the day. Sitting for six or more hours a day appears to increase mortality rates even among people who run or swim for an hour a day, every day, seven days a week.[22]

I'm not saying we should all quit our desk jobs, but there are other options. For instance, try switching to a standing desk, which elevates the heart rate and may burn as many as fifty extra calories per hour. This may not seem like a lot, but simply standing for three hours a day at work equates to about thirty thousand extra calories burned per year—the equivalent of running ten marathons.[23] Whether you're at the office, reading the newspaper at home, or, yes, even watching TV, why not find a way to stand while doing it? In fact, most of this book was written while I was walking fifteen miles a day on a treadmill underneath my standing desk. Prebuilt treadmill desks are expensive, but thrift stores are often awash with old exercise equipment. My treadmill "desk" is just a treadmill stuck under some cheap plastic shelving.

If you have been sedentary for a long time, start out slowly. I'm sure you've heard the familiar refrain: "Before starting this or any other exercise program, be sure to check with your doctor." This is definitely true for vigorous exercise, but most people can safely start to take up walking ten or fifteen minutes a few times a day. If, however, you are unsteady on your feet, prone to dizzy spells, or have a chronic or unstable health condition, it really is best to first consult with a health professional.

What If You Really Have to Sit All Day?

Why is sitting around so bad for you? One reason may be endothelial dysfunction, the inability of the inner lining of your blood vessels to signal your arteries to relax normally in response to blood flow. Just as your muscles atrophy if you don't use them, "use it or lose it" may apply to arterial function as well. Increased blood flow promotes a healthy endothelium.[24] Blood flow is what maintains the stability and integrity of the inner lining of your arteries. Without that constant tugging flow with each heartbeat of exertion, you can end up a sitting duck for arterial dysfunction diseases.

What if sitting all day is part of your job? Research suggests treadmill desks may improve the health of office workers without detracting from work performance,[25] but your office might not accommodate a standing desk. Preliminary evidence from observational[26] as well as interventional[27] studies suggests that regular interruptions in sitting time can be beneficial. And they don't have to be long. Breaks could be as short as one minute and not necessarily entail strenuous exercise—just walking up and down stairs may be enough. Another option at a sedentary workplace is to opt for "walking meetings" rather than traditional sit-downs.

What if you have a sitting job in which you can't take frequent breaks, like truck driving? Is there any way to improve your endothelial function sitting on your butt? First you need to get rid of any butts—cigarette butts, that is. Smoking a single cigarette can significantly impair endothelial function.[28] Diet-wise, drinking green tea every two hours can help keep your endothelium functional,[29] as can eating meals with greens and other nitrate-rich vegetables. (See chapter 7.)

Turmeric may also help. One head-to-head study found that daily ingestion of the turmeric component curcumin can improve endothelial

continued

function just as well as up to an hour a day of aerobic exercise.[30] Does that mean you can just be a couch potato as long as you eat curried potatoes? No, you still need to move around as much as possible—the combination of curcumin *and* exercise appears to work even better than either option alone.[31]

Treating Sore Muscles with Plants

Optimizing recovery from exercise is considered the holy grail of exercise science.[32] Anyone who works out regularly knows about sore muscles. There's the burning sensation during strenuous exercise, which may be related to the buildup of lactic acid in your muscles, and then there's delayed-onset muscle soreness, the kind you get in the days following extreme physical activity. Delayed soreness is likely the result of inflammation caused by microtears in your muscles and can adversely affect athletic performance in the days following a heavy workout. If you're suffering from an inflammatory reaction, might anti-inflammatory phytonutrients help? The bioflavonoids in citrus can help with the lactic acid buildup,[33] but you may need to ramp up to the anthocyanin flavonoids in berries to deal with the inflammation.

Muscle biopsies of athletes have confirmed that eating blueberries, for example, can significantly reduce exercise-induced inflammation.[34] Studies using cherries show that this anti-inflammatory effect can translate into faster recovery time, reducing the strength loss from excessive bicep curling from 22 percent down to only 4 percent in male college students over the subsequent four days.[35] The muscle-soothing effects of berries don't only work for weight lifters; follow-up studies have shown that cherries can also help reduce muscle pain in long-distance runners[36] and aid in recovery from marathons.[37]

Eating two cups of watermelon prior to intense physical activity was also found to significantly reduce muscle soreness. The researchers concluded that functional compounds in fruits and vegetables can "play a key role in the design of new natural and functional products" like beverages, juices, and energy bars.[38] But why design *new* products when nature has already designed everything you need?

Preventing Exercise-Induced Oxidative Stress

As discussed in part 1, when you use oxygen to burn fuel in your body, free radicals can be produced, just as cars burning fuel produce combustion by-products out the exhaust. This happens even if you're just idling, living your day-to-day life. What if you rev things up, start exercising, and really start burning fuel? Might you create more oxidative stress and therefore need to eat even more antioxidant-rich foods?

Studies have demonstrated that ultramarathoners show evidence of DNA damage in about 10 percent of their cells tested during[39] and up to two weeks following[40] a race. But most of us aren't ultramarathoners. Might short bouts of exercise still damage your DNA?

Yes. After just five minutes of moderate or intense cycling, you can get an uptick in DNA damage.[41] Never ones to miss an opportunity, pharmaceutical and supplement companies have investigated ways to block exercise-induced oxidative damage with antioxidant pills, but, ironically, this may lead to a state of *pro*-oxidation. For example, guys doing arm curls taking about 1,000 mg of vitamin C ended up with *more* muscle damage and oxidative stress.[42]

Instead of using supplements, what about using antioxidant-rich foods to douse the free radicals? Researchers led subjects onto treadmills and cranked up the intensity until they nearly collapsed. While a spike in free-radical levels was witnessed in the control group, subjects who loaded up on watercress two hours before exercising actually ended up with fewer free radicals after the treadmill test than when they started. After two months of eating a daily serving of watercress, no DNA damage resulted, no matter how much it seemed the subjects were punished on the treadmill.[43] So, with a healthy diet, you can get the best of both worlds—all the benefits of strenuous exercise without excess free-radical damage. As a review in the *Journal of Sports Sciences* put it, those who eat plant-based diets may naturally "have an enhanced antioxidant defence system to counter exercise-induced oxidative stress."[44] Whether it's about training longer or living longer, the science seems clear. Your quality and quantity of life improves when you choose green-light foods.

How Much Should You Exercise?

The current official physical activity guidelines recommend adults get at least 150 minutes a week of moderate aerobic exercise, which comes out to a little more than 20 minutes a day.[45] That's actually down from previous recommendations from the surgeon general,[46] the CDC, and the American College of Sports Medicine,[47] which recommended at least 30 minutes each day. The exercise authorities seem to have fallen into the same trap as the nutrition authorities, recommending what they think may be achievable, rather than simply informing you what the science says and letting you make up your own mind. They already emphasize that any physical activity is better than none,[48] so why not stop patronizing the public and just tell everyone the truth?

It is true that walking 150 minutes a week is better than walking 60 minutes a week. Following the current recommendations for 150 minutes appears to reduce your overall mortality rate by 7 percent compared to being sedentary. Walking for only 60 minutes a week only drops your mortality rate about 3 percent. But walking 300 minutes a week drops overall mortality by *14 percent*.[49] So walking twice as long—40 minutes a day compared to the recommended 20—yields twice the benefit. And an hour-long walk each day may reduce mortality by 24 percent![50] (I use walking as an example because it's an exercise nearly everyone can do, but the same goes for other moderate-intensity activities, such as gardening or cycling.[51])

A meta-analysis of physical activity dose and longevity found that the equivalent of about an hour a day of brisk (4 mph) walking was good, but 90 minutes was even better.[52] What about more than 90 minutes? Unfortunately, so few people exercise that much every day that there weren't enough studies to compile a higher category. If we know 90 minutes of exercise a day is better than 60 minutes is better than 30 minutes, why is the recommendation only 20 minutes? I understand that only about half of Americans even make the recommended 20 minutes a day,[53] so the authorities are just hoping to nudge people in the right direction. It's like the dietary guidelines advising us to "eat less candy." If only they'd just give it to us straight.

That's what I've tried to do in this book.

Conclusion

My friend Art was one of those guys you just wanted to be around. Successful, generous, kind, and hilarious, he was more than the public face of the natural foods business empire that he had started. He truly walked the walk, or rather, ran the run. An avid snowboarder and mountain biker, Art ate a whole-food, plant-based diet for more than two decades. He was one of the healthiest guys I ever met.

He died while I was writing this book.

At just forty-six years old, he was found dead in the shower of a health retreat he owned. My heart couldn't deal with the grief of losing my friend, so my head took over, my mind spinning with possible causes of his death. I thought that if I could figure out what had happened, I could give his family some closure.

I considered all the rare congenital heart disorders that can cause sudden death in young athletes. Maybe it was Brugada syndrome? I remembered there was a case of a marathon runner who had collapsed due to this rare genetic disorder,[1] which can be triggered by heat.[2] I looked it up, and indeed, there was a previous case tied to a hot bath,[3] so it seemed plausible that this was what took Art's life.

The heat of the water was indeed the reason he'd died, but not in the way I had suspected. The sheriff called later that week to inform us that others had collapsed in the very same shower. These victims were medevaced to a nearby hospital and, thankfully, they survived.

It turned out that Art had died of carbon monoxide poisoning. A newly installed hot-water heater must not have been vented properly. It was an unbearable tragedy. I haven't been able to stop thinking about him.

Art's passing made me realize that no matter how well we eat or how well we live, we can always get hit by a bus—metaphorically or literally. We need to make sure to look both ways in life and before crossing the street. We need to take care of ourselves. We need to wear seat belts and bike helmets and practice safer sex. (After all, practice makes perfect!)

And we need to make each day count by filling it with fresh air, laughter, and love—love for ourselves, for others, and for whatever we are doing with our one precious life. That's what Art taught me.

In Pursuit of Pleasure

The idea of preventive health is that you do something now so that nothing bad happens later. You floss your teeth not because it makes you feel better but because, by doing so, one day you won't feel worse. You could consider the healthy habits described in this book to be preventive—you eat a healthier diet now to avoid disease later.

A healthy diet, however, does more than that.

The food industries bank their billions by manipulating the pleasure centers within your brain, the so-called dopamine reward system. Dopamine is the neurotransmitter the brain evolved to reward you for good behavior, helping to motivate your drive for things like food, water, and sex—all necessary for the perpetuation of our species. This natural response has been and continues to be perverted for profit.

The food industry, like the tobacco companies and other drug lords, has been able to come up with products that tap into the same dopamine reward system that keeps people smoking cigarettes and snorting cocaine. People have chewed coca leaves for at least eight thousand years without any evidence of addiction,[4] but a problem arises when certain components are isolated and concentrated into cocaine—when the coca leaves are *processed*. The same may be true for sugar. After all, few people binge on bananas. The isolation of sugar from the whole food may be the reason you're more likely to supersize soda than sweet potatoes or why you're unlikely to eat too much corn on the cob but can't seem to get enough high-fructose corn syrup.

The overconsumption of sugar-sweetened foods has often been compared to drug addiction. Until very recently, this parallel was based more on anecdotal evidence than on solid scientific grounds. But now we have PET scans, imaging technology that allows doctors to measure brain activity in real time. It all started with a study that showed decreased dopamine sensitivity in obese individuals. The more the individual being studied weighed, the less responsive to dopamine he or she appeared to be.[5] We see the same reduction in sensitivity in cocaine addicts and alcoholics.[6] The brain gets so overstimulated that it ends up trying to turn down the volume.

It was healthy and adaptive for our primate brains to drive us to eat that banana when there wasn't much food around, but now that fruit is available in fruit *loop* form, this evolutionary adaptation has become a liability.[7] The original Coca-Cola formulation actually included coca leaf, but now, perhaps, its sugar content may be the addictive stand-in.

The brain responds similarly to fat. Within thirty minutes of being fed yogurt packed with butterfat, research subjects exhibited similar brain activity[8] to those who drank straight sugar water.[9] People who regularly eat ice cream (sugar *and* fat) have a deadened dopamine response in their brains when drinking a milkshake. It's comparable to the way drug abusers have to use more and more drugs to obtain the same high. A neuroimaging study found that frequent ice cream consumption "is related to a reduction in reward-region [pleasure center] responsivity in humans, paralleling the tolerance observed in drug addiction." Once you've so dulled your dopamine response, you may subsequently overeat in an effort to achieve the degree of gratification experienced previously, contributing to unhealthy weight gain.[10]

What do fatty and sugary foods have in common? They are both energy dense. It may be less about the number of calories than their concentration. Consumption of green-light foods, which are naturally calorie dilute, doesn't lead to a deadened dopamine response, but a calorie-dense diet with the same number of calories does.[11] It's like the difference between cocaine and crack: It's the same stuff chemically, but by smoking crack cocaine, a user can deliver a higher dose more quickly to his or her brain.

Given our new understanding of the biological basis of food addiction, there have been calls to include obesity as an official mental disorder.[12] After all, both obesity and addiction share the inability to restrain behavior in spite of an awareness of detrimental health consequences, one of the defining criteria of substance abuse (a phenomenon referred to as the "pleasure trap").[13] Of course, redefining obesity as an addiction would be a boon to the pharmaceutical companies that are already working on a whole array of drugs to muck with your brain chemistry.[14]

For example, when researchers tried giving an opiate blocker to binge eaters (similar to how heroin addicts are sometimes treated with opiate blockers to minimize the narcotic's effects), the binge eaters ate significantly fewer fatty and sugary snacks—the snacks just didn't seem to do as much for them when their opiate receptors were blocked.[15] In addition to new drugs, addiction specialists have urged that the food industry "should be given incentives to develop low calorie foods that are more attractive, palatable and affordable so that people can adhere to diet programs for a long time."[16] No need—Mother Nature beat them to it. That's what the produce aisle is for.

Rather than taking drugs, you can prevent the numbing of your pleasure center in the first place by sticking to green-light foods. This can help return your dopamine sensitivity to normal levels so that you can again derive the same pleasure from the simplest of foods. When you regularly eat calorie-dense animal products and junk foods like ice cream, it's not just your taste buds that change but your brain chemistry. After eating a bunch of candy bars, not only may a ripe peach no longer taste as sweet on your tongue but your brain downregulates dopamine receptors to compensate for the repeated jolts of fat and sugar. In fact, an overly rich diet could cause you to experience less enjoyment from other activities as well.

There is a reason cocaine addicts appear to have an impaired neurological capacity for sexual stimulation[17] and why smokers have an impaired ability to respond to positive stimuli.[18] Related brain circuits wire all these sensations. Since they all involve overlapping dopamine pathways, what you put into your body—what you eat and what you drink—can affect how you experience all of life's pleasures. Try it and see. Try it and *feel*.

Do you see where I'm going with this?

Eating a whole-food, plant-based diet and returning your brain's dopamine sensitivity to its healthy, normal levels can help you live life to the fullest and allow you to experience greater joy, satisfaction, and pleasure from all the things you do—not just what you eat.

Let Me Help

I hope I've been able to persuade you that nutrition is not the stale, lifeless subject your middle school home-economics class may have led you to believe. It's vibrant and overflowing with opportunity for the betterment of your life. This abundance can create a problem, though. Over the last year alone, more than twenty-five thousand articles on nutrition were published in the medical literature. Who has time to sift through them all?

Every year, my team and I read through every issue of every English-language nutrition journal in the world so you don't have to. Then I compile all the most interesting, groundbreaking, and practical findings we can uncover to create new videos and articles every day for my nonprofit site, NutritionFacts.org.

Everything on NutritionFacts.org is provided absolutely free of charge. There's no special member area where you pay a fee to get extra lifesaving information. What membership websites seem to be saying, in essence, is that if you don't give them money, they'll withhold information that could make your family healthier. That's unacceptable to me. Advances in health sciences should be freely available and accessible to all.

Since we refuse to sell products, advertisements, or endorsements, how do the bills get paid? NutritionFacts.org is a 501(c)(3) nonprofit organization that thrives on the Wikipedia model of simply accepting donations from visitors who appreciate the content. We reach so many millions of people that if even one in one thousand makes a small, tax-deductible contribution, we are able to pay for all the staff and server costs. (I personally don't accept any compensation for my work on NutritionFacts.org; I'm privileged to be able to donate my time as a labor of love.) The hope is to offer a public service so valuable that viewers will feel moved to support it and keep this life-changing, life-*saving* resource free for everyone for all time.

I welcome you to come and make NutritionFacts.org a part of your life. I've got new videos and articles *every day* on the latest in evidence-based nutrition. You can sign up for daily, weekly, or monthly e-mails highlighting all the new, fun, juicy information. It warms my heart to hear it's become a Sunday ritual for many families. It exists to serve you.

Taking Responsibility

My goal is to give you the information to empower and inspire you to make healthy changes in your life, but in the end, it's all up to you. Know, however, that there is only one way of eating that's ever been proven to reverse heart disease in the majority of patients, a diet centered around whole plant foods. Anytime anyone tries to sell you on some new diet, ask just one simple question: "Has it been proven to reverse heart disease?" (You know, the most likely cause of death for you and everyone you love?) If it hasn't, why would you even consider it?

If that's all a whole-food, plant-based diet could do—reverse our number-one killer—then shouldn't that be the default diet until proven otherwise? And the fact that it can also be effective in preventing, treating, and arresting other leading killers would seem to make the case for eating this way overwhelming. Please give it a try.

It could save your life.

How Not to Die may seem to you a strange title for a book. After all, everyone is going to die eventually. It's about how not to die *prematurely*. If there is one takeaway message, it's that you have tremendous power over your health destiny. The vast majority of premature deaths can be prevented with simple changes in what you eat and how you live.

In other words, a long and healthy life is largely a matter of choice. In 2015, Dr. Kim Williams became president of the American College of Cardiology. He was asked why he chose to eat a strictly plant-based diet. "I don't mind dying," Dr. Williams said. "I just don't want it to be my fault."[19]

That's what this book is about: taking responsibility for your and your family's health.

Acknowledgments

There are many thanks I'd like to express: to my cowriters and editors, Gene, Jennifer, Miranda, Miyun, Nick, and Whitney, who helped turn my bite-sized chunks of science into a coherent, four-course narrative meal; to my fact-checkers, Alissa, Allison, Frances, Helena, Martin, Michelle, Seth, Stephanie, and Valerie; and to all the NutritionFacts.org volunteers who helped with the book: Brad, Cassie, Emily, Giang, Jerold, Kari, Kimberley, Laura, Lauren, Luis, Tracy, and especially Jennifer—no physician has ever known a better PA or a better friend. Also, much appreciation to Brenda and Vesanto for their keen insights and vast knowledge.

This book would not have been possible without my wonderful staff—Joe, Katie, Liz, and Tommasina—and everyone at HSUS who supported me on the work front, and Andrea, my partner in life, and our beloved family, who supported me on the home front. NutritionFacts.org would not have even been possible without the Jesse & Julie Rasch Foundation, the design and coding genius of Christi Richards, and the thousands who have donated to enable my work to reach millions.

Though it was my grandmother who made me the doctor I am today, it was my mother who made me the person I am today. I love you, Mom!

Supplements

By getting your nutrients from green-light foods, not only will you minimize exposure to harmful food components, such as sodium, saturated fat, and cholesterol, but you will maximize your intake of nearly every required nutrient: vitamin A carotenoids; vitamin C; vitamin E; the B vitamins, including thiamin, riboflavin, and folate; as well as magnesium, iron, and potassium, not to mention fiber.[1] Dietary quality rating scales consistently rank the most-plant-based diets as the healthiest.[2]

That said, because of the way we live in our modern world, there are important shortfalls that need to be corrected.

For example, vitamin B12 is not made by plants; it's made by microbes that blanket the earth. But in this sanitized modern world, we now chlorinate the water supply to kill off any bacteria. While you don't get much B12 in the water anymore, you don't get much cholera, either—that's a good thing! Similarly, we evolved to make all the vitamin D we need from the sun, but most of us are no longer running around naked in equatorial Africa. You may be covered up, inside, at a high northern latitude and therefore need to supplement your diet with this "sunshine vitamin." Thus, these two vitamins must be addressed.

2,500 mcg (µg) Vitamin B12 (Cyanocobalamin) at Least Once a Week

Given modern sanitary standards, a regular, reliable source of vitamin B12 is *critical* for anyone eating a plant-based diet.[3] Though deficiency for those starting out with adequate stores may take years to develop,[4] the results of B12 deficiency can be devastating, with cases reported of paralysis,[5] psychosis,[6] blindness,[7] and even death.[8] Newborn infants of mothers who eat a plant-based diet and who fail to supplement can develop deficiency much more rapidly with disastrous results.[9]

For adults under age sixty-five, the easiest way to get B12 is to take at least one 2,500 mcg supplement each week. If you take too much, you merely get expensive pee. Well, not all that expensive: A five-year supply of vitamin B12 can cost less than twenty dollars.[10] If you'd rather get into the habit of taking it daily, the once-a-day dosing is 250 mcg.[11] Note that these doses are specific to cyanocobalamin, the preferred supplemental form of vitamin B12, as there is insufficient evidence to support the efficacy of the other forms, like methylcobalamin.[12]

As you age, your ability to absorb vitamin B12 may decline.[13] For those over sixty-five who eat plant-based diets, the supplementation should probably be increased from at least 2,500 mcg a week (or 250 mcg a day) up to 1,000 mcg of cyanocobalamin each day.[14,15]

Instead of taking B12 supplements, it's possible to get sufficient amounts from B12-fortified foods, but you would have to eat three servings a day of foods providing at least 25 percent of the Daily Value (on the Nutrition Facts label),[16] with each serving eaten at least four to six hours after the last.[17] The only green-light source I'm aware of is B12-fortified nutritional yeast, for which two teaspoons three times a day would suffice. For most people, though, it would probably be cheaper and more convenient to just take a supplement.

My other supplement recommendations in this section can be considered conditional, but getting enough vitamin B12 is absolutely nonnegotiable for those centering their diets around green-light foods.

Vitamin D from Sun or Supplements

I recommend that people unable to get sufficient sun take one 2,000 IU vitamin D3 supplement each day,[18] ideally with the largest meal of the day.[19]

In the northern hemisphere, below approximately 30° latitude (south of Los Angeles, Dallas, or Atlanta), fifteen minutes each day of midday sun on the forearms and face without sunblock should produce sufficient vitamin D for Caucasians under the age of sixty. Those who have darker skin[20] or who are older[21] may require thirty minutes or more.

Farther north, at 40° latitude (Portland, Chicago, or New York City), the sun's rays are at such an angle during the months of November through February that vitamin D may not be produced. No matter how long you might sunbathe naked in Times Square on New Year's Day, you won't make any vitamin D.[22]

Above 50° latitude (around London, Berlin, Moscow, and Edmonton, Canada), this "vitamin D winter" may extend for as long as six months of the year.

Vitamin D supplements are therefore recommended for people at higher latitudes during the winter months and year-round for those not getting enough midday sun, regardless of location. This may also apply to those living in smoggy cities, such as Los Angeles or San Diego.[23]

I do not recommend tanning beds. They can be both ineffective[24] and dangerous.[25] The lamps emit mostly UVA,[26] which increases melanoma skin cancer risk without producing vitamin D.[27]

Eat Iodine-Rich Foods

Iodine, a mineral essential for thyroid function, is found predominantly in the ocean and in variable amounts in the soils of the world. To ensure everyone was getting enough, table salt was fortified with the mineral starting in the 1920s. So if you do add salt to your food, use iodized salt (*not* sea salt or "natural" salt, which contains about sixty times less iodine[28]). Given that sodium is considered the second-leading dietary killer in the world,[29] however, iodized salt should be considered a red-light source.

There are two yellow-light sources of iodine: seafood and dairy milk. (Iodine leaches into the milk from iodine-containing antiseptic chemicals used to disinfect the cow's teats to prevent mastitis.[30]) The most concentrated green-light source is seaweed, which has the iodine of seafood without the fat-soluble pollutants that build up in the aquatic food chain.

Sea vegetables are the underwater dark-green leafies. I encourage you to experiment with ways to include them in your diet. The recommended daily intake of iodine is 150 mcg, which is what is in about two sheets of nori,[31] the seaweed that's used to make sushi. There are all sorts of seaweed snacks on the market now, but most, if not all of them, seem to have added red-light ingredients. So I buy plain nori and season the sheets myself by brushing them with jarred pickled ginger juice and lightly sprinkling on wasabi powder before recrisping them at 300°F for about five minutes.

Sprinkling just a half teaspoon of the seaweeds arame or dulse onto dishes you're preparing may also get you your iodine for the day. Dulse is sold as pretty purple flakes you can just shake onto your food. I do caution *against* hijiki[32] (also spelled hiziki), because it has been found to be contaminated with arsenic. I also caution against kelp, which may have *too much* iodine; just a half teaspoon of kelp could exceed the daily upper limit. For the same reason, you shouldn't get into a regular habit of eating more than fifteen sheets of nori or more than a tablespoon of arame or dulse a day.[33] Too much iodine can cause excessive thyroid gland activity.[34]

For those who don't like seaweed, Eden brand's canned beans have a tiny amount of kelp added such that iodine levels average between 36.3 mcg per half-cup serving (great northern beans) to 71.2 mcg (navy beans).[35] Not only are those levels safe—you'd have to eat about twenty cans a day to get too much—but checkmarking my three legume servings a day with Eden's beans would fulfill your daily iodine requirement.

One last note about iodine: Although people who avoid seafood and dairy products do not appear to have impaired thyroid function,[36,37] I would not leave it to chance during pregnancy, where iodine is critical for proper brain development.[38] I agree with the American Thyroid Association's recommendation that all North American pregnant and breast-feeding women receive a prenatal vitamin containing 150 mcg of iodine daily.[39]

Consider Taking 250 mg of Pollutant-Free (Yeast- or Algae-Derived) Long-Chain Omega-3s Daily

According to two of the most credible nutrition authorities, the World Health Organization and the European Food Safety Authority, you should get at least a half a percent of your calories from the short-chain omega-3 ALA.[40] That's easy—the one Daily Dozen tablespoon of ground flaxseeds takes care of that. Your body can then take the short-chain omega-3 from flaxseeds (or chia seeds or walnuts) and elongate it into the long-chain omega-3s EPA and DHA found in fish fat. The question, however, is whether the body can make enough for optimal brain health.[41,42] Until we know more, I recommend taking 250 mg of pollutant-free long-chain omega-3s directly.

I don't recommend fish oil, since even purified ("distilled") fish oil has been found to be contaminated with considerable amounts of PCBs and other pollutants, so much so that taken as directed, salmon, herring, and tuna oils would exceed the tolerable daily intake of toxicity.[43] This may help explain the studies that found adverse effects of fish consumption on cognitive function in both adults and children. But many of those studies either were done downstream of a gold-mining area contaminated with mercury, which is used in the mining process,[44] or included people who ate whale meat or fish caught next to chemical plants or toxic spills.[45] What about fish you'd just get at a restaurant or grocery store?

An elite group of Floridians (mostly corporate executives) was studied. They ate so much seafood that at least 43 percent exceeded the U.S. Environmental Protection Agency's safety limit for mercury, and it appeared to have an effect. The researchers found that excessive seafood intake, which they defined as more than around three to four servings per month of such fish as tuna or snapper, elevates mercury levels and appeared to cause cognitive dysfunction. The effect wasn't large—only about a 5 percent drop in cognitive performance—but "a decrement [in executive function] that no one, let alone a health-conscious and achievement-oriented person, is likely to welcome."[46]

Thankfully, you can get the benefits without the risks by getting long-chain omega-3s from algae instead,[47] which is where the fish primarily get it from to begin with.[48] By cutting out the middle-fish and getting EPA and DHA directly from the source at the bottom of the food chain, you don't have to worry about pollutant contamination. In fact, the algae used for supplements are just grown in tanks and never even come in contact with the ocean.[49] That's why I recommend a contaminant-free source to get the best of both worlds, omega-3 levels associated with brain preservation[50] and minimized exposure to industrial pollutants.

What About . . . ?

All the other vitamins, minerals, and nutrients should be taken care of by the mountains of nutrition you'll be getting by centering your diet around whole plant foods. And many of those nutrients are ones Americans normally don't get in sufficient quantity—namely, vitamins A, C, and E and the minerals magnesium and potassium, along with fiber.[51] Ninety-three percent of Americans don't get enough vitamin E. Ninety-seven percent of American adults don't get enough fiber.[52] *Ninety-eight* percent of American diets are deficient in potassium.[53] You, my friend, are going to be the one in a thousand who does it right.

If you have a specific question about some obscure nutrient—like, "What about my molybdenum or menaquinones?"—rather than have me bore everyone else with minutiae, allow me to refer you to the best reference book available on plant-based nutrition by the preeminent dietitians Brenda Davis and Vesanto Melina.[54] The authors go into great detail and even have chapters on pregnancy, breast-feeding, and raising bouncing boys and girls.

Vitamin B12-fortified plant-based diets can offer health benefits for all stages of the life cycle.[55] Dr. Benjamin Spock, the most esteemed pediatrician of all time, wrote perhaps the bestselling American book of the twentieth century: *The Common Sense Book of Baby and Child Care.* In the seventh edition, the final one before Dr. Spock died at ninety-four, he advocated children be raised on a plant-based diet with no exposure to meat or dairy products. Dr. Spock had lived long enough to see the beginnings of the childhood obesity epidemic. "Children who grow up getting their nutrition from plant foods," he wrote, "have a tremendous health advantage and are much less likely to develop health problems as the years go by."[56]

Notes

Preface

1. Monte T, Pritikin I. *Pritikin: The Man Who Healed America's Heart*. Emmaus, PA: Rodale Press; 1988.
2. Gould KL, Ornish D, Scherwitz L, et al. Changes in myocardial perfusion abnormalities by positron emission tomography after long-term, intense risk factor modification. *JAMA*. 1995;274: 894–901.
3. Ornish D, Scherwitz L, Billings J, et al. Intensive lifestyle changes for reversal of coronary heart disease. Five-year follow-up of the Lifestyle Heart Trial. *JAMA*. 1998;280:2001–7.
4. Ornish DM, Scherwitz LW, Doody RS, et al. Effects of stress management training and dietary changes in treating ischemic heart disease. *JAMA*. 1983;249:54–9.
5. Ornish D. Intensive lifestyle changes and health reform. *Lancet Oncol*. 2009;10(7):638–9.
6. Adams KM, Kohlmeier M, Zeisel SH. Nutrition education in U.S. medical schools: latest update of a national survey. *Acad Med*. 2010;85(9):1537–42.
7. Jamal A, Dube SR, Malarcher AM, Shaw L, Engstrom MC. Tobacco use screening and counseling during physician office visits among adults. National Ambulatory Medical Care Survey and National Health Interview Survey, United States, 2005–2009. *MMWR Morb Mortal Wkly Rep*. 2012; 61 Suppl:38–45.

Introduction

1. Berzlanovich AM, Keil W, Waldhoer T, Sim E, Fasching P, Fazeny-Dörner B. Do centenarians die healthy? An autopsy study. *J Gerontol A Biol Sci Med Sci*. 2005;60(7):862–5.
2. Kohn RR. Cause of death in very old people. *JAMA*. 1982;247(20):2793–7.
3. Berzlanovich AM, Keil W, Waldhoer T, Sim E, Fasching P, Fazeny-Dörner B. Do centenarians die healthy? An autopsy study. *J Gerontol A Biol Sci Med Sci*. 2005;60(7):862–5.
4. Lenders C, Gorman K, Milch H, et al. A novel nutrition medicine education model: the Boston University experience. *Adv Nutr*. 2013;4(1):1–7.
5. Murray CJ, Atkinson C, Bhalla K, et al. The state of US health, 1990–2010: burden of diseases, injuries, and risk factors. *JAMA*. 2013;310(6):591–608.
6. Kris-Etherton PM, Akabas SR, Bales CW, et al. The need to advance nutrition education in the

training of health care professionals and recommended research to evaluate implementation and effectiveness. *Am J Clin Nutr.* 2014;99(5 Suppl):1153S–66S.

7. Swift CS. Nutrition trends: implications for diabetes health care professionals. *Diabetes Spectr.* 2009;29(1):23–5.

8. Vetter ML, Herring SJ, Sood M, Shah NR, Kalet AL. What do resident physicians know about nutrition? An evaluation of attitudes, self-perceived proficiency and knowledge. *J Am Coll Nutr.* 2008;27(2):287–98.

9. Lazarus K, Weinsier RL, Boker JR. Nutrition knowledge and practices of physicians in a family-practice residency program: the effect of an education program provided by a physician nutrition specialist. *Am J Clin Nutr.* 1993;58(3):319–25.

10. Senate Committee on Business, Professions and Economic Development. Bill Analysis on SB 380. http://www.leginfo.ca.gov/pub/11-12/bill/sen/sb_0351-0400/sb_380_cfa_20110421 _125358_sen_comm.html. Hearing held April 25, 2011. Accessed March 31, 2015.

11. The Medical Board of California. Continuing Medical Education. http://www.mbc.ca.gov /Licensees/Continuing_Education/. Nd. Accessed March 31, 2015.

12. Wizard Edison says doctors of future will give no medicine. *Newark Advocate.* January 2, 1903.

13. Stange KC, Zyzanski SJ, Jaén CR, et al. Illuminating the "black box." A description of 4454 patient visits to 138 family physicians. *J Fam Pract.* 1998;46(5):377–89.

14. Aitken M, Johns Hopkins Bloomberg School of Public Health. The trillion dollar market for medicines: characteristics, dynamics and outlook. http://www.jhsph.edu/research/centers-and -institutes/center-for-drug-safety-and-effectiveness/academic-training/seminar-series /MUrray%20Aikten.pdf. February 24, 2014. Accessed March 29, 2015.

15. Willett WC. Balancing life-style and genomics research for disease prevention. *Science.* 2002;296(5568):695–8.

16. Willett WC. Balancing life-style and genomics research for disease prevention. *Science.* 2002;296(5568):695–8.

17. Robertson TL, Kato H, Rhoads GG, et al. Epidemiologic studies of coronary heart disease and stroke in Japanese men living in Japan, Hawaii and California. Incidence of myocardial infarction and death from coronary heart disease. *Am J Cardiol.* 1977;39(2):239–43.

18. Mayo Clinic News Network. Nearly 7 in 10 Americans take prescription drugs, Mayo Clinic, Olmsted Medical Center Find. http://newsnetwork.mayoclinic.org/discussion/nearly-7-in-10 -americans-take-prescription-drugs-mayo-clinic-olmsted-medical-center-find/. June 19, 2013. Accessed March 31, 2015.

19. Murray CJ, Atkinson C, Bhalla K, et al. The state of US health, 1990–2010: burden of diseases, injuries, and risk factors. *JAMA.* 2013;310(6):591–608.

20. Crimmins EM, Beltrán-Sánchez H. Mortality and morbidity trends: is there compression of morbidity? *J Gerontol B Psychol Sci Soc Sci.* 2011;66(1):75–86.

21. Crimmins EM, Beltrán-Sánchez H. Mortality and morbidity trends: is there compression of morbidity? *J Gerontol B Psychol Sci Soc Sci.* 2011;66(1):75–86.

22. Olshansky SJ, Passaro DJ, Hershow RC, et al. A potential decline in life expectancy in the United States in the 21st century. *N Engl J Med.* 2005;352(11):1138–45.

23. Offord DR. Selection of levels of prevention. *Addict Behav.* 2000;25(6):833–42.

24. Gofrit ON, Shemer J, Leibovici D, Modan B, Shapira SC. Quaternary prevention: a new look at an old challenge. *Isr Med Assoc J.* 2000;2(7):498–500.

25. Strasser T. Reflections on cardiovascular diseases. *Interdiscip Sci Rev.* 1978;3(3):225–30.

26. Lloyd-Jones DM, Hong Y, Labarthe D, et al. Defining and setting national goals for cardiovascular health promotion and disease reduction: the American Heart Association's strategic Impact Goal through 2020 and beyond. *Circulation.* 2010;121(4):586–613.

27. Yancy CW. Is ideal cardiovascular health attainable? *Circulation.* 2011;123(8):835–7.

28. Lloyd-Jones DM, Hong Y, Labarthe D, et al. Defining and setting national goals for cardiovascular health promotion and disease reduction: the American Heart Association's strategic Impact Goal through 2020 and beyond. *Circulation.* 2010;121(4):586–613.

29. Yusuf S, Hawken S, Ounpuu S, et al. Effect of potentially modifiable risk factors associated with myocardial infarction in 52 countries (the INTERHEART study): case-control study. *Lancet.* 2004;364(9438):937–52.

30. Lloyd-Jones DM, Hong Y, Labarthe D, et al. Defining and setting national goals for cardiovascular health promotion and disease reduction: the American Heart Association's strategic Impact Goal through 2020 and beyond. *Circulation.* 2010;121(4):586–613.

31. Shay CM, Ning H, Allen NB, et al. Status of cardiovascular health in US adults: prevalence estimates from the National Health and Nutrition Examination Surveys (NHANES) 2003–2008. *Circulation.* 2012;125(1):45–56.

32. Shay CM, Ning H, Allen NB, et al. Status of cardiovascular health in US adults: prevalence estimates from the National Health and Nutrition Examination Surveys (NHANES) 2003–2008. *Circulation.* 2012;125(1):45–56.

33. Omran AR. The epidemiologic transition. A theory of the epidemiology of population change. *Milbank Mem Fund Q.* 1971;49(4):509–38.

34. US Centers for Disease Control and Prevention. Leading causes of death, 1900–1998. http://www.cdc.gov/nchs/data/dvs/lead1900_98.pdf. Accessed April 29, 2015.

35. Kochanek KD, Murphy SL, Xu J, Arias E. Mortality in the United States, 2013. NCHS Data Brief 2014;178.

36. Lim SS, Vos T, Flaxman AD, et al. A comparative risk assessment of burden of disease and injury attributable to 67 risk factors and risk factor clusters in 21 regions, 1990–2010: a systematic analysis for the Global Burden of Disease Study 2010. *Lancet.* 2012;380(9859):2224–60.

37. Popkin BM. Global nutrition dynamics: the world is shifting rapidly toward a diet linked with noncommunicable diseases. *Am J Clin Nutr.* 2006;84(2):289–98.

38. Zhai F, Wang H, Du S, et al. Prospective study on nutrition transition in China. *Nutr Rev.* 2009;67 Suppl 1:S56–61.

39. Singh PN, Arthur KN, Orlich MJ, et al. Global epidemiology of obesity, vegetarian dietary patterns, and noncommunicable disease in Asian Indians. *Am J Clin Nutr.* 2014;100 Suppl 1:359S–64S.

40. Singh PN, Arthur KN, Orlich MJ, et al. Global epidemiology of obesity, vegetarian dietary patterns, and noncommunicable disease in Asian Indians. *Am J Clin Nutr.* 2014;100 Suppl 1:359S–64S.

41. McCarty MF. Proposal for a dietary "phytochemical index." *Med Hypotheses.* 2004;63(5):813–7.

42. Mirmiran P, Bahadoran Z, Golzarand M, Shiva N, Azizi F. Association between dietary phytochemical index and 3-year changes in weight, waist circumference and body adiposity index in adults: Tehran Lipid and Glucose study. *Nutr Metab* (Lond). 2012;9(1):108.

43. Mirmiran P, Bahadoran Z, Golzarand M, Shiva N, Azizi F. Association between dietary phytochemical index and 3-year changes in weight, waist circumference and body adiposity index in adults: Tehran Lipid and Glucose study. *Nutr Metab* (Lond). 2012;9(1):108.

44. Golzarand M, Bahadoran Z, Mirmiran P, Sadeghian-Sharif S, Azizi F. Dietary phytochemical index is inversely associated with the occurrence of hypertension in adults: a 3-year follow-up (the Tehran Lipid and Glucose Study). *Eur J Clin Nutr.* 2015;69(3):392–8.

45. Golzarand M, Mirmiran P, Bahadoran Z, Alamdari S, Azizi F. Dietary phytochemical index and subsequent changes of lipid profile: a 3-year follow-up in Tehran Lipid and Glucose Study in Iran. *ARYA Atheroscler.* 2014;10(4):203–10.

46. Bahadoran Z, Karimi Z, Houshiar-Rad A, Mirzayi HR, Rashidkhani B. Dietary phytochemical index and the risk of breast cancer: a case control study in a population of Iranian women. *Asian Pac J Cancer Prev.* 2013;14(5):2747–51.

47. U.S. Department of Agriculture Economic Research Service. Loss-adjusted food availability. http://www.ers.usda.gov/datafiles/Food_Availabily_Per_Capita_Data_System/LossAdjusted _Food_Availability/calories.xls. September 30, 2014. Accessed April 29, 2015.

48. Wansink B, Kniffin KM, Shimizu M. Death row nutrition. Curious conclusions of last meals. *Appetite.* 2012;59(3):837–43.

49. Bambs C, Kip KE, Dinga A, Mulukutla SR, Aiyer AN, Reis SE. Low prevalence of "ideal cardiovascular health" in a community-based population: the heart strategies concentrating on risk evaluation (Heart SCORE) study. *Circulation.* 2011;123(8):850–7.

50. Yancy CW. Is ideal cardiovascular health attainable? *Circulation.* 2011;123(8):835–7.

51. Ford ES, Bergmann MM, Krord J, Schienkiewitz A, Weikert C, Boeing H. Healthy living is the best revenge: findings from the European Prospective Investigation Into Cancer and Nutrition-Potsdam study. *Arch Intern Med.* 2009;169(15):1355–62.

52. Platz EA, Willett WC, Colditz GA, Rimm EB, Spiegelman D, Giovannucci E. Proportion of colon cancer risk that might be preventable in a cohort of middle-aged US men. *Cancer Causes Control.* 2000;11(7):579–88.

53. Wahls TL. The seventy percent solution. *J Gen Intern Med.* 2011;26(10):1215–6.

54. Ford ES, Bergmann MM, Boeing H, Li C, Capewell S. Healthy lifestyle behaviors and all-cause mortality among adults in the United States. *Prev Med.* 2012;55(1):23–7.

55. Khaw KT, Wareham N, Bingham S, Welch A, Luben R, Day N. Combined impact of health behaviours and mortality in men and women: the EPIC-Norfolk prospective population study. *PLoS Med.* 2008;5(1):e12.

56. Jiang H, Ju Z, Rudolph KL. Telomere shortening and ageing. *Z Gerontol Geriatr.* 2007;40(5): 314–24.

57. Mather KA, Jorm AF, Parslow RA, Christensen H. Is telomere length a biomarker of aging? A review. *J Gerontol A Biol Sci Med Sci.* 2011;66(2):202–13.

58. Tsuji A, Ishiko A, Takasaki T, Ikeda N. Estimating age of humans based on telomere shortening. *Forensic Sci Int.* 2002;126(3):197–9.

59. Shammas MA. Telomeres, lifestyle, cancer, and aging. *Curr Opin Clin Nutr Metab Care.* 2011; 14(1):28–34.

60. Huzen J, Wong LS, van Veldhuisen DJ, et al. Telomere length loss due to smoking and metabolic traits. *J Intern Med.* 2014;275(2):155–63.

61. Hou L, Savage SA, Blaser MJ, et al. Telomere length in peripheral leukocyte DNA and gastric cancer risk. *Cancer Epidemiol Biomarkers Prev.* 2009;18(11):3103–9.

62. Gu Y, Honig LS, Schupf N, et al. Mediterranean diet and leukocyte telomere length in a multiethnic elderly population. *Age* (Dordr). 2015;37(2):9758.

63. García-Calzón S, Moleres A, Martínez-González MA, et al. Dietary total antioxidant capacity is associated with leukocyte telomere length in a children and adolescent population. *Clin Nutr.* 2014;S0261–5614(14):00191–5.

64. García-Calzón S, Moleres A, Martínez-González MA, et al. Dietary total antioxidant capacity is associated with leukocyte telomere length in a children and adolescent population. *Clin Nutr.* 2014;S0261–5614(14):00191–5.

65. Leung CW, Laraia BA, Needham BL, et al. Soda and cell aging: associations between sugar-sweetened beverage consumption and leukocyte telomere length in healthy adults from the National Health and Nutrition Examination Surveys. *Am J Public Health.* 2014;104(12):2425–31.

66. Nettleton JA, Diez-Roux A, Jenny NS, Fitzpatrick AL, Jacobs DR. Dietary patterns, food

groups, and telomere length in the Multi-Ethnic Study of Atherosclerosis (MESA). *Am J Clin Nutr.* 2008;88(5):1405–12.

67. Gu Y, Honig LS, Schupf N, et al. Mediterranean diet and leukocyte telomere length in a multi-ethnic elderly population. *Age* (Dordr). 2015;37(2):9758.

68. Flanary BE, Kletetschka G. Analysis of telomere length and telomerase activity in tree species of various life-spans, and with age in the bristlecone pine Pinus longaeva. *Biogerontology.* 2005; 6(2):101–11.

69. Ornish D, Lin J, Daubenmier J, et al. Increased telomerase activity and comprehensive lifestyle changes: a pilot study. *Lancet Oncol.* 2008;9(11):1048–57.

70. Skordalakes E. Telomerase and the benefits of healthy living. *Lancet Oncol.* 2008;9(11):1023–4.

71. Ornish D, Lin J, Chan JM, et al. Effect of comprehensive lifestyle changes on telomerase activity and telomere length in men with biopsy-proven low-risk prostate cancer: 5-year follow-up of a descriptive pilot study. *Lancet Oncol.* 2013;14(11):1112–20.

72. Mason C, Risques RA, Xiao L, et al. Independent and combined effects of dietary weight loss and exercise on leukocyte telomere length in postmenopausal women. *Obesity* (Silver Spring). 2013;21(12):E549–54.

73. Ornish D, Lin J, Daubenmier J, et al. Increased telomerase activity and comprehensive lifestyle changes: a pilot study. *Lancet Oncol.* 2008;9(11):1048–57.

74. Ornish D, Lin J, Chan JM, et al. Effect of comprehensive lifestyle changes on telomerase activity and telomere length in men with biopsy-proven low-risk prostate cancer: 5-year follow-up of a descriptive pilot study. *Lancet Oncol.* 2013;14(11):1112–20.

75. Artandi SE, Depinho RA. Telomeres and telomerase in cancer. *Carcinogenesis.* 2010;31(1): 9–18.

76. Mozaffarian D, Benjamin EJ, Go AS, et al. Heart disease and stroke statistics—2015 update: a report from the American Heart Association. *Circulation.* 2015;131(4):e29–322.

77. American Cancer Society. Cancer Facts & Figures 2015. Atlanta: American Cancer Society; 2015.

78. NHLBI Fact Book, Fiscal Year 2012. National Heart, Lung, and Blood Institute, NIH. http://www.nhlbi.nih.gov/files/docs/factbook/FactBook2012.pdf. February 2013. Accessed March 31, 2015.

79. Mozaffarian D, Benjamin EJ, Go AS, et al. Heart disease and stroke statistics—2015 update: a report from the American Heart Association. *Circulation.* 2015;131(4):e29–322.

80. Centers for Disease Control and Prevention. Deaths: final data for 2013 table 10. Number of deaths from 113 selected causes. National Vital Statistics Report 2016;64(2).

81. American Cancer Society. Cancer Facts & Figures 2015. Atlanta: American Cancer Society; 2015.

82. Centers for Disease Control and Prevention. Deaths: final data for 2013 table 10. Number of deaths from 113 selected causes. National Vital Statistics Report 2016;64(2).

83. Centers for Disease Control and Prevention. Deaths: final data for 2013 table 10. Number of deaths from 113 selected causes. National Vital Statistics Report 2016;64(2).

84. Mozaffarian D, Benjamin EJ, Go AS, et al. Heart disease and stroke statistics—2015 update: a report from the American Heart Association. *Circulation.* 2015;131(4):e29–322.

85. Centers for Disease Control and Prevention. Deaths: final data for 2013 table 10. Number of deaths from 113 selected causes. National Vital Statistics Report 2016;64(2).

86. American Cancer Society. Cancer Facts & Figures 2015. Atlanta: American Cancer Society; 2015.

87. Centers for Disease Control and Prevention. Deaths: final data for 2013 table 10. Number of deaths from 113 selected causes. National Vital Statistics Report 2016;64(2).

88. Centers for Disease Control and Prevention. Deaths: final data for 2013 table 10. Number of deaths from 113 selected causes. *National Vital Statistics Report* 2016;64(2).

89. Centers for Disease Control and Prevention. Deaths: final data for 2013 table 10. Number of deaths from 113 selected causes. *National Vital Statistics Report* 2016;64(2).

90. Centers for Disease Control and Prevention. Deaths: final data for 2013 table 10. Number of deaths from 113 selected causes. *National Vital Statistics Report* 2016;64(2).

91. Centers for Disease Control and Prevention. Deaths: final data for 2013 table 10. Number of deaths from 113 selected causes. *National Vital Statistics Report* 2016;64(2).

92. Tuso PJ, Ismail MH, Ha BP, Bartolotto C. Nutritional update for physicians: plant-based diets. *Perm J.* 2013;17(2):61–6.

93. Egger GJ, Binns AF, Rossner SR. The emergence of "lifestyle medicine" as a structured approach for management of chronic disease. *Med J Aust.* 2009;190(3):143–5.

94. Hyman MA, Ornish D, Roizen M. Lifestyle medicine: treating the causes of disease. *Altern Ther Health Med.* 2009;15(6):12–4.

95. Willett WC. Balancing life-style and genomics research for disease prevention. *Science.* 2002;296(5568):695–8.

96. Hyman MA, Ornish D, Roizen M. Lifestyle medicine: treating the causes of disease. *Altern Ther Health Med.* 2009;15(6):12–4.

97. Allen J, Anderson DR, Baun B, et al. Reflections on developments in health promotion in the past quarter century from founding members of the American Journal of Health Promotion Editorial Board. *Am J Health Promot.* 2011;25(4):ei–eviii.

98. Tuso PJ, Ismail MH, Ha BP, Bartolotto C. Nutritional update for physicians: plant-based diets. *Perm J.* 2013;17(2):61–6.

99. Tuso PJ, Ismail MH, Ha BP, Bartolotto C. Nutritional update for physicians: plant-based diets. *Perm J.* 2013;17(2):61–6.

100. Tuso PJ, Ismail MH, Ha BP, Bartolotto C. Nutritional update for physicians: plant-based diets. *Perm J.* 2013;17(2):61–6.

101. Kono S. Secular trend of colon cancer incidence and mortality in relation to fat and meat intake in Japan. *Eur J Cancer Prev.* 2004;13(2):127–32.

102. Willett WC. Balancing life-style and genomics research for disease prevention. *Science.* 2002;296(5568):695–8.

103. Kono S. Secular trend of colon cancer incidence and mortality in relation to fat and meat intake in Japan. *Eur J Cancer Prev.* 2004;13(2):127–32.

104. Kulshreshtha A, Goyal A, Veledar E, et al. Association between ideal cardiovascular health and carotid intima-media thickness: a twin study. *J Am Heart Assoc.* 2014;3(1):e000282.

105. Corona M, Velarde RA, Remolina S, et al. Vitellogenin, juvenile hormone, insulin signaling, and queen honey bee longevity. *Proc Natl Acad Sci USA.* 2007;104(17):7128–33.

106. Kucharski R, Maleszka J, Foret S, Maleszka R. Nutritional control of reproductive status in honeybees via DNA methylation. *Science.* 2008;319(5871):1827–30.

107. Gnyszka A, Jastrzebski Z, Flis S. DNA methyltransferase inhibitors and their emerging role in epigenetic therapy of cancer. *Anticancer Res.* 2013;33(8):2989–96.

108. Joven J, Micol V, Segura-Carretero A, Alonso-Villaverde C, Menéndez JA. Polyphenols and the modulation of gene expression pathways: can we eat our way out of the danger of chronic disease? *Crit Rev Food Sci Nutr.* 2014;54(8):985–1001.

109. Fang MZ, Wang Y, Ai N, et al. Tea polyphenol (-)-epigallocatechin-3-gallate inhibits DNA methyltransferase and reactivates methylation-silenced genes in cancer cell lines. *Cancer Res.* 2003;63(22):7563–70.

110. Myzak MC, Tong P, Dashwood WM, Dashwood RH, Ho E. Sulforaphane retards the growth

of human PC-3 xenografts and inhibits HDAC activity in human subjects. *Exp Biol Med* (Maywood). 2007;232(2):227–34.

111. Dashwood RH, Ho E. Dietary histone deacetylase inhibitors: from cells to mice to man. *Semin Cancer Biol.* 2007;17(5):363–9.

112. Gryder BE, Sodji QH, Oyelere AK. Targeted cancer therapy: giving histone deacetylase inhibitors all they need to succeed. *Future Med Chem.* 2012;4(4):505–24.

113. Ornish D, Magbanua MJ, Weidner G, et al. Changes in prostate gene expression in men undergoing an intensive nutrition and lifestyle intervention. *Proc Natl Acad Sci USA.* 2008; 105(24):8369–74.

PART 1

1. How Not to Die from Heart Disease

1. Myerburg RJ, Junttila MJ. 2012. Sudden cardiac death caused by coronary heart disease. *Circulation.* 28;125(8):1043–52.

2. Campbell TC, Parpia B, Chen J. Diet, lifestyle, and the etiology of coronary artery disease: the Cornell China study. *Am J Cardiol.* 1998;82(10B):18T-21T.

3. Shaper AG, Jones KW. Serum-cholesterol, diet, and coronary heart-disease in Africans and Asians in Uganda: 1959. *Int J Epidemiol.* 2012;41(5):1221–5.

4. Thomas WA, Davies JN, O'Neal RM, Dimakulangan AA. Incidence of myocardial infarction correlated with venous and pulmonary thrombosis and embolism. A geographic study based on autopsies in Uganda, East Africa and St. Louis, U.S.A. *Am J Cardiol.* 1960;5:41–7.

5. Benfante R. Studies of cardiovascular disease and cause-specific mortality trends in Japanese-American men living in Hawaii and risk factor comparisons with other Japanese populations in the Pacific region: a review. *Hum Biol.* 1992;64(6):791–805.

6. Chen J, Campbell TC, Li J, Peto R. Diet, life-style and mortality in China: A study of the characteristics of 65 Chinese counties. New York: Oxford University Press; 1990.

7. Shaper AG, Jones KW. Serum-cholesterol, diet, and coronary heart-disease in Africans and Asians in Uganda: 1959. *Int J Epidemiol.* 2012;41(5):1221–5.

8. De Biase SG, Fernandes SF, Gianini RJ, Duarte JL. Vegetarian diet and cholesterol and triglycerides levels. *Arq Bras Cardiol.* 2007;88(1):35–9.

9. Stoy PJ. Dental disease and civilization. *Ulster Med J.* 1951;20(2):144–58.

10. Kris-Etherton PM, Harris WS, Appel LJ, Nutrition Committee. Fish consumption, fish oil, omega-3 fatty acids, and cardiovascular disease. *Arterioscler Thromb Vasc Biol.* 2003;23(2):e20–30.

11. Shepherd CJ, Jackson AJ. Global fishmeal and fish-oil supply: inputs, outputs and markets. *J Fish Biol.* 2013;83(4):1046–66.

12. Rizos EC, Ntzani EE, Bika E, Kostapanos MS, Elisaf MS. Association between omega-3 fatty acid supplementation and risk of major cardiovascular disease events: a systematic review and meta-analysis. *JAMA.* 2012;308(10):1024–33.

13. Kwak SM, Myung SK, Lee YJ, Seo HG. Efficacy of omega-3 fatty acid supplements (eicosapentaenoic acid and docosahexaenoic acid) in the secondary prevention of cardiovascular disease: a meta-analysis of randomized, double-blind, placebo-controlled trials. *Arch Intern Med.* 2012;172(9):686–94.

14. Fodor JG, Helis E, Yazdekhasti N, Vohnout B. "Fishing" for the origins of the "Eskimos and heart disease" story: facts or wishful thinking? *Can J Cardiol.* 2014;30(8):864–8.

15. Burr ML, Fehily AM, Gilbert JF, et al. Effects of changes in fat, fish, and fibre intakes on death and myocardial reinfarction: diet and reinfarction trial (DART). *Lancet.* 1989;2(8666):757–61.

16. Burr ML. Secondary prevention of CHD in UK men: the Diet and Reinfarction Trial and its sequel. *Proc Nutr Soc.* 2007;66(1):9–15.

17. Burr ML, Ashfield-Watt PAL, Dunstan FDJ, et al. Lack of benefit of dietary advice to men with angina: results of a controlled trial. *Eur J Clin Nutr.* 2003;57(2):193–200.

18. Rizos EC, Ntzani EE, Bika E, Kostapanos MS, Elisaf MS. Association between omega-3 fatty acid supplementation and risk of major cardiovascular disease events: a systematic review and meta-analysis. *JAMA.* 2012;308(10):1024–33.

19. Smith DA. ACP Journal Club. Review: omega-3 polyunsaturated fatty acid supplements do not reduce major cardiovascular events in adults. *Ann Intern Med.* 2012;157(12):JC6–5.

20. Enos WF, Holmes RH, Beyer J. Coronary disease among United States soldiers killed in action in Korea; preliminary report. *JAMA.* 1953;152(12):1090–3.

21. Strong JP. Landmark perspective: Coronary atherosclerosis in soldiers. A clue to the natural history of atherosclerosis in the young. *JAMA.* 1986;256(20):2863–6.

22. Voller RD, Strong WB. Pediatric aspects of atherosclerosis. *Am Heart J.* 1981;101(6):815–36.

23. Napoli C, D'Armiento FP, Mancini FP, et al. Fatty streak formation occurs in human fetal aortas and is greatly enhanced by maternal hypercholesterolemia. Intimal accumulation of low density lipoprotein and its oxidation precede monocyte recruitment into early atherosclerotic lesions. *J Clin Invest.* 1997;100(11):2680–90.

24. Benjamin MM, Roberts WC. Facts and principles learned at the 39th Annual Williamsburg Conference on Heart Disease. *Proc* (Bayl Univ Med Cent). 2013;26(2):124–36.

25. McMahan CA, Gidding SS, Malcom GT, et al. Pathobiological determinants of atherosclerosis in youth risk scores are associated with early and advanced atherosclerosis. *Pediatrics.* 2006; 118(4):1447–55.

26. Trumbo PR, Shimakawa T. Tolerable upper intake levels for trans fat, saturated fat, and cholesterol. *Nutr Rev.* 2011;69(5):270–8.

27. Roberts WC. It's the cholesterol, stupid! *Am J Cardiol.* 2010;106(9):1364–6.

28. O'Keefe JH, Cordain L, Harris WH, Moe RM, Vogel R. Optimal low-density lipoprotein is 50 to 70 mg/dl: lower is better and physiologically normal. *J Am Coll Cardiol.* 2004;43(11): 2142–6.

29. Esselstyn CB. In cholesterol lowering, moderation kills. *Cleve Clin J Med.* 2000;67(8):560–4.

30. Roberts WC. The cause of atherosclerosis. *Nutr Clin Pract.* 2008;23(5):464–7.

31. Roberts WC. The cause of atherosclerosis. *Nutr Clin Pract.* 2008;23(5):464–7.

32. King S. The best selling drugs since 1996 - why AbbVie's Humira is set to eclipse Pfizer's Lipitor. http://www.forbes.com/sites/simonking/2013/07/15/the-best-selling-drugs-since-1996-why -abbvies-humira-is-set-to-eclipse-pfizers-lipitor/. July 15, 2013. Accessed May 1, 2015.

33. Ginter E, Kajaba I, Sauša M. Addition of statins into the public water supply? Risks of side effects and low cholesterol levels. *Cas Lek Cesk.* 2012;151(5):243–7.

34. Ferenczi EA, Asaria P, Hughes AD, Chaturvedi N, Francis DP. Can a statin neutralize the cardiovascular risk of unhealthy dietary choices? *Am J Cardiol.* 2010;106(4):587–92.

35. Draeger A, Monastyrskaya K, Mohaupt M, et al. Statin therapy induces ultrastructural damage in skeletal muscle in patients without myalgia. *J Pathol.* 2006;210(1):94–102.

36. Scott D, Blizzard L, Fell J, Jones G. Statin therapy, muscle function and falls risk in community-dwelling older adults. *QJM.* 2009;102(9):625–33.

37. Jefferson E. FDA announces safety changes in labeling for some cholesterol-lowering drugs. US Food and Drug Administration website. http://www.fda.gov/NewsEvents/Newsroom/Press Announcements/ucm293623.htm. February 28, 2012. Accessed February 14, 2015.

38. McDougall JA, Malone KE, Daling JR, Cushing-Haugen KL, Porter PL, Li CI. Long-term statin use and risk of ductal and lobular breast cancer among women 55 to 74 years of age. *Cancer Epidemiol Biomarkers Prev.* 2013;22(9):1529–37.

39. Jenkins DJ, Kendall CW, Marchie A, et al. The Garden of Eden—plant based diets, the genetic drive to conserve cholesterol and its implications for heart disease in the 21st century. *Comp Biochem Physiol, Part A Mol Integr Physiol.* 2003;136(1):141–51.

40. Esselstyn CB. Is the present therapy for coronary artery disease the radical mastectomy of the twenty-first century? *Am J Cardiol.* 2010;106(6):902–4.

41. Kadoch MA. The power of nutrition as medicine. *Prev Med.* 2012;55(1):80.

42. Wakai K, Marugame T, Kuriyama S, et al. Decrease in risk of lung cancer death in Japanese men after smoking cessation by age at quitting: pooled analysis of three large-scale cohort studies. *Cancer Sci.* 2007;98(4):584–9.

43. Vogel RA, Corretti MC, Plotnick GD. Effect of a single high-fat meal on endothelial function in healthy subjects. *Am J Cardiol.* 1997;79(3):350–4.

44. Erridge C. The capacity of foodstuffs to induce innate immune activation of human monocytes in vitro is dependent on food content of stimulants of Toll-like receptors 2 and 4. *Br J Nutr.* 2011;105(1):15–23.

45. Ornish D, Scherwitz LW, Billings JH, et al. Intensive lifestyle changes for reversal of coronary heart disease. *JAMA.* 1998;280(23):2001–7.

46. Ornish D, Scherwitz LW, Doody RS, et al. Effects of stress management training and dietary changes in treating ischemic heart disease. *JAMA.* 1983;249(1):54–9.

47. Ornish D, Scherwitz LW, Billings JH, et al. Intensive lifestyle changes for reversal of coronary heart disease. *JAMA.* 1998;280(23):2001–7.

48. Ellis FR, Sanders TA. Angina and vegan diet. *Am Heart J.* 1977;93(6):803–5.

49. Sweeney M. Effects of very low-fat diets on anginal symptoms. *Med Hypotheses.* 2004;63(3):553.

50. Savarese G, Rosano G, D'amore C, et al. Effects of ranolazine in symptomatic patients with stable coronary artery disease. A systematic review and meta-analysis. *Int J Cardiol.* 2013; 169(4):262–70.

51. Colpo E, Vilanova CD, Brenner Reetz LG, et al. A single consumption of high amounts of the Brazil nuts improves lipid profile of healthy volunteers. *J Nutr Metab.* 2013;2013:1–7.

52. Stern RH, Yang BB, Hounslow NJ, et al. Pharmacodynamics and pharmacokinetic-pharmacodynamic relationships of atorvastatin, an HMG-CoA reductase Inhibitor. *J Clin Pharmacol.* 2000;40(6):616–3.

53. Hegsted M. Dietary Guidelines. Food Politics website. www.foodpolitics.com/wp-content/uploads/Hegsted.pdf. nd. Accessed February 14, 2015.

54. Campbell TC. *The Low-Carb Fraud.* Dallas, TX: BenBella Books, Inc.; 2014.

55. Herman J. Saving U.S. dietary advice from conflicts of interest. *Food and Drug Law Journal* 2010; 65(20):285–316.

56. Herman J. Saving U.S. dietary advice from conflicts of interest. *Food and Drug Law Journal* 2010; 65(20):285–316.

57. Goodwin JS, Goodwin JM. The tomato effect. Rejection of highly efficacious therapies. *JAMA.* 1984;251(18):2387–90.

58. Adams KM, Kohlmeier M, Zeisel SH. Nutrition education in U.S. medical schools: latest update of a national survey. *Acad Med.* 2010;85(9):1537–42.

59. Hearing of California Senate Bill 380. Vimeo website. http://vimeo.com/23744792. April 25, 2011. Accessed February 14, 2015.

60. Murray JL. Coke and the AAFP—the real thing or a dangerous liaison? *Fam Med.* 2010; 42(1):57–8.

61. Blum A. AAFP-Coke editorial was music to [our] ears. *J Fam Pract*. 2010;59(2):74.

62. Brownell KD, Warner KE. The perils of ignoring history: Big Tobacco played dirty and millions died. How similar is Big Food? *Milbank Q*. 2009;87(1):259–94.

63. Brownell KD, Warner KE. The perils of ignoring history: Big Tobacco played dirty and millions died. How similar is Big Food? *Milbank Q*. 2009;87(1):259–94.

64. Simon, M. AND now a word from our sponsors. Eat Drinks Politics website. http://www .eatdrinkpolitics.com/wp-content/uploads/AND_Corporate_Sponsorship_Report.pdf. January 22, 2013. Accessed February 14, 2015.

65. Bruckert E, Pouchain D, Auboiron S, Mulet C. Cross-analysis of dietary prescriptions and adherence in 356 hypercholesterolaemic patients. *Arch Cardiovasc Dis*. 2012;105(11): 557–65.

66. Barnard ND. The physician's role in nutrition-related disorders: from bystander to leader. *Virtual Mentor*. 2013;15(4):367–72.

2. How Not to Die from Lung Diseases

1. American Cancer Society. Cancer Facts & Figures 2015. Atlanta: American Cancer Society; 2015.

2. Howlader N, Noone AM, Krapcho M, et al., eds. SEER Cancer Statistics Review, 1975–2011, National Cancer Institute. http://seer.cancer.gov/csr/1975_2011/. April 2014. Accessed February 27, 2015.

3. American Lung Association. Lung Cancer Fact Sheet. http://www.lung.org/lung-disease/lung -cancer/resources/facts-figures/lung-cancer-fact-sheet.html. 2015. Accessed February 14, 2015.

4. Moodie R, Stuckler D, Monteiro C, et al. Profits and pandemics: prevention of harmful effects of tobacco, alcohol, and ultra-processed food and drink industries. *Lancet*. 2013;381(9867): 670–9.

5. American Cancer Society. When smokers quit—what are the benefits over time? http://www .cancer.org/healthy/stayawayfromtobacco/guidetoquittingsmoking/guide-to-quitting-smoking -benefits. 6 February 2015. Accessed February 26, 2015.

6. US Department of Health and Human Services. A Report of the Surgeon General. How Tobacco Smoke Causes Disease: What It Means to You. Atlanta: US Department of Health and Human Services, Centers for Disease Control and Prevention, National Center for Chronic Disease Prevention and Health Promotion, Office on Smoking and Health, 2010.

7. Riso P, Martini D, Møller P, et al. DNA damage and repair activity after broccoli intake in young healthy smokers. *Mutagenesis*. 2010;25(6):595–602.

8. Gupta GP, Massagué J. Cancer metastasis: building a framework. *Cell*. 2006;127(4):679–95.

9. Wu X, Zhu Y, Yan H, et al. Isothiocyanates induce oxidative stress and suppress the metastasis potential of human non-small cell lung cancer cells. *BMC Cancer*. 2010;10:269.

10. Kim SY, Yoon S, Kwon SM, Park KS, Lee-Kim YC. Kale juice improves coronary artery disease risk factors in hypercholesterolemic men. *Biomed Environ Sci*. 2008;21(2):91–7.

11. Dressendorfer RH, Wade CE, Hornick C, Timmis GC. High-density lipoprotein-cholesterol in marathon runners during a 20-day road race. *JAMA*. 1982;247(12):1715–7.

12. Park W, Amin AR, Chen ZG, Shin DM. New perspectives of curcumin in cancer prevention. *Cancer Prev Res* (Phila). 2013;6(5):387–400.

13. Park W, Amin AR, Chen ZG, Shin DM. New perspectives of curcumin in cancer prevention. *Cancer Prev Res* (Phila). 2013;6(5):387–400.

14. Nagabhushan M, Amonkar AJ, Bhide SV. In vitro antimutagenicity of curcumin against environmental mutagens. *Food Chem Toxicol.* 1987;25(7):545–7.

15. Polasa K, Raghuram TC, Krishna TP, Krishnaswamy K. Effect of turmeric on urinary mutagens in smokers. *Mutagenesis.* 1992;7(2):107–9.

16. Ravindran J, Prasad S, Aggarwal BB. Curcumin and cancer cells: how many ways can curry kill tumor cells selectively? *AAPS J.* 2009;11(3):495–510.

17. Wu SH, Hang LW, Yang JS, et al. Curcumin induces apoptosis in human non-small cell lung cancer NCI-H460 cells through ER stress and caspase cascade- and mitochondria-dependent pathways. *Anticancer Res.* 2010;30(6):2125–33.

18. Su CC, Lin JG, Li TM, et al. Curcumin-induced apoptosis of human colon cancer colo 205 cells through the production of ROS, Ca2+ and the activation of caspase-3. *Anticancer Res.* 2006; 26(6B):4379–89.

19. Ravindran J, Prasad S, Aggarwal BB. Curcumin and cancer cells: how many ways can curry kill tumor cells selectively? *AAPS J.* 2009;11(3):495–510.

20. Ravindran J, Prasad S, Aggarwal BB. Curcumin and cancer cells: how many ways can curry kill tumor cells selectively? *AAPS J.* 2009;11(3):495–510.

21. Pallis AG, Syrigos KN. Lung cancer in never smokers: disease characteristics and risk factors. *Crit Rev Oncol Hematol.* 2013;88(3):494–503.

22. Chiang TA, Wu PF, Wang LF, Lee H, Lee CH, Ko YC. Mutagenicity and polycyclic aromatic hydrocarbon content of fumes from heated cooking oils produced in Taiwan. *Mutat Res.* 1997;381(2):157–61.

23. Katragadda HR, Fullana A, Sidhu S, Carbonell-Barrachina AA. Emissions of volatile aldehydes from heated cooking oils. *Food Chem.* 2010;120(1):59–65.

24. Jin ZY, Wu M, Han RQ, et al. Household ventilation may reduce effects of indoor air pollutants for prevention of lung cancer: a case-control study in a Chinese population. *PLoS ONE.* 2014;9(7):e102685.

25. Seow A, Poh WT, Teh M, et al. Fumes from meat cooking and lung cancer risk in Chinese women. *Cancer Epidemiol Biomarkers Prev.* 2000;9(11):1215–21.

26. Jedrychowski W, Perera FP, Tang D, et al. Impact of barbecued meat consumed in pregnancy on birth outcomes accounting for personal prenatal exposure to airborne polycyclic aromatic hydrocarbons: birth cohort study in Poland. *Nutrition.* 2012;28(4):372–7.

27. Perera FP, Li Z, Whyatt R, et al. Prenatal airborne polycyclic aromatic hydrocarbon exposure and child IQ at age 5 years. *Pediatrics.* 2009;124(2):e195–202.

28. Chen JW, Wang SL, Hsieh DP, Yang HH, Lee HL. Carcinogenic potencies of polycyclic aromatic hydrocarbons for back-door neighbors of restaurants with cooking emissions. *Sci Total Environ.* 2012;417–418:68–75.

29. Yang SC, Jenq SN, Kang ZC, Lee H. Identification of benzo[a]pyrene 7,8-diol 9,10-epoxide N2-deoxyguanosine in human lung adenocarcinoma cells exposed to cooking oil fumes from frying fish under domestic conditions. *Chem Res Toxicol.* 2000;13(10):1046–50.

30. Chen JW, Wang SL, Hsieh DP, Yang HH, Lee HL. Carcinogenic potencies of polycyclic aromatic hydrocarbons for back-door neighbors of restaurants with cooking emissions. *Sci Total Environ.* 2012 Feb 15;417–418:68–75.

31. Lijinsky W. N-Nitroso compounds in the diet. *Mutat Res.* 1999 Jul 15;443(1–2):129–38.

32. Thiébaud HP, Knize MG, Kuzmicky PA, Hsieh DP, Felton JS. Airborne mutagens produced by frying beef, pork and a soy-based food. *Food Chem Toxicol.* 1995;33(10):821–8.

33. Thiébaud HP, Knize MG, Kuzmicky PA, Hsieh DP, Felton JS. Airborne mutagens produced by frying beef, pork and a soy-based food. *Food Chem Toxicol.* 1995;33(10):821–8.

34. Mitsakou C, Housiadas C, Eleftheriadis K, Vratolis S, Helmis C, Asimakopoulos D. Lung deposition

of fine and ultrafine particles outdoors and indoors during a cooking event and a no activity period. *Indoor Air*. 2007;17(2):143–52.

35. COPD Statistics across America. COPD Foundation website. http://www.copdfoundation.org /What-is-COPD/COPD-Facts/Statistics.aspx. 2015. Accessed February 14, 2015.

36. Tabak C, Smit HA, Räsänen L, et al. Dietary factors and pulmonary function: a cross sectional study in middle aged men from three European countries. *Thorax*. 1999;54(11):1021–6.

37. Walda IC, Tabak C, Smit HA, et al. Diet and 20-year chronic obstructive pulmonary disease mortality in middle-aged men from three European countries. *Eur J Clin Nutr*. 2002;56(7):638–43.

38. Varraso R, Jiang R, Barr RG, Willett WC, Camargo CA, Jr. Prospective study of cured meats consumption and risk of chronic obstructive pulmonary disease in men. *Am J Epidemiol*. 2007 Dec 15;166(12):1438–45.

39. Jiang R, Paik DC, Hankinson JL, Barr RG. Cured meat consumption, lung function, and chronic obstructive pulmonary disease among United States adults. *Am J Respir Crit Care Med*. 2007 Apr 15;175(8):798–804.

40. Jiang R, Camargo CA, Varraso R, Paik DC, Willett WC, Barr RG. Consumption of cured meats and prospective risk of chronic obstructive pulmonary disease in women. *Am J Clin Nutr*. 2008; 87(4):1002–8.

41. Keranis E, Makris D, Rodopoulou P, et al. Impact of dietary shift to higher-antioxidant foods in COPD: a randomised trial. *Eur Respir J*. 2010;36(4):774–80.

42. Warner JO. Worldwide variations in the prevalence of atopic symptoms: what does it all mean? *Thorax*. 1999;54 Suppl 2:S46–51.

43. What Is Asthma? National Heart, Lung, and Blood Institute. http://www.nhlbi.nih.gov/health /health-topics/topics/asthma/. August 4, 2014. Accessed February 14, 2015.

44. Warner JO. Worldwide variations in the prevalence of atopic symptoms: what does it all mean? *Thorax*. 1999;54 Suppl 2:S46–51.

45. Aït-Khaled N, Pearce N, Anderson HR, et al. Global map of the prevalence of symptoms of rhinoconjunctivitis in children: The International Study of Asthma and Allergies in Childhood (ISAAC) Phase Three. *Allergy*. 2009;64(1):123–48.

46. Asher MI, Stewart AW, Mallol J, et al. Which population level environmental factors are associated with asthma, rhinoconjunctivitis and eczema? Review of the ecological analyses of ISAAC Phase One. *Respir Res*. 2010;11:8.

47. Ellwood P, Asher MI, Björkstén B, Burr M, Pearce N, Robertson CF. Diet and asthma, allergic rhinoconjunctivitis and atopic eczema symptom prevalence: an ecological analysis of the International Study of Asthma and Allergies in Childhood (ISAAC) data. ISAAC Phase One Study Group. *Eur Respir J*. 2001;17(3):436–43.

48. Protudjer JL, Sevenhuysen GP, Ramsey CD, Kozyrskyj AL, Becker AB. Low vegetable intake is associated with allergic asthma and moderate-to-severe airway hyperresponsiveness. *Pediatr Pulmonol*. 2012;47(12):1159–69.

49. Bime C, Wei CY, Holbrook J, Smith LJ, Wise RA. Association of dietary soy genistein intake with lung function and asthma control: a post-hoc analysis of patients enrolled in a prospective multicentre clinical trial. *Prim Care Respir J*. 2012;21(4):398–404.

50. Agrawal S, Pearce N, Ebrahim S. Prevalence and risk factors for self-reported asthma in an adult Indian population: a cross-sectional survey. *Int J Tuberc Lung Dis*. 2013 17(2):275–82.

51. Tsai HJ, Tsai AC. The association of diet with respiratory symptoms and asthma in schoolchildren in Taipei, Taiwan. *J Asthma*. 2007;44(8):599–603.

52. Yusoff NA, Hampton SM, Dickerson JW, Morgan JB. The effects of exclusion of dietary egg and milk in the management of asthmatic children: a pilot study. *J R Soc Promot Health*. 2004; 124(2):74–80.

53. Wood LG, Garg ML, Blake RJ, Garcia-Caraballo S, Gibson PG. Airway and circulating levels of carotenoids in asthma and healthy controls. *J Am Coll Nutr.* 2005;24(6):448–55.

54. Miller ER, Appel LJ, Risby TH. Effect of dietary patterns on measures of lipid peroxidation: results from a randomized clinical trial. *Circulation.* 1998;98(22):2390–5.

55. Wood LG, Garg ML, Smart JM, Scott HA, Barker D, Gibson PG. Manipulating antioxidant intake in asthma: a randomized controlled trial. *Am J Clin Nutr.* 2012;96(3):534–43.

56. Wood LG, Garg ML, Smart JM, Scott HA, Barker D, Gibson PG. Manipulating antioxidant intake in asthma: a randomized controlled trial. *Am J Clin Nutr.* 2012;96(3):534–43.

57. Patel S, Murray CS, Woodcock A, Simpson A, Custovic A. Dietary antioxidant intake, allergic sensitization and allergic diseases in young children. *Allergy.* 2009;64(12):1766–72.

58. Troisi RJ, Willett WC, Weiss ST, Trichopoulos D, Rosner B, Speizer FE. A prospective study of diet and adult-onset asthma. *Am J Respir Crit Care Med.* 1995;151(5):1401–8.

59. Wood LG, Garg ML, Smart JM, Scott HA, Barker D, Gibson PG. Manipulating antioxidant intake in asthma: a randomized controlled trial. *Am J Clin Nutr.* 2012;96(3):534–43.

60. Lindahl O, Lindwall L, Spångberg A, Stenram A, Ockerman PA. Vegan regimen with reduced medication in the treatment of bronchial asthma. *J Asthma.* 1985;22(1):45–55.

61. Lindahl O, Lindwall L, Spångberg A, Stenram A, Ockerman PA. Vegan regimen with reduced medication in the treatment of bronchial asthma. *J Asthma.* 1985;22(1):45–55.

62. Lindahl O, Lindwall L, Spångberg A, Stenram A, Ockerman PA. Vegan regimen with reduced medication in the treatment of bronchial asthma. *J Asthma.* 1985;22(1):45–55.

3. How Not to Die from Brain Diseases

1. Mozaffarian D, Benjamin EJ, Go AS, et al. Heart disease and stroke statistics—2015 update: a report from the American Heart Association. *Circulation.* 2015;131(4):e29–322.

2. Centers for Disease Control and Prevention. Deaths: final data for 2013 table 10. Number of deaths from 113 selected causes. National Vital Statistics Report 2016;64(2).

3. Mozaffarian D, Benjamin EJ, Go AS, et al. Heart disease and stroke statistics—2015 update: a report from the American Heart Association. *Circulation.* 2015;131(4):e29–322.

4. Grau-Olivares M, Arboix A. Mild cognitive impairment in stroke patients with ischemic cerebral small-vessel disease: a forerunner of vascular dementia? *Expert Rev Neurother.* 2009; 9(8):1201–17.

5. Aune D, Chan DS, Lau R, et al. Dietary fibre, whole grains, and risk of colorectal cancer: systematic review and dose-response meta-analysis of prospective studies. *BMJ.* 2011;343:d6617.

6. Aune D, Chan DS, Greenwood DC, et al. Dietary fiber and breast cancer risk: a systematic review and meta-analysis of prospective studies. *Ann Oncol.* 2012;23(6):1394–402.

7. Yao B, Fang H, Xu W, et al. Dietary fiber intake and risk of type 2 diabetes: a dose-response analysis of prospective studies. *Eur J Epidemiol.* 2014;29(2):79–88.

8. Threapleton DE, Greenwood DC, Evans CE, et al. Dietary fibre intake and risk of cardiovascular disease: systematic review and meta-analysis. *BMJ.* 2013;347:f6879.

9. Maskarinec G, Takata Y, Pagano I, et al. Trends and dietary determinants of overweight and obesity in a multiethnic population. *Obesity* (Silver Spring). 2006;14(4):717–26.

10. Kim Y, Je Y. Dietary fiber intake and total mortality: a meta-analysis of prospective cohort studies. *Am J Epidemiol.* 2014;180(6):565–73.

11. Threapleton DE, Greenwood DC, Evans CE, et al. Dietary fiber intake and risk of first stroke: a systematic review and meta-analysis. *Stroke.* 2013;44(5):1360–8.

12. Clemens R, Kranz S, Mobley AR, et al. Filling America's fiber intake gap: summary of a

roundtable to probe realistic solutions with a focus on grain-based foods. *J Nutr.* 2012;142(7):1390S –401S.

13. Threapleton DE, Greenwood DC, Evans CE, et al. Dietary fiber intake and risk of first stroke: a systematic review and meta-analysis. *Stroke.* 2013;44(5):1360–8.

14. Whitehead A, Beck EJ, Tosh S, Wolever TM. Cholesterol-lowering effects of oat β-glucan: a meta-analysis of randomized controlled trials. *Am J Clin Nutr.* 2014;100(6):1413–21.

15. Silva FM, Kramer CK, De Almeida JC, Steemburgo T, Gross JL, Azevedo MJ. Fiber intake and glycemic control in patients with type 2 diabetes mellitus: a systematic review with meta-analysis of randomized controlled trials. *Nutr Rev.* 2013;71(12):790–801.

16. Streppel MT, Arends LR, van 't Veer P, Grobbee DE, Geleijnse JM. Dietary fiber and blood pressure: a meta-analysis of randomized placebo-controlled trials. *Arch Intern Med.* 2005; 165(2):150–6.

17. Centers for Disease Control and Prevention. Deaths: final data for 2013 table 10. Number of deaths from 113 selected causes. National Vital Statistics Report 2016;64(2).

18. van de Laar RJ, Stehouwer CDA, van Bussel BCT, et al. Lower lifetime dietary fiber intake is associated with carotid artery stiffness: the Amsterdam Growth and Health Longitudinal Study. *Am J Clin Nutr.* 2012;96(1):14–23.

19. van de Laar RJ, Stehouwer CDA, van Bussel BCT, et al. Lower lifetime dietary fiber intake is associated with carotid artery stiffness: the Amsterdam Growth and Health Longitudinal Study. *Am J Clin Nutr.* 2012;96(1):14–23.

20. Casiglia E, Tikhonoff V, Caffi S, et al. High dietary fiber intake prevents stroke at a population level. *Clin Nutr.* 2013;32(5):811–8.

21. Tikhonoff V, Palatini P, Casiglia E. Letter by Tikhonoff et al regarding article, "Dietary fiber intake and risk of first stroke: a systematic review and meta-analysis," *Stroke.* 2013;44(9): e109.

22. Threapleton DE, Greenwood DC, Burley VJ. Response to letter regarding article, "Dietary fiber intake and risk of first stroke: a systematic review and meta-analysis," *Stroke.* 2013; 44(9):e110.

23. Eaton SB, Konner M. Paleolithic nutrition. A consideration of its nature and current implications. *N Engl J Med.* 1985;312(5):283–9.

24. Cogswell ME, Zhang Z, Carriquiry AL, et al. Sodium and potassium intakes among US adults: NHANES 2003–2008. *Am J Clin Nutr.* 2012;96(3):647–57.

25. Cogswell ME, Zhang Z, Carriquiry AL, et al. Sodium and potassium intakes among US adults: NHANES 2003–2008. *Am J Clin Nutr.* 2012;96(3):647–57.

26. D'Elia L, Barba G, Cappuccio FP, et al. Potassium intake, stroke, and cardiovascular disease a meta-analysis of prospective studies. *J Am Coll Cardiol.* 2011;57(10):1210–9.

27. U.S. Department of Agriculture. USDA National Nutrient Database for Standard Reference. http://ndb.nal.usda.gov/ndb/nutrients/index?fg=&nutrient1=306&nutrient2=&nutrient3= &subset=0&sort=c&totCount=0&offset=0&measureby=g. 2011. Accessed April 1, 2015.

28. U.S. Department of Agriculture Dietary Guidelines for Americans 2005. Appendix B-1. Food sources of potassium. http://www.health.gov/dietaryguidelines/dga2005/document/html /appendixb.htm. July 9, 2008. Accessed May 1, 2015.

29. Hu D, Huang J, Wang Y, Zhang D, Qu Y. Fruits and vegetables consumption and risk of stroke: a meta-analysis of prospective cohort studies. *Stroke.* 2014;45(6):1613–9.

30. Morand C, Dubray C, Milenkovic D, et al. Hesperidin contributes to the vascular protective effects of orange juice: a randomized crossover study in healthy volunteers. *Am J Clin Nutr.* 2011;93(1):73–80.

31. Takumi H, Nakamura H, Simizu T, et al. Bioavailability of orally administered water-

dispersible hesperetin and its effect on peripheral vasodilatation in human subjects: implication of endothelial functions of plasma conjugated metabolites. *Food Funct.* 2012;3(4):389–98.

32. Patyar S, Patyar RR. Correlation between sleep duration and risk of stroke. *J Stroke Cerebrovasc Dis.* 2015;24(5):905–11.

33. Ikehara S, Iso H, Date C, et al; JACC Study Group. Association of sleep duration with mortality from cardiovascular disease and other causes for Japanese men and women: the JACC study. *Sleep.* 2009;32(3):295–301.

34. Fang J, Wheaton AG, Ayala C. Sleep duration and history of stroke among adults from the USA. *J Sleep Res.* 2014;23(5):531–7.

35. von Ruesten A, Weikert C, Fietze I, et al. Association of sleep duration with chronic diseases in the European Prospective Investigation into Cancer and Nutrition (EPIC)-Potsdam study. *PLoS ONE.* 2012;7(1):e30972.

36. Pan A, De Silva DA, Yuan JM, et al. Sleep duration and risk of stroke mortality among Chinese adults: Singapore Chinese health study. *Stroke.* 2014;45(6):1620–5.

37. Leng Y, Cappuccio FP, Wainwright NW, et al. Sleep duration and risk of fatal and nonfatal stroke: a prospective study and meta-analysis. *Neurology.* 2015;84(11):1072–9.

38. Sansevero TB. *The Profit Machine.* Madrid: Cultiva Libros. 2009;59.

39. Harman D. The biologic clock: the mitochondria? *J Am Geriatr Soc.* 1972;20(4):145–7.

40. Chance B, Sies H, Boveris A. Hydroperoxide metabolism in mammalian organs. *Physiol Rev.* 1979;59(3):527–605.

41. Emerit I. Reactive oxygen species, chromosome mutation, and cancer: possible role of clastogenic factors in carcinogenesis. *Free Radic Biol Med.* 1994;16(1):99–109.

42. Rautiainen S, Larsson S, Virtamo J, et al. Total antioxidant capacity of diet and risk of stroke: a population-based prospective cohort of women. *Stroke.* 2012;43(2):335–40.

43. Del Rio D, Agnoli C, Pellegrini N, et al. Total antioxidant capacity of the diet is associated with lower risk of ischemic stroke in a large Italian cohort. *J Nutr.* 2011;141(1):118–23.

44. Satia JA, Littman A, Slatore CG, Galanko JA, White E. Long-term use of beta-carotene, retinol, lycopene, and lutein supplements and lung cancer risk: results from the VITamins And Lifestyle (VITAL) study. *Am J Epidemiol.* 2009;169(7):815–28.

45. Hankey GJ. Vitamin supplementation and stroke prevention. *Stroke.* 2012;43(10):2814–8.

46. Carlsen MH, Halvorsen BL, Holte K, et al. The total antioxidant content of more than 3100 foods, beverages, spices, herbs and supplements used worldwide. *Nutr J.* 2010 Jan 22;9:3.

47. Yang M, Chung SJ, Chung CE, et al. Estimation of total antioxidant capacity from diet and supplements in US adults. *Br J Nutr.* 2011;106(2):254–63.

48. Carlsen MH, Halvorsen BL, Holte K, et al. The total antioxidant content of more than 3100 foods, beverages, spices, herbs and supplements used worldwide. *Nutr J.* 2010 Jan 22;9:3.

49. Bastin S, Henken K. Water Content of Fruits and Vegetables. ENRI-129. University of Kentucky College of Agriculture Cooperative Extension Service. http://www2.ca.uky.edu/enri /pubs/enri129.pdf. December 1997. Accessed March 3, 2015.

50. Carlsen MH, Halvorsen BL, Holte K, et al. The total antioxidant content of more than 3100 foods, beverages, spices, herbs and supplements used worldwide. *Nutr J.* 2010 Jan 22;9:3.

51. Carlsen MH, Halvorsen BL, Holte K, et al. The total antioxidant content of more than 3100 foods, beverages, spices, herbs and supplements used worldwide. *Nutr J.* 2010 Jan 22;9:3.

52. Kelly PJ, Morrow JD, Ning M, et al. Oxidative stress and matrix metalloproteinase-9 in acute ischemic stroke: the Biomarker Evaluation for Antioxidant Therapies in Stroke (BEAT-Stroke) study. *Stroke.* 2008;39(1):100–4.

53. Lilamand M, Kelaiditi E, Guyonnet S, et al. Flavonoids and arterial stiffness: promising perspectives. *Nutr Metab Cardiovasc Dis.* 2014;24(7):698–704.

54. Santhakumar AB, Bulmer AC, Singh I. A review of the mechanisms and effectiveness of dietary polyphenols in reducing oxidative stress and thrombotic risk. *J Hum Nutr Diet.* 2014;27(1):1–21.

55. Stoclet JC, Chataigneau T, Ndiaye M, et al. Vascular protection by dietary polyphenols. *Eur J Pharmacol.* 2004;500(1–3):299–313.

56. Moylan S, Berk M, Dean OM, et al. Oxidative & nitrosative stress in depression: why so much stress?. *Neurosci Biobehav Rev.* 2014;45:46–62.

57. Watzl B. Anti-inflammatory effects of plant-based foods and of their constituents. *Int J Vitam Nutr Res.* 2008;78(6):293–8.

58. Franzini L, Ardigò D, Valtueña S, et al. Food selection based on high total antioxidant capacity improves endothelial function in a low cardiovascular risk population. *Nutr Metab Cardiovasc Dis.* 2012;22(1):50–7.

59. Alzheimer's Association factsheet. http://www.alz.org/documents_custom/2013_facts _figures_fact_sheet.pdf. March 2013. Accessed April 3, 2015.

60. de la Torre JC. A turning point for Alzheimer's disease? *Biofactors.* 2012;38(2):78–83.

61. de la Torre JC. Alzheimer's disease is incurable but preventable. *J Alzheimers Dis.* 2010; 20(3):861–70.

62. Barnes DE, Yaffe K. The projected effect of risk factor reduction on Alzheimer's disease prevalence. *Lancet Neurol.* 2011;10(9):819–28.

63. Singh-Manoux A, Kivimaki M, Glymour MM, et al. Timing of onset of cognitive decline: results from Whitehall II prospective cohort study. *BMJ.* 2012;344:d7622.

64. Roher AE, Tyas SL, Maarouf CL, et al. Intracranial atherosclerosis as a contributing factor to Alzheimer's disease dementia. *Alzheimers Dement.* 2011;7(4):436–44.

65. Barnard ND, Bush AI, Ceccarelli A, et al. Dietary and lifestyle guidelines for the prevention of Alzheimer's disease. *Neurobiol Aging.* 2014;35 Suppl 2:S74–8.

66. Ramirez-Bermudez J. Alzheimer's disease: critical notes on the history of a medical concept. *Arch Med Res.* 2012;43(8):595–9.

67. Alzheimer A, Stelzmann RA, Schnitzlein HN, Murtagh FR. An English translation of Alzheimer's 1907 paper, "Uber eine eigenartige Erkankung der Hirnrinde." *Clin Anat.* 1995;8(6):429–31.

68. Kovacic JC, Fuster V. Atherosclerotic risk factors, vascular cognitive impairment, and Alzheimer disease. *Mt Sinai J Med.* 2012;79:664–73.

69. Cardiogenic Dementia. *Lancet.* 1977;1(8001):27–8.

70. Roher AE, Tyas SL, Maarouf CL, et al. Intracranial atherosclerosis as a contributing factor to Alzheimer's disease dementia. *Alzheimers Dement.* 2011;7(4):436–44.

71. Roher AE, Tyas SL, Maarouf CL, et al. Intracranial atherosclerosis as a contributing factor to Alzheimer's disease dementia. *Alzheimers Dement.* 2011;7(4):436–44.

72. Yarchoan M, Xie SX, Kling MA, et al. Cerebrovascular atherosclerosis correlates with Alzheimer pathology in neurodegenerative dementias. *Brain.* 2012;135(Pt 12):3749–56.

73. Honig LS, Kukull W, Mayeux R. Atherosclerosis and AD: analysis of data from the US National Alzheimer's Coordinating Center. *Neurology.* 2005;64(3):494–500.

74. de la Torre JC. Vascular risk factors: a ticking time bomb to Alzheimer's disease. *Am J Alzheimers Dis Other Demen.* 2013;28(6):551–9.

75. Roher AE, Tyas SL, Maarouf CL, et al. Intracranial atherosclerosis as a contributing factor to Alzheimer's disease dementia. *Alzheimers Dement.* 2011;7(4):436–44.

76. de la Torre JC. Vascular basis of Alzheimer's pathogenesis. *Ann N Y Acad Sci.* 2002;977:196–215.

77. Zhu J, Wang Y, Li J, et al. Intracranial artery stenosis and progression from mild cognitive impairment to Alzheimer disease. *Neurology.* 2014;82(10):842–9.

78. Deschaintre Y, Richard F, Leys D, Pasquier F. Treatment of vascular risk factors is associated with slower decline in Alzheimer disease. *Neurology.* 2009;73(9):674–80.

79. Mizuno T, Nakata M, Naiki H, et al. Cholesterol-dependent generation of a seeding amyloid beta-protein in cell culture. *J Biol Chem.* 1999;274(21):15110–4.

80. Trumbo PR, Shimakawa T. Tolerable upper intake levels for trans fat, saturated fat, and cholesterol. *Nutr Rev.* 2011;69(5):270–8.

81. Benjamin MM, Roberts WC. Facts and principles learned at the 39th Annual Williamsburg Conference on Heart Disease. *Proc* (Bayl Univ Med Cent). 2013;26(2):124–36.

82. Corsinovi L, Biasi F, Poli G, et al. Dietary lipids and their oxidized products in Alzheimer's disease. *Mol Nutr Food Res.* 2011;55 Suppl 2:S161–72.

83. Harris JR, Milton NGN. Cholesterol in Alzheimer's disease and other amyloidogenic disorders. *Subcell Biochem.* 2010;51:47–75.

84. Puglielli L, Tanzi RE, Kovacs DM. Alzheimer's disease: the cholesterol connection. *Nat Neurosci.* 2003;6(4):345–51.

85. Harris JR, Milton NGN. Cholesterol in Alzheimer's disease and other amyloidogenic disorders. *Subcell Biochem.* 2010;51:47–75.

86. Reed B, Villeneuve S, Mack W, et al. Associations between serum cholesterol levels and cerebral amyloidosis. *JAMA Neurol.* 2014;71(2):195–200.

87. US Food and Drug Administration. Important safety label changes to cholesterol-lowering statin drugs. Silver Spring, MD: US Department of Health and Human Services; 2012. http://www.fda.gov/Drugs/DrugSafety/ucm293101.htm. July 7, 2012. Accessed April 2, 2015.

88. Rojas-Fernandez CH, Cameron JC. Is statin-associated cognitive impairment clinically relevant? A narrative review and clinical recommendations. *Ann Pharmacother.* 2012;46(4):549–57.

89. Grant WB. Dietary links to Alzheimer's disease. *Alzheimer Dis Rev.* 1997;2:42–55.

90. Chandra V, Pandav R, Dodge HH, et al. Incidence of Alzheimer's disease in a rural community in India: the Indo-US study. *Neurology.* 2001;57(6):985–9.

91. White L, Petrovitch H, Ross GW, et al. Prevalence of dementia in older Japanese-American men in Hawaii: The Honolulu-Asia aging study. *JAMA.* 1996;276(12):955–60.

92. Grant WB. Dietary links to Alzheimer's disease. *Alzheimer Dis Rev.* 1997;2:42–55.

93. Grant WB. Trends in diet and Alzheimer's disease during the nutrition transition in Japan and developing countries. *J Alzheimers Dis.* 2014;38(3):611–20.

94. Chan KY, Wang W, Wu JJ, et al. Epidemiology of Alzheimer's disease and other forms of dementia in China, 1990–2010: A systematic review and analysis. *Lancet.* 2013;381(9882):2016–23.

95. Grant WB. Trends in diet and Alzheimer's disease during the nutrition transition in Japan and developing countries. *J Alzheimers Dis.* 2014;38(3):611–20.

96. Chandra V, Ganguli M, Pandav R, et al. Prevalence of Alzheimer's disease and other dementias in rural India: the Indo-US study. *Neurology.* 1998;51(4):1000–8.

97. Shetty PS. Nutrition transition in India. *Public Health Nutr.* 2002;5(1A):175–82.

98. Giem P, Beeson WL, Fraser GE. The incidence of dementia and intake of animal products: preliminary findings from the Adventist Health Study. *Neuroepidemiology.* 1993;12(1):28–36.

99. Roses AD, Saunders AM. APOE is a major susceptibility gene for Alzheimer's disease. *Curr Opin Biotechnol.* 1994;5(6):663–7.

100. Puglielli L, Tanzi RE, Kovacs DM. Alzheimer's disease: the cholesterol connection. *Nat Neurosci.* 2003;6(4):345–51.

101. Chen X, Hui L, Soliman ML, Geiger JD. Altered cholesterol intracellular trafficking and the development of pathological hallmarks of sporadic AD. *J Parkinsons Dis Alzheimers Dis.* 2014;1(1).

102. Sepehrnia B, Kamboh MI, Adams-Campbell LL, et al. Genetic studies of human apolipoproteins.X.

The effect of the apolipoprotein E polymorphism on quantitative levels of lipoproteins in Nigerian blacks. *Am J Hum Genet*. 1989;45(4):586–91.

103. Grant WB. Dietary links to Alzheimer's disease. *Alzheimer Dis Rev*. 1997;2:42–55.

104. Sepehrnia B, Kamboh MI, Adams-Campbell LL, et al. Genetic studies of human apolipoproteins. X. The effect of the apolipoprotein E polymorphism on quantitative levels of lipoproteins in Nigerian blacks. *Am J Hum Genet*. 1989;45(4):586–91.

105. Hendrie HC, Murrell J, Gao S, Unverzagt FW, Ogunniyi A, Hall KS. International studies in dementia with particular emphasis on populations of African origin. *Alzheimer Dis Assoc Disord*. 2006;20(3 Suppl 2):S42–6.

106. Kivipelto M, Helkala EL, Laakso MP, et al. Apolipoprotein E epsilon4 allele, elevated midlife total cholesterol level, and high midlife systolic blood pressure are independent risk factors for late-life Alzheimer disease. *Ann Intern Med*. 2002;137(3):149–55.

107. Kivipelto M, Helkala EL, Laakso MP, et al. Apolipoprotein E epsilon4 allele, elevated midlife total cholesterol level, and high midlife systolic blood pressure are independent risk factors for late-life Alzheimer disease. *Ann Intern Med*. 2002;137(3):149–55.

108. Jost BC, Grossberg GT. The natural history of Alzheimer's disease: a brain bank study. *J Am Geriatr Soc*. 1995;43(11):1248–55.

109. Del Tredici K, Braak H. Neurofibrillary changes of the Alzheimer type in very elderly individuals: neither inevitable nor benign: Commentary on 'No disease in the brain of a 115-year-old woman.' *Neurobiol Aging*. 2008;29(8):1133–6.

110. Barnard ND, Bush AI, Ceccarelli A, et al. Dietary and lifestyle guidelines for the prevention of Alzheimer's disease. *Neurobiol Aging*. 2014;35 Suppl 2:S74–8.

111. Lourida I, Soni M, Thompson-Coon J, et al. Mediterranean diet, cognitive function, and dementia: a systematic review. *Epidemiology*. 2013;24(4):479–89.

112. Roberts RO, Geda YE, Cerhan JR, et al. Vegetables, unsaturated fats, moderate alcohol intake, and mild cognitive impairment. *Dementia and Geriatric Cognitive Disorders*. 2010;29(5):413–23.

113. Okereke OI, Rosner BA, Kim DH, et al. Dietary fat types and 4-year cognitive change in community-dwelling older women. *Ann Neurol*. 2012;72(1):124–34.

114. Parletta N, Milte CM, Meyer BJ. Nutritional modulation of cognitive function and mental health. *J Nutr Biochem*. 2013;24(5):725–43.

115. Essa MM, Vijayan RK, Castellano-Gonzalez G, Memon MA, Braidy N, Guillemin GJ. Neuroprotective effect of natural products against Alzheimer's disease. *Neurochem Res*. 2012; 37(9):1829–42.

116. Shukitt-Hale B. Blueberries and neuronal aging. *Gerontology*. 2012;58(6):518–23.

117. Cherniack EP. A berry thought-provoking idea: the potential role of plant polyphenols in the treatment of age-related cognitive disorders. *Br J Nutr*. 2012;108(5):794–800.

118. Johnson EJ. A possible role for lutein and zeaxanthin in cognitive function in the elderly. *Am J Clin Nutr*. 2012;96(5):1161S–5S.

119. Krikorian R, Shidler MD, Nash TA, et al. Blueberry supplementation improves memory in older adults. *J Agric Food Chem*. 2010;58(7):3996–4000.

120. Devore EE, Kang JH, Breteler MMB, et al. Dietary intakes of berries and flavonoids in relation to cognitive decline. *Ann Neurol*. 2012;72(1):135–43.

121. Dai Q, Borenstein AR, Wu Y, et al. Fruit and vegetable juices and Alzheimer's disease: the Kame Project. *Am J Med*. 2006;119(9):751–9.

122. Krikorian R, Nash TA, Shidler MD, Shukitt-Hale B, Joseph JA. Concord grape juice supplementation improves memory function in older adults with mild cognitive impairment. *Br J Nutr*. 2010;103(5):730–4.

123. Nurk E, Refsum H, Drevon CA, et al. Cognitive performance among the elderly in relation to the intake of plant foods. The Hordaland Health Study. *Br J Nutr.* 2010;104(8):1190–201.

124. Mullen W, Marks SC, Crozier A. Evaluation of phenolic compounds in commercial fruit juices and fruit drinks. *J Agric Food Chem.* 2007;55(8):3148–57.

125. Tarozzi A, Morroni F, Merlicco A, et al. Neuroprotective effects of cyanidin 3-O-glucopyranoside on amyloid beta (25–35) oligomer-induced toxicity. *Neurosci Lett.* 2010;473(2):72–6.

126. Hattori M, Sugino E, Minoura K, et al. Different inhibitory response of cyanidin and methylene blue for filament formation of tau microtubule-binding domain. *Biochem Biophys Res Commun.* 2008;374(1):158–63.

127. Mandel SA, Weinreb O, Amit T, Youdim MB. Molecular mechanisms of the neuroprotective/neurorescue action of multi-target green tea polyphenols. *Front Biosci* (Schol Ed). 2012; 4:581–98.

128. Ward RJ, Zucca FA, Duyn JH, Crichton RR, Zecca L. The role of iron in brain ageing and neurodegenerative disorders. *Lancet Neurol.* 2014;13(10):1045–60.

129. Hishikawa N, Takahashi Y, Amakusa Y, et al. Effects of turmeric on Alzheimer's disease with behavioral and psychological symptoms of dementia. *Ayu.* 2012;33(4):499–504.

130. Akhondzadeh S, Sabet MS, Harirchian MH, et al. Saffron in the treatment of patients with mild to moderate Alzheimer's disease: a 16-week, randomized and placebo-controlled trial. *J Clin Pharm Ther.* 2010;35(5):581–8.

131. Akhondzadeh S, Shafiee Sabet M, Harirchian MH, et al. A 22-week, multicenter, randomized, double-blind controlled trial of Crocus sativus in the treatment of mild-to-moderate Alzheimer's disease. *Psychopharmacology* (Berl). 2010;207(4):637–43.

132. Hyde C, Peters J, Bond M, et al. Evolution of the evidence on the effectiveness and cost-effectiveness of acetylcholinesterase inhibitors and memantine for Alzheimer's disease: systematic review and economic model. *Age Ageing.* 2013;42(1):14–20.

133. US Food and Drug Administation. ARICEPT® (Donepezil Hydrochloride Tablets) package insert. http://www.fda.gov/downloads/Drugs/GuidanceComplianceRegulatoryInformation/Surveillance/DrugMarketingAdvertisingandCommunications/UCM368444.pdf. Accessed April 2, 2015.

134. Toledo C, Saltsman K. Genetics by the Numbers. Inside Life Science, Bethesda, MD: National Institute of General Medical Sciences. http://publications.nigms.nih.gov/insidelifescience/genetics-numbers.html. June 11, 2012. Accessed March 3, 2015.

135. Mostoslavsky R, Esteller M, Vaquero A. At the crossroad of lifespan, calorie restriction, chromatin and disease: meeting on sirtuins. *Cell Cycle.* 2010;9(10):1907–12.

136. Julien C, Tremblay C, Emond V, et al. Sirtuin 1 reduction parallels the accumulation of tau in Alzheimer disease. *J Neuropathol Exp Neurol.* 2009;68(1):48–58.

137. Cai W, Uribarri J, Zhu L, et al. Oral glycotoxins are a modifiable cause of dementia and the metabolic syndrome in mice and humans. *Proc Natl Acad Sci USA.* 2014;111(13):4940–5.

138. Cai W, Uribarri J, Zhu L, et al. Oral glycotoxins are a modifiable cause of dementia and the metabolic syndrome in mice and humans. *Proc Natl Acad Sci USA.* 2014;111(13):4940–5.

139. Rahmadi A, Steiner N, Münch G. Advanced glycation endproducts as gerontotoxins and biomarkers for carbonyl-based degenerative processes in Alzheimer's disease. *Clin Chem Lab Med.* 2011;49(3):385–91.

140. Semba RD, Nicklett EJ, Ferrucci L. Does accumulation of advanced glycation end products contribute to the aging phenotype? *J Gerontol A Biol Sci Med Sci.* 2010;65(9):963–75.

141. Srikanth V, Westcott B, Forbes J, et al. Methylglyoxal, cognitive function and cerebral atrophy in older people. *J Gerontol A Biol Sci Med Sci.* 2013;68(1):68–73.

142. Cai W, Uribarri J, Zhu L, et al. Oral glycotoxins are a modifiable cause of dementia and the metabolic syndrome in mice and humans. *Proc Natl Acad Sci USA*. 2014;111(13):4940–5.

143. Beeri MS, Moshier E, Schmeidler J, et al. Serum concentration of an inflammatory glycotoxin, methylglyoxal, is associated with increased cognitive decline in elderly individuals. *Mech Ageing Dev*. 2011;132(11–12):583–7.

144. Yaffe K, Lindquist K, Schwartz AV, et al. Advanced glycation end product level, diabetes, and accelerated cognitive aging. *Neurology*. 2011;77(14):1351–6.

145. Angeloni C, Zambonin L, Hrelia S. Role of methylglyoxal in Alzheimer's disease. *Biomed Res Int*. 2014;2014:238485.

146. Vlassara H, Cai W, Goodman S, et al. Protection against loss of innate defenses in adulthood by low advanced glycation end products (AGE) intake: role of the antiinflammatory AGE receptor-1. *J Clin Endocrinol Metab*. 2009;94(11):4483–91.

147. Cerami C, Founds H, Nicholl I, et al. Tobacco smoke is a source of toxic reactive glycation products. *Proc Natl Acad Sci USA*. 1997;94(25):13915–20.

148. Uribarri J, Cai W, Sandu O, Peppa M, Goldberg T, Vlassara H. Diet-derived advanced glycation end products are major contributors to the body's AGE pool and induce inflammation in healthy subjects. *Ann N Y Acad Sci*. 2005;1043:461–6.

149. Uribarri J, Cai W, Sandu O, Peppa M, Goldberg T, Vlassara H. Diet-derived advanced glycation end products are major contributors to the body's AGE pool and induce inflammation in healthy subjects. *Ann N Y Acad Sci*. 2005;1043:461–6.

150. Uribarri J, Woodruff S, Goodman S, et al. Advanced glycation end products in foods and a practical guide to their reduction in the diet. *J Am Diet Assoc*. 2010;110(6):911–6.e12.

151. Uribarri J, Woodruff S, Goodman S, et al. Advanced glycation end products in foods and a practical guide to their reduction in the diet. *J Am Diet Assoc*. 2010;110(6):911–6.e12.

152. Uribarri J, Woodruff S, Goodman S, et al. Advanced glycation end products in foods and a practical guide to their reduction in the diet. *J Am Diet Assoc*. 2010;110(6):911–6.e12.

153. Cai W, Uribarri J, Zhu L, et al. Oral glycotoxins are a modifiable cause of dementia and the metabolic syndrome in mice and humans. *Proc Natl Acad Sci USA*. 2014;111(13):4940–5.

154. Baker LD, Frank LL, Foster-Schubert K, et al. Effects of aerobic exercise on mild cognitive impairment: a controlled trial. *Arch Neurol*. 2010;67(1):71–9.

155. Baker LD, Frank LL, Foster-Schubert K, et al. Effects of aerobic exercise on mild cognitive impairment: a controlled trial. *Arch Neurol*. 2010;67(1):71–9.

156. Erickson KI, Voss MW, Prakash RS, et al. Exercise training increases size of hippocampus and improves memory. *Proc Natl Acad Sci USA*. 2011;108(7):3017–22.

157. ten Brinke LF, Bolandzadeh N, Nagamatsu LS, et al. Aerobic exercise increases hippocampal volume in older women with probable mild cognitive impairment: a 6-month randomised controlled trial. *Br J Sports Med*. 2015;49(4):248–54.

4. How Not to Die from Digestive Cancers

1. Liu PH, Wang JD, Keating NL. Expected years of life lost for six potentially preventable cancers in the United States. *Prev Med*. 2013;56(5):309–13.

2. Bertram JS, Kolonel LN, Meyskens FL. Rationale and strategies for chemoprevention of cancer in humans. *Cancer Res*. 1987;47(11):3012–31.

3. Hasleton PS. The internal surface area of the adult human lung. *J Anat*. 1972;112(Pt 3):391–400.

4. Macdonald TT, Monteleone G. Immunity, inflammation, and allergy in the gut. *Science*. 2005;307(5717):1920–5.

5. What are the key statistics about colorectal cancer? American Cancer Society website. http://www.cancer.org/cancer/colonandrectumcancer/detailedguide/colorectal-cancer-key-statistics. Accessed March 3, 2015.

6. What are the key statistics about pancreatic cancer? American Cancer Society website. http://www.cancer.org/cancer/pancreaticcancer/detailedguide/pancreatic-cancer-key-statistics. Accessed March 3, 2015.

7. American Cancer Society. Cancer Facts & Figures 2014. Atlanta: American Cancer Society; 2014.

8. What are the key statistics about colorectal cancer? American Cancer Society website. http://www.cancer.org/cancer/colonandrectumcancer/detailedguide/colorectal-cancer-key-statistics. Accessed March 3, 2015.

9. American Cancer Society. Cancer Facts & Figures 2014. Atlanta: American Cancer Society; 2014.

10. Screening for Colorectal Cancer. US Preventive Services Task Force website. http://www.uspreventiveservicestaskforce.org/Home/GetFile/1/467/colcancsumm/pdf. Accessed March 3, 2015.

11. International Monetary Fund. World Economic Outlook Database. http://bit.ly/1bNdlWu. April 2015. Accessed May 2, 2015.

12. World Bank. World Development Indicators. http://data.worldbank.org/country/india. 2011. Accessed May 2, 2015.

13. Bengmark S, Mesa MD, Gill A. Plant-derived health: the effects of turmeric and curcuminoids. *Nutr Hosp*. 2009;24(3):273–81.

14. Hutchins-Wolfbrandt A, Mistry AM. Dietary turmeric potentially reduces the risk of cancer. *Asian Pac J Cancer Prev*. 2011;12(12):3169–73.

15. Sharma RA, Euden SA, Platton SL, et al. Phase I clinical trial of oral curcumin: biomarkers of systemic activity and compliance. *Clin Cancer Res*. 2004;10(20):6847–54.

16. Carroll RE, Benya RV, Turgeon DK, et al. Phase IIa clinical trial of curcumin for the prevention of colorectal neoplasia. *Cancer Prev Res* (Phila). 2011;4(3):354–64.

17. Cruz-Correa M, Shoskes DA, Sanchez P, et al. Combination treatment with curcumin and quercetin of adenomas in familial adenomatous polyposis. *Clin Gastroenterol Hepatol*. 2006;4(8):1035–8.

18. Sharma RA, McLelland HR, Hill KA, et al. Pharmacodynamic and pharmacokinetic study of oral Curcuma extract in patients with colorectal cancer. *Clin Cancer Res*. 2001;7(7):1894–900.

19. Singh S. From exotic spice to modern drug? *Cell*. 2007;130(5):765–8.

20. International Institute for Population Sciences & Macro International: National Family Health Survey (NFHS-3), 2005–06: India: Vol. I. Mumbai: IIPS; 2007.

21. Cummings JH, Bingham SA, Heaton KW, Eastwood MA. Fecal weight, colon cancer risk, and dietary intake of nonstarch polysaccharides (dietary fiber). *Gastroenterology*. 1992;103(6):1783–9.

22. Gear JS, Brodribb AJ, Ware A, Mann JI. Fibre and bowel transit times. *Br J Nutr*. 1981;45(1):77–82.

23. Burkitt DP, Walker AR, Painter NS. Effect of dietary fibre on stools and the transit-times, and its role in the causation of disease. *Lancet*. 1972;2(7792):1408–12.

24. Sonnenberg A, Koch TR. Physician visits in the United States for constipation: 1958 to 1986. *Dig Dis Sci*. 1989;34(4):606–11.

25. Burkitt DP. A deficiency of dietary fiber may be one cause of certain colonic and venous disorders. *Am J Dig Dis*. 1976;21(2):104–8.

26. Fox A, Tietze PH, Ramakrishnan K. Anorectal conditions: anal fissure and anorectal fistula. *FP Essent*. 2014;419:20–7.

27. Burkitt DP. A deficiency of dietary fiber may be one cause of certain colonic and venous disorders. *Am J Dig Dis.* 1976;21(2):104–8.

28. Sanjoaquin MA, Appleby PN, Spencer EA, Key TJ. Nutrition and lifestyle in relation to bowel movement frequency: a cross-sectional study of 20630 men and women in EPIC-Oxford. *Public Health Nutr.* 2004;7(1):77–83.

29. What are the key statistics about colorectal cancer? American Cancer Society website. http://www.cancer.org/cancer/colonandrectumcancer/detailedguide/colorectal-cancer-key-statistics. Accessed March 3, 2015.

30. Doll R. The geographical distribution of cancer. *Br J Cancer.* 1969;23(1):1–8.

31. Lipski E. Traditional non-Western diets. *Nutr Clin Pract.* 2010;25(6):585–93.

32. Burkitt DP. Epidemiology of cancer of the colon and rectum.1971. *Dis. Colon Rectum.* 1993; 36(11):1071–82.

33. Shaper AG, Jones KW. Serum-cholesterol, diet, and coronary heart-disease in Africans and Asians in Uganda: 1959. *Int J Epidemiol.* 2012;41(5):1221–5.

34. Malila N, Hakulinen T. Epidemiological trends of colorectal cancer in the Nordic countries. *Scand J Surg.* 2003;92(1):5–9.

35. Englyst HN, Bingham SA, Wiggins HS, et al. Nonstarch polysaccharide consumption in four Scandinavian populations. *Nutr Cancer.* 1982;4(1):50–60.

36. Graf E, Eaton JW. Dietary suppression of colonic cancer. Fiber or phytate? *Cancer.* 1985;56(4): 717–8.

37. Fonseca-Nunes A, Jakszyn P, Agudo A. Iron and cancer risk—a systematic review and meta-analysis of the epidemiological evidence. *Cancer Epidemiol Biomarkers Prev.* 2014;23(1):12–31.

38. Mellanby E. The rickets-producing and anti-calcifying action of phytate. *J Physiol.* 1949; 109(3–4):488–533.

39. House WA, Welch RM, Van Campen DR. Effect of phytic acid on the absorption, distribution, and endogenous excretion of zinc in rats. *J Nutr.* 1982;112(5):941–53.

40. Urbano G, López-Jurado M, Aranda P, Vidal-Valverde C, Tenorio E, Porres J. The role of phytic acid in legumes: antinutrient or beneficial function? *J Physiol Biochem.* 2000;56(3):283–94.

41. López-González AA, Grases F, Roca P, Mari B, Vicente-Herrero MT, Costa-Bauzá A. Phytate (myo-inositol hexaphosphate) and risk factors for osteoporosis. *J Med Food.* 2008;11(4): 747–52.

42. López-González AA, Grases F, Monroy N, et al. Protective effect of myo-inositol hexa-phosphate (phytate) on bone mass loss in postmenopausal women. *Eur J Nutr.* 2013;52(2): 717–26.

43. Arriero Mdel M, Ramis JM, Perelló J, Monjo M. Inositol hexakisphosphate inhibits osteoclas-togenesis on RAW 264.7 cells and human primary osteoclasts. *PLoS ONE.* 2012;7(8):e43187.

44. Khosla S, Burr D, Cauley J, et al. Bisphosphonate-associated osteonecrosis of the jaw: report of a task force of the American Society for Bone and Mineral Research. *J Bone Miner Res.* 2007; 22(10):1479–91.

45. Singh PN, Fraser GE. Dietary risk factors for colon cancer in a low-risk population. *Am J Epidemiol.* 1998;148(8):761–74.

46. Manousos O, Day NE, Trichopoulos D, Gerovassilis F, Tzonou A, Polychronopoulou A. Diet and colorectal cancer: A case-control study in Greece. *Int J Cancer.* 1983;32(1):1–5.

47. Lanza E, Hartman TJ, Albert PS, et al. High dry bean intake and reduced risk of advanced colorectal adenoma recurrence among participants in the polyp prevention trial. *J Nutr.* 2006; 136(7):1896–1903.

48. Vucenik I, Shamsuddin AM. Protection against cancer by dietary IP6 and inositol. *Nutr Cancer.* 2006;55(2):109–25.

49. Vucenik I, Shamsuddin AM. Cancer inhibition by inositol hexaphosphate (IP6) and inositol: from laboratory to clinic. *J Nutr.* 2003;133(11-Suppl-1):3778S–84S.

50. Ogawa S, Kobayashi H, Amada S, et al. Sentinel node detection with (99m)Tc phytate alone is satisfactory for cervical cancer patients undergoing radical hysterectomy and pelvic lymphadenectomy. *Int J Clin Oncol.* 2010;15(1):52–8.

51. Vucenik I, Shamsuddin AM. Protection against cancer by dietary IP6 and inositol. *Nutr Cancer.* 2006;55(2):109–25.

52. Vucenik I, Passaniti A, Vitolo MI, Tantivejkul K, Eggleton P, Shamsuddin AM. Anti-angiogenic activity of inositol hexaphosphate (IP6). *Carcinogenesis.* 2004;25(11):2115–23.

53. Wang H, Khor TO, Shu L, et al. Plants vs. cancer: a review on natural phytochemicals in preventing and treating cancers and their druggability. *Anticancer Agents Med Chem.* 2012;12(10):1281–305.

54. Yang GY, Shamsuddin AM. IP6-induced growth inhibition and differentiation of HT-29 human colon cancer cells: involvement of intracellular inositol phosphates. *Anticancer Res.* 1995;15(6B):2479–87.

55. Shamsuddin AM, Yang GY, Vucenik I. Novel anti-cancer functions of IP6: growth inhibition and differentiation of human mammary cancer cell lines in vitro. *Anticancer Res.* 1996;16(6A):3287–92.

56. Vucenik I, Tantivejkul K, Zhang ZS, Cole KE, Saied I, Shamsuddin AM. IP6 in treatment of liver cancer. I. IP6 inhibits growth and reverses transformed phenotype in HepG2 human liver cancer cell line. *Anticancer Res.* 1998;18(6A):4083–90.

57. Shamsuddin AM, Yang GY. Inositol hexaphosphate inhibits growth and induces differentiation of PC-3 human prostate cancer cells. *Carcinogenesis.* 1995;16(8):1975–9.

58. Shamsuddin AM. Anti-cancer function of phytic acid. *Int J Food Sci Tech.* 2002;37(7):769–82.

59. Sun J, Chu YF, Wu X, Liu RH. Antioxidant and antiproliferative activities of common fruits. *J Agric Food Chem.* 2002;50(25):7449–54.

60. Olsson ME, Andersson CS, Oredsson S, Berglund RH, Gustavsson KE. Antioxidant levels and inhibition of cancer cell proliferation in vitro by extracts from organically and conventionally cultivated strawberries. *J Agric Food Chem.* 2006;54(4):1248–55.

61. Graham DJ, Campen D, Hui R, et al. Risk of acute myocardial infarction and sudden cardiac death in patients treated with cyclo-oxygenase 2 selective and non-selective non-steroidal anti-inflammatory drugs: nested case-control study. *Lancet.* 2005;365(9458):475–81.

62. Wang LS, Burke CA, Hasson H, et al. A phase Ib study of the effects of black raspberries on rectal polyps in patients with familial adenomatous polyposis. *Cancer Prev Res* (Phila). 2014;7(7):666–74.

63. Wang LS, Burke CA, Hasson H, et al. A phase Ib study of the effects of black raspberries on rectal polyps in patients with familial adenomatous polyposis. *Cancer Prev Res* (Phila). 2014;7(7):666–74.

64. Pan A, Sun Q, Bernstein AM, et al. Red meat consumption and mortality: Results from 2 prospective cohort studies. *Arch Intern Med.* 2012;172(7):555–63.

65. Sinha R, Cross AJ, Graubard BI, Leitzmann MF, Schatzkin A. Meat intake and mortality: a prospective study of over half a million people. *Arch Intern Med.* 2009;169(6):562–71.

66. Popkin BM. Reducing meat consumption has multiple benefits for the world's health. *Arch Intern Med.* 2009;169(6):543.

67. Dixon SJ, Stockwell BR. The role of iron and reactive oxygen species in cell death. *Nat Chem Biol.* 2014;10(1):9–17.

68. Hurrell R, Egli I. Iron bioavailability and dietary reference values. *Am J Clin Nutr.* 2010;91(5):1461S–7S.

69. Cook JD. Adaptation in iron metabolism. *Am J Clin Nutr.* 1990;51(2):301–8.

70. Fonseca-Nunes A, Jakszyn P, Agudo A. Iron and cancer risk—a systematic review and meta-analysis of the epidemiological evidence. *Cancer Epidemiol Biomarkers Prev.* 2014;23(1):12–31.

71. Yang W, Li B, Dong X, et al. Is heme iron intake associated with risk of coronary heart disease? A meta-analysis of prospective studies. *Eur J Nutr.* 2014;53(2):395–400.

72. Bao W, Rong Y, Rong S, Liu L. Dietary iron intake, body iron stores, and the risk of type 2 diabetes: a systematic review and meta-analysis. *BMC Med.* 2012;10:119.

73. Zacharski LR, Chow BK, Howes PS, et al. Decreased cancer risk after iron reduction in patients with peripheral arterial disease: results from a randomized trial. *J Natl Cancer Inst.* 2008;100(14):996–1002.

74. Edgren G, Nyrén O, Melbye M. Cancer as a ferrotoxic disease: are we getting hard stainless evidence? *J Natl Cancer Inst.* 2008;100(14):976–7.

75. Corpet DE. Red meat and colon cancer: should we become vegetarians, or can we make meat safer? *Meat Sci.* 2011;89(3):310–6.

76. Farmer B, Larson BT, Fulgoni VL 3rd, Rainville AJ, Liepa GU. A vegetarian dietary pattern as a nutrient-dense approach to weight management: an analysis of the national health and nutrition examination survey 1999–2004. *J Am Diet Assoc.* 2011;111(6):819–27.

77. Iron deficiency—United States, 1999–2000. MMWR Morb Mortal Wkly Rep. 2002;51(40):897–9.

78. Craig WJ, Mangels AR. Position of the American Dietetic Association: vegetarian diets. *J Am Diet Assoc.* 2009;109(7):1266–82.

79. Tiwari AK, Mahdi AA, Chandyan S, et al. Oral iron supplementation leads to oxidative imbalance in anemic women: a prospective study. *Clin Nutr.* 2011;30(2):188–93.

80. Saunders AV, Craig WJ, Baines SK, Posen JS. Iron and vegetarian diets. *Med J Aust.* 2013;199(4 Suppl):S11–6.

81. American Cancer Society. Cancer Facts & Figures 2014. Atlanta: American Cancer Society; 2014.

82. Iodice S, Gandini S, Maisonneuve P, Lowenfels AB. Tobacco and the risk of pancreatic cancer: a review and meta-analysis. *Langenbecks Arch Surg.* 2008;393(4):535–45.

83. Kolodecik T, Shugrue C, Ashat M, Thrower EC. Risk factors for pancreatic cancer: underlying mechanisms and potential targets. *Front Physiol.* 2013;4:415.

84. Thiébaut AC, Jiao L, Silverman DT, et al. Dietary fatty acids and pancreatic cancer in the NIH-AARP diet and health study. *J Natl Cancer Inst.* 2009;101(14):1001–11.

85. Landrigan PJ. Preface. *Ann N Y Acad Sci.* 1991;643:xv–xvi.

86. Weiner R, Rees D, Lunga FJ, Felix MA. Third wave of asbestos-related disease from secondary use of asbestos. A case report from industry. *S Afr Med J.* 1994;84(3):158–60.

87. Johnson ES, Zhou Y, Lillian Yau C, et al. Mortality from malignant diseases-update of the Baltimore union poultry cohort. *Cancer Causes Control.* 2010;21(2):215–21.

88. Felini M, Johnson E, Preacely N, Sarda V, Ndetan H, Bangara S. A pilot case-cohort study of liver and pancreatic cancers in poultry workers. *Ann Epidemiol.* 2011;21(10):755–66.

89. Lynch SM, Vrieling A, Lubin JH, et al. Cigarette smoking and pancreatic cancer: a pooled analysis from the pancreatic cancer cohort consortium. *Am J Epidemiol.* 2009;170(4):403–13.

90. Rohrmann S, Linseisen J, Nöthlings U, et al. Meat and fish consumption and risk of pancreatic cancer: results from the European Prospective Investigation into Cancer and Nutrition. *Int J Cancer.* 2013;132(3):617–24.

91. Rohrmann S, Linseisen J, Jakobsen MU, et al. Consumption of meat and dairy and lymphoma

risk in the European Prospective Investigation into Cancer and Nutrition. *Int J Cancer.* 2011; 128(3):623–34.

92. Lotti M, Bergamo L, Murer B. Occupational toxicology of asbestos-related malignancies. *Clin Toxicol* (Phila). 2010;48(6):485–96.

93. Marvisi M, Balzarini L, Mancini C, Mouzakiti P. A new type of hypersensitivity pneumonitis: salami brusher's disease. *Monaldi Arch Chest Dis.* 2012;77(1):35–7.

94. Yang ZY, Yuan JQ, Di MY, et al. Gemcitabine plus erlotinib for advanced pancreatic cancer: a systematic review with meta-analysis. *PLoS ONE.* 2013;8(3):e57528.

95. Li L, Aggarwal BB, Shishodia S, Abbruzzese J, Kurzrock R. Nuclear factor-kappaB and Ikap-paB kinase are constitutively active in human pancreatic cells, and their down-regulation by curcumin (diferuloylmethane) is associated with the suppression of proliferation and the induction of apoptosis. *Cancer.* 2004;101(10):2351–62.

96. Dhillon N, Aggarwal BB, Newman RA, et al. Phase II trial of curcumin in patients with advanced pancreatic cancer. *Clin Cancer Res.* 2008;14(14):4491–9.

97. Bosetti C, Bravi F, Turati F, et al. Nutrient-based dietary patterns and pancreatic cancer risk. *Ann Epidemiol.* 2013;23(3):124–8.

98. Mills PK, Beeson WL, Abbey DE, Fraser GE, Phillips RL. Dietary habits and past medical history as related to fatal pancreas cancer risk among Adventists. *Cancer.* 1988;61(12):2578–85.

99. American Cancer Society. Cancer Facts & Figures 2014. Atlanta: American Cancer Society; 2014.

100. Bagnardi V, Rota M, Botteri E, et al. Light alcohol drinking and cancer: a meta-analysis. *Ann Oncol.* 2013;24(2):301–8.

101. Rubenstein JH, Chen JW. Epidemiology of gastroesophageal reflux disease. *Gastroenterol Clin North Am.* 2014;43(1):1–14.

102. Lagergren J, Bergström R, Lindgren A, Nyrén O. Symptomatic gastroesophageal reflux as a risk factor for esophageal adenocarcinoma. *N Engl J Med.* 1999;340(11):825–31.

103. Pohl H, Welch HG. The role of overdiagnosis and reclassification in the marked increase of esophageal adenocarcinoma incidence. *J Natl Cancer Inst.* 2005;97(2):142–6.

104. Parasa S, Sharma P. Complications of gastro-oesophageal reflux disease. *Best Pract Res Clin Gastroenterol.* 2013;27(3):433–42.

105. El-Serag HB. Time trends of gastroesophageal reflux disease: a systematic review. *Clin Gastroenterol Hepatol.* 2007;5(1):17–26.

106. De Ceglie A, Fisher DA, Filiberti R, Blanchi S, Conio M. Barrett's esophagus, esophageal and esophagogastric junction adenocarcinomas: the role of diet. *Clin Res Hepatol Gastroenterol.* 2011;35(1):7–16.

107. Navarro Silvera SA, Mayne ST, Risch H, et al. Food group intake and risk of subtypes of esophageal and gastric cancer. *Int J Cancer.* 2008;123(4):852–60.

108. Nebel OT, Castell DO. Lower esophageal sphincter pressure changes after food ingestion. *Gastroenterology.* 1972;63(5):778–83.

109. Becker DJ, Sinclair J, Castell DO, Wu WC. A comparison of high and low fat meals on postprandial esophageal acid exposure. *Am J Gastroenterol.* 1989;84(7):782–6.

110. Charlton KE, Tapsell LC, Batterham MJ, et al. Pork, beef and chicken have similar effects on acute satiety and hormonal markers of appetite. *Appetite.* 2011;56(1):1–8.

111. Mitsukawa T, Takemura J, Ohgo S, et al. Gallbladder function and plasma cholecystokinin levels in diabetes mellitus. *Am J Gastroenterol.* 1990;85(8):981–5.

112. Matsuki N, Fujita T, Watanabe N, et al. Lifestyle factors associated with gastroesophageal reflux disease in the Japanese population. *J Gastroenterol.* 2013;48(3):340–9.

113. Jung JG, Kang HW, Hahn SJ, et al. Vegetarianism as a protective factor for reflux esophagitis:

a retrospective, cross-sectional study between Buddhist priests and general population. *Dig Dis Sci.* 2013;58(8):2244–52.

114. Fashner J, Gitu AC. Common gastrointestinal symptoms: risks of long-term proton pump inhibitor therapy. *FP Essent.* 2013;413:29–39.

115. Terry P, Lagergren J, Ye W, Nyrén O, Wolk A. Antioxidants and cancers of the esophagus and gastric cardia. *Int J Cancer.* 2000;87(5):750–4.

116. Ekström AM, Serafini M, Nyrén O, Hansson LE, Ye W, Wolk A. Dietary antioxidant intake and the risk of cardia cancer and noncardia cancer of the intestinal and diffuse types: a population-based case-control study in Sweden. *Int J Cancer.* 2000;87(1):133–40.

117. Nilsson M, Johnsen R, Ye W, Hveem K, Lagergren J. Lifestyle related risk factors in the aetiology of gastro-oesophageal reflux. *Gut.* 2004;53(12):1730–5.

118. Coleman HG, Murray LJ, Hicks B, et al. Dietary fiber and the risk of precancerous lesions and cancer of the esophagus: a systematic review and meta-analysis. *Nutr Rev.* 2013;71(7):474–82.

119. Burkitt DP. Hiatus hernia: is it preventable? *Am J Clin Nutr.* 1981;34(3):428–31.

120. Burkitt DP, James PA. Low-residue diets and hiatus hernia. *Lancet.* 1973;2(7821):128–30.

121. Burkitt DP, James PA. Low-residue diets and hiatus hernia. *Lancet.* 1973;2(7821):128–30.

122. Burkitt DP. Two blind spots in medical knowledge. *Nurs Times.* 1976;72(1):24–7.

123. Burkitt DP. Hiatus hernia: is it preventable? *Am J Clin Nutr.* 1981;34(3):428–31.

124. American Cancer Society. Cancer Facts & Figures 2014. Atlanta: American Cancer Society; 2014.

125. Polednak AP. Trends in survival for both histologic types of esophageal cancer in US surveillance, epidemiology and end results areas. *Int J Cancer.* 2003;105(1):98–100.

126. Chen T, Yan F, Qian J, et al. Randomized phase II trial of lyophilized strawberries in patients with dysplastic precancerous lesions of the esophagus. *Cancer Prev Res* (Phila). 2012;5(1):41–50.

127. Chen T, Yan F, Qian J, et al. Randomized phase II trial of lyophilized strawberries in patients with dysplastic precancerous lesions of the esophagus. *Cancer Prev Res* (Phila). 2012;5(1):41–50.

128. Eaton SB, Konner M, Shostak M. Stone agers in the fast lane: chronic degenerative diseases in evolutionary perspective. *Am J Med.* 1988;84(4):739–49.

129. King DE, Mainous AG, Lambourne CA. Trends in dietary fiber intake in the United States, 1999–2008. *J Acad Nutr Diet.* 2012;112(5):642–8.

130. Zhang N, Huang C, Ou S. In vitro binding capacities of three dietary fibers and their mixture for four toxic elements, cholesterol, and bile acid. *J Hazard Mater.* 2011;186(1):236–9.

131. Moshfegh A, Goldman J, Cleveland l. *What We Eat in America, NHANES 2001–2002: Usual Nutrient Intakes from Food Compared to Dietary Reference Intakes.* Washington, D.C.: US Department of Agriculture Agricultural Research Service; 2005.

5. How Not to Die from Infections

1. Civil Practice And Remedies Code. Title 4. Liability in Tort. Chapter 96. False Disparagement of Perishable Food Products. Texas Constitution and Statutes. http://www.statutes.legis.state.tx.us/Docs/CP/htm/CP.96.htm. Accessed March 3, 2015.

2. Civil Practice and Remedies Code. Title 4. Liability in Tort. Chapter 96. False Disparagement of Perishable Food Products. Texas Constitution and Statutes. http://www.statutes.legis.state.tx.us/Docs/CP/htm/CP.96.htm. Accessed March 3, 2015.

3. Oppel Jr RA. Taping of farm cruelty is becoming the crime. *New York Times*. http://www .nytimes.com/2013/04/07/us/taping-of-farm-cruelty-is-becoming-the-crime.html. April 6, 2013. Accessed March 3, 2015.

4. Shrestha SS, Swerdlow DL, Borse RH, et al. Estimating the burden of 2009 pandemic influenza A (H1N1) in the United States (April 2009–April 2010). *Clin Infect Dis*. 2011;52 Suppl 1:S75–82.

5. Woolhouse ME, Gowtage-Sequeria S. Host range and emerging and reemerging pathogens. *Emerging Infect Dis*. 2005;11(12):1842–7.

6. Epstein PR, Chivian E, Frith K. Emerging diseases threaten conservation. *Environ Health Perspect*. 2003;111(10):A506–7.

7. Espinosa de los Monteros LE, Galán JC, Gutiérrez M, et al. Allele-specific PCR method based on pncA and oxyR sequences for distinguishing Mycobacterium bovis from Mycobacterium tuberculosis: intraspecific M. bovis pncA sequence polymorphism. *J Clin Microbiol*. 1998;36(1): 239–42.

8. Esmail H, Barry CE, Young DB, Wilkinson RJ. The ongoing challenge of latent tuberculosis. *Philos Trans R Soc Lond, B, Biol Sci*. 2014;369(1645):20130437.

9. Daszak P, Cunningham AA. Emerging infectious diseases: a key role for conservation medicine. In: Aguirre AA, Ostfeld RS, Tabor GM, et al. *Conservation Medicine: Ecological Health in Practice*. Oxford: Oxford University Press; 2002:40–61.

10. McMichael AJ. *Human Frontiers, Environments and Disease, Past Patterns, Uncertain Futures*. Cambridge: Cambridge University Press; 2001.

11. Torrey EF, Yolken RH. *Beasts of the Earth, Animals, Humans, and Disease*. New Brunswick, NJ: Rutgers University Press; 2005.

12. McMichael AJ. *Human Frontiers, Environments and Disease, Past Patterns, Uncertain Futures*. Cambridge: Cambridge University Press; 2001.

13. Van Heuverswyn F, Peeters M. The origins of HIV and implications for the global epidemic. *Curr Infect Dis Rep*. 2007;9(4):338–46.

14. Whon TW, Kim MS, Roh SW, Shin NR, Lee HW, Bae JW. Metagenomic characterization of airborne viral DNA diversity in the near-surface atmosphere. *J Virol*. 2012;86(15):8221–31.

15. USDA. Microbiological testing of AMS purchased meat, poultry and egg commodities. http:// www.ams.usda.gov/AMSv1.0/ams.fetchTemplateData.do?template=TemplateA&navID= MicrobialTestingofCommodities&rightNav1=MicrobialTestingofCommodities&topNav= &leftNav=&page=FPPMicroDataReports&resultType=&acct=lsstd. Accessed March 3, 2015.

16. Centers for Disease Control and Prevention. Deaths: final data for 2013 table 10. Number of deaths from 113 selected causes. National Vital Statistics Report. 2016;64(2).

17. Barker J, Stevens D, and Bloomfield SF. Spread and prevention of some common viral infections in community facilities and domestic homes. *J Appl Microbiol*. 2001;91(1):7–21.

18. Boone SA, Gerba CP. The occurrence of influenza A virus on household and day care center fomites. *J Infect*. 2005;51(2):103–9.

19. World Health Organization. WHO Guidelines on Hand Hygiene in Health Care. Geneva: World Health Organization; 2009. http://www.ncbi.nlm.nih.gov/books/n/whohand/pdf/. Accessed April 4, 2015.

20. How does the immune system work? PubMed Health. http://www.ncbi.nlm.nih.gov /pubmedhealth/PMH0010386/. Accessed March 3, 2015.

21. U.S. Centers for Disease Control and Prevention. Prevention of pneumococcal disease: recommendations of the Advisory Committee on Immunization Practices (ACIP). MMWR 1997; 46(RR-08):1–24.

22. Gibson A, Edgar J, Neville C, et al. Effect of fruit and vegetable consumption on immune function in older people: a randomized controlled trial. *Am J Clin Nutr*. 2012;96(6):1429–36.

23. USDA. Food availability (per capita) Data System. Fresh kale: per capita availability adjusted for loss. http://www.ers.usda.gov/datafiles/Food_Availabily_Per_Capita_Data_System/Loss Adjusted_Food_Availability/veg.xls. Accessed March 3, 2015.

24. Nishi K, Kondo A, Okamoto T, et al. Immunostimulatory in vitro and in vivo effects of a water-soluble extract from kale. *Biosci Biotechnol Biochem.* 2011;75(1):40–6.

25. Nishi K, Kondo A, Okamoto T, et al. Immunostimulatory in vitro and in vivo effects of a water-soluble extract from kale. *Biosci Biotechnol Biochem.* 2011;75(1):40–6.

26. Macdonald TT, Monteleone G. Immunity, inflammation, and allergy in the gut. *Science.* 2005;307(5717):1920–5.

27. United States Census Bureau. Median and average square feet of floor area in new single-family houses completed by location. https://www.census.gov/const/C25Ann/sftotalmedavgsqft.pdf. Accessed April 3, 2015.

28. Sheridan BS, Lefrançois L. Intraepithelial lymphocytes: To serve and protect. *Curr Gastroenterol Rep.* 2010;12(6):513–21.

29. Hooper LV. You AhR what you eat: linking diet and immunity. *Cell.* 2011;147(3):489–91.

30. Esser C. Biology and function of the aryl hydrocarbon receptor: report of an international and interdisciplinary conference. *Arch Toxicol.* 2012;86(8):1323–9.

31. Veldhoen M. Direct interactions between intestinal immune cells and the diet. *Cell Cycle.* 2012 Feb 1;11(3):426–7.

32. Hooper LV. You AhR what you eat: linking diet and immunity. *Cell.* 2011;147(3):489–91.

33. Savouret JF, Berdeaux A, Casper RF. The aryl hydrocarbon receptor and its xenobiotic ligands: A fundamental trigger for cardiovascular diseases. *Nutr Metab Cardiovasc Dis.* 2003;13(2):104–13.

34. Ashida H, Fukuda I, Yamashita T, Kanazawa K. Flavones and flavonols at dietary levels inhibit a transformation of aryl hydrocarbon receptor induced by dioxin. *FEBS Lett.* 2000;476(3):213–7.

35. Ashida H, Fukuda I, Yamashita T, Kanazawa K. Flavones and flavonols at dietary levels inhibit a transformation of aryl hydrocarbon receptor induced by dioxin. *FEBS Lett.* 2000;476(3): 213–7.

36. Alhaider AA, El Gendy MAM, Korashy HM, El-Kadi AOS. Camel urine inhibits the cytochrome P450 1a1 gene expression through an AhR-dependent mechanism in Hepa 1c1c7 cell line. *J Ethnopharmacol.* 2011;133(1):184–90.

37. Watts AR, Lennard MS, Mason SL, Tucker GT, Woods HF. Beeturia and the biological fate of beetroot pigments. *Pharmacogenetics.* 1993;3(6):302–11.

38. Yalindag-Ozturk N, Ozdamar M, Cengiz P. Trial of garlic as an adjunct therapy for multidrug resistant Pseudomonas aeruginosa pneumonia in a critically ill infant. *J Altern Complement Med.* 2011;17(4):379–80. Epub 2011 Apr 11.

39. Seeram NP. Recent trends and advances in berry health benefits research. *J Agric Food Chem.* 2010;58(7):3869–70.

40. Seeram NP. Berry fruits for cancer prevention: Current status and future prospects. *J Agric Food Chem.* 2008;56(3):630–5.

41. Caligiuri MA. Human natural killer cells. *Blood.* 2008;112(3):461–9.

42. McAnulty LS, Nieman DC, Dumke CL, et al. Effect of blueberry ingestion on natural killer cell counts, oxidative stress, and inflammation prior to and after 2. 5 H of running. *Appl Physiol Nutr Metab.* 2011;36(6):976–84.

43. Majdalawieh AF, Carr RI. In vitro investigation of the potential immunomodulatory and anti-cancer activities of black pepper (Piper nigrum) and cardamom (Elettaria cardamomum). *J Med Food.* 2010;13(2):371–81.

44. Bager P, Wohlfahrt J, Westergaard T. Caesarean delivery and risk of atopy and allergic disease: Meta-analyses. *Clin Exp Allergy.* 2008;38(4):634–42

45. Benn CS, Thorsen P, Jensen JS, et al. Maternal vaginal microflora during pregnancy and the risk of asthma hospitalization and use of antiasthma medication in early childhood. *J Allergy Clin Immunol*. 2002;110(1):72–7

46. Sheih YH, Chiang BL, Wang LH, Liao CK, Gill HS. Systemic immunity-enhancing effects in healthy subjects following dietary consumption of the lactic acid bacterium Lactobacillus rhamnosus HN001. *J Am Coll Nutr*. 2001;20(Suppl 2):149–56

47. Berggren A, Lazou Ahrhiang BL, Wang LH, Liao G. Randomised, double-blind and placebo-controlled study using new probiotic lactobacilli for strengthening the body immune defence against viral infections. *Eur J Nutr*. 2011;50(3):203–10.

48. Hao Q, Lu Z, Dong BR, Huang CQ, Wu T. Probiotics for preventing acute upper respiratory tract infections. *Cochrane Database Syst Rev*. 2011;9:1–42

49. Homayoni Rad A, Akbarzadeh F, Mehrabany EV. Which are more important: prebiotics or probiotics? *Nutrition*. 2012;28(11–12):1196–7.

50. Vitali B, Minervini G, Rizzello CG, et al. Novel probiotic candidates for humans isolated from raw fruits and vegetables. *Food Microbiol*. 2012;31(1):116–25.

51. Nieman DC. Moderate exercise improves immunity and decreases illness rates. *Am J Lifestyle Med*. 2011;5(4):338–45.

52. Schwindt CD, Zaldivar F, Wilson L, et al. Do circulating leucocytes and lymphocyte subtypes increase in response to brief exercise in children with and without asthma? *Br J Sports Med*. 2007;41(1):34–40.

53. Nieman DC, Henson DA, Gusewitch G, et al. Physical activity and immune function in elderly women. *Med Sci Sports Exerc*. 1993;25(7):823–31.

54. Neville V, Gleeson M, Folland JP. Salivary IgA as a risk factor for upper respiratory infections in elite professional athletes. *Med Sci Sports Exerc*. 2008;40(7):1228–36.

55. Otsuki T, Shimizu K, Iemitsu M, Kono I. Salivary secretory immunoglobulin A secretion increases after 4-weeks ingestion of chlorella-derived multicomponent supplement in humans: a randomized cross over study. *Nutr J*. 2011 Sep 9;10:91.

56. Klentrou P, Cieslak T, MacNeil M, Vintinner A, Plyley M. Effect of moderate exercise on salivary immunoglobulin A and infection risk in humans. *Eur J Appl Physiol*. 2002;87(2):153–8.

57. Nieman DC. Moderate exercise improves immunity and decreases illness rates. *Am J Lifestyle Med*. 2011;5(4):338–46.

58. Walsh NP, Gleeson M, Shephard RJ, et al. Position statement. Part one: immune function and exercise. *Exerc Immunol Rev*. 2011;17:6–63.

59. Akimoto T, Nakahori C, Aizawa K, Kimura F, Fukubayashi T, Kono I. Acupuncture and responses of immunologic and endocrine markers during competition. *Med Sci Sports Exerc*. 2003;35(8):1296–302.

60. Neville V, Gleeson M, Folland JP. Salivary IgA as a risk factor for upper respiratory infections in elite professional athletes. *Med Sci Sports Exerc*. 2008;40(7):1228–36.

61. Nieman DC. Exercise effects on systemic immunity. *Immunol Cell Biol*. 2000;78(5):496–501.

62. Otsuki T, Shimizu K, Iemitsu M, Kono I. Salivary secretory immunoglobulin A secretion increases after 4-weeks ingestion of chlorella-derived multicomponent supplement in humans: a randomized cross over study. *Nutr J*. 2011 Sep 9;10:91.

63. Halperin SA, Smith B, Nolan C, Shay J, Kralovec J. Safety and immunoenhancing effect of a Chlorella-derived dietary supplement in healthy adults undergoing influenza vaccination: randomized, double-blind, placebo-controlled trial. *CMAJ*. 2003 Jul 22;169(2):111–7.

64. Otsuki T, Shimizu K, Iemitsu M, Kono I. Chlorella intake attenuates reduced salivary SIgA secretion in kendo training camp participants. *Nutr J*. 2012 Dec 11;11:103.

65. Selvaraj V, Singh H, Ramaswamy S. Chlorella-induced psychosis. *Psychosomatics*. 2013;54(3): 303–4.

66. Selvaraj V, Singh H, Ramaswamy S. Chlorella-induced psychosis. *Psychosomatics*. 2013;54(3): 303–4.

67. Carpenter KC, Breslin WL, Davidson T, Adams A, McFarlin BK. Baker's yeast β-glucan supplementation increases monocytes and cytokines post-exercise: implications for infection risk? *Br J Nutr*. 2013;109(3):478–86.

68. Carpenter KC, Breslin WL, Davidson T, Adams A, McCarlin BK. Baker's yeast β-glucan supplementation increases monocytes and cytokines post-exercise: implications for infection risk? *Br J Nutr*. 2013;109(3):478–86.

69. Talbott S, Talbott J. Effect of BETA 1, 3/1, 6 GLUCAN on upper respiratory tract infection symptoms and mood state in marathon athletes. *J Sports Sci Med*. 2009 Dec 1;8(4):509–15.

70. Merrill RM, Isakson RT, Beck RE. The association between allergies and cancer: what is currently known? *Ann Allergy Asthma Immunol*. 2007;99(2):102–16.

71. Wakchaure GC. Production and marketing of mushrooms: global and national scenario. In: Singh M, ed. *Mushrooms: Cultivation, Marketing and Consumption*. Indian Council of Agricultural Research Directorate of Mushroom Research; 2011.

72. Jeong SC, Koyyalamudi SR, Pang G. Dietary intake of Agaricus bisporus white button mushroom accelerates salivary immunoglobulin A secretion in healthy volunteers. *Nutrition*. 2012; 28(5):527–31.

73. Jeong SC, Koyyalamudi SR, Pang G. Dietary intake of Agaricusbisporus white button mushroom accelerates salivary immunoglobulin A secretion in healthy volunteers. *Nutrition*. 2012; 28(5):527–31.

74. Moro C, Palacios I, Lozano M, et al. Anti-inflammatory activity of methanolic extracts from edible mushrooms in LPS activated RAW 264. 7 macrophages. *Food Chemistry*. 2012; 130:350–5.

75. Jesenak M, Hrubisko M, Majtan J, Rennerova Z, Banovcin P. Anti-allergic effect of Pleuran (β-glucan from Pleurotus ostreatus) in children with recurrent respiratory tract infections. *Phytother Res*. 2014;28(3):471–4.

76. Centers for Disease Control and Prevention. Estimates of foodborne illness in the United States. http://www.cdc.gov/foodborneburden/. Accessed March 3, 2015.

77. Batz MB, Hoffmann S, Morris Jr JG. Ranking the disease burden of 14 pathogens in food sources in the United States using attribution data from outbreak investigations and expert elicitation. *J Food Prot*. 2012;75(7):1278–91.

78. Park S, Navratil S, Gregory A, et al. Multifactorial effects of ambient temperature, precipitation, farm management, and environmental factors determine the level of generic Escherichia coli contamination on preharvested spinach. *Appl Environ Microbiol*. 2015;81(7): 2635–50.

79. Hoffmann S, Batz MB, Morris Jr JG. Annual cost of illness and quality-adjusted life year losses in the United States due to 14 foodborne pathogens. *J Food Prot*. 2012;75(7):1292–302.

80. Chai SJ, White PL. Salmonella enterica Serotype Enteritidis: increasing incidence of domestically acquired infections. *Clin Infect Dis*. 2012;54(Sup5): 488–97.

81. Salmonella. Centers for Disease Control and Prevention. http://www.cdc.gov/salmonella/. Accessed March 3, 2015.

82. Baura GD. The incredible inedible egg. *IEEE Pulse*. 2010 Nov–Dec;1(3):56, 62.

83. Krouse B. Opposing view on food safety: committed to safety. *USA Today*. http://usatoday 30.usatoday.com/news/opinion/editorials/2010-08-30-editorial30_ST1_N.htm. Accessed March 3, 2015.

84. Davis AL, Curtis PA, Conner DE, McKee SR, Kerth LK. Validation of cooking methods using shell eggs inoculated with Salmonella serotypes Enteritidis and Heidelberg. *Poult Sci.* 2008; 87(8):1637–42.

85. Stadelman WJ, Muriana PM, Schmieder H. The effectiveness of traditional egg-cooking practices for elimination of Salmonella enteritidis. *Poult Sci.* 1995;74(s1):119.

86. Humphrey TJ, Greenwood M, Gilbert RJ, Rowe B, Chapman PA. The survival of salmonellas in shell eggs cooked under simulated domestic conditions. *Epidemiol Infect.* 1989;103:35–45.

87. U.S. Food and Drug Administration. Playing it safe with eggs. http://www.fda.gov/food /resourcesforyou/Consumers/ucm077342.htm. Accessed March 3, 2015.

88. Batz MB, Hoffmann S, Morris Jr JG. Ranking the disease burden of 14 pathogens in food sources in the United States using attribution data from outbreak investigations and expert elicitation. *J Food Prot.* 2012;75(7):1278–91.

89. Centers for Disease Control and Prevention. Multistate outbreak of multidrug-resistant Salmonella Heidelberg infections linked to Foster Farms brand chicken. http://www.cdc.gov /salmonella/heidelberg-10-13/. Accessed March 3, 2015.

90. USDA. Notice of Intended Enforcement. http://www.marlerblog.com/files/2013/10/foster -farms-est-6137a-p1.pdf. Accessed March 3, 2015.

91. Voetsch AC, Van Gilder TJ, Angulo FJ, et al. FoodNet estimate of the burden of illness caused by nontyphoidal Salmonella infections in the United States. *Clin Infect Dis.* 2004;38(Supplement-3):S127–S134.

92. USDA. Notice of Intended Enforcement. http://www.marlerblog.com/files/2013/10/foster -farms-est-6137a-p1.pdf. Accessed March 3, 2015.

93. Pierson D. Mexico blocks Foster Farms chicken imports amid salmonella fears. *LA Times.* http://articles. latimes.com/2013/oct/24/business/la-fi-foster-farms-mexico-20131025. Accessed March 3, 2015.

94. Supreme Beef Processors, Inc v United States Dept. of Agriculture, 275 F. 3d 432 (5th Cir 2001).

95. Fravalo P, Laisney MJ, Gillard MO, Salvat G, Chemaly M. Campylobacter transfer from naturally contaminated chicken thighs to cutting boards is inversely related to initial load. *J Food Prot.* 2009;72(9):1836–40.

96. Guyard-Nicodème M, Tresse O, Houard E, et al. Characterization of Campylobacter spp. transferred from naturally contaminated chicken legs to cooked chicken slices via a cutting board. *Int J Food Microbiol.* 2013 Jun 3;164(1):7–14.

97. Foster Farms Provides Food Safety Update. Close Up Media Website. http://closeupmedia .com/food/Foster-Farms-Provides-Food-Safety-Update.html. 2013. Accessed March 5, 2015.

98. Hoffmann S, Batz MB, Morris Jr JG. Annual cost of illness and quality-adjusted life year losses in the United States due to 14 foodborne pathogens. *J Food Prot.* 2012;75(7):1292–302.

99. Karapetian A. Model EU. *Meatingplace.* March 2010:91.

100. The high cost of cheap chicken. *Consumer Reports.* http://www.consumerreports.org/cro/magazine /2014/02/the-high-cost-of-cheap-chicken/index.htm. February 2014. Accessed March 5, 2015.

101. Antibiotic Resistance Threats in the United States, 2013. Centers for Disease Control and Prevention. http://www. cdc. gov/drugresistance/threat-report-2013/pdf/ar-threats-2013-508.pdf. Accessed March 3, 2015.

102. Mayo Clinic Staff. Salmonella infection. The Mayo Clinic. http://www.mayoclinic.org /diseases-conditions/salmonella/basics/causes/con-20029017. Accessed March 3, 2015.

103. U.S. Food and Drug Administration. NARMS 2011 retail meat annual report. http://www.fda .gov/downloads/AnimalVeterinary/SafetyHealth/AntimicrobialResistance/NationalAnti microbialResistanceMonitoringSystem/UCM334834.pdf. Accessed April 3, 2015.

104. U.S. Food and Drug Administration. NARMS 2011 retail meat annual report. http://www.fda .gov/downloads/AnimalVeterinary/SafetyHealth/AntimicrobialResistance/NationalAnti microbialResistanceMonitoringSystem/UCM334834.pdf. Accessed April 3, 2015.

105. NA. Vital signs: incidence and trends of infection with pathogens transmitted commonly through food—foodborne diseases active surveillance network, 10 U.S. Sites, 1996–2010. *MMWR Morb Mortal Wkly Rep.* 2011;60(22):749–55.

106. Chai SJ, White PL, Lathrop SL, et al. Salmonella enterica serotype Enteritidis: increasing incidence of domestically acquired infections. *Clin Infect Dis.* 2012;54-Suppl-5(NA): S488–97.

107. Hoffmann S, Batz MB, Morris Jr JG. Annual cost of illness and quality-adjusted life year losses in the United States due to 14 foodborne pathogens. *J Food Prot.* 2012;75(7):1292–302.

108. 511 F. 2d 331-American Public Health Association v. Butz. http://openjurist.org/511/f2d/331 /american-public-health-association-v-butz. Accessed March 3, 2015.

109. Supreme Beef Processors v. U.S. Dept. of Agriculture. United States Court of Appeals, Fifth Circuit. http://www.leagle.com/decision/2001707275F3d432_1672. Accessed March 3, 2015.

110. Stamey TA, Timothy M, Millar M, Mihara G. Recurrent urinary infections in adult women. The role of introital enterobacteria. *Calif Med.* 1971;115(1):1–19.

111. Yamamoto S, Tsukamoto T, Terai A, Kurazono H, Takeda Y, Yoshida O. Genetic evidence supporting the fecal-perineal-urethral hypothesis in cystitis caused by Escherichia coli. *J Urol.* 1997;157(3):1127–9.

112. Bergeron CR, Prussing C, Boerlin P, et al. Chicken as reservoir for extraintestinal pathogenic Escherichia coli in humans, Canada. *Emerging Infect Dis.* 2012;18(3):415–21.

113. Jakobsen L, Garneau P, Bruant G, et al. Is Escherichia coli urinary tract infection a zoonosis? Proof of direct link with production animals and meat. *Eur J Clin Microbiol Infect Dis.* 2012;31(6): 1121–9.

114. Foxman B, Barlow R, D'arcy H, Gillespie B, Sobel JD. Urinary tract infection: self-reported incidence and associated costs. *Ann Epidemiol.* 2000;10(8):509–15.

115. Platell JL, Johnson JR, Cobbold RN, Trott DJ. Multidrug-resistant extraintestinal pathogenic Escherichia coli of sequence type ST131 in animals and foods. *Vet Microbiol.* 2011;153(1–2): 99–108.

116. Linton AH, Howe K, Bennett PM, Richmond MH, Whiteside EJ. The colonization of the human gut by antibiotic resistant Escherichia coli from chickens. *J Appl Bacteriol.* 1977;43(3): 465–9.

117. Linton AH, Howe K, Bennett PM, Richmond MH, Whiteside EJ. The colonization of the human gut by antibiotic resistant Escherichia coli from chickens. *J Appl Bacteriol.* 1977;43(3): 465–9.

118. Rusin P, Orosz-Coughlin P, Gerba C. Reduction of faecal coliform, coliform and heterotrophic plate count bacteria in the household kitchen and bathroom by disinfection with hypochlorite cleaners. *J Appl Microbiol.* 1998;85(5):819–28.

119. Cogan TA, Bloomfield SF, Humphrey TJ. The effectiveness of hygiene procedures for prevention of cross-contamination from chicken carcases in the domestic kitchen. *Lett Appl Microbiol.* 1999;29(5):354–8.

120. Cogan TA, Bloomfield SF, Humphrey TJ. The effectiveness of hygiene procedures for prevention of cross-contamination from chicken carcases in the domestic kitchen. *Lett Appl Microbiol.* 1999;29(5):354–8.

121. Cogan TA, Bloomfield SF, Humphrey TJ. The effectiveness of hygiene procedures for preven-

tion of cross-contamination from chicken carcases in the domestic kitchen. *Lett Appl Microbiol.* 1999;29(5):354–8.

122. Linton AH, Howe K, Bennett PM, Richmond MH, Whiteside EJ. The colonization of the human gut by antibiotic resistant Escherichia coli from chickens. *J Appl Bacteriol.* 1977;43(3): 465–9.

123. Scallan E, Hoekstra RM, Angulo FJ, et al. Foodborne illness acquired in the United States— major pathogens. *Emerging Infect Dis.* 2011;17:7–15.

124. Batz MB, Hoffmann S, Morris Jr JG. Ranking the disease burden of 14 pathogens in food sources in the United States using attribution data from outbreak investigations and expert elicitation. *J Food Prot.* 2012;75:1278 91.

125. Zheng H, Sun Y, Lin S, Mao Z, Jiang B. Yersinia enterocolitica infection in diarrheal patients. *Eur J Clin Microbiol Infect Dis.* 2008;27:741–52.

126. Bari ML, Hossain MA, Isshiki K, Ukuku D. Behavior of Yersinia enterocolitica in foods. *J Pathog.* 2011;2011:420732.

127. Ternhag A, Törner A, Svensson A, Ekdahl K, Giesecke J. Short- and long-term effects of bacterial gastrointestinal infections. *Emerging Infect Dis.* 2008;14:143–8.

128. Brix TH, Hansen PS, Hegedüs L, Wenzel BE. Too early to dismiss Yersinia enterocolitica infection in the aetiology of Graves' disease: evidence from a twin case-control study. *Clin Endocrinol* (Oxf). 2008;69:491–6.

129. What's in that pork? *Consumer Reports.* http://www.consumerreports.org/cro/magazine /2013/01/what-s-in-that-pork/index.htm. Accessed March 3, 2015.

130. Bari ML, Hossain MA, Isshiki K, Ukuku D. Behavior of Yersinia enterocolitica in foods. *J Pathog.* 2011;2011:420732.

131. Crowding pigs pays—if it's managed properly. *National Hog Farmer.* November 15, 1993;62.

132. Poljak Z, Dewey CE, Martin SW, et al. Prevalence of Yersinia enterocolitica shedding and bioserotype distribution in Ontario finisher pig herds in 2001, 2002, and 2004. *Prev Vet Med.* 2010;93:110–20.

133. Hoffmann S, Batz MB, Morris Jr JG. Annual cost of illness and quality-adjusted life year losses in the United States due to 14 foodborne pathogens. *J Food Prot.* 2012;75:1292–1302.

134. Centers for Disease Control and Prevention. Antibiotic Resistance Threats in the United States, 2013. http://www.cdc.gov/drugresistance/pdf/ar-threats-2013-508.pdf. Accessed March 3, 2015.

135. Eyre DW, Cule ML, Wilson DJ, et al. Diverse sources of C. difficile infection identified on whole-genome sequencing. *N Engl J Med.* 2013 Sep 26;369(13):1195–205.

136. Songer JG, Trinh HT, Killgore GE, Thompson AD, McDonald LC, Limbago BM. Clostridium difficile in retail meat products, USA, 2007. *Emerg Infect Dis.* 2009;15(5):819–21.

137. Rupnik M, Songer JG. Clostridium difficile: its potential as a source of foodborne disease. *Adv Food Nutr Res.* 2010;60:53–66.

138. Rodriguez-Palacios A, Borgmann S, Kline TR, LeJeune JT. Clostridium difficile in foods and animals: history and measures to reduce exposure. *Anim Health Res Rev.* 2013;14(1):11–29.

139. Hensgrens MPM, Keessen EC, Squire MM, et al. European Society of Clinical Microbiology and Infectious Diseases Study Group for Clostridium difficile (ESGCD). Clostridium difficile infection in the community: a zoonotic disease? *Clin Microbiol Infect.* 2012;18(7):635–45.

140. Rupnik M, Songer JG. Clostridium difficile: its potential as a source of foodborne disease. *Adv Food Nutr Res.* 2010;60:53–66.

141. Sayedy L, Kothari D, Richards RJ. Toxic megacolon associated Clostridium difficile colitis. *World J Gastrointest Endosc.* 2010;2(8):293–7.

142. Gweon TG, Lee KJ, Kang DH, et al. A case of toxic megacolon caused by Clostridium difficile infection and treated with fecal microbiota transplantation. *Gut Liver*. 2015;9(2):247–50.

143. Weese JS. Clostridium difficile in food—innocent bystander or serious threat? *Clin Microbiol Infect*. 2010;16:3–10.

144. Jabbar U, Leischner J, Kasper D, et al. Effectiveness of alcohol-based hand rubs for removal of Clostridium difficile spores from hands. *Infect Control Hosp Epidemiol*. 2010;31(6):565–70.

145. Bhargava K, Wang X, Donabedian S, Zervos M, de Rocha L, Zhang Y. Methicillin-resistant Staphylococcus aureus in retail meat, Detroit, Michigan, USA. *Emerging Infect Dis*. 2011;17(6): 1135–7.

146. Reinberg S. Scientists find MRSA germ in supermarket meats. http://usatoday30.usatoday .com/news/health/medical/health/medical/story/2011/05/Scientists-find-MRSA-germ-in -supermarket-meats/47105974/1. May 12, 2011. Accessed April 4, 2015.

147. Chan M. Antimicrobial resistance in the European Union and the world. Talk presented at: Conference on combating antimicrobial resistance: time for action. March 14, 2012; Copen-hagen, Denmark. http://www.who.int/dg/speeches/2012/amr_20120314/en/. Accessed March 6, 2015.

148. Love DC, Halden RU, Davis MF, Nachman KE. Feather meal: a previously unrecognized route for reentry into the food supply of multiple pharmaceuticals and personal care products (PPCPs). *Environ Sci Technol*. 2012;46(7):3795–802.

149. Ji K, Kho Y, Park C, et al. Influence of water and food consumption on inadvertent antibiotics intake among general population. *Environ Res*. 2010;110(7):641–9.

150. Ji K, Lim Kho YL, Park Y, Choi K. Influence of a five-day vegetarian diet on urinary levels of antibiotics and phthalate metabolites: a pilot study with "Temple Stay" participants. *Environ Res*. 2010;110(4):375–82.

151. Keep Antibiotics Working. http://www.keepantibioticsworking.com/new/indepth_groups. php. Accessed March 3, 2015.

152. Hayes DJ, Jenson HH. Technology choice and the economic effects of a ban on the use of anti-microbial feed additives in swine rations. *Food Control*. 2002;13(2):97–101.

153. Rival diet doc leaks Atkins death report. http://www.thesmokinggun.com/file/rival-diet-doc-leaks-atkins-death-report?page=3. Accessed March 3, 2015.

154. Corporate Threat. http://www.atkinsexposed.org/Corporate_Threat.htm. Accessed June 14, 2015.

6. How Not to Die from Diabetes

1. Matthews DR, Matthews PC. Banting Memorial Lecture 2010. Type 2 diabetes as an 'infec-tious' disease: is this the Black Death of the 21st century? *Diabet Med*. 2011;28(1):2–9.

2. Centers for Disease Control and Prevention. Number (in millions) of civilian, noninstitution-alized persons with diagnosed diabetes, United States, 1980–2011. http://www.cdc.gov/dia betes/statistics/prev/national/figpersons.htm. March 28, 2013. Accessed May 3, 2015.

3. Boyle JP, Thompson TJ, Gregg EW, Barker LE, Williamson DF. Projection of the year 2050 burden of diabetes in the US adult population: dynamic modeling of incidence, mortality, and prediabetes prevalence. *Popul Health Metr*. 2010;8:29.

4. Centers for Disease Control and Prevention. National Diabetes Statistics Report: Estimates of Diabetes and Its Burden in the United States, 2014. Atlanta, GA: U.S. Department of Health and Human Services; 2014.

5. Centers for Disease Control and Prevention. Deaths: final data for 2013 table 10. Number of deaths from 113 selected causes. National Vital Statistics Report 2016;64(2).

6. 2014 Statistics Report. Centers for Disease Control and Prevention. http://www.cdc.gov/diabetes/data/statistics/2014StatisticsReport.html. Updated October 24, 2014. Accessed March 3, 2015.

7. Lempainen J, Tauriainen S, Vaarala O, et al. Interaction of enterovirus infection and cow's milk-based formula nutrition in type 1 diabetes-associated autoimmunity. *Diabetes Metab Res Rev.* 2012;28(2):177–85.

8. 2014 Statistics Report. Centers for Disease Control and Prevention. http://www.cdc.gov/diabetes/data/statistics/2014StatisticsReport.html. Updated October 24, 2014. Accessed March 3, 2015.

9. Rachek LI. Free fatty acids and skeletal muscle insulin resistance. *Prog Mol Biol Transl Sci.* 2014;121:267–92.

10. 2014 Statistics Report. Centers for Disease Control and Prevention. http://www.cdc.gov/diabetes/data/statistics/2014StatisticsReport.html. Updated October 24, 2014. Accessed March 3, 2015.

11. Sweeney JS. Dietary factors that influence the dextrose tolerance test. *Arch Intern Med.* 1927; 40(6):818–30.

12. Roden M, Price TB, Perseghin G, et al. Mechanism of free fatty acid-induced insulin resistance in humans. *J Clin Invest.* 1996;97(12):2859–65.

13. Roden M, Krssak M, Stingl H, et al. Rapid impairment of skeletal muscle glucose transport/phosphorylation by free fatty acids in humans. *Diabetes.* 1999;48(2):358–64.

14. Santomauro AT, Boden G, Silva ME, et al. Overnight lowering of free fatty acids with Acipimox improves insulin resistance and glucose tolerance in obese diabetic and nondiabetic subjects. *Diabetes.* 1999;48(9):1836–41.

15. Krssak M, Falk Petersen K, Dresner A, et al. Intramyocellular lipid concentrations are correlated with insulin sensitivity in humans: a ¹H NMR spectroscopy study. *Diabetologia.* 1999;42(1):113–6.

16. Lee S, Boesch C, Kuk JL, Arslanian S. Effects of an overnight intravenous lipid infusion on intramyocellular lipid content and insulin sensitivity in African-American versus Caucasian adolescents. *Metab Clin Exp.* 2013;62(3):417–23.

17. Roden M, Krssak M, Stingl H, et al. Rapid impairment of skeletal muscle glucose transport/phosphorylation by free fatty acids in humans. *Diabetes.* 1999;48(2):358–64.

18. Himsworth HP. Dietetic factors influencing the glucose tolerance and the activity of insulin. *J Physiol* (Lond). 1934;81(1):29–48.

19. Tabák AG1, Herder C, Rathmann W, Brunner EJ, Kivimäki M. Prediabetes: a high-risk state for diabetes. *Lancet.* 2012;379(9833):2279–90.

20. Pratley RE. The early treatment of type 2 diabetes. *Am J Med.* 2013;126(9 Suppl 1):S2–9.

21. Reinehr T. Type 2 diabetes mellitus in children and adolescents. *World J Diabetes.* 2013;4(6):270–81.

22. Pihoker C, Scott CR, Lensing SY, Cradock MM, Smith J. Non-insulin dependent diabetes mellitus in African-American youths of Arkansas. *Clin Pediatr* (Phila). 1998;37(2):97–102.

23. Dean H, Flett B. Natural history of type 2 diabetes diagnosed in childhood: long term follow-up in young adult years. *Diabetes.* 2002;51(s1):A24.

24. Hannon TS, Rao G, Arslanian SA. Childhood obesity and type 2 diabetes mellitus. *Pediatrics.* 2005;116(2):473–80.

25. Rocchini AP. Childhood obesity and a diabetes epidemic. *N Engl J Med.* 2002;346(11):854–5.

26. Lifshitz F. Obesity in children. *J Clin Res Pediatr Endocrinol.* 2008;1(2):53–60.

27. Must A, Jacques PF, Dallal GE, Bajema CJ, Dietz WH. Long-term morbidity and mortality of

overweight adolescents. A follow-up of the Harvard Growth Study of 1922 to 1935. *N Engl J Med.* 1992;327(19):1350–5.

28. Sabaté J, Wien M. Vegetarian diets and childhood obesity prevention. *Am J Clin Nutr.* 2010; 91(5):1525S–1529S.

29. Tonstad S, Butler T, Yan R, Fraser GE. Type of vegetarian diet, body weight, and prevalence of type 2 diabetes. *Diabetes Care.* 2009;32(5):791–6.

30. Sabaté J, Lindsted KD, Harris RD, Sanchez A. Attained height of lacto-ovo vegetarian children and adolescents. *Eur J Clin Nutr.* 1991;45(1):51–8.

31. Sabaté J, Wien M. Vegetarian diets and childhood obesity prevention. *Am J Clin Nutr.* 2010; 91(5):1525S–1529S.

32. Cali AM, Caprio S. Prediabetes and type 2 diabetes in youth: an emerging epidemic disease? *Curr Opin Endocrinol Diabetes Obes.* 2008;15(2):123–7.

33. Ginter E, Simko V. Type 2 diabetes mellitus, pandemic in 21st century. *Adv Exp Med Biol.* 2012;771:42–50.

34. Spalding KL, Arner E, Westermark PO, et al. Dynamics of fat cell turnover in humans. *Nature.* 2008;453(7196):783–7.

35. Roden M. How free fatty acids inhibit glucose utilization in human skeletal muscle. *News Physiol Sci.* 2004;19:92–6.

36. Fraser GE. Vegetarian diets: what do we know of their effects on common chronic diseases? *Am J Clin Nutr.* 2009;89(5):1607S–1612S.

37. Tonstad S, Stewart K, Oda K, Batech M, Herring RP, Fraser GE. Vegetarian diets and incidence of diabetes in the Adventist Health Study-2. *Nutr Metab Cardiovasc Dis.* 2013;23(4):292–9.

38. Nolan CJ, Larter CZ. Lipotoxicity: why do saturated fatty acids cause and monounsaturates protect against it? *J Gastroenterol Hepatol.* 2009;24(5):703–6.

39. Evans WJ. Oxygen-carrying proteins in meat and risk of diabetes mellitus. *JAMA Intern Med.* 2013;173(14):1335–6.

40. Egnatchik RA, Leamy AK, Jacobson DA, Shiota M, Young JD. ER calcium release promotes mitochondrial dysfunction and hepatic cell lipotoxicity in response to palmitate overload. *Mol Metab.* 2014;3(5):544–53.

41. Estadella D, da Penha Oller do Nascimento CM, Oyama LM, Ribeiro EB, Dâmaso AR, de Piano A. Lipotoxicity: effects of dietary saturated and transfatty acids. *Mediators Inflamm.* 2013; 2013:137579.

42. Perseghin G, Scifo P, De Cobelli F, et al. Intramyocellular triglyceride content is a determinant of in vivo insulin resistance in humans: a 1H-13C nuclear magnetic resonance spectroscopy assessment in offspring of type 2 diabetic parents. *Diabetes.* 1999;48(8):1600–6.

43. Nolan CJ, Larter CZ. Lipotoxicity: why do saturated fatty acids cause and monounsaturates protect against it? *J Gastroenterol Hepatol.* 2009;24(5):703–6.

44. Goff LM, Bell JD, So PW, Dornhorst A, Frost GS. Veganism and its relationship with insulin resistance and intramyocellular lipid. *Eur J Clin Nutr.* 2005;59(2):291–8.

45. Gojda J, Patková J, Jaček M, et al. Higher insulin sensitivity in vegans is not associated with higher mitochondrial density. *Eur J Clin Nutr.* 2013;67(12):1310–5.

46. Goff LM, Bell JD, So PW, Dornhorst A, Frost GS. Veganism and its relationship with insulin resistance and intramyocellular lipid. *Eur J Clin Nutr.* 2005;59(2):291–8.

47. Papanikolaou Y, Fulgoni VL. Bean consumption is associated with greater nutrient intake, reduced systolic blood pressure, lower body weight, and a smaller waist circumference in adults: results from the National Health and Nutrition Examination Survey 1999–2002. *J Am Coll Nutr.* 2008;27(5):569–76.

48. Mollard RC, Luhovyy BL, Panahi S, Nunez M, Hanley A, Anderson GH. Regular consumption

of pulses for 8 weeks reduces metabolic syndrome risk factors in overweight and obese adults. *Br J Nutr.* 2012;108 Suppl 1:S111–22.

49. Cnop M, Hughes SJ, Igoillo-Esteve M, et al. The long lifespan and low turnover of human islet beta cells estimated by mathematical modelling of lipofuscin accumulation. *Diabetologia.* 2010;53(2):321–30.

50. Taylor R. Banting Memorial lecture 2012: reversing the twin cycles of type 2 diabetes. *Diabet Med.* 2013;30(3):267–75.

51. Cunha DA, Igoillo-Esteve M, Gurzov EN, et al. Death protein 5 and p53-upregulated modulator of apoptosis mediate the endoplasmic reticulum stress-mitochondrial dialog triggering lipotoxic rodent and human β-cell apoptosis. *Diabetes.* 2012;61(11):2763–75.

52. Cnop M, Hannaert JC, Grupping AY, Pipeleers DG. Low density lipoprotein can cause death of islet beta-cells by its cellular uptake and oxidative modification. *Endocrinology.* 2002;143(9): 3449–53.

53. Maedler K, Oberholzer J, Bucher P, Spinas GA, Donath MY. Monounsaturated fatty acids prevent the deleterious effects of palmitate and high glucose on human pancreatic beta-cell turnover and function. *Diabetes.* 2003;52(3):726–33.

54. Xiao C, Giacca A, Carpentier A, Lewis GF. Differential effects of monounsaturated, polyunsaturated and saturated fat ingestion on glucose-stimulated insulin secretion, sensitivity and clearance in overweight and obese, non-diabetic humans. *Diabetologia.* 2006;49(6):1371–9.

55. Wang L, Folsom AR, Zheng ZJ, Pankow JS, Eckfeldt JH. Plasma fatty acid composition and incidence of diabetes in middle-aged adults: the Atherosclerosis Risk in Communities (ARIC) Study. *Am J Clin Nutr.* 2003;78(1):91–8.

56. Cunha DA, Igoillo-Esteve M, Gurzov EN, et al. Death protein 5 and p53-upregulated modulator of apoptosis mediate the endoplasmic reticulum stress-mitochondrial dialog triggering lipotoxic rodent and human β-cell apoptosis. *Diabetes.* 2012;61(11):2763–75.

57. Welch RW. Satiety: have we neglected dietary non-nutrients? *Proc Nutr Soc.* 2011;70(2):145–54.

58. Barnard ND, Cohen J, Jenkins DJ, et al. A low-fat vegan diet improves glycemic control and cardiovascular risk factors in a randomized clinical trial in individuals with type 2 diabetes. *Diabetes Care.* 2006;29(8):1777–83.

59. Trapp CB, Barnard ND. Usefulness of vegetarian and vegan diets for treating type 2 diabetes. *Curr Diab Rep.* 2010;10(2):152–8.

60. Pratley RE. The early treatment of type 2 diabetes. *Am J Med.* 2013;126(9 Suppl 1):S2–9.

61. Juutilainen A, Lehto S, Rönnemaa T, Pyörälä K, Laakso M. Type 2 diabetes as a "coronary heart disease equivalent": an 18-year prospective population-based study in Finnish subjects. *Diabetes Care.* 2005;28(12):2901–7.

62. Kahleova H, Matoulek M, Malinska H, et al. Vegetarian diet improves insulin resistance and oxidative stress markers more than conventional diet in subjects with type 2 diabetes. *Diabet Med.* 2011;28(5):549–59.

63. Ornish D. Statins and the soul of medicine. *Am J Cardiol.* 2002;89(11):1286–90.

64. Kahleova H, Hrachovinova T, Hill M, et al. Vegetarian diet in type 2 diabetes—improvement in quality of life, mood and eating behaviour. *Diabet Med.* 2013;30(1):127–9.

65. Chiu THT, Huang HY, Chiu YF, et al. Taiwanese vegetarians and omnivores: dietary composition, prevalence of diabetes and IFG. *PLoS One.* 2014;9(2):e88547.

66. Chiu THT, Huang HY, Chiu YF, et al. Taiwanese vegetarians and omnivores: dietary composition, prevalence of diabetes and IFG. *PLoS One.* 2014;9(2):e88547.

67. Magliano DJ, Loh VHY, Harding JL, et al. Persistent organic pollutants and diabetes: a review of the epidemiological evidence. *Diabetes Metab.* 2014;40(1):1–14.

68. Lee DH, Lee IK, Song K, et al. A strong dose-response relation between serum concentrations

of persistent organic pollutants and diabetes: results from the National Health and Examination Survey 1999–2002. *Diabetes Care*. 2006;29(7):1638–44.

69. Wu H, Bertrand KA, Choi AL, et al. Persistent organic pollutants and type 2 diabetes: a prospective analysis in the Nurses' Health Study and meta-analysis. *Environ Health Perspect*. 2013; 121(2):153–61.

70. Schecter A, Colacino J, Haffner D, et al. Perfluorinated compounds, polychlorinated biphenyls, and organochlorine pesticide contamination in composite food samples from Dallas, Texas, USA. *Environ Health Perspect*. 2010;118(6):796–802.

71. Crinnion WJ. The role of persistent organic pollutants in the worldwide epidemic of type 2 diabetes mellitus and the possible connection to farmed Atlantic salmon (Salmo salar). *Altern Med Rev*. 2011;16(4):301–13.

72. Lee DH, Lee IK, Song K, et al. A strong dose-response relation between serum concentrations of persistent organic pollutants and diabetes: results from the National Health and Examination Survey 1999–2002. *Diabetes Care*. 2006;29(7):1638–44.

73. Crinnion WJ. The role of persistent organic pollutants in the worldwide epidemic of type 2 diabetes mellitus and the possible connection to farmed Atlantic salmon (Salmo salar). *Altern Med Rev*. 2011;16(4):301–13.

74. Farmer B, Larson BT, Fulgoni VL III, et al. A vegetarian dietary pattern as a nutrient-dense approach to weight management: an analysis of the National Health and Nutrition Examination Survey 1999–2004. *J Am Diet Assoc*. 2011;111(6):819–27.

75. Farmer B, Larson BT, Fulgoni VL III, et al. A vegetarian dietary pattern as a nutrient-dense approach to weight management: an analysis of the National Health and Nutrition Examination Survey 1999–2004. *J Am Diet Assoc*. 2011;111(6):819–27.

76. Toth MJ, Poehlman ET. Sympathetic nervous system activity and resting metabolic rate in vegetarians. *Metabolism*. 1994;43(5):621–5.

77. Karlic H, Schuster D, Varga F, et al. Vegetarian diet affects genes of oxidative metabolism and collagen synthesis. *Ann Nutr Metab*. 2008;53(1):29–32.

78. Vergnaud AC, Norat T, Romaguera D, et al. Meat consumption and prospective weight change in participants of the EPIC-PANACEA study. *Am J Clin Nutr*. 2010;92(2):398–407.

79. The Action to Control Cardiovascular Risk in Diabetes Study Group, Gerstein HC, Miller ME, et al. Effects of intensive glucose lowering in type 2 diabetes. *N Engl J Med*. 2008;358(24): 2545–59.

80. The Action to Control Cardiovascular Risk in Diabetes Study Group, Gerstein HC, Miller ME, et al. Effects of intensive glucose lowering in type 2 diabetes. *N Engl J Med*. 2008;358(24): 2545–59.

81. Luan FL, Nguyen K. Intensive glucose control in type 2 diabetes. *N Engl J Med*. 2008;359(14): 1519–20.

82. Blagosklonny MV. Prospective treatment of age-related diseases by slowing down aging. *Am J Pathol*. 2012;181(4):1142–6.

83. Madonna R, Pandolfi A, Massaro M, et al. Insulin enhances vascular cell adhesion molecule-1 expression in human cultured endothelial cells through a pro-atherogenic pathway mediated by p38 mitogen-activated protein-kinase. *Diabetologia*. 2004;47(3):532–6.

84. Lingvay I, Guth E, Islam A, et al. Rapid improvement in diabetes after gastric bypass surgery: is it the diet or surgery? *Diabetes Care*. 2013;36(9):2741–7.

85. Lingvay I, Guth E, Islam A, et al. Rapid improvement in diabetes after gastric bypass surgery: is it the diet or surgery? *Diabetes Care*. 2013;36(9):2741–7.

86. Taylor R. Type 2 diabetes: etiology and reversibility. *Diabetes Care*. 2013;36(4):1047–55.

87. Lim EL, Hollingsworth KG, Aribisala BS, Chen MJ, Mathers JC, Taylor R. Reversal of type 2

diabetes: normalisation of beta cell function in association with decreased pancreas and liver triacylglycerol. *Diabetologia*. 2011;54(10):2506–14.

88. Taheri S, Tahrani A, Barnett A. Bariatric surgery: a cure for diabetes? *Pract Diabetes Int.* 2009;26:356–8.

89. Vergnaud AC, Norat T, Romaguera D, et al. Meat consumption and prospective weight change in participants of the EPIC-PANACEA study. *Am J Clin Nutr.* 2010;92(2):398–407.

90. Gilsing AM, Weijenberg MP, Hughes LA, et al. Longitudinal changes in BMI in older adults are associated with meat consumption differentially, by type of meat consumed. *J Nutr.* 2012;142(2):340–9.

91. Wang Y, Lchanc C, Ghebremeskel K, et al. Modern organic and broiler chickens sold for human consumption provide more energy from fat than protein. *Public Health Nutr.* 2010;13(3):400–8.

92. National Cattlemen's Beef Association, Young MK, Redson BA. New USDA data show 29 beef cuts now meet government guidelines for lean. http://www.beef.org/udocs/29leancuts.pdf. 2005. Accessed March 6, 2015.

93. Steven S, Lim EL, Taylor R. Dietary reversal of type 2 diabetes motivated by research knowledge. *Diabet Med.* 2010;27(6):724–5.

94. Taylor R. Pathogenesis of type 2 diabetes: tracing the reverse route from cure to cause. *Diabetologia*. 2008;51(10):1781–9.

95. American Diabetes Association. Standards of medical care in diabetes—2015. *Diabetes Care*. 2015;38(suppl 1):S1–S93.

96. Dunaief DM, Fuhrman J, Dunaief JL, et al. Glycemic and cardiovascular parameters improved in type 2 diabetes with the high nutrient density (HND) diet. *Open Journal of Preventive Medicine*. 2012;2(3):364–71.

97. Lim EL, Hollingsworth KG, Aribisala BS, Chen MJ, Mathers JC, Taylor R. Reversal of type 2 diabetes: normalisation of beta cell function in association with decreased pancreas and liver triacylglycerol. *Diabetologia*. 2011;54(10):2506–14.

98. Steven S, Lim EL, Taylor R. Population response to information on reversibility of Type 2 diabetes. *Diabet Med.* 2013;30(4):e135–8.

99. Dunaief DM, Fuhrman J, Dunaief JL, et al. Glycemic and cardiovascular parameters improved in type 2 diabetes with the high nutrient density (HND) diet. *Open J Prev Med.* 2012;2(3):364–71.

100. Anderson JW, Ward K. High-carbohydrate, high-fiber diets for insulin-treated men with diabetes mellitus. *Am J Clin Nutr.* 1979;32(11):2312–21.

101. Anderson JW, Ward K. High-carbohydrate, high-fiber diets for insulin-treated men with diabetes mellitus. *Am J Clin Nutr.* 1979;32(11):2312–21.

102. Callaghan BC, Cheng H, Stables CL, et al. Diabetic neuropathy: clinical manifestations and current treatments. *Lancet Neurol.* 2012;11(6):521–34.

103. Said G. Diabetic neuropathy—a review. *Nat Clin Pract Neurol.* 2007;3(6):331–40.

104. Crane MG, Sample C. Regression of diabetic neuropathy with total vegetarian (vegan) diet. *J Nutr Med.* 1994;4(4):431–9.

105. Crane MG, Sample C. Regression of diabetic neuropathy with total vegetarian (vegan) diet. *J Nutr Med.* 1994;4(4):431–9.

106. Rabinowitch IM. Effects of the high carbohydrate-low calorie diet upon carbohydrate tolerance in diabetes mellitus. *Can Med Assoc J.* 1935;33(2):136–44.

107. Newborg B, Kempner W. Analysis of 177 cases of hypertensive vascular disease with papilledema; one hundred twenty-six patients treated with rice diet. *Am J Med.* 1955;19(1):33–47.

108. Crane MG, Sample C. Regression of diabetic neuropathy with total vegetarian (vegan) diet. *J Nutr Med.* 1994;4(4):431–9.

109. Crane MG, Sample C. Regression of diabetic neuropathy with total vegetarian (vegan) diet. *J Nutr Med*. 1994;4(4):431–9.

110. Crane MG, Sample C. Regression of diabetic neuropathy with total vegetarian (vegan) diet. *J Nutr Med*. 1994;4(4):431–9.

111. Crane MG, Zielinski R, Aloia R. Cis and trans fats in omnivores, lacto-ovo vegetarians and vegans. *Am J Clin Nutr*. 1988;48:920.

112. Tesfaye S, Chaturvedi N, Eaton SEM, et al. Vascular risk factors and diabetic neuropathy. *N Engl J Med*. 2005;352(4):341–50.

113. Newrick PG, Wilson AJ, Jakubowski J, et al. Sural nerve oxygen tension in diabetes. *Br Med J* (Clin Res Ed). 1986;293(6554):1053–4.

114. McCarty MF. Favorable impact of a vegan diet with exercise on hemorheology: implications for control of diabetic neuropathy. *Med Hypotheses*. 2002;58(6):476–86.

115. Kempner W, Peschel RL, Schlayer C. Effect of rice diet on diabetes mellitus associated with vascular disease. *Postgrad Med*. 1958;24(4):359–71.

116. McCarty MF. Favorable impact of a vegan diet with exercise on hemorheology: implications for control of diabetic neuropathy. *Med Hypotheses*. 2002;58(6):476–86.

117. Browning LM, Hsieh SD, Ashwell M. A systematic review of waist-to-height ratio as a screening tool for the prediction of cardiovascular disease and diabetes: 0·5 could be a suitable global boundary value. *Nutr Res Rev*. 2010;23(2):247–69.

118. Bigaard J, Tjønneland A, Thomsen BL, Overvad K, Heitmann BL, S, Sørensen TI. Waist circumference, BMI, smoking, and mortality in middle-aged men and women. *Obes Res*. 2003; 11(7):895–903.

119. Bigaard J, Tjønneland A, Thomsen BL, Overvad K, Heitmann BL, S, Sørensen TI. Waist circumference, BMI, smoking, and mortality in middle-aged men and women. *Obes Res*. 2003; 11(7):895–903.

120. Leitzmann MF, Moore SC, Koster A, et al. Waist circumference as compared with body-mass index in predicting mortality from specific causes. *PLoS One*. 2011;6(4):e18582.

121. Browning LM, Hsieh SD, Ashwell M. A systematic review of waist-to-height ratio as a screening tool for the prediction of cardiovascular disease and diabetes: 0·5 could be a suitable global boundary value. *Nutr Res Rev*. 2010;23(2):247–69.

122. Centers for Disease Control and Prevention. National Diabetes Statistics Report: Estimates of Diabetes and Its Burden in the United States, 2014. Atlanta, GA: U.S. Department of Health and Human Services; 2014. http://www.cdc.gov/diabetes/data/statistics/2014StatisticsReport.html. Updated October 24, 2014. Accessed March 6, 2015.

123. Nathan DM, Davidson MB, Defronzo RA, et al. Impaired fasting glucose and impaired glucose tolerance: implications for care. *Diabetes Care*. 2007;30(3):753–9.

124. Karve A, Hayward RA. Prevalence, diagnosis, and treatment of impaired fasting glucose and impaired glucose tolerance in nondiabetic U.S. adults. *Diabetes Care*. 2010;33(11):2355–9.

125. Cardona-Morrell M, Rychetnik L, Morrell SL, Espinel PT, Bauman A. Reduction of diabetes risk in routine clinical practice: are physical activity and nutrition interventions feasible and are the outcomes from reference trials replicable? A systematic review and meta-analysis. *BMC Public Health*. 2010;10:653.

126. Holman H. Chronic disease—the need for a new clinical education. *JAMA*. 2004;292(9):1057–9.

127. Institute of Medicine. Crossing the Quality Chasm: A New Health System for the 21st Century. Washington, D.C.: The National Academies Press, 2001:213. http://www.iom.edu/Reports/2001/Crossing-the-Quality-Chasm-A-New-Health-System-for-the-21st-Century.aspx.

7. How Not to Die from High Blood Pressure

1. Lozano R, Naghavi M, Foreman K, et al. Global and regional mortality from 235 causes of death for 20 age groups in 1990 and 2010: a systematic analysis for the Global Burden of Disease Study 2010. *Lancet.* 2012;380(9859):2095–128.

2. Das P, Samarasekera U. The story of GBD 2010: a "super-human" effort. *Lancet.* 2012;380 (9859):2067–70.

3. Lim SS, Vos T, Flaxman AD, et al. A comparative risk assessment of burden of disease and injury attributable to 67 risk factors and risk factor clusters in 21 regions, 1990–2010: a systematic analysis for the Global Burden of Disease Study 2010. *Lancet.* 2012;380(9859):2224–60.

4. Lim SS, Vos T, Flaxman AD, et al. A comparative risk assessment of burden of disease and injury attributable to 67 risk factors and risk factor clusters in 21 regions, 1990–2010: a systematic analysis for the Global Burden of Disease Study 2010. *Lancet.* 2012;380(9859):2224–60.

5. Lim SS, Vos T, Flaxman AD, et al. A comparative risk assessment of burden of disease and injury attributable to 67 risk factors and risk factor clusters in 21 regions, 1990–2010: a systematic analysis for the Global Burden of Disease Study 2010. *Lancet.* 2012;380(9859):2224–60.

6. Bromfield S, Muntner P. High blood pressure: the leading global burden of disease risk factor and the need for worldwide prevention programs. *Curr Hypertens Rep.* 2013;15(3):134–6.

7. Lim SS, Vos T, Flaxman AD, et al. A comparative risk assessment of burden of disease and injury attributable to 67 risk factors and risk factor clusters in 21 regions, 1990–2010: a systematic analysis for the Global Burden of Disease Study 2010. *Lancet.* 2012;380(9859):2224–60.

8. American Heart Association. Understanding Blood Pressure Readings. http://www.heart.org/HEARTORG/Conditions/HighBloodPressure/AboutHighBloodPressure/Understanding-Blood-Pressure-Readings_UCM_301764_Article.jsp. March 11, 2015. Accessed March 11, 2015.

9. Go AS, Bauman MA, Coleman King SM, et al. An effective approach to high blood pressure control: a science advisory from the American Heart Association, the American College of Cardiology, and the Centers for Disease Control and Prevention. *J Am Coll Cardiol.* 2014;63(12):1230–8.

10. Nwankwo T, Yoon SS, Burt V, Gu Q. Hypertension among adults in the United States: National Health and Nutrition Examination Survey, 2011–2012. *NCHS Data Brief.* 2013;(133):1–8.

11. Walker AR, Walker BF. High high-density-lipoprotein cholesterol in African children and adults in a population free of coronary heart diseae. *Br Med J.* 1978;2(6148):1336–7.

12. Donnison CP. Blood pressure in the African native. *Lancet.* 1929;213(5497):6–7.

13. Macmahon S, Neal B, Rodgers A. Hypertension—time to move on. *Lancet.* 2005;365(9464):1108–9.

14. Law MR, Morris JK, Wald NJ. Use of blood pressure lowering drugs in the prevention of cardiovascular disease: meta-analysis of 147 randomised trials in the context of expectations from prospective epidemiological studies. *BMJ.* 2009;338:b1665.

15. Donnison CP. Blood pressure in the African native. *Lancet.* 1929;213(5497):6–7.

16. Lim SS, Vos T, Flaxman AD, et al. A comparative risk assessment of burden of disease and injury attributable to 67 risk factors and risk factor clusters in 21 regions, 1990–2010: a systematic analysis for the Global Burden of Disease Study 2010. *Lancet.* 2012;380(9859):2224–60.

17. Lim SS, Vos T, Flaxman AD, et al. A comparative risk assessment of burden of disease and injury attributable to 67 risk factors and risk factor clusters in 21 regions, 1990–2010: a systematic analysis for the Global Burden of Disease Study 2010. *Lancet.* 2012;380(9859):2224–60.

18. Karppanen H, Mervaala E. Sodium intake and hypertension. *Prog Cardiovasc Dis.* 2006;49(2):59–75.

19. Delahaye F. Should we eat less salt? *Arch Cardiovasc Dis.* 2013;106(5):324–32.

20. Jenkins DJ, Kendall CW. The garden of Eden: plant-based diets, the genetic drive to store fat and conserve cholesterol, and implications for epidemiology in the 21st century. *Epidemiology.* 2006;17(2):128–30.

21. Roberts WC. High salt intake, its origins, its economic impact, and its effect on blood pressure. *Am J Cardiol.* 2001;88(11):1338–46.

22. Roberts WC. High salt intake, its origins, its economic impact, and its effect on blood pressure. *Am J Cardiol.* 2001;88(11):1338–46.

23. Celermajer DS, Neal B. Excessive sodium intake and cardiovascular disease: a-salting our vessels. *J Am Coll Cardiol.* 2013;61(3):344–5.

24. Whelton PK, Appel LJ, Sacco RL, et al. Sodium, blood pressure, and cardiovascular disease: further evidence supporting the American Heart Association sodium reduction recommendations. *Circulation.* 2012;126(24):2880–9.

25. Centers for Disease Control and Prevention. Sodium intake among adults - United States, 2005–2006. *MMWR Morb Mortal Wkly Rep.* 2010;59(24):746–9.

26. Beaglehole R, Bonita R, Horton R, et al. Priority actions for the non-communicable disease crisis. *Lancet.* 2011;377(9775):1438–47.

27. Law MR, Frost CD, Wald NJ. By how much does dietary salt reduction lower blood pressure? III—Analysis of data from trials of salt reduction. *BMJ.* 1991;302(6780):819–24.

28. Bibbins-Domingo K, Chertow GM, Coxson PG, et al. Projected effect of dietary salt reductions on future cardiovascular disease. *N Engl J Med.* 2010 Feb 18;362(7):590–9.

29. MacGregor GA, Markandu ND, Best FE, et al. Double-blind randomised crossover trial of moderate sodium restriction in essential hypertension. *Lancet.* 1982;1(8268):351–5.

30. MacGregor GA, Markandu ND, Sagnella GA, Singer DR, Cappuccio FP. Double-blind study of three sodium intakes and long-term effects of sodium restriction in essential hypertension. *Lancet.* 1989;2(8674):1244–7.

31. MacGregor GA, Markandu ND, Sagnella GA, Singer DR, Cappuccio FP. Double-blind study of three sodium intakes and long-term effects of sodium restriction in essential hypertension. *Lancet.* 1989;2(8674):1244–7.

32. Rudelt A, French S, Harnack L. Fourteen-year trends in sodium content of menu offerings at eight leading fast-food restaurants in the USA. *Public Health Nutr.* 2014;17(8):1682–8.

33. Suckling RJ, He FJ, Markandu ND, MacGregor GA. Dietary salt influences postprandial plasma sodium concentration and systolic blood pressure. *Kidney Int.* 2012;81(4):407–11.

34. He FJ, Li J, MacGregor GA. Effect of longer term modest salt reduction on blood pressure: Cochrane systematic review and meta-analysis of randomised trials. *BMJ.* 2013;346:f1325.

35. Celermajer DS, Neal B. Excessive sodium intake and cardiovascular disease: a-salting our vessels. *J Am Coll Cardiol.* 2013;61(3):344–5.

36. Oliver WJ, Cohen EL, Neel JV. Blood pressure, sodium intake, and sodium related hormones in the Yanomamo Indians, a "no-salt" culture. *Circulation.* 1975;52(1):146–51.

37. Mancilha-Carvalho J de J, de Souza e Silva NA. The Yanomami Indians in the INTERSALT Study. *Arq Bras Cardiol.* 2003;80(3):289–300.

38. Celermajer DS, Neal B. Excessive sodium intake and cardiovascular disease: a-salting our vessels. *J Am Coll Cardiol.* 2013;61(3):344–5.

39. Mancilha-Carvalho J de J, de Souza e Silva NA. The Yanomami Indians in the INTERSALT Study. *Arq Bras Cardiol.* 2003;80(3):289–300.

40. Mancilha-Carvalho J de J, Crews DE. Lipid profiles of Yanomamo Indians of Brazil. *Prev Med.* 1990;19(1):66–75.

41. Kempner W. Treatment of heart and kidney disease and of hypertensive and arteriosclerotic vascular disease with the rice diet. *Ann Intern Med*. 1949;31(5):821–56.

42. Klemmer P, Grim CE, Luft FC. Who and what drove Walter Kempner? The rice diet revisited. *Hypertension*. 2014;64(4):684–8.

43. Kempner W. Treatment of heart and kidney disease and of hypertensive and arteriosclerotic vascular disease with the rice diet. *Ann Intern Med*. 1949;31(5):821–56.

44. Roberts WC. High salt intake, its origins, its economic impact, and its effect on blood pressure. *Am J Cardiol*. 2001;88(11):1338–46.

45. Dickinson KM, Clifton PM, Keogh JB. Endothelial function is impaired after a high-salt meal in healthy subjects. *Am J Clin Nutr*. 2011;93(3):500–5.

46. DuPont JJ, Greaney JL, Wenner MM, et al. High dietary sodium intake impairs endothelium-dependent dilation in healthy salt-resistant humans. *J Hypertens*. 2013;31(3):530–6.

47. Dickinson KM, Clifton PM, Keogh JB. Endothelial function is impaired after a high-salt meal in healthy subjects. *Am J Clin Nutr*. 2011;93(3):500–5.

48. Greaney JL, DuPont JJ, Lennon-Edwards SL, Sanders PW, Edwards DG, Farquhar WB. Dietary sodium loading impairs microvascular function independent of blood pressure in humans: role of oxidative stress. *J Physiol* (Lond). 2012;590(Pt 21):5519–28.

49. Jablonski KL, Racine ML, Geolfos CJ, et al. Dietary sodium restriction reverses vascular endothelial dysfunction in middle-aged/older adults with moderately elevated systolic blood pressure. *J Am Coll Cardiol*. 2013;61(3):335–43.

50. McCord JM. Analysis of superoxide dismutase activity. *Curr Protoc Toxicol*. 1999;Chapter 7: Unit 7.3.

51. Dickinson KM, Clifton PM, Burrell LM, Barrett PHR, Keogh JB. Postprandial effects of a high salt meal on serum sodium, arterial stiffness, markers of nitric oxide production and markers of endothelial function. *Atherosclerosis*. 2014;232(1):211–6.

52. *Huang Ti Nei Ching Su Wua* [*The Yellow Emperor's Classic of Internal Medicine*] (Veith I, Trans.) Oakland, CA: University of California Press; 1972:141.

53. Hanneman RL, Satin M. Comments to the Dietary Guidelines Committee on behalf of the Salt Institute. Comment ID: 000447. April 23, 2009.

54. Vital signs: food categories contributing the most to sodium consumption - United States, 2007–2008. *MMWR Morb Mortal Wkly Rep*. 2012;61(5):92–8.

55. Miller GD. Comments to the Dietary Guidelines Committee on behalf of the National Dairy Council, July 27, 2009.

56. Roberts WC. High salt intake, its origins, its economic impact, and its effect on blood pressure. *Am J Cardiol*. 2001;88(11):1338–46.

57. MacGregor G, de Wardener HE. Salt, blood pressure and health. *Int J Epidemiol*. 2002; 31(2):320–7.

58. Appel LJ, Anderson CAM. Compelling evidence for public health action to reduce salt intake. *N Engl J Med*. 2010;362(7):650–2.

59. Roberts WC. High salt intake, its origins, its economic impact, and its effect on blood pressure. *Am J Cardiol*. 2001;88(11):1338–46.

60. Buying this chicken? *Consum Rep*. June 2008;7.

61. Drewnowski A, Rehm CD. Sodium intakes of US children and adults from foods and beverages by location of origin and by specific food source. *Nutrients*. 2013;5(6):1840–55.

62. U.S. Department of Agriculture, Agricultural Research Service. 2014. USDA National Nutrient Database for Standard Reference, Release 27. Pizza Hut 14" pepperoni pizza, pan crust. http://ndb.nal.usda.gov/ndb/foods/show/6800. Accessed March 22, 2015.

63. Drewnowski A, Rehm CD. Sodium intakes of US children and adults from foods and beverages by location of origin and by specific food source. *Nutrients*. 2013;5(6):1840–55.

64. Blais CA, Pangborn RM, Borhani NO, Ferrell MF, Prineas RJ, Laing B. Effect of dietary sodium restriction on taste responses to sodium chloride: a longitudinal study. *Am J Clin Nutr*. 1986;44(2):232–43.

65. Tucker RM, Mattes RD. Are free fatty acids effective taste stimuli in humans? Presented at the symposium "The Taste for Fat: New Discoveries on the Role of Fat in Sensory Perception, Metabolism, Sensory Pleasure and Beyond" held at the Institute of Food Technologists 2011 Annual Meeting, New Orleans, LA, June 12, 2011. *J Food Sci*. 2012;77(3):S148–51.

66. Grieve FG, Vander Weg MW. Desire to eat high- and low-fat foods following a low-fat dietary intervention. *J Nutr Educ Behav*. 2003;35(2):98–102.

67. Stewart JE, Newman LP, Keast RS. Oral sensitivity to oleic acid is associated with fat intake and body mass index. *Clin Nutr*. 2011;30(6):838–44.

68. Stewart JE, Keast RS. Recent fat intake modulates fat taste sensitivity in lean and overweight subjects. *Int J Obes* (Lond). 2012;36(6):834–42.

69. Roberts WC. High salt intake, its origins, its economic impact, and its effect on blood pressure. *Am J Cardiol*. 2001;88(11):1338–46.

70. Newson RS, Elmadfa I, Biro G, et al. Barriers for progress in salt reduction in the general population. An international study. *Appetite*. 2013;71:22–31.

71. Cappuccio FP, Capewell S, Lincoln P, McPherson K. Policy options to reduce population salt intake. *BMJ*. 2011;343:d4995.

72. Toldrá F, Barat JM. Strategies for salt reduction in foods. *Recent Pat Food Nutr Agric*. 2012; 4(1):19–25.

73. Lin B-H, Guthrie J. Nutritional Quality of Food Prepared at Home and Away from Home, 1977–2008. USDA, Economic Research Service, December 2012.

74. Newson RS, Elmadfa I, Biro G, et al. Barriers for progress in salt reduction in the general population. An international study. *Appetite*. 2013;71:22–31.

75. Roberts WC. High salt intake, its origins, its economic impact, and its effect on blood pressure. *Am J Cardiol*. 2001;88(11):1338–46.

76. U.S. Department of Agriculture and U.S. Department of Health and Human Services. Dietary Guidelines for Americans, 2010. 7th Edition, Washington, D.C.: US Government Printing Office, December 2010.

77. Karppanen H, Mervaala E. Sodium intake and hypertension. *Prog Cardiovasc Dis*. 2006;49(2): 59–75.

78. Law MR, Morris JK, Wald NJ. Use of blood pressure lowering drugs in the prevention of cardiovascular disease: meta-analysis of 147 randomised trials in the context of expectations from prospective epidemiological studies. *BMJ*. 2009;338:b1665.

79. Tighe P, Duthie G, Vaughan N, et al. Effect of increased consumption of whole-grain foods on blood pressure and other cardiovascular risk markers in healthy middle-aged persons: a randomized controlled trial. *Am J Clin Nutr*. 2010;92(4):733–40.

80. Diaconu CC, Balaceanu A, Bartos D. Diuretics, first-line antihypertensive agents: are they always safe in the elderly? *Rom J Intern Med*. 2014;52(2):87–90.

81. Li CI, Daling JR, Tang MT, Haugen KL, Porter PL, Malone KE. Use of antihypertensive medications and breast cancer risk among women aged 55 to 74 years. *JAMA Intern Med*. 2013; 173(17):1629–37.

82. Kaiser EA, Lotze U, Schiser HH. Increasing complexity: which drug class to choose for treatment of hypertension in the elderly? *Clin Interv Aging*. 2014;9:459–75.

83. Rasmussen ER, Mey K, Bygum A. Angiotensin-converting enzyme inhibitor-induced angio-edema—a dangerous new epidemic. *Acta Derm Venereol*. 2014;94(3):260–4.

84. Tinetti ME, Han L, Lee DS, et al. Antihypertensive medications and serious fall injuries in a nationally representative sample of older adults. *JAMA Intern Med*. 2014;174(4):588–95.

85. Ye EQ, Chacko SA, Chou EL, Kugizaki M, Liu S. Greater whole-grain intake is associated with lower risk of type 2 diabetes, cardiovascular disease, and weight gain. *J Nutr*. 2012;142(7): 1304–13.

86. Aune D, Chan DS, Lau R, et al. Dietary fibre, whole grains, and risk of colorectal cancer: systematic review and dose-response meta-analysis of prospective studies. *BMJ*. 2011;343:d6617.

87. Tighe P, Duthie G, Vaughan N, et al. Effect of increased consumption of whole-grain foods on blood pressure and other cardiovascular risk markers in healthy middle-aged persons: a randomized controlled trial. *Am J Clin Nutr*. 2010;92(4):733–40.

88. Sun Q, Spiegelman D, van Dam RM, et al. White rice, brown rice, and risk of type 2 diabetes in US men and women. *Arch Intern Med*. 2010;170(11):961–9.

89. Ye EQ, Chacko SA, Chou EL, Kugizaki M, Liu S. Greater whole-grain intake is associated with lower risk of type 2 diabetes, cardiovascular disease, and weight gain. *J Nutr*. 2012;142(7):1304–13.

90. Mellen PB, Liese AD, Tooze JA, Vitolins MZ, Wagenknecht LE, Herrington DM. Whole-grain intake and carotid artery atherosclerosis in a multiethnic cohort: the Insulin Resistance Atherosclerosis Study. *Am J Clin Nutr*. 2007;85(6):1495–502.

91. Erkkilä AT, Herrington DM, Mozaffarian D, et al. Cereal fiber and whole-grain intake are associated with reduced progression of coronary-artery atherosclerosis in postmenopausal women with coronary artery disease. *Am Heart J*. 2005;150(1):94–101.

92. Go AS, Bauman MA, Coleman King SM, et al. An effective approach to high blood pressure control: a science advisory from the American Heart Association, the American College of Cardiology, and the Centers for Disease Control and Prevention. *J Am Coll Cardiol*. 2014;63(12):1230–8.

93. Mahmud A, Feely J. Low-dose quadruple antihypertensive combination: more efficacious than individual agents—a preliminary report. *Hypertension*. 2007;49(2):272–5.

94. Kronish IM, Woodward M, Sergie Z, Ogedegbe G, Falzon L, Mann DM. Meta-analysis: impact of drug class on adherence to antihypertensives. *Circulation*. 2011;123(15):1611–21.

95. Messerli FH, Bangalore S. Half a century of hydrochlorothiazide: facts, fads, fiction, and follies. *Am J Med*. 2011;124(10):896–9.

96. Law MR, Morris JK, Wald NJ. Use of blood pressure lowering drugs in the prevention of cardiovascular disease: meta-analysis of 147 randomised trials in the context of expectations from prospective epidemiological studies. *BMJ*. 2009;338:b1665.

97. Donnison CP. Blood pressure in the African native. *Lancet*. 1929;213(5497):6–7.

98. Morse WR, McGill MD, Beh YT. Blood pressure amongst aboriginal ethnic groups of Szechwan Province, West China. *Lancet*. 1937;229(5929):966–8.

99. Sacks FM, Kass EH. Low blood pressure in vegetarians: effects of specific foods and nutrients. *Am J Clin Nutr*. 1988;48(3 Suppl):795–800.

100. Go AS, Bauman MA, Coleman King SM, et al. An effective approach to high blood pressure control: a science advisory from the American Heart Association, the American College of Cardiology, and the Centers for Disease Control and Prevention. *J Am Coll Cardiol*. 2014; 63(12):1230–8.

101. Sharma AM, Schorr U. Dietary patterns and blood pressure. *N Engl J Med*. 1997;337(9):637.

102. Chen Q, Turban S, Miller ER, Appel LJ. The effects of dietary patterns on plasma renin activity: results from the Dietary Approaches to Stop Hypertension trial. *J Hum Hypertens*. 2012; 26(11):664–9.

103. Sacks FM, Rosner B, Kass EH. Blood pressure in vegetarians. *Am J Epidemiol*. 1974;100(5): 390–8.

104. Donaldson AN. The relation of protein foods to hypertension. *Cal West Med*. 1926;24(3):328–31.

105. Appel LJ, Brands MW, Daniels SR, et al. Dietary approaches to prevent and treat hypertension: a scientific statement from the American Heart Association. *Hypertension*. 2006;47(2): 296–308.

106. Sacks FM, Obarzanek E, Windhauser MM, et al. Rationale and design of the Dietary Approaches to Stop Hypertension trial (DASH). A multicenter controlled-feeding study of dietary patterns to lower blood pressure. *Ann Epidemiol*. 1995;5(2):108–18.

107. Karanja NM, Obarzanek E, Lin PH, et al. Descriptive characteristics of the dietary patterns used in the Dietary Approaches to Stop Hypertension trial. DASH Collaborative Research Group. *J Am Diet Assoc*. 1999;99(8 Suppl):S19–27.

108. Sacks FM, Kass EH. Low blood pressure in vegetarians: effects of specific foods and nutrients. *Am J Clin Nutr*. 1988;48(3 Suppl):795–800.

109. de Paula TP, Steemburgo T, de Almeida JC, Dall'Alba V, Gross JL, de Azevedo MJ. The role of Dietary Approaches to Stop Hypertension (DASH) diet food groups in blood pressure in type 2 diabetes. *Br J Nutr*. 2012;108(1):155–62.

110. Yokoyama Y, Nishimura K, Barnard ND, et al. Vegetarian diets and blood pressure: a meta-analysis. *JAMA Intern Med*. 2014;174(4):577–87.

111. Le LT, Sabaté J. Beyond meatless, the health effects of vegan diets: findings from the Adventist cohorts. *Nutrients*. 2014;6(6):2131–47.

112. Fraser GE. Vegetarian diets: what do we know of their effects on common chronic diseases? *Am J Clin Nutr*. 2009;89(5):1607S–1612S.

113. Tonstad S, Stewart K, Oda K, Batech M, Herring RP, Fraser GE. Vegetarian diets and incidence of diabetes in the Adventist Health Study-2. *Nutr Metab Cardiovasc Dis*. 2013;23(4):292–9.

114. Fraser GE. Vegetarian diets: what do we know of their effects on common chronic diseases? *Am J Clin Nutr*. 2009;89(5):1607S–1612S.

115. Fontana L, Meyer TE, Klein S, Holloszy JO. Long-term low-calorie low-protein vegan diet and endurance exercise are associated with low cardiometabolic risk. *Rejuvenation Res*. 2007;10(2):225–34.

116. Rodriguez-Leyva D, Weighell W, Edel AL, et al. Potent antihypertensive action of dietary flaxseed in hypertensive patients. *Hypertension*. 2013;62(6):1081–9.

117. Cornelissen VA, Buys R, Smart NA. Endurance exercise beneficially affects ambulatory blood pressure: a systematic review and meta-analysis. *J Hypertens*. 2013;31(4):639–48.

118. Geleijnse JM. Relation of raw and cooked vegetable consumption to blood pressure: the INTERMAP study. *J Hum Hypertens*. 2014;28(6):343–4.

119. Jayalath VH, de Souza RJ, Sievenpiper JL, et al. Effect of dietary pulses on blood pressure: a systematic review and meta-analysis of controlled feeding trials. *Am J Hypertens*. 2014;27(1): 56–64.

120. Chiva-Blanch G, Urpi-Sarda M, Ros E, et al. Dealcoholized red wine decreases systolic and diastolic blood pressure and increases plasma nitric oxide: short communication. *Circ Res*. 2012;111(8):1065–8.

121. Figueroa A, Sanchez-Gonzalez MA, Wong A, Arjmandi BH. Watermelon extract supplementation reduces ankle blood pressure and carotid augmentation index in obese adults with prehypertension or hypertension. *Am J Hypertens*. 2012;25(6):640–3.

122. Gammon CS, Kruger R, Brown SJ, Conlon CA, von Hurst PR, Stonehouse W. Daily kiwifruit consumption did not improve blood pressure and markers of cardiovascular function in men with hypercholesterolemia. *Nutr Res*. 2014;34(3):235–40.

123. Anderson JW, Weiter KM, Christian AL, Ritchey MB, Bays HE. Raisins compared with other snack effects on glycemia and blood pressure: a randomized, controlled trial. *Postgrad Med.* 2014;126(1):37–43.

124. Akhtar S, Ismail T, Riaz M. Flaxseed - a miraculous defense against some critical maladies. *Pak J Pharm Sci.* 2013;26(1):199–208.

125. Rodriguez-Leyva D, Weighell W, Edel AL, et al. Potent antihypertensive action of dietary flaxseed in hypertensive patients. *Hypertension.* 2013;62(6):1081–9.

126. Ninomiya T, Perkovic V, Turnbull F, et al. Blood pressure lowering and major cardiovascular events in people with and without chronic kidney disease: meta-analysis of randomised controlled trials. *BMJ.* 2013;347:f5680.

127. Goyal A, Sharma V, Upadhyay N, Gill S, Sihag M. Flax and flaxseed oil: an ancient medicine & modern functional food. *J Food Sci Technol.* 2014;51(9):1633–53.

128. Carlsen MH, Halvorsen BL, Holte K, et al. The total antioxidant content of more than 3100 foods, beverages, spices, herbs and supplements used worldwide. *Nutr J.* 2010;9:3.

129. Frank T, Netzel G, Kammerer DR, et al. Consumption of Hibiscus sabdariffa L. aqueous extract and its impact on systemic antioxidant potential in healthy subjects. *J Sci Food Agric.* 2012;92(10):2207–18.

130. Chang HC, Peng CH, Yeh DM, Kao ES, Wang CJ. Hibiscus sabdariffa extract inhibits obesity and fat accumulation, and improves liver steatosis in humans. *Food Funct.* 2014;5(4):734–9.

131. Mozaffari-Khosravi H, Jalali-Khanabadi BA, Afkhami-Ardekani M, Fatehi F. Effects of sour tea (Hibiscus sabdariffa) on lipid profile and lipoproteins in patients with type II diabetes. *J Altern Complement Med.* 2009;15(8):899–903.

132. Aziz Z, Wong SY, Chong NJ. Effects of Hibiscus sabdariffa L. on serum lipids: a systematic review and meta-analysis. *J Ethnopharmacol.* 2013;150(2):442–50.

133. Lin T-L. Lin H-H, Chen C-C, et al. Hibiscus sabdariffa extract reduces serum cholesterol in men and women. *Nutr Res.* 2007;27:140–5.

134. Hopkins AL, Lamm MG, Funk JL, Ritenbaugh C. Hibiscus sabdariffa L. in the treatment of hypertension and hyperlipidemia: a comprehensive review of animal and human studies. *Fitoterapia.* 2013;85:84–94.

135. McKay DL, Chen CY, Saltzman E, Blumberg JB. Hibiscus sabdariffa L. tea (tisane) lowers blood pressure in prehypertensive and mildly hypertensive adults. *J Nutr.* 2010;140(2):298–303.

136. Chobanian AV, Bakris GL, Black HR, et al. Seventh report of the Joint National Committee on Prevention, Detection, Evaluation, and Treatment of High Blood Pressure. *Hypertension.* 2003;42(6):1206–52.

137. McKay DL, Chen CY, Saltzman E, Blumberg JB. Hibiscus sabdariffa L. tea (tisane) lowers blood pressure in prehypertensive and mildly hypertensive adults. *J Nutr.* 2010;140(2):298–303.

138. Herrera-Arellano A, Flores-Romero S, Chávez-Soto MA, Tortoriello J. Effectiveness and tolerability of a standardized extract from Hibiscus sabdariffa in patients with mild to moderate hypertension: a controlled and randomized clinical trial. *Phytomedicine.* 2004;11(5): 375–82.

139. US Food and Drug Administration. CAPOTEN® (Captopril Tablets, USP) http://www.accessdata.fda.gov/drugsatfda_docs/label/2012/018343s084lbl.pdf. Accessed March 19, 2015.

140. Hendricks JL, Marshall TA, Harless JD, Hogan MM, Qian F, Wefel JS. Erosive potentials of brewed teas. *Am J Dent.* 2013;26(5):278–82.

141. Malik J, Frankova A, Drabek O, Szakova J, Ash C, Kokoska L. Aluminium and other elements in selected herbal tea plant species and their infusions. *Food Chem.* 2013;139(1–4):728–34.

142. Förstermann U. Janus-faced role of endothelial NO synthase in vascular disease: uncoupling

of oxygen reduction from NO synthesis and its pharmacological reversal. *Biol Chem*. 2006; 387(12):1521–33.

143. Franzini L, Ardigò D, Valtueña S, et al. Food selection based on high total antioxidant capacity improves endothelial function in a low cardiovascular risk population. *Nutr Metab Cardiovasc Dis*. 2012;22(1):50–7.

144. Webb AJ, Patel N, Loukogeorgakis S, et al. Acute blood pressure lowering, vasoprotective, and antiplatelet properties of dietary nitrate via bioconversion to nitrite. *Hypertension*. 2008;51(3):784–90.

145. Smith RE, Ashiya M. Antihypertensive therapies. *Nat Rev Drug Discov*. 2007;6(8):597–8.

146. Kapil V, Khambata RS, Robertson A, Caulfield MJ, Ahluwalia A. Dietary nitrate provides sustained blood pressure lowering in hypertensive patients: a randomized, phase 2, double-blind, placebo-controlled study. *Hypertension*. 2015;65(2):320–7.

147. Wylie LJ, Kelly J, Bailey SJ, et al. Beetroot juice and exercise: pharmacodynamic and dose-response relationships. *J Appl Physiol*. 2013;115(3):325–36.

148. European Food Safety Authority. Nitrate in vegetables: scientific opinion of the panel on contaminants in the food chain. *EFSA J*. 2008;689:1–79.

149. Murphy M, Eliot K, Heuertz RM, Weiss E. Whole beetroot consumption acutely improves running performance. *J Acad Nutr Diet*. 2012;112(4):548–52.

150. Clements WT, Lee SR, Bloomer RJ. Nitrate ingestion: a review of the health and physical performance effects. *Nutrients*. 2014;6(11):5224–64.

151. Hord NG, Tang Y, Bryan NS. Food sources of nitrates and nitrites: the physiologic context for potential health benefits. *Am J Clin Nutr*. 2009;90(1):1–10.

152. Bhupathiraju SN, Wedick NM, Pan A, et al. Quantity and variety in fruit and vegetable intake and risk of coronary heart disease. *Am J Clin Nutr*. 2013;98(6):1514–23.

153. Tamakoshi A, Tamakoshi K, Lin Y, Yagyu K, Kikuchi S. Healthy lifestyle and preventable death: findings from the Japan Collaborative Cohort (JACC) Study. *Prev Med*. 2009;48(5):486–92.

154. Wang F, Dai S, Wang M, Morrison H. Erectile dysfunction and fruit/vegetable consumption among diabetic Canadian men. *Urology*. 2013;82(6):1330–5.

155. Presley TD, Morgan AR, Bechtold E, et al. Acute effect of a high nitrate diet on brain perfusion in older adults. *Nitric Oxide*. 2011;24(1):34–42.

156. Engan HK, Jones AM, Ehrenberg F, Schagatay E. Acute dietary nitrate supplementation improves dry static apnea performance. *Respir Physiol Neurobiol*. 2012;182(2–3):53–9.

157. Bailey SJ, Winyard P, Vanhatalo A, et al. Dietary nitrate supplementation reduces the O2 cost of low-intensity exercise and enhances tolerance to high-intensity exercise in humans. *J Appl Physiol*. 2009;107(4):1144–55.

158. Murphy M, Eliot K, Heuertz RM, Weiss E. Whole beetroot consumption acutely improves running performance. *J Acad Nutr Diet*. 2012;112(4):548–52.

159. Lidder S, Webb AJ. Vascular effects of dietary nitrate (as found in green leafy vegetables and beetroot) via the nitrate-nitrite-nitric oxide pathway. *Br J Clin Pharmacol*. 2013;75(3):677–96.

160. Wylie LJ, Kelly J, Bailey SJ, et al. Beetroot juice and exercise: pharmacodynamic and dose-response relationships. *J Appl Physiol*. 2013;115(3):325–36.

8. How Not to Die from Liver Diseases

1. Chiras, DD. *Human Biology*. Burlington, MA: Jones & Bartlett Learning; 2015.

2. Centers for Disease Control and Prevention. Deaths: final data for 2013 table 10. Number of deaths from 113 selected causes. National Vital Statistics Report 2016;64(2).

3. National Cancer Institute Surveillance, Epidemiology, and End Results Program. SEER stat fact sheets: liver and intrahepatic bile duct cancer. http://seer.cancer.gov/statfacts/html/livibd.html. Accessed May 3, 2015.

4. Holubek WJ, Kalman S, Hoffman RS. Acetaminophen-induced acute liver failure: results of a United States multicenter, prospective study. *Hepatology.* 2006;43(4):880.

5. Mokdad AH, Marks JS, Stroup DF, Gerberding JL. Actual causes of death in the United States, 2000. *JAMA.* 2004;291(10):1238–45.

6. CDC Morbidity and Mortality Weekly Report. Alcohol-attributable deaths and years of potential life l—United States, 2001. http://www.cdc.gov/mmwr/preview/mmwrhtml/mm5337a2 .htm. September 24, 2004. Accessed March 2, 2015.

7. Centers for Disease Control and Prevention. Fact sheets - alcohol use and your health. http://www.cdc.gov/alcohol/fact-sheets/alcohol-use.htm. November 7, 2014. Accessed March 2, 2015.

8. Schwartz JM, Reinus JF. Prevalence and natural history of alcoholic liver disease. *Clin Liver Dis.* 2012;16(4):659–66.

9. Lane BP, Lieber CS. Ultrastructural alterations in human hepatocytes following ingestion of ethanol with adequate diets. *Am J Pathol.* 1966;49(4):593–603.

10. Mendenhall CL. Anabolic steroid therapy as an adjunct to diet in alcoholic hepatic steatosis. *Am J Dig Dis.* 1968;13(9):783–91.

11. O'Shea RS, Dasarathy S, McCullough AJ. Alcoholic liver disease. *Hepatology.* 2010;51(1):307–28.

12. Mandayam S, Jamal MM, Morgan TR. Epidemiology of alcoholic liver disease. *Semin Liver Dis.* 2004;24(3):217–32.

13. Galambos JT. Natural history of alcoholic hepatitis. 3. Histological changes. *Gastroenterology.* 1972;63(6):1026–35.

14. Woerle S, Roeber J, Landen MG. Prevalence of alcohol dependence among excessive drinkers in New Mexico. *Alcohol Clin Exp Res.* 2007;31(2):293–8.

15. Kaskutas LA. Alcoholics anonymous effectiveness: faith meets science. *J Addict Dis.* 2009;28(2):145–57.

16. Grønbaek M. The positive and negative health effects of alcohol and the public health implications. *J Intern Med.* 2009;265(4):407–20.

17. Britton A, Marmot MG, Shipley M. Who benefits most from the cardioprotective properties of alcohol consumption—health freaks or couch potatoes? *J Epidemiol Community Health.* 2008;62(10):905–8.

18. Agarwal DP. Cardioprotective effects of light-moderate consumption of alcohol: a review of putative mechanisms. *Alcohol Alcohol.* 2002;37(5):409–15.

19. Britton A, Marmot MG, Shipley M. Who benefits most from the cardioprotective properties of alcohol consumption—health freaks or couch potatoes? *J Epidemiol Community Health.* 2008;62(10):905–8.

20. Britton A, Marmot MG, Shipley M. Who benefits most from the cardioprotective properties of alcohol consumption—health freaks or couch potatoes? *J Epidemiol Community Health.* 2008;62(10):905–8.

21. Kechagias S, Ernersson Å, Dahlqvist O, et al. Fast-food-based hyper-alimentation can induce rapid and profound elevation of serum alanine aminotransferase in healthy subjects. *Gut.* 2008;57(5):649–54.

22. McCarthy EM, Rinella ME. The role of diet and nutrient composition in nonalcoholic fatty liver disease. *J Acad Nutr Diet.* 2012;112(3):401–9.

23. Silverman JF, Pories WJ, Caro JF. Liver pathology in diabetes mellitus and morbid obesity: clinical, pathological and biochemical considerations. *Pathol Annu.* 1989;24:275–302.

24. Singh S, Allen AM, Wang Z, Prokop LJ, Murad MH, Loomba R. Fibrosis progression in nonalcoholic fatty liver vs nonalcoholic steatohepatitis: a systematic review and meta-analysis of paired-biopsy studies. *Clin Gastroenterol Hepatol.* 2014;S1542–3565(14):00602–8.

25. Zelber-Sagi S, Nitzan-Kaluski D, Goldsmith R, et al. Long term nutritional intake and the risk for non-alcoholic fatty liver disease (NAFLD): a population based study. *J Hepatol.* 2007; 47(5):711–7.

26. Zelber-Sagi S, Nitzan-Kaluski D, Goldsmith R, et al. Long term nutritional intake and the risk for non-alcoholic fatty liver disease (NAFLD): a population based study. *J Hepatol.* 2007; 47(5):711–7.

27. Longato L. Non-alcoholic fatty liver disease (NAFLD): a tale of fat and sugar? *Fibrogenesis Tissue Repair.* 2013;6(1):14.

28. Musso G, Gambino R, De Michieli F, et al. Dietary habits and their relations to insulin resistance and postprandial lipemia in nonalcoholic steatohepatitis. *Hepatology.* 2003;37(4):909–16.

29. Kontogianni MD, Tileli N, Margariti A, et al. Adherence to the Mediterranean diet is associated with the severity of non-alcoholic fatty liver disease. *Clin Nutr.* 2014;33(4):678–83.

30. Kim EJ, Kim BH, Seo HS, et al. Cholesterol-induced non-alcoholic fatty liver disease and atherosclerosis aggravated by systemic inflammation. *PLoS ONE.* 2014;9(6):e97841.

31. Yasutake K, Nakamuta M, Shima Y, et al. Nutritional investigation of non-obese patients with non-alcoholic fatty liver disease: the significance of dietary cholesterol. *Scand J Gastroenterol.* 2009;44(4):471–7.

32. Duewell P, Kono H, Rayner KJ, et al. NLRP3 inflammasomes are required for atherogenesis and activated by cholesterol crystals that form early in disease. *Nature.* 2010;464(7293): 1357–61.

33. Ioannou GN, Haigh WG, Thorning D, Savard C. Hepatic cholesterol crystals and crown-like structures distinguish NASH from simple steatosis. *J Lipid Res.* 2013;54(5):1326–34.

34. U.S. Department of Agriculture Agricultural Research Service. National Nutrient Database for Standard Reference Release 27. Basic Report: 21359, McDonald's, sausage McMuffin with egg. http://ndb.nal.usda.gov/ndb/foods/show/6845. Accessed March 2, 2015.

35. Ioannou GN, Morrow OB, Connole ML, Lee SP. Association between dietary nutrient composition and the incidence of cirrhosis or liver cancer in the United States population. *Hepatology.* 2009;50(1):175–84.

36. National Institute of Diabetes and Digestive and Kidney Diseases. Liver transplantation. http://www.niddk.nih.gov/health-information/health-topics/liver-disease/liver-transplant /Pages/facts.aspx. June 2010. Accessed March 2, 2015.

37. Kwak JH, Baek SH, Woo Y, et al. Beneficial immunostimulatory effect of short-term Chlorella supplementation: enhancement of natural killer cell activity and early inflammatory response (randomized, double-blinded, placebo-controlled trial). *Nutr J.* 2012;11:53.

38. Azocar J, Diaz A. Efficacy and safety of Chlorella supplementation in adults with chronic hepatitis C virus infection. *World J Gastroenterol.* 2013 Feb 21;19(7):1085–90.

39. Goozner M. Why Sovaldi shouldn't cost $84,000. *Mod Healthc.* 2014;44(18):26.

40. Lock G, Dirscherl M, Obermeier F, et al. Hepatitis C - contamination of toothbrushes: myth or reality? *J Viral Hepat.* 2006;13(9):571–3.

41. Bocket L, Chevaliez S, Talbodec N, Sobaszek A, Pawlotsky JM, Yazdanpanah Y. Occupational transmission of hepatitis C virus resulting from use of the same supermarket meat slicer. *Clin Microbiol Infect.* 2011;17(2):238–41.

42. Teo CG. Much meat, much malady: changing perceptions of the epidemiology of hepatitis E. *Clin Microbiol Infect.* 2010;16(1):24–32.

43. Yazaki Y, Mizuo H, Takahashi M, et al. Sporadic acute or fulminant hepatitis E in Hokkaido,

Japan, may be food-borne, as suggested by the presence of hepatitis E virus in pig liver as food. *J Gen Virol*. 2003;84(Pt 9):2351–7.

44. Feagins AR, Opriessnig T, Guenette DK, Halbur PG, Meng XJ. Detection and characterization of infectious Hepatitis E virus from commercial pig livers sold in local grocery stores in the USA. *J Gen Virol*. 2007;88(Pt 3):912–7.

45. Feagins AR, Opriessnig T, Guenette DK, Halbur PG, Meng XJ. Detection and characterization of infectious Hepatitis E virus from commercial pig livers sold in local grocery stores in the USA. *J Gen Virol*. 2007;88(Pt 3):912–7.

46. Dalton HR, Bendall RP, Pritchard C, Henley W, Melzer D. National mortality rates from chronic liver disease and consumption of alcohol and pig meat. *Epidemiol Infect*. 2010;138(2): 174–82.

47. Emerson SU, Arankalle VA, Purcell RH. Thermal stability of hepatitis E virus. *J Infect Dis*. 2005 Sep 1;192(5):930–3.

48. Centers for Disease Control and Prevention. What can you do to protect yourself and your family from food poisoning? http://www.cdc.gov/foodsafety/prevention.html. September 6, 2013. Accessed March 11, 2015.

49. Shinde NR, Patil TB, Deshpande AS, Gulhane RV, Patil MB, Bansod YV. Clinical profile, maternal and fetal outcomes of acute hepatitis E in pregnancy. *Ann Med Health Sci Res*. 2014; 4(Suppl 2):S133–9.

50. Navarro VJ, Barnhart H, Bonkovsky HL, et al. Liver injury from herbals and dietary supplements in the U.S. Drug-Induced Liver Injury Network. *Hepatology*. 2014;60(4):1399–408.

51. Yu EL, Sivagnanam M, Ellis L, Huang JS. Acute hepatotoxicity after ingestion of Morinda citrifolia (Noni Berry) juice in a 14-year-old boy. *J Pediatr Gastroenterol Nutr*. 2011;52(2):222–4.

52. Licata A, Craxt A. Considerations regarding the alleged association between Herbalife products and cases of hepatotoxicity: a rebuttal. *Intern Emerg Med*. 2014;9(5):601–2.

53. Lobb AL. Science in liquid dietary supplement promotion: the misleading case of mangosteen juice. *Hawaii J Med Public Health*. 2012;71(2):46–8.

54. Lobb AL. Science in liquid dietary supplement promotion: the misleading case of mangosteen juice. *Hawaii J Med Public Health*. 2012;71(2):46–8.

55. Boozer CN, Nasser JA, Heymsfield SB, Wang V, Chen G, Solomon JL. An herbal supplement containing Ma Huang-Guarana for weight loss: a randomized, double-blind trial. *Int J Obes Relat Metab Disord*. 2001;25(3):316–24.

56. US Government Accountability Office. Dietary Supplements Containing Ephedra: Health Risks and FDA's Oversight. http://www.gao.gov/assets/120/110228.pdf. July 23, 2003. Accessed March 2, 2015.

57. Preuss HG, Bagchi D, Bagchi M, Rao CV, Dey DK, Satyanarayana S. Effects of a natural extract of (-)-hydroxycitric acid (HCA-SX) and a combination of HCA-SX plus niacin-bound chromium and Gymnema sylvestre extract on weight loss. *Diabetes Obes Metab*. 2004;6(3):171–80.

58. Fong TL, Klontz KC, Canas-Coto A, et al. Hepatotoxicity due to hydroxycut: a case series. *Am J Gastroenterol*. 2010;105(7):1561–6.

59. Ye EQ, Chacko SA, Chou EL, Kugizaki M, Liu S. Greater whole-grain intake is associated with lower risk of type 2 diabetes, cardiovascular disease, and weight gain. *J Nutr*. 2012;142(7):1304–13.

60. Karl JP, Saltzman E. The role of whole grains in body weight regulation. *Adv Nutr*. 2012; 3(5):697–707.

61. Ye EQ, Chacko SA, Chou EL, Kugizaki M, Liu S. Greater whole-grain intake is associated with lower risk of type 2 diabetes, cardiovascular disease, and weight gain. *J Nutr*. 2012;142(7): 1304–13.

62. Chang H-C, Huang C-N, Yeh D-M, Wang S-J, Peng C-H, Wang C-J. Oat prevents obesity and

abdominal fat distribution, and improves liver function in humans. *Plant Foods Hum Nutr.* 2013;68(1):18–23.

63. Chang H-C, Huang C-N, Yeh D-M, Wang S-J, Peng C-H, Wang C-J. Oat prevents obesity and abdominal fat distribution, and improves liver function in humans. *Plant Foods Hum Nutr.* 2013;68(1):18–23.

64. Georgoulis M, Kontogianni MD, Tileli N, et al. The impact of cereal grain consumption on the development and severity of non-alcoholic fatty liver disease. *Eur J Nutr.* 2014;53(8):1727–35.

65. Valenti L, Riso P, Mazzocchi A, Porrini M, Fargion S, Agostoni C. Dietary anthocyanins as nutritional therapy for nonalcoholic fatty liver disease. *Oxid Med Cell Longev.* 2013;2013:145421.

66. Suda I, Ishikawa F, Hatakeyama M, et al. Intake of purple sweet potato beverage affects on serum hepatic biomarker levels of healthy adult men with borderline hepatitis. *Eur J Clin Nutr.* 2008;62(1):60–7.

67. Sun J, Chu YF, Wu X, Liu RH. Antioxidant and antiproliferative activities of common fruits. *J Agric Food Chem.* 2002;50(25):7449–54.

68. Ferguson PJ, Kurowska EM, Freeman DJ, Chambers AF, Koropatnick J. In vivo inhibition of growth of human tumor lines by flavonoid fractions from cranberry extract. *Nutr Cancer.* 2006;56(1):86–94.

69. Sun J, Hai Liu R. Cranberry phytochemical extracts induce cell cycle arrest and apoptosis in human MCF-7 breast cancer cells. *Cancer Lett.* 2006;241(1):124–34.

70. Ferguson PJ, Kurowska EM, Freeman DJ, Chambers AF, Koropatnick J. In vivo inhibition of growth of human tumor lines by flavonoid fractions from cranberry extract. *Nutr Cancer.* 2006; 56(1):86–94.

71. Kresty LA, Howell AB, Baird M. Cranberry proanthocyanidins mediate growth arrest of lung cancer cells through modulation of gene expression and rapid induction of apoptosis. *Molecules.* 2011;16(3):2375–90.

72. Seeram NP, Adams LS, Zhang Y, et al. Blackberry, black raspberry, blueberry, cranberry, red raspberry, and strawberry extracts inhibit growth and stimulate apoptosis of human cancer cells in vitro. *J Agric Food Chem.* 2006;54(25):9329–39.

73. Kim KK, Singh AP, Singh RK, et al. Anti-angiogenic activity of cranberry proanthocyanidins and cytotoxic properties in ovarian cancer cells. *Int J Oncol.* 2012;40(1):227–35.

74. Déziel B, MacPhee J, Patel K, et al. American cranberry (Vaccinium macrocarpon) extract affects human prostate cancer cell growth via cell cycle arrest by modulating expression of cell cycle regulators. *Food Funct.* 2012;3(5):556–64.

75. Liu M, Lin LQ, Song BB, et al. Cranberry phytochemical extract inhibits SGC-7901 cell growth and human tumor xenografts in Balb/c nu/nu mice. *J Agric Food Chem.* 2009;57(2):762–8.

76. Seeram NP, Adams LS, Hardy ML, Heber D. Total cranberry extract versus its phytochemical constituents: antiproliferative and synergistic effects against human tumor cell lines. *J Agric Food Chem.* 2004;52(9):2512–7.

77. Grace MH, Massey AR, Mbeunkui F, Yousef GG, Lila MA. Comparison of health-relevant flavonoids in commonly consumed cranberry products. *J Food Sci.* 2012;77(8):H176–83.

78. Grace MH, Massey AR, Mbeunkui F, Yousef GG, Lila MA. Comparison of health-relevant flavonoids in commonly consumed cranberry products. *J Food Sci.* 2012;77(8):H176–83.

79. Vinson JA, Bose P, Proch J, Al Kharrat H, Samman N. Cranberries and cranberry products: powerful in vitro, ex vivo, and in vivo sources of antioxidants. *J Agric Food Chem.* 2008; 56(14):5884–91.

80. White BL, Howard LR, Prior RL. Impact of different stages of juice processing on the anthocyanin, flavonol, and procyanidin contents of cranberries. *J Agric Food Chem.* 2011;59(9):4692–8.

81. Arnesen E, Huseby N-E, Brenn T, Try K. The Tromse heart study: distribution of, and deter-

minants for, gamma-glutamyltransferase in a free-living population. *Scand J Clin Lab Invest.* 1986;46(1):63–70.

82. Ruhl CE, Everhart JE. Coffee and tea consumption are associated with a lower incidence of chronic liver disease in the United States. *Gastroenterology.* 2005;129(6):1928–36.

83. Salgia R, Singal AG. Hepatocellular carcinoma and other liver lesions. *Med Clin North Am.* 2014;98(1):103–18.

84. Sang LX, Chang B, Li X-H, Jiang M. Consumption of coffee associated with reduced risk of liver cancer: a meta-analysis. *BMC Gastroenterol.* 2013;13:34.

85. Lai GY, Weinstein SJ, Albanes D, et al. The association of coffee intake with liver cancer incidence and chronic liver disease mortality in male smokers. *Br J Cancer.* 2013;109(5):1344–51.

86. Fujita Y, Shibata A, Ogimoto I, et al. The effect of interaction between hepatitis C virus and cigarette smoking on the risk of hepatocellular carcinoma. *Br J Cancer.* 2006;94(5):737–9.

87. Danielsson J, Kangastupa P, Laatikainen T, Aalto M, Niemelä O. Dose- and gender-dependent interactions between coffee consumption and serum GGT activity in alcohol consumers. *Alcohol Alcohol.* 2013;48(3):303–7.

88. Bravi F, Bosetti C, Tavani A, Gallus S, La Vecchia C. Coffee reduces risk for hepatocellular carcinoma: an meta-analysis. *Clin Gastroenterol Hepatol.* 2013;11(11):1413–21.e1.

89. Browning JD, Szczepaniak LS, Dobbins R, et al. Prevalence of hepatic steatosis in an urban population in the United States: impact of ethnicity. *Hepatology.* 2004;40(6):1387–95.

90. Cardin R, Piciocchi M, Martines D, Scribano L, Petracco M, Farinati F. Effects of coffee consumption in chronic hepatitis C: a randomized controlled trial. *Dig Liver Dis.* 2013;45(6): 499–504.

91. Torres DM, Harrison SA. Is it time to write a prescription for coffee? Coffee and liver disease. *Gastroenterology.* 2013;144(4):670–2.

92. Ng V, Saab S. Can daily coffee consumption reduce liver disease-related mortality? *Clin Gastroenterol Hepatol.* 2013;11(11):1422–3.

93. Torres DM, Harrison SA. Is it time to write a prescription for coffee? Coffee and liver disease. *Gastroenterology.* 2013;144(4):670–2.

94. Juliano LM, Griffiths RR. A critical review of caffeine withdrawal: empirical validation of symptoms and signs, incidence, severity, and associated features. *Psychopharmacology* (Berl). 2004; 176(1):1–29.

95. O'Keefe JH, Bhatti SK, Patil HR, DiNicolantonio JJ, Lucan SC, Lavie CJ. Effects of habitual coffee consumption on cardiometabolic disease, cardiovascular health, and all-cause mortality. *J Am Coll Cardiol.* 2013;62(12):1043–51.

9. How Not to Die from Blood Cancers

1. Hunger SP, Lu X, Devidas M, et al. Improved survival for children and adolescents with acute lymphoblastic leukemia between 1990 and 2005: a report from the children's oncology group. *J Clin Oncol.* 2012;30(14):1663–9.

2. National Cancer Institute Surveillance, Epidemiology, and End Results Program. SEER Stat Fact Sheets: Leukemia. http://seer.cancer.gov/statfacts/html/leuks.html. Accessed June 15, 2015.

3. American Cancer Society. Cancer Facts & Figures 2014. Atlanta: American Cancer Society; 2014.

4. American Cancer Society. Cancer Facts & Figures 2014. Atlanta: American Cancer Society; 2014.

5. American Cancer Society. Cancer Facts & Figures 2014. Atlanta: American Cancer Society; 2014.

6. Key TJ, Appleby PN, Spencer EA, et al. Cancer incidence in British vegetarians. *Br J Cancer.* 2009;101(1):192–7.

7. Vegetarians less likely to develop cancer than meat eaters [news release]. London, UK: *British Journal of Cancer*; July 1, 2009. http://www.nature.com/bjc/press_releases/p_r_jul09_6605098 .html. Accessed March 11, 2015.

8. Suppipat K, Park CS, Shen Y, Zhu X, Lacorazza HD. Sulforaphane induces cell cycle arrest and apoptosis in acute lymphoblastic leukemia cells. *PLoS One.* 2012;7(12):e51251.

9. Han X, Zheng T, Foss F, et al. Vegetable and fruit intake and non-Hodgkin lymphoma survival in Connecticut women. *Leuk Lymphoma.* 2010;51(6):1047–54.

10. Thompson CA, Cerhan JR. Fruit and vegetable intake and survival from non-Hodgkin lymphoma: does an apple a day keep the doctor away? *Leuk Lymphoma.* 2010;51(6):963–4.

11. Thompson CA, Habermann TM, Wang AH, et al. Antioxidant intake from fruits, vegetables and other sources and risk of non-Hodgkin's lymphoma: the Iowa Women's Health Study. *Int J Cancer.* 2010;126(4):992–1003.

12. Holtan SG, O'Connor HM, Fredericksen ZS, et al. Food-frequency questionnaire-based estimates of total antioxidant capacity and risk of non-Hodgkin lymphoma. *Int J Cancer.* 2012; 131(5):1158–68.

13. Holtan SG, O'Connor HM, Fredericksen ZS, et al. Food-frequency questionnaire-based estimates of total antioxidant capacity and risk of non-Hodgkin lymphoma. *Int J Cancer.* 2012; 131(5):1158–68.

14. Thompson CA, Habermann TM, Wang AH, et al. Antioxidant intake from fruits, vegetables and other sources and risk of non-Hodgkin's lymphoma: the Iowa Women's Health Study. *Int J Cancer.* 2010;126(4):992–1003.

15. Bjelakovic G, Nikolova D, Simonetti RG, Gluud C. Antioxidant supplements for prevention of gastrointestinal cancers: a systematic review and meta-analysis. *Lancet.* 2004;364(9441):1219–28.

16. Jacobs DR, Tapsell LC. Food synergy: the key to a healthy diet. *Proc Nutr Soc.* 2013;72(2):200–6.

17. Elsayed RK, Glisson JK, Minor DS. Rhabdomyolysis associated with the use of a mislabeled "acai berry" dietary supplement. *Am J Med Sci.* 2011;342(6):535–8.

18. Zhang Y, Wang D, Lee RP, Henning SM, Heber D. Absence of pomegranate ellagitannins in the majority of commercial pomegranate extracts: implications for standardization and quality control. *J Agric Food Chem.* 2009;57(16):7395–400.

19. Zhang Y, Krueger D, Durst R, et al. International multidimensional authenticity specification (IMAS) algorithm for detection of commercial pomegranate juice adulteration. *J Agric Food Chem.* 2009;57(6):2550–7.

20. Del Pozo-Insfran D, Percival SS, Talcott ST. Açai (Euterpe oleracea Mart.) polyphenolics in their glycoside and aglycone forms induce apoptosis of HL-60 leukemia cells. *J Agric Food Chem.* 2006;54(4):1222–9.

21. Schauss AG, Wu X, Prior RL, et al. Antioxidant capacity and other bioactivities of the freeze-dried Amazonian palm berry, Euterpe oleraceae mart. (aSch). *J Agric Food Chem.* 2006; 54(22):8604–10.

22. Jensen GS, Ager DM, Redman KA, Mitzner MA, Benson KF, Schauss AG. Pain reduction and improvement in range of motion after daily consumption of an açai (Euterpe oleracea Mart.) pulp-fortified polyphenolic-rich fruit and berry juice blend. *J Med Food.* 2011;14(7–8):702–11.

23. Udani JK, Singh BB, Singh VJ, Barrett ML. Effects of açai (Euterpe oleracea Mart.) berry preparation on metabolic parameters in a healthy overweight population: a pilot study. *Nutr J.* 2011;10:45.

24. Haytowitz DB, Bhagwat SA. USDA database for the oxygen radical capacity (ORAC) of selected foods, release 2. Washington, D.C.: United States Department of Agriculture; 2010.

25. American Cancer Society. Cancer Facts & Figures 2014. Atlanta: American Cancer Society; 2014.

26. Landgren O, Kyle RA, Pfeiffer RM, et al. Monoclonal gammopathy of undetermined significance (MGUS) consistently precedes multiple myeloma: a prospective study. Blood. 2009; 113(22):5412–7.

27. Landgren O, Kyle RA, Pfeiffer RM, et al. Monoclonal gammopathy of undetermined significance (MGUS) consistently precedes multiple myeloma: a prospective study. Blood. 2009; 113(22):5412–7.

28. Greenberg AJ, Vachon CM, Rajkumar SV. Disparities in the prevalence, pathogenesis and progression of monoclonal gammopathy of undetermined significance and multiple myeloma between blacks and whites. Leukemia. 2012;26(4):609–14.

29. Kyle RA, Therneau TM, Rajkumar SV, et al. A long-term study of prognosis in monoclonal gammopathy of undetermined significance. N Engl J Med. 2002;346(8):564–9.

30. Bharti AC, Donato N, Singh S, Aggarwal BB. Curcumin (diferuloylmethane) down-regulates the constitutive activation of nuclear factor-kappa B and IkappaBalpha kinase in human multiple myeloma cells, leading to suppression of proliferation and induction of apoptosis. Blood. 2003; 101(3):1053–62.

31. Golombick T, Diamond TH, Badmaev V, Manoharan A, Ramakrishna R. The potential role of curcumin in patients with monoclonal gammopathy of undefined significance—its effect on paraproteinemia and the urinary N-telopeptide of type I collagen bone turnover marker. Clin Cancer Res. 2009;15(18):5917–22.

32. Golombick T, Diamond TH, Manoharan A, Ramakrishna R. Monoclonal gammopathy of undetermined significance, smoldering multiple myeloma, and curcumin: a randomized, double-blind placebo-controlled cross-over 4g study and an open-label 8g extension study. Am J Hematol. 2012;87(5):455–60.

33. Key TJ, Appleby PN, Spencer EA, et al. Cancer incidence in British vegetarians. Br J Cancer. 2009;101(1):192–7.

34. Rohrmann S, Linseisen J, Jakobsen MU, et al. Consumption of meat and dairy and lymphoma risk in the European Prospective Investigation into Cancer and Nutrition. Int J Cancer. 2011; 128(3):623–34.

35. U.S. Department of Agriculture Agricultural Research Service. National Nutrient Database for Standard Reference Release 27. Basic Report: 05358, Chicken, broiler, rotisserie, BBQ, breast meat and skin. http://ndb.nal.usda.gov/ndb/foods/show/1058. Accessed March 2, 2015.

36. Rohrmann S, Linseisen J, Jakobsen MU, et al. Consumption of meat and dairy and lymphoma risk in the European Prospective Investigation into Cancer and Nutrition. Int J Cancer. 2011; 128(3):623–34.

37. Chiu BC, Cerhan JR, Folsom AR, et al. Diet and risk of non-Hodgkin lymphoma in older women. JAMA. 1996;275(17):1315–21.

38. Daniel CR, Sinha R, Park Y, et al. Meat intake is not associated with risk of non-Hodgkin lymphoma in a large prospective cohort of U.S. men and women. J Nutr. 2012;142(6):1074–80.

39. Puangsombat K, Gadgil P, Houser TA, Hunt MC, Smith JS. Occurrence of heterocyclic amines in cooked meat products. Meat Sci. 2012;90(3):739–46.

40. 't Mannetje A, Eng A, Pearce N. Farming, growing up on a farm, and haematological cancer mortality. Occup Environ Med. 2012;69(2):126–32.

41. Johnson ES, Zhou Y, Yau LC, et al. Mortality from malignant diseases-update of the Baltimore union poultry cohort. Cancer Causes Control. 2010;21(2):215–21.

42. Neasham D, Sifi A, Nielsen KR, et al. Occupation and risk of lymphoma: a multicentre prospective cohort study (EPIC). *Occup Environ Med.* 2011;68(1):77–81.

43. Kalland KH, Ke XS, Øyan AM. Tumour virology—history, status and future challenges. *APMIS.* 2009;117(5–6):382–99.

44. Centers for Disease Control and Prevention. Human Orf virus infection from household exposures—United States, 2009–2011. *MMWR Morb Mortal Wkly Rep.* 2012;61(14):245–8.

45. Benton EC. Warts in butchers—a cause for concern? *Lancet.* 1994;343(8906):1114.

46. Gubéran, Usel M, Raymond L, Fioretta G. Mortality and incidence of cancer among a cohort of self employed butchers from Geneva and their wives. *Br J Ind Med.* 1993;50(11):1008–16.

47. Johnson ES, Zhou Y, Yau LC, et al. Mortality from malignant diseases-update of the Baltimore union poultry cohort. *Cancer Causes Control.* 2010;21(2):215–21.

48. Johnson ES, Ndetan H, Lo KM. Cancer mortality in poultry slaughtering/processing plant workers belonging to a union pension fund. *Environ Res.* 2010;110(6):588–94.

49. Choi KM, Johnson ES. Occupational exposure assessment using antibody levels: exposure to avian leukosis/sarcoma viruses in the poultry industry. *Int J Environ Health Res.* 2011;21(4): 306–16.

50. Choi KM, Johnson ES. Industrial hygiene assessment of reticuloendotheliosis viruses exposure in the poultry industry. *Int Arch Occup Environ Health.* 2011;84(4):375–82.

51. Choi KM, Johnson ES. Industrial hygiene assessment of reticuloendotheliosis viruses exposure in the poultry industry. *Int Arch Occup Environ Health.* 2011;84(4):375–82.

52. Johnson ES, Ndetan H, Lo KM. Cancer mortality in poultry slaughtering/processing plant workers belonging to a union pension fund. *Environ Res.* 2010;110(6):588–94.

53. 't Mannetje A, Eng A, Pearce N. Farming, growing up on a farm, and haematological cancer mortality. *Occup Environ Med.* 2012;69(2):126–32.

54. Tranah GJ, Bracci PM, Holly EA. Domestic and farm-animal exposures and risk of non-Hodgkin's lymphoma in a population-based study in the San Francisco Bay Area. *Cancer Epidemiol Biomarkers Prev.* 2008;17(9):2382–7.

55. Buehring GC, Philpott SM, Choi KY. Humans have antibodies reactive with Bovine leukemia virus. *AIDS Res Hum Retroviruses.* 2003;19(12):1105–13.

56. U.S. Department of Agriculture Animal and Plant Health Inspection Service. Bovine Leukosis Virus (BLV) on U.S. Dairy Operations, 2007. http://www.aphis.usda.gov/animal_health/nahms/dairy/downloads/dairy07/Dairy07_is_BLV.pdf. October 2008. Accessed March 2, 2015.

57. Buehring GC, Shen HM, Jensen HM, Choi KY, Sun D, Nuovo G. Bovine leukemia virus DNA in human breast tissue. *Emerging Infect Dis.* 2014;20(5):772–82.

58. Tranah GJ, Bracci PM, Holly EA. Domestic and farm-animal exposures and risk of non-Hodgkin's lymphoma in a population-based study in the San Francisco Bay Area. *Cancer Epidemiol Biomarkers Prev.* 2008;17(9):2382–7.

59. Schernhammer ES, Bertrand KA, Birmann BM, Sampson L, Willett WC, Feskanich D. Consumption of artificial sweetener- and sugar-containing soda and risk of lymphoma and leukemia in men and women. *Am J Clin Nutr.* 2012;96(6):1419–28.

60. Lim U, Subar AF, Mouw T, et al. Consumption of aspartame-containing beverages and incidence of hematopoietic and brain malignancies. *Cancer Epidemiol Biomarkers Prev.* 2006;15(9): 1654–9.

61. McCullough ML, Teras LR, Shah R, Diver WR, Gaudet MM, Gapstur SM. Artificially and sugar-sweetened carbonated beverage consumption is not associated with risk of lymphoid neoplasms in older men and women. *J Nutr.* 2014;144(12):2041–9.

10. How Not to Die from Kidney Disease

1. Stokes JB. Consequences of frequent hemodialysis: comparison to conventional hemodialysis and transplantation. *Trans Am Clin Climatol Assoc.* 2011;122:124–36.
2. Coresh J, Selvin E, Stevens LA, et al. Prevalence of chronic kidney disease in the United States. *JAMA.* 2007;298(17):2038–47.
3. Stevens LA, Li S, Wang C, et al. Prevalence of CKD and comorbid illness in elderly patients in the United States: results from the Kidney Early Evaluation Program (KEEP). *Am J Kidney Dis.* 2010;55(3 Suppl 2):S23–33.
4. Ryan TP, Sloand JA, Winters PC, Corsetti JP, Fisher SG. Chronic kidney disease prevalence and rate of diagnosis. *Am J Med.* 2007;120(11):981–6.
5. Hoerger TJ, Simpson SA, Yarnoff BO, et al. The future burden of CKD in the United States: a simulation model for the CDC CKD Initiative. *Am J Kidney Dis.* 2015;65(3):403–11.
6. Dalrymple LS, Katz R, Kestenbaum B, et al. Chronic kidney disease and the risk of end-stage renal disease versus death. *J Gen Intern Med.* 2011;26(4):379–85.
7. Kumar S, Bogle R, Banerjee D. Why do young people with chronic kidney disease die early? *World J Nephrol.* 2014;3(4):143–55.
8. Lin J, Hu FB, Curhan GC. Associations of diet with albuminuria and kidney function decline. *Clin J Am Soc Nephrol.* 2010;5(5):836–43.
9. Lin J, Hu FB, Curhan GC. Associations of diet with albuminuria and kidney function decline. *Clin J Am Soc Nephrol.* 2010;5(5):836–43.
10. Virchow, R. Cellular Pathology as Based upon Physiological and Pathological Histology. Twenty Lectures Delivered in the Pathological Institute of Berlin During the Months of February, March and April, 1858. Philadelpia, PA: J. B. Lippincott and Co.; 1863.
11. Moorhead JF, Chan MK, El-Nahas M, Varghese Z. Lipid nephrotoxicity in chronic progressive glomerular and tubulo-interstitial disease. *Lancet.* 1982;2(8311):1309–11.
12. Hartroft WS. Fat emboli in glomerular capillaries of choline-deficient rats and of patients with diabetic glomerulosclerosis. *Am J Pathol.* 1955;31(3):381–97.
13. Gyebi L, Soltani Z, Reisin E. Lipid nephrotoxicity: new concept for an old disease. *Curr Hypertens Rep.* 2012;14(2):177–81.
14. US Burden of Disease Collaborators. The state of US health, 1990–2010: burden of diseases, injuries, and risk factors. *JAMA.* 2013 Aug 14;310(6):591–608.
15. Odermatt A. The Western-style diet: a major risk factor for impaired kidney function and chronic kidney disease. *Am J Physiol Renal Physiol.* 2011;301(5):F919–31.
16. van den Berg E, Hospers FA, Navis G, et al. Dietary acid load and rapid progression to end-stage renal disease of diabetic nephropathy in Westernized South Asian people. *J Nephrol.* 2011;24(1):11–7.
17. Piccoli GB, Vigotti FN, Leone F, et al. Low-protein diets in CKD: how can we achieve them? A narrative, pragmatic review. *Clin Kidney J.* 2015;8(1):61–70.
18. Brenner BM, Meyer TW, Hostetter TH. Dietary protein intake and the progressive nature of kidney disease: the role of hemodynamically mediated glomerular injury in the pathogenesis of progressive glomerular sclerosis in aging, renal ablation, and intrinsic renal disease. *N Engl J Med.* 1982 Sep 9;307(11):652–9.
19. Wiseman MJ, Hunt R, Goodwin A, Gross JL, Keen H, Viberti GC. Dietary composition and renal function in healthy subjects. *Nephron.* 1987;46(1):37–42.
20. Nakamura H, Takasawa M, Kashara S, et al. Effects of acute protein loads of different sources on renal function of patients with diabetic nephropathy. *Tohoku J Exp Med.* 1989;159(2):153–62.
21. Simon AH, Lima PR, Almerinda M, Alves VF, Bottini PV, de Faria JB. Renal haemodynamic

responses to a chicken or beef meal in normal individuals. *Nephrol Dial Transplant*. 1998;13(9): 2261–4.

22. Kontessis P, Jones S, Dodds R, et al. Renal, metabolic and hormonal responses to ingestion of animal and vegetable proteins. *Kidney Int*. 1990;38(1):136–44.

23. Nakamura H, Takasawa M, Kashara S, et al. Effects of acute protein loads of different sources on renal function of patients with diabetic nephropathy. *Tohoku J Exp Med*. 1989;159(2):153–62.

24. Azadbakht L, Shakerhosseini R, Atabak S, Jamshidian M, Mehrabi Y, Esmaill-Zadeh A. Beneficiary effect of dietary soy protein on lowering plasma levels of lipid and improving kidney function in type II diabetes with nephropathy. *Eur J Clin Nutr*. 2003;57(10):1292–4.

25. Kontessis PA, Bossinakou I, Sarika L, et al. Renal, metabolic, and hormonal responses to proteins of different origin in normotensive, nonproteinuric type I diabetic patients. *Diabetes Care*. 1995;18(9):1233–40.

26. Teixeira SR, Tappenden KA, Carson L, et al. Isolated soy protein consumption reduces urinary albumin excretion and improves the serum lipid profile in men with type 2 diabetes mellitus and nephropathy. *J Nutr*. 2004;134(8):1874–80.

27. Stephenson TJ, Setchell KD, Kendall CW, Jenkins DJ, Anderson JW, Fanti P. Effect of soy protein-rich diet on renal function in young adults with insulin-dependent diabetes mellitus. *Clin Nephrol*. 2005;64(1):1–11.

28. Jibani MM, Bloodworth LL, Foden E, Griffiths KD, Galpin OP. Predominantly vegetarian diet in patients with incipient and early clinical diabetic nephropathy: effects on albumin excretion rate and nutritional status. *Diabet Med*. 1991;8(10):949–53.

29. Bosch JP, Saccaggi A, Lauer A, Ronco C, Belledonne M, Glabman S. Renal functional reserve in humans. Effect of protein intake on glomerular filtration rate. *Am J Med*. 1983;75(6):943–50.

30. Liu ZM, Ho SC, Chen YM, Tang N, Woo J. Effect of whole soy and purified isoflavone daidzein on renal function—a 6-month randomized controlled trial in equol-producing postmenopausal women with prehypertension. *Clin Biochem*. 2014;47(13–14):1250–6.

31. Fioretto P, Trevisan R, Valerio A, et al. Impaired renal response to a meat meal in insulin-dependent diabetes: role of glucagon and prostaglandins. *Am J Physiol*. 1990;258(3 Pt 2): F675–83.

32. Frassetto L, Morris RC, Sellmeyer DE, Todd K, Sebastian A. Diet, evolution and aging—the pathophysiologic effects of the post-agricultural inversion of the potassium-to-sodium and base-to-chloride ratios in the human diet. *Eur J Nutr*. 2001;40(5):200–13.

33. Banerjee T, Crews DC, Wesson DE, et al. Dietary acid load and chronic kidney disease among adults in the United States. *BMC Nephrol*. 2014 Aug 24;15:137.

34. Sebastian A, Frassetto LA, Sellmeyer DE, Merriam RL, Morris RC. Estimation of the net acid load of the diet of ancestral preagricultural Homo sapiens and their hominid ancestors. *Am J Clin Nutr*. 2002;76(6):1308–16.

35. van den Berg E, Hospers FA, Navis G, et al. Dietary acid load and rapid progression to end-stage renal disease of diabetic nephropathy in Westernized South Asian people. *J Nephrol*. 2011;24(1):11–7.

36. Uribarri J, Oh MS. The key to halting progression of CKD might be in the produce market, not in the pharmacy. *Kidney Int*. 2012;81(1):7–9.

37. Cohen E, Nardi Y, Krause I, et al. A longitudinal assessment of the natural rate of decline in renal function with age. *J Nephrol*. 2014;27(6):635–41.

38. Brenner BM, Meyer TW, Hostetter TH. Dietary protein intake and the progressive nature of kidney disease: the role of hemodynamically mediated glomerular injury in the pathogenesis of progressive glomerular sclerosis in aging, renal ablation, and intrinsic renal disease. *N Engl J Med*. 1982 Sep 9;307(11):652–9.

39. Frassetto LA, Todd KM, Morris RC, Sebastian A. Estimation of net endogenous noncarbonic acid production in humans from diet potassium and protein contents. *Am J Clin Nutr*. 1998;68(3): 576–83.

40. Wiseman MJ, Hunt R, Goodwin A, Gross JL, Keen H, Viberti GC. Dietary composition and renal function in healthy subjects. *Nephron*. 1987;46(1):37–42.

41. Kempner W. Treatment of heart and kidney disease and of hypertensive and arteriosclerotic vascular disease with the rice diet. *Ann Intern Med*. 1949;31(5):821–56.

42. Barsotti G, Morelli E, Cupisti A, Meola M, Dani L, Giovannetti S. A low-nitrogen low-phosphorus vegan diet for patients with chronic renal failure. *Nephron*. 1996;74(2):390–4.

43. Deriemaeker P, Aerenhouts D, Hebbelinck M, Clarys P. Nutrient based estimation of acid-base balance in vegetarians and non-vegetarians. *Plant Foods Hum Nutr*. 2010;65(1):77–82.

44. Goraya N, Simoni J, Jo C, Wesson DE. Dietary acid reduction with fruits and vegetables or bicarbonate attenuates kidney injury in patients with a moderately reduced glomerular filtration rate due to hypertensive nephropathy. *Kidney Int*. 2012;81(1):86–93.

45. Yaqoob MM. Treatment of acidosis in CKD. *Clin J Am Soc Nephrol*. 2013;8(3):342–3.

46. Goraya N, Simoni J, Jo C, Wesson DE. Dietary acid reduction with fruits and vegetables or bicarbonate attenuates kidney injury in patients with a moderately reduced glomerular filtration rate due to hypertensive nephropathy. *Kidney Int*. 2012;81(1):86–93.

47. Wright JA, Cavanaugh KL. Dietary sodium in chronic kidney disease: a comprehensive approach. *Semin Dial*. 2010;23(4):415–21.

48. Uribarri J, Oh MS. The key to halting progression of CKD might be in the produce market, not in the pharmacy. *Kidney Int*. 2012;81(1):7–9.

49. Goldfarb S. Dietary factors in the pathogenesis and prophylaxis of calcium nephrolithiasis. *Kidney Int*. 1988;34(4):544–55.

50. Scales CD Jr, Smith AC, Hanley JM, Saigal CS; Urologic Diseases in America Project. Prevalence of kidney stones in the United States. *Eur Urol*. 2012;62(1):160–5.

51. Robertson WG, Peacock M, Hodgkinson A. Dietary changes and the incidence of urinary calculi in the U.K. between 1958 and 1976. *J Chronic Dis*. 1979;32(6):469–76.

52. Robertson WG, Heyburn PJ, Peacock M, Hanes FA, Swaminathan R. The effect of high animal protein intake on the risk of calcium stone-formation in the urinary tract. *Clin Sci* (Lond). 1979;57(3):285–8.

53. Robertson WG, Heyburn PJ, Peacock M, Hanes FA, Swaminathan R. The effect of high animal protein intake on the risk of calcium stone-formation in the urinary tract. *Clin Sci* (Lond). 1979; 57(3):285–8.

54. Robertson WG, Peacock M, Heyburn PJ, et al. Should recurrent calcium oxalate stone formers become vegetarians? *Br J Urol*. 1979;51(6):427–31.

55. Turney BW, Appleby PN, Reynard JM, Noble JG, Key TJ, Allen NE. Diet and risk of kidney stones in the Oxford cohort of the European Prospective Investigation into Cancer and Nutrition (EPIC). *Eur J Epidemiol*. 2014;29(5):363–9.

56. Tracy CR, Best S, Bagrodia A, et al. Animal protein and the risk of kidney stones: A comparative metabolic study of animal protein sources. *J Urol*. 2014 Feb 8;192:137–41.

57. Bushinsky DA. Recurrent hypercalciuric nephrolithiasis—does diet help? *N Engl J Med*. 2002 Jan 10;346(2):124–5.

58. Borghi L, Schianchi T, Meschi T, et al. Comparison of two diets for the prevention of recurrent stones in idiopathic hypercalciuria. *N Engl J Med*. 2002 Jan 10;346(2):77–84.

59. Sorensen MD, Hsi RS, Chi T, et al. Dietary intake of fiber, fruit and vegetables decreases the risk of incident kidney stones in women: a Women's Health Initiative report. *J Urol*. 2014; 192(6):1694–9.

60. Mehta TH, Goldfarb DS. Uric acid stones and hyperuricosuria. *Adv Chronic Kidney Dis.* 2012;19(6):413–8.

61. de Vries A, Frank M, Liberman UA, Sperling O. Allopurinol in the prophylaxis of uric acid stones. *Ann Rheum Dis.* 1966;25(6 Suppl):691–3.

62. Siener R, Hesse A. The effect of a vegetarian and different omnivorous diets on urinary risk factors for uric acid stone formation. *Eur J Nutr.* 2003;42(6):332–7.

63. Siener R, Hesse A. The effect of a vegetarian and different omnivorous diets on urinary risk factors for uric acid stone formation. *Eur J Nutr.* 2003;42(6):332–7.

64. Trinchieri A. Development of a rapid food screener to assess the potential renal acid load of diet in renal stone formers (LAKE score). *Arch Ital Urol Androl.* 2012;84(1):36–8.

65. Chae JY, Kim JW, Kim JW, et al. Increased fluid intake and adequate dietary modification may be enough for the successful treatment of uric acid stone. *Urolithiasis.* 2013;41(2):179–82.

66. Deriemaeker P, Aerenhouts D, Hebbelinck M, Clarys P. Nutrient based estimation of acid-base balance in vegetarians and non-vegetarians. *Plant Foods Hum Nutr.* 2010;65(1):77–82.

67. Adeva MM, Souto G. Diet-induced metabolic acidosis. *Clin Nutr.* 2011;30(4):416–21.

68. Dawson-Hughes B, Harris SS, Ceglia L. Alkaline diets favor lean tissue mass in older adults. *Am J Clin Nutr.* 2008;87(3):662–5.

69. Ritz E, Hahn K, Ketteler M, Kuhlmann MK, Mann J. Phosphate additives in food—a health risk. *Dtsch Arztebl Int.* 2012;109(4):49–55.

70. Ritz E, Hahn K, Ketteler M, Kuhlmann MK, Mann J. Phosphate additives in food—a health risk. *Dtsch Arztebl Int.* 2012;109(4):49–55.

71. Calvo MS, Uribarri J. Public health impact of dietary phosphorus excess on bone and cardiovascular health in the general population. *Am J Clin Nutr.* 2013;98(1):6–15.

72. Moe SM, Zidehsarai MP, Chambers MA, et al. Vegetarian compared with meat dietary protein source and phosphorus homeostasis in chronic kidney disease. *Clin J Am Soc Nephrol.* 2011; 6(2):257–64.

73. Fukagawa M, Komaba H, Miyamoto K. Source matters: from phosphorus load to bioavailability. *Clin J Am Soc Nephrol.* 2011;6(2):239–40.

74. Murphy-Gutekunst L, Uribarri J. Hidden phosphorus-enhanced meats: Part 3. *J Ren Nutr.* 2005 15(4):E1–E4.

75. Ritz E, Hahn K, Ketteler M, Kuhlmann MK, Mann J. Phosphate additives in food—a health risk. *Dtsch Arztebl Int.* 2012;109(4):49–55.

76. Karp H, Ekholm P, Kemi V, et al. Differences among total and in vitro digestible phosphorus content of plant foods and beverages. *J Ren Nutr.* 2012;22(4):416–22.

77. Karp H, Ekholm P, Kemi V, Hirvonen T, Lamberg-Allardt C. Differences among total and in vitro digestible phosphorus content of meat and milk products. *J Ren Nutr.* 2012;22(3):344–9.

78. Karp H, Ekholm P, Kemi V, et al. Differences among total and in vitro digestible phosphorus content of plant foods and beverages. *J Ren Nutr.* 2012;22(4):416–22.

79. Murphy-Gutekunst L, Uribarri J. Hidden phosphorus-enhanced meats: Part 3. *J Ren Nutr.* 2005 15(4):E1–E4.

80. Sherman RA, Mehta O. Phosphorus and potassium content of enhanced meat and poultry products: implications for patients who receive dialysis. *Clin J Am Soc Nephrol.* 2009;4(8):1370–3.

81. Benini O, D'Alessandro C, Gianfaldoni D, Cupisti A. Extra-phosphate load from food additives in commonly eaten foods: a real and insidious danger for renal patients. *J Ren Nutr.* 2011;21(4): 303–8.

82. Sherman RA, Mehta O. Phosphorus and potassium content of enhanced meat and poultry products: implications for patients who receive dialysis. *Clin J Am Soc Nephrol.* 2009;4(8): 1370–3.

83. Benini O, D'Alessandro C, Gianfaldoni D, Cupisti A. Extra-phosphate load from food additives in commonly eaten foods: a real and insidious danger for renal patients. *J Ren Nutr.* 2011;21(4):303–8.

84. Shroff R. Phosphate is a vascular toxin. *Pediatr Nephrol.* 2013;28(4):583–93.

85. Shuto E, Taketani Y, Tanaka R, et al. Dietary phosphorus acutely impairs endothelial function. *J Am Soc Nephrol.* 2009;20(7):1504–12.

86. Gunther NW, He Y, Fratamico P. Effects of polyphosphate additives on the pH of processed chicken exudates and the survival of Campylobacter. *J Food Prot.* 2011;74(10):1735–40.

87. Sherman RA, Mehta O. Dietary phosphorus restriction in dialysis patients: potential impact of processed meat, poultry, and fish products as protein sources. *Am J Kidney Dis.* 2009;54(1): 18–23.

88. Sherman RA, Mehta O. Dietary phosphorus restriction in dialysis patients: potential impact of processed meat, poultry, and fish products as protein sources. *Am J Kidney Dis.* 2009;54(1): 18–23.

89. Sullivan CM, Leon JB, Sehgal AR. Phosphorus-containing food additives and the accuracy of nutrient databases: implications for renal patients. *J Ren Nutr.* 2007;17(5):350–4.

90. Food and Drug Administration, Department of Health and Human Services. Final Determination Regarding Partially Hydrogenated Oils. Docket No. FDA-2013-N-1317. https://s3.amazonaws .com/public-inspection.federalregister.gov/2015-14883.pdf. June 16, 2015. Accessed June 16, 2015.

91. Food and Drug Administration, Department of Health and Human Services. Tentative determination regarding partially hydrogenated oils; request for comments and for scientific data and information. Federal Register Docket No. D78 FR 67169-75. https://www.federalregister.gov /articles/2013/11/08/2013-26854/tentative-determination-regarding-partially-hydrogenated -oils-request-for-comments-and-for. November 8, 2013. Accessed March 2, 2015.

92. Food and Drug Administration, Department of Health and Human Services. Tentative determination regarding partially hydrogenated oils; request for comments and for scientific data and information. Federal Register Docket No. D78 FR 67169-75. https://www.federalregister.gov /articles/2013/11/08/2013-26854/tentative-determination-regarding-partially-hydrogenated -oils-request-for-comments-and-for. November 8, 2013. Accessed March 2, 2015.

93. Neltner TG, Kulkami NR, Alger HM, et al. Navigating the U.S. food additive regulatory program. *Compr Rev Food Sci Food Saf.* 2011;10(6):342–68.

94. Neltner TG, Alger HM, O'Reilly JT, Krimsky S, Bero LA, Maffini MV. Conflicts of interest in approvals of additives to food determined to be generally recognized as safe: out of balance. *JAMA Intern Med.* 2013;173(22):2032–6.

95. Stuckler D, Basu S, McKee M. Commentary: UN high level meeting on non-communicable diseases: an opportunity for whom? *BMJ.* 2011;343:d5336.

96. Moodie R, Stuckler D, Monteiro C, et al. Profits and pandemics: prevention of harmful effects of tobacco, alcohol, and ultra-processed food and drink industries. *Lancet.* 2013;381(9867):670–9.

97. American Cancer Society. Cancer Facts & Figures 2014. Atlanta: American Cancer Society; 2014.

98. Kirkali Z, Cal C. Renal Cell Carcinoma: Overview. In Nargund VH, Raghavan D, Sandler HM, eds. *Urological Oncology.* London, UK: Springer; 2008:263–80.

99. Kirkali Z, Cal C. Renal Cell Carcinoma: Overview. In Nargund VH, Raghavan D, Sandler HM, eds. *Urological Oncology.* London, UK: Springer; 2008:263–80.

100. Ramírez N, Özel MZ, Lewis AC, Marcé RM, Borrull F, Hamilton JF. Exposure to nitrosamines in thirdhand tobacco smoke increases cancer risk in non-smokers. *Environ Int.* 2014; 71:139–47.

101. Schick SF, Farraro KF, Perrino C, et al. Thirdhand cigarette smoke in an experimental

chamber: evidence of surface deposition of nicotine, nitrosamines and polycyclic aromatic hydrocarbons and de novo formation of NNK. *Tob Control*. 2014;23(2):152–9.

102. Hecht SS. It is time to regulate carcinogenic tobacco-specific nitrosamines in cigarette tobacco. *Cancer Prev Res* (Phila). 2014;7(7):639–47.

103. Rodgman A, Perfetti TA. *The Chemical Components of Tobacco and Tobacco Smoke*. Boca Raton, FL: CRC Press, Taylor & Francis Group; 2009.

104. Haorah J, Zhou L, Wang X, Xu G, Mirvish SS. Determination of total N-nitroso compounds and their precursors in frankfurters, fresh meat, dried salted fish, sauces, tobacco, and tobacco smoke particulates. *J Agric Food Chem*. 2001;49(12):6068–78.

105. Rohrmann S, Overvad K, Bueno-de-Mesquita HB, et al. Meat consumption and mortality—results from the European Prospective Investigation into Cancer and Nutrition. *BMC Med*. 2013;11:63.

106. Sinha R, Cross AJ, Graubard BI, Leitzmann MF, Schatzkin A. Meat intake and mortality: a prospective study of over half a million people. *Arch Intern Med*. 2009;169(6):562–71.

107. American Institute for Cancer Research. Recommendations for Cancer Prevention. http://www.aicr.org/reduce-your-cancer-risk/recommendations-for-cancer-prevention/recommendations_05_red_meat.html. April 17, 2011. Accessed March 2, 2015.

108. USDA. Additives in meat and poultry products. http://www.fsis.usda.gov/wps/portal/fsis/topics/food-safety-education/get-answers/food-safety-fact-sheets/food-labeling/additives-in-meat-and-poultry-products/additives-in-meat-and-poultry-products. March 24, 2015. Accessed May 3, 2015.

109. Sebranek JG, Jackson-Davis AL, Myers KL, Lavieri NA. Beyond celery and starter culture: advances in natural/organic curing processes in the United States. *Meat Sci*. 2012;92(3):267–73.

110. Dellavalle CT, Daniel CR, Aschebrook-Kilfoy B, et al. Dietary intake of nitrate and nitrite and risk of renal cell carcinoma in the NIH-AARP Diet and Health Study. *Br J Cancer*. 2013;108(1):205–12.

111. Bartsch H, Ohshima H, Pignatelli B. Inhibitors of endogenous nitrosation. Mechanisms and implications in human cancer prevention. *Mutat Res*. 1988;202(2):307–24.

112. Dellavalle CT, Daniel CR, Aschebrook-Kilfoy B, et al. Dietary intake of nitrate and nitrite and risk of renal cell carcinoma in the NIH-AARP Diet and Health Study. *Br J Cancer*. 2013;108(1):205–12.

113. Liu B, Mao Q, Wang X, et al. Cruciferous vegetables consumption and risk of renal cell carcinoma: a meta-analysis. *Nutr Cancer*. 2013;65(5):668–76.

11. How Not to Die from Breast Cancer

1. American Cancer Society. Breast Cancer Facts & Figures 2013–2014. http://www.cancer.org/acs/groups/content/@research/documents/document/acspc-042725.pdf. 2013. Accessed March 10, 2015.

2. Sanders ME, Schuyler PA, Dupont WD, Page DL. The natural history of low-grade ductal carcinoma in situ of the breast in women treated by biopsy only revealed over 30 years of long-term follow-up. *Cancer*. 2005;103(12):2481–4.

3. Nielsen M, Thomsen JL, Primdahl S, Dyreborg U, Andersen JA. Breast cancer and atypia among young and middle-aged women: a study of 110 medicolegal autopsies. *Br J Cancer*. 1987;56(6):814–9.

4. Soto AM, Brisken C, Schaeberle C, Sonnenschein C. Does cancer start in the womb? Altered

mammary gland development and predisposition to breast cancer due to in utero exposure to endocrine disruptors. *J Mammary Gland Biol Neoplasia*. 2013;18(2):199–208.

5. Del Monte U. Does the cell number 10(9) still really fit one gram of tumor tissue? *Cell Cycle*. 2009;8(3):505–6.

6. Black WC, Welch HG. Advances in diagnostic imaging and overestimations of disease prevalence and the benefits of therapy. *N Engl J Med*. 1993;328(17):1237–43.

7. Friberg S, Mattson S. On the growth rates of human malignant tumors: implications for medical decision making. *J Surg Oncol*. 1997;65(4):284–97.

8. Philippe E, Le Gal Y. Growth of seventy-eight recurrent mammary cancers. Quantitative study. *Cancer*. 1968;21(3):461–7.

9. Kuroishi T, Tominaga S, Morimoto T, et al. Tumor growth rate and prognosis of breast cancer mainly detected by mass screening. *Jpn J Cancer Res*. 1990;81(5):454–62.

10. American Association for Cancer Research. Studies weigh cost, effectiveness of mammography. *Cancer Discov*. 2014;4(5):OF5.

11. Nielsen M, Thomsen JL, Primdahl S, Dyreborg U, Andersen JA. Breast cancer and atypia among young and middle-aged women: a study of 110 medicolegal autopsies. *Br J Cancer*. 1987;56(6): 814–9.

12. American Institute for Cancer Research. Recommendations for Cancer Prevention. http://www.aicr.org/reduce-your-cancer-risk/recommendations-for-cancer-prevention/. September 12, 2014. Accessed March 10, 2015.

13. American Institute for Cancer Research. AICR, the China Study, and Forks Over Knives. http://www.aicr.org/about/advocacy/the-china-study.html. January 9, 2015. Accessed March 10, 2015.

14. Hastert TA, Beresford SAA, Patterson RE, Kristal AR, White E. Adherence to WCRF/AICR cancer prevention recommendations and risk of postmenopausal breast cancer. *Cancer Epidemiol Biomarkers Prev*. 2013;22(9):1498–508.

15. Barnard RJ, Gonzalez JH, Liva ME, Ngo TH. Effects of a low-fat, high-fiber diet and exercise program on breast cancer risk factors in vivo and tumor cell growth and apoptosis in vitro. *Nutr Cancer*. 2006;55(1):28–34.

16. Ngo TH, Barnard RJ, Tymchuk CN, Cohen P, Aronson WJ. Effect of diet and exercise on serum insulin, IGF-I, and IGFBP-1 levels and growth of LNCaP cells in vitro (United States). *Cancer Causes Control*. 2002;13(10):929–35.

17. Allen NE, Appleby PN, Davey GK, Kaaks R, Rinaldi S, Key TJ. The associations of diet with serum insulin-like growth factor I and its main binding proteins in 292 women meat-eaters, vegetarians, and vegans. *Cancer Epidemiol Biomarkers Prev*. 2002;11(11):1441–8.

18. IARC. IARC Monographs on the Evaluation of Carcinogenic Risks to Humans, Vol 96, Alcohol Consumption and Ethyl Carbamate. Lyon, France: International Agency for Research on Cancer; 2010.

19. Stewart BW, Wild CP, eds. *World Cancer Report 2014*. Lyon, France: International Agency for Research on Cancer; 2014.

20. Bagnardi V, Rota M, Botteri E, et al. Light alcohol drinking and cancer: a meta-analysis. *Ann Oncol*. 2013;24(2):301–8.

21. Linderborg K, Salaspuro M, Väkeväinen S. A single sip of a strong alcoholic beverage causes exposure to carcinogenic concentrations of acetaldehyde in the oral cavity. *Food Chem Toxicol*. 2011;49(9):2103–6.

22. Lachenmeier DW, Gumbel-Mako S, Sohnius EM, Keck-Wilhelm A, Kratz E, Mildau G. Salivary acetaldehyde increase due to alcohol-containing mouthwash use: a risk factor for oral cancer. *Int J Cancer*. 2009;125(3):730–5.

23. Chen WY, Rosner B, Hankinson SE, Colditz GA, Willett WC. Moderate alcohol consumption during adult life, drinking patterns, and breast cancer risk. *JAMA*. 2011;306(17): 1884–90.

24. Shufelt C, Merz CN, Yang Y, et al. Red versus white wine as a nutritional aromatase inhibitor in premenopausal women: a pilot study. *J Womens Health* (Larchmt). 2012;21(3):281–4.

25. Eng ET, Williams D, Mandava U, Kirma N, Tekmal RR, Chen S. Anti-aromatase chemicals in red wine. *Ann N Y Acad Sci*. 2002;963:239–46.

26. Shufelt C, Merz CN, Yang Y, et al. Red versus white wine as a nutritional aromatase inhibitor in premenopausal women: a pilot study. *J Womens Health* (Larchmt). 2012;21(3):281–4.

27. Chen S, Sun XZ, Kao YC, Kwon A, Zhou D, Eng E. Suppression of breast cancer cell growth with grape juice. *Pharmaceutical Biology*. 1998;36(Suppl 1):53–61.

28. Chen S, Sun XZ, Kao YC, Kwon A, Zhou D, Eng E. Suppression of breast cancer cell growth with grape juice. *Pharmaceutical Biology*. 1998;36(Suppl 1):53–61.

29. Adams LS, Zhang Y, Seeram NP, Heber D, Chen S. Pomegranate ellagitannin-derived compounds exhibit anti-proliferative and anti-aromatase activity in breast cancer cells in vitro. *Cancer Prev Res* (Phila). 2010;3(1):108–13.

30. Chen S, Oh SR, Phung S, et al. Anti-aromatase activity of phytochemicals in white button mushrooms (Agaricus bisporus). *Cancer Res*. 2006;66(24):12026–34.

31. Mishal AA. Effects of different dress styles on vitamin D levels in healthy young Jordanian women. *Osteoporos Int*. 2001;12(11):931–5.

32. Cardinali DP, Pévet P. Basic aspects of melatonin action. *Sleep Med Rev*. 1998;2(3):175–90.

33. Blask DE, Dauchy RT, Sauer LA. Putting cancer to sleep at night: the neuroendocrine/circadian melatonin signal. *Endocrine*. 2005;27(2):179–88.

34. Flynn-Evans EE, Stevens RG, Tabandeh H, Schernhammer ES, Lockley SW. Total visual blindness is protective against breast cancer. *Cancer Causes Control*. 2009;20(9):1753–6.

35. He C, Anand ST, Ebell MH, Vena JE, Robb SW. Circadian disrupting exposures and breast cancer risk: a meta-analysis. *Int Arch Occup Environ Health*. 2015 Jul;88(5):533–47.

36. Hurley S, Goldberg D, Nelson D, et al. Light at night and breast cancer risk among California teachers. *Epidemiology*. 2014;25(5):697–706.

37. Bauer SE, Wagner SE, Burch J, Bayakly R, Vena JE. A case-referent study: light at night and breast cancer risk in Georgia. *Int J Health Geogr*. 2013;12:23.

38. Kloog I, Haim A, Stevens RG, Barchana M, Portnov BA. Light at night co-distributes with incident breast but not lung cancer in the female population of Israel. *Chronobiol Int*. 2008;25(1):65–81.

39. Li Q, Zheng T, Holford TR, Boyle P, Zhang Y, Dai M. Light at night and breast cancer risk: results from a population-based case-control study in Connecticut, USA. *Cancer Causes Control*. 2010;21(12):2281–5.

40. Basler M, Jetter A, Fink D, Seifert B, Kullak-Ublick GA, Trojan A. Urinary excretion of melatonin and association with breast cancer: meta-analysis and review of the literature. *Breast Care* (Basel). 2014;9(3):182–7.

41. Nagata C, Nagao Y, Shibuya C, Kashiki Y, Shimizu H. Association of vegetable intake with urinary 6-sulfatoxymelatonin level. *Cancer Epidemiol Biomarkers Prev*. 2005;14(5):1333–5.

42. Schernhammer ES, Feskanich D, Niu C, Dopfel R, Holmes MD, Hankinson SE. Dietary correlates of urinary 6-sulfatoxymelatonin concentrations in the Nurses' Health Study cohorts. *Am J Clin Nutr*. 2009;90(4):975–85.

43. Gonçalves AK, Dantas Florencio GL, Maisonnette de Atayde Silva MJ, Cobucci RN, Giraldo PC, Cote NM. Effects of physical activity on breast cancer prevention: a systematic review. *J Phys Act Health*. 2014;11(2):445–54.

44. Friedenreich CM, Woolcott CG, McTiernan A, et al. Alberta physical activity and breast cancer prevention trial: sex hormone changes in a year-long exercise intervention among postmenopausal women. *J Clin Oncol.* 2010;28(9):1458–66.

45. Kossman DA, Williams NI, Domchek SM, Kurzer MS, Stopfer JE, Schmitz KH. Exercise lowers estrogen and progesterone levels in premenopausal women at high risk of breast cancer. *J Appl Physiol.* 2011;111(6):1687–93.

46. Thune I, Furberg AS. Physical activity and cancer risk: dose-response and cancer, all sites and site-specific. *Med Sci Sports Exerc.* 2001;33(6 Suppl):S530–50.

47. Carpenter CL, Ross RK, Paganini-Hill A, Bernstein L. Lifetime exercise activity and breast cancer risk among post-menopausal women. *Br J Cancer.* 1999;80(11):1852–8.

48. Peters TM, Moore SC, Gierach GL, et al. Intensity and timing of physical activity in relation to postmenopausal breast cancer risk: the prospective NIH-AARP diet and health study. *BMC Cancer.* 2009;9:349.

49. Friedenreich CM, Cust AE. Physical activity and breast cancer risk: impact of timing, type and dose of activity and population subgroup effects. *Br J Sports Med.* 2008;42(8):636–47.

50. Hildebrand JS, Gapstur SM, Campbell PT, Gaudet MM, Patel AV. Recreational physical activity and leisure-time sitting in relation to postmenopausal breast cancer risk. *Cancer Epidemiol Biomarkers Prev.* 2013;22(10):1906–12.

51. Widmark, EMP. Presence of cancer-producing substances in roasted food. *Nature.* 1939;143:984.

52. National Cancer Institute. Chemicals in Meat Cooked at High Temperatures and Cancer Risk. http://www.cancer.gov/cancertopics/factsheet/Risk/cooked-meats. Reviewed October 15, 2010. Accessed March 10, 2015.

53. Shaughnessy DT, Gangarosa LM, Schliebe B, et al. Inhibition of fried meat-induced colorectal DNA damage and altered systemic genotoxicity in humans by crucifera, chlorophyllin, and yogurt. *PLoS ONE.* 2011;6(4):e18707.

54. Zaidi R, Kumar S, Rawat PR. Rapid detection and quantification of dietary mutagens in food using mass spectrometry and ultra performance liquid chromatography. *Food Chem.* 2012; 135(4):2897–903.

55. Thiébaud HP, Knize MG, Kuzmicky PA, Hsieh DP, Felton JS. Airborne mutagens produced by frying beef, pork and a soy-based food. *Food Chem Toxicol.* 1995;33(10):821–8.

56. Zheng W, Lee SA. Well-done meat intake, heterocyclic amine exposure, and cancer risk. *Nutr Cancer.* 2009;61(4):437–46.

57. Goldfinger SE. By the way, doctor. In your May issue you say that eating medium or well-done beef increases one's risk for stomach cancer. But what about the dangers of eating rare beef?. *Harv Health Lett.* 1999;24(5):7.

58. Frandsen H, Frederiksen H, Alexander J. 2-Amino-1-methyl-6-(5-hydroxy-)phenylimidazo [4,5-b]pyridine (5-OH-PhIP), a biomarker for the genotoxic dose of the heterocyclic amine, 2-amino-1-methyl-6-phenylimidazo[4,5-b]pyridine (PhIP). *Food Chem Toxicol.* 2002;40(8): 1125–30.

59. Frandsen H. Biomonitoring of urinary metabolites of 2-amino-1-methyl-6-phenylimidazo[4,5 -b]pyridine (PhIP) following human consumption of cooked chicken. *Food Chem Toxicol.* 2008; 46(9):3200–5.

60. Steck SE, Gaudet MM, Eng SM, et al. Cooked meat and risk of breast cancer—lifetime versus recent dietary intake. *Epidemiology.* 2007;18(3):373–82.

61. Zheng W, Gustafson DR, Sinha R, et al. Well-done meat intake and the risk of breast cancer. *J Natl Cancer Inst.* 1998;90(22):1724–9.

62. Rohrmann S, Lukas Jung SU, Linseisen J, Pfau W. Dietary intake of meat and meat-derived heterocyclic aromatic amines and their correlation with DNA adducts in female breast tissue. *Mutagenesis.* 2009;24(2):127–32.

63. Santella RM, Gammon M, Terry M, et al. DNA adducts, DNA repair genotype/phenotype and cancer risk. *Mutat Res.* 2005;592(1–2):29–35.

64. Lauber SN, Ali S, Gooderham NJ. The cooked food derived carcinogen 2-amino-1-methyl-6-phenylimidazo[4,5-b] pyridine is a potent oestrogen: a mechanistic basis for its tissue-specific carcinogenicity. *Carcinogenesis.* 2004;25(12):2509–17.

65. Debruin LS, Martos PA, Josephy PD. Detection of PhIP (2-amino-1-methyl-6-phenylimidazo [4,5-b]pyridine) in the milk of healthy women. *Chem Res Toxicol.* 2001;14(11):1523–8.

66. Lauber SN, Ali S, Gooderham NJ. The cooked food derived carcinogen 2-amino-1-methyl-6-phenylimidazo[4,5-b] pyridine is a potent oestrogen: a mechanistic basis for its tissue-specific carcinogenicity. *Carcinogenesis.* 2004;25(12):2509–17.

67. Debruin LS, Martos PA, Josephy PD. Detection of PhIP (2-amino-1-methyl-6-phenylimidazo [4,5-b]pyridine) in the milk of healthy women. *Chem Res Toxicol.* 2001;14(11):1523–8.

68. Bessette EE, Yasa I, Dunbar D, Wilkens LR, Le Marchand L, Turesky RJ. Biomonitoring of carcinogenic heterocyclic aromatic amines in hair: a validation study. *Chem Res Toxicol.* 2009; 22(8):1454–63.

69. Grose KR, Grant JL, Bjeldanes LF, et al. Isolation of the carcinogen IQ from fried egg patties. *J Agric Food Chem.* 1986;34(2):201–2.

70. Holland RD, Gehring T, Taylor J, Lake BG, Gooderham NJ, Turesky RJ. Formation of a mutagenic heterocyclic aromatic amine from creatinine in urine of meat eaters and vegetarians. *Chem Res Toxicol.* 2005;18(3):579–90.

71. Magagnotti C, Orsi F, Bagnati R, et al. Effect of diet on serum albumin and hemoglobin adducts of 2-amino-1-methyl-6-phenylimidazo[4,5-b]pyridine (PhIP) in humans. *Int J Cancer.* 2000; 88(1):1–6.

72. Lauber SN, Gooderham NJ. The cooked meat-derived mammary carcinogen 2-amino-1-methyl -6-phenylimidazo[4,5-b]pyridine promotes invasive behaviour of breast cancer cells. *Toxicology.* 2011;279(1–3):139–45.

73. Lauber SN, Gooderham NJ. The cooked meat-derived mammary carcinogen 2-amino-1-methyl -6-phenylimidazo[4,5-b]pyridine promotes invasive behaviour of breast cancer cells. *Toxicology.* 2011;279(1–3):139–45.

74. Vergnaud AC, Romaguera D, Peeters PH, et al. Adherence to the World Cancer Research Fund/ American Institute for Cancer Research guidelines and risk of death in Europe: results from the European Prospective Investigation into Nutrition and Cancer cohort study. *Am J Clin Nutr.* 2013;97(5):1107–20.

75. Danilo C, Frank PG. Cholesterol and breast cancer development. *Current Opinion in Pharmacology.* 2012;12(6):677.

76. Firestone RA. Low-density lipoprotein as a vehicle for targeting antitumor compounds to cancer cells. *Bioconjug Chem.* 1994 5(2):105–13.

77. Rudling MJ, Ståhle L, Peterson CO, Skoog L. Content of low density lipoprotein receptors in breast cancer tissue related to survival of patients. *Br Med J* (Clin Res Ed). 1986;292(6520): 580–2.

78. Danilo C, Frank PG. Cholesterol and breast cancer development. *Current Opinion in Pharmacology.* 2012;12(6):677–82.

79. Antalis CJ, Arnold T, Rasool T, Lee B, Buhman KK, Siddiqui RA. High ACAT1 expression in estrogen receptor negative basal-like breast cancer cells is associated with LDL-induced proliferation. *Breast Cancer Res Treat.* 2010;122(3):661–70.

80. Firestone RA. Low-density lipoprotein as a vehicle for targeting antitumor compounds to cancer cells. *Bioconjug Chem.* 1994;5(2):105–13.

81. Kitahara CM, Berrington de González A, Freedman ND, et al. Total cholesterol and cancer risk in a large prospective study in Korea. *J Clin Oncol.* 2011;29(12):1592–8.

82. Undela K, Srikanth V, Bansal D. Statin use and risk of breast cancer: a meta-analysis of observational studies. *Breast Cancer Res Treat.* 2012;135(1):261–9.

83. McDougall JA, Malone KE, Daling JR, Cushing-Haugen KL, Porter PL, Li CI. Long-term statin use and risk of ductal and lobular breast cancer among women 55 to 74 years of age. *Cancer Epidemiol Biomarkers Prev.* 2013;22(9):1529–37.

84. Centers for Disease Control and Prevention. Data table for Figure 17. Statin drug use in the past 30 days among adults 45 years of age and over, by sex and age: United States, 1988–1994, 1999–2002, and 2005–2008. National Health and Nutrition Examination Survey. Chartbook: Centers for Disease Control; 2010. http://www.cdc.gov/nchs/data/hus/2010/fig17.pdf. Accessed March 25, 2015.

85. Maunsell E, Drolet M, Brisson J, Robert J, Deschell L. Dietary change after breast cancer: extent, predictors, and relation with psychological distress. *J Clin Oncol.* 2002;20(4):1017–25.

86. Pierce JP, Stefanick ML, Flatt SW, et al. Greater survival after breast cancer in physically active women with high vegetable-fruit intake regardless of obesity. *J Clin Oncol.* 2007;25(17):2345–51.

87. Li Q, Holford TR, Zhang Y, et al. Dietary fiber intake and risk of breast cancer by menopausal and estrogen receptor status. *Eur J Nutr.* 2013;52(1):217–23.

88. Li Q, Holford TR, Zhang Y, et al. Dietary fiber intake and risk of breast cancer by menopausal and estrogen receptor status. *Eur J Nutr.* 2013;52(1):217–23.

89. Howe GR, Hirohata T, Hislop TG, et al. Dietary factors and risk of breast cancer: combined analysis of 12 case-control studies. *J Natl Cancer Inst.* 1990;82(7):561–9.

90. Dong J-Y, He K, Wang P, Qin LQ. Dietary fiber intake and risk of breast cancer: a meta-analysis of prospective cohort studies. *Am J Clin Nutr.* 2011;94(3):900–5.

91. Aune D, Chan DS, Greenwood DC, et al. Dietary fiber and breast cancer risk: a systematic review and meta-analysis of prospective studies. *Ann Oncol.* 2012;23(6):1394–402.

92. Clemens R, Kranz S, Mobley AR, et al. Filling America's fiber intake gap: summary of a roundtable to probe realistic solutions with a focus on grain-based foods. *J Nutr.* 2012;142(7):1390S–401S.

93. Farmer B, Larson BT, Fulgoni VL, Rainville AJ, Liepa GU. A vegetarian dietary pattern as a nutrient-dense approach to weight management: an analysis of the National Health and Nutrition Examination Survey 1999–2004. *J Am Diet Assoc.* 2011;111(6):819–27.

94. Rizzo NS, Jaceldo-Siegl K, Sabate J, Fraser GE. Nutrient profiles of vegetarian and nonvegetarian dietary patterns. *J Acad Nutr Diet.* 2013;113(12):1610–9.

95. Dewell A, Weidner G, Sumner MD, Chi CS, Ornish D. A very-low-fat vegan diet increases intake of protective dietary factors and decreases intake of pathogenic dietary factors. *J Am Diet Assoc.* 2008;108(2):347–56.

96. Gallus S, Talamini R, Giacosa A, et al. Does an apple a day keep the oncologist away? *Ann Oncol.* 2005;16(11):1841–4.

97. Wolfe K, Wu X, Liu RH. Antioxidant activity of apple peels. *J Agric Food Chem.* 2003;51(3):609–14.

98. Sun J, Liu RH. Apple phytochemical extracts inhibit proliferation of estrogen-dependent and estrogen-independent human breast cancer cells through cell cycle modulation. *J Agric Food Chem.* 2008;56(24):11661–7.

99. Wolfe K, Wu X, Liu RH. Antioxidant activity of apple peels. *J Agric Food Chem.* 2003;51(3): 609–14.

100. Reagan-Shaw S, Eggert D, Mukhtar H, Ahmad N. Antiproliferative effects of apple peel extract against cancer cells. *Nutr Cancer.* 2010;62(4):517–24.

101. Steck SE, Gaudet MM, Eng SM, et al. Cooked meat and risk of breast cancer—lifetime versus recent dietary intake. *Epidemiology.* 2007;18(3):373–82.

102. Murray S, Lake BG, Gray S, et al. Effect of cruciferous vegetable consumption on heterocyclic aromatic amine metabolism in man. *Carcinogenesis.* 2001;22(9):1413–20.

103. Murray S, Lake BG, Gray S, et al. Effect of cruciferous vegetable consumption on heterocyclic aromatic amine metabolism in man. *Carcinogenesis.* 2001;22(9):1413–20.

104. Murray S, Lake BG, Gray S, et al. Effect of cruciferous vegetable consumption on heterocyclic aromatic amine metabolism in man. *Carcinogenesis.* 2001;22(9):1413–20.

105. Thiébaud HP, Knize MG, Kuzmicky PA, Hsieh DP, Felton JS. Airborne mutagens produced by frying beef, pork and a soy-based food. *Food Chem Toxicol.* 1995;33(10):821–8.

106. Boggs DA, Palmer JR, Wise LA, et al. Fruit and vegetable intake in relation to risk of breast cancer in the Black Women's Health Study. *Am J Epidemiol.* 2010;172(11):1268–79.

107. Boggs DA, Palmer JR, Wise LA, et al. Fruit and vegetable intake in relation to risk of breast cancer in the Black Women's Health Study. *Am J Epidemiol.* 2010;172(11):1268–79.

108. Tiede B, Kang Y. From milk to malignancy: the role of mammary stem cells in development, pregnancy and breast cancer. *Cell Res.* 2011;21(2):245–57.

109. Clevers H. The cancer stem cell: premises, promises and challenges. *Nat Med.* 2011;17(3):313–9.

110. Karrison TG, Ferguson DJ, Meier P. Dormancy of mammary carcinoma after mastectomy. *J Natl Cancer Inst.* 1999;91(1):80–5.

111. Aguirre-Ghiso JA. Models, mechanisms and clinical evidence for cancer dormancy. *Nat Rev Cancer.* 2007;7(11):834–46.

112. Clevers H. The cancer stem cell: premises, promises and challenges. *Nat Med.* 2011;17(3):313–9.

113. Li Y, Zhang T, Korkaya H, et al. Sulforaphane, a dietary component of broccoli/broccoli sprouts, inhibits breast cancer stem cells. *Clin Cancer Res.* 2010;16(9):2580–90.

114. Cornblatt BS, Ye L, Dinkova-Kostova AT, et al. Preclinical and clinical evaluation of sulforaphane for chemoprevention in the breast. *Carcinogenesis.* 2007;28(7):1485–90.

115. Fahey JW, Zhang Y, Talalay P. Broccoli sprouts: an exceptionally rich source of inducers of enzymes that protect against chemical carcinogens. *Proc Natl Acad Sci USA.* 1997;94(19): 10367–72.

116. Goyal A, Sharma V, Upadhyay N, Gill S, Sihag M. Flax and flaxseed oil: an ancient medicine & modern functional food. *J Food Sci Technol.* 2014;51(9):1633–53.

117. Smeds AI, Eklund PC, Sjöholm RE, et al. Quantification of a broad spectrum of lignans in cereals, oilseeds, and nuts. *J Agric Food Chem.* 2007;55(4):1337–46.

118. Rosolowich V, Saettler E, Szuck B, et al. Mastalgia. *J Obstet Gynaecol Can.* 2006;170:49–57.

119. Phipps WR, Martini MC, Lampe JW, Slavin JL, Kurzer MS. Effect of flax seed ingestion on the menstrual cycle. *J Clin Endocrinol Metab.* 1993;77(5):1215–9.

120. Kelsey JL, Gammon MD, John EM. Reproductive factors and breast cancer. *Epidemiol Rev.* 1993;15(1):36–47.

121. Knekt P, Adlercreutz H, Rissanen H, Aromaa A, Teppo L, Heliövaara M. Does antibacterial treatment for urinary tract infection contribute to the risk of breast cancer? *Br J Cancer.* 2000;82(5):1107–10.

122. Buck K, Zaineddin AK, Vrieling A, Linseisen J, Chang-Claude J. Meta-analyses of lignans and enterolignans in relation to breast cancer risk. *Am J Clin Nutr.* 2010;92(1):141–53.

123. Abarzua S, Serikawa T, Szewczyk M, Richter DU, Piechulla B, Briese V. Antiproliferative activity of lignans against the breast carcinoma cell lines MCF 7 and BT 20. *Arch Gynecol Obstet.* 2012;285(4):1145–51.

124. Fabian CJ, Kimler BF, Zalles CM, et al. Reduction in Ki-67 in benign breast tissue of high-risk women with the lignan secoisolariciresinol diglycoside. *Cancer Prev Res* (Phila). 2010;3(10):1342–50.

125. Buck K, Vrieling A, Zaineddin AK, et al. Serum enterolactone and prognosis of postmenopausal breast cancer. *J Clin Oncol.* 2011;29(28):3730–8.

126. Guglielmini P, Rubagotti A, Boccardo F. Serum enterolactone levels and mortality outcome in women with early breast cancer: a retrospective cohort study. *Breast Cancer Res Treat.* 2012;132(2):661–8.

127. McCann SE, Thompson LU, Nie J, et al. Dietary lignan intakes in relation to survival among women with breast cancer: the Western New York Exposures and Breast Cancer (WEB) Study. *Breast Cancer Res Treat.* 2010;122(1):229–35.

128. Åberg UW, Saarinen N, Abrahamsson A, Nurmi T, Engblom S, Dabrosin C. Tamoxifen and flaxseed alter angiogenesis regulators in normal human breast tissue in vivo. *PLoS ONE.* 2011;6(9):e25720.

129. Thompson LU, Chen JM, Li T, Strasser-Weippl K, Goss PE. Dietary flaxseed alters tumor biological markers in postmenopausal breast cancer. *Clin Cancer Res.* 2005;11(10):3828–35.

130. Mueller SO, Simon S, Chae K, Metzler M, Korach KS. Phytoestrogens and their human metabolites show distinct agonistic and antagonistic properties on estrogen receptor alpha (ERalpha) and ERbeta in human cells. *Toxicol Sci.* 2004;80(1):14–25.

131. Oseni T, Patel R, Pyle J, Jordan VC. Selective estrogen receptor modulators and phytoestrogens. *Planta Med.* 2008;74(13):1656–65.

132. Oseni T, Patel R, Pyle J, Jordan VC. Selective estrogen receptor modulators and phytoestrogens. *Planta Med.* 2008;74(13):1656–65.

133. Nagata C, Mizoue T, Tanaka K, et al. Soy intake and breast cancer risk: an evaluation based on a systematic review of epidemiologic evidence among the Japanese population. *Jpn J Clin Oncol.* 2014;44(3):282–95.

134. Chen MN, Lin CC, Liu CF. Efficacy of phytoestrogens for menopausal symptoms: a meta-analysis and systematic review. *Climacteric.* 2015;18(2):260–9.

135. Chi F, Wu R, Zeng YC, Xing R, Liu Y, Xu ZG. Post-diagnosis soy food intake and breast cancer survival: a meta-analysis of cohort studies. *Asian Pac J Cancer Prev.* 2013;14(4):2407–12.

136. Bhagwat S, Haytowitz DB, Holden JM. USDA Database for the Isoflavone Content of Selected Foods, Release 2.0. http://www.ars.usda.gov/SP2UserFiles/Place/12354500/Data/isoflav/Isoflav_R2.pdf. September 2008. Accessed March 26, 2015.

137. Nechuta SJ, Caan BJ, Chen WY, et al. Soy food intake after diagnosis of breast cancer and survival: an in-depth analysis of combined evidence from cohort studies of US and Chinese women. *Am J Clin Nutr.* 2012;96(1):123–32.

138. Chi F, Wu R, Zeng YC, Xing R, Liu Y, Xu ZG. Post-diagnosis soy food intake and breast cancer survival: a meta-analysis of cohort studies. *Asian Pac J Cancer Prev.* 2013;14(4):2407–12.

139. Kang HB, Zhang YF, Yang JD, Lu KL. Study on soy isoflavone consumption and risk of breast cancer and survival. *Asian Pac J Cancer Prev.* 2012;13(3):995–8.

140. Bosviel R, Dumollard E, Déchelotte P, Bignon YJ, Bernard-Gallon D. Can soy phytoestrogens decrease DNA methylation in BRCA1 and BRCA2 oncosuppressor genes in breast cancer? *OMICS.* 2012;16(5):235–44.

141. National Breast Cancer Coalition. National Breast Cancer Coalition survey reveals that heightened breast cancer awareness has insufficient impact on knowledge. http://www .prnewswire.com/news-releases/national-breast-cancer-coalition-survey-reveals-that-heightened-breast-cancer-awareness-has-insufficient-impact-on-knowledge-58248962. html. October 1, 2007. Accessed March 23, 2015.

142. Colditz GA, Willett WC, Hunter DJ, et al. Family history, age, and risk of breast cancer. Prospective data from the Nurses' Health Study. *JAMA*. 1993;270(3):338–43.

143. Bal A, Verma S, Joshi K, et al. BRCA1-methylated sporadic breast cancers are BRCA-like in showing a basal phenotype and absence of ER expression. *Virchows Arch*. 2012;461(3): 305–12.

144. Bosviel R, Dumollard E, Déchelotte P, Bignon YJ, Bernard-Gallon D. Can soy phytoestrogens decrease DNA methylation in BRCA1 and BRCA2 oncosuppressor genes in breast cancer? *OMICS*. 2012;16(5):235–44.

145. Magee PJ, Rowland I. Soy products in the management of breast cancer. *Curr Opin Clin Nutr Metab Care*. 2012;15(6):586–91.

146. Parkin DM, Fernández LM. Use of statistics to assess the global burden of breast cancer. *Breast J*. 2006;12 Suppl 1:S70–80.

147. Wu AH, Butler LM. Green tea and breast cancer. *Mol Nutr Food Res*. 2011;55(6):921–30.

148. Korde LA, Wu AH, Fears T, et al. Childhood soy intake and breast cancer risk in Asian American women. *Cancer Epidemiol Biomarkers Prev*. 2009;18(4):1050–9.

149. Wakchaure GC. Chapter 3: Production and marketing of mushrooms: Global and national scenario. In : Mushrooms: Singh N, Cijay B, Kamal S, Wakchaure GC, eds. *Cultivation, Marketing and Consumption*. Himachal Pradesh-173213, India: Directorate of Mushroom Research; 2014:15–22.

150. Zhang M, Huang J, Xie X, Holman CD. Dietary intakes of mushrooms and green tea combine to reduce the risk of breast cancer in Chinese women. *Int J Cancer*. 2009;124(6):1404–8.

151. Ganz PA. A teachable moment for oncologists: cancer survivors, 10 million strong and growing! *J Clin Oncol*. 2005;23(24):5458–60.

152. Ganz PA. A teachable moment for oncologists: cancer survivors, 10 million strong and growing! *J Clin Oncol*. 2005;23(24):5458–60.

12. How Not to Die from Suicidal Depression

1. Centers for Disease Control and Prevention. National Center for Health Statistics. Deaths: Final Data for 2013, table 18. http://www.cdc.gov/nchs/data/nvsr/nvsr64/nvsr64_02.pdf. Accessed March 20, 2015.

2. Sartorius N. The economic and social burden of depression. *J Clin Psychiatry*. 2001;62 Suppl 15: 8–11.

3. Preamble to the Constitution of the World Health Organization as adopted by the International Health Conference, New York, 19–22 June 1946; signed on 22 July 1946 by the representatives of 61 States (Official Records of the World Health Organization, no. 2, p. 100) and entered into force on 7 April 1948.

4. Kessler RC, Chiu WT, Demler O, Merikangas KR, Walters EE. Prevalence, severity, and comorbidity of 12-month DSM-IV disorders in the National Comorbidity Survey Replication. *Arch Gen Psychiatry*. 2005;62(6):617–27.

5. Chida Y, Steptoe A. Positive psychological well-being and mortality: a quantitative review of prospective observational studies. *Psychosom Med*. 2008;70(7):741–56.

6. Chida Y, Steptoe A. Positive psychological well-being and mortality: a quantitative review of prospective observational studies. *Psychosom Med.* 2008;70(7):741–56.

7. Grant N, Wardle J, Steptoe A. The relationship between life satisfaction and health behavior: a cross-cultural analysis of young adults. *Int J Behav Med.* 2009;16(3):259–68.

8. Cohen S, Doyle WJ, Turner RB, Alper CM, Skoner DP. Emotional style and susceptibility to the common cold. *Psychosom Med.* 2003;65(4):652–7.

9. Cohen S, Alper CM, Doyle WJ, Treanor JJ, Turner RB. Positive emotional style predicts resistance to illness after experimental exposure to rhinovirus or influenza A virus. *Psychosom Med.* 2006;68(6):809–15.

10. Beezhold BL, Johnston CS, Daigle DR. Vegetarian diets are associated with healthy mood states: a cross-sectional study in Seventh Day Adventist adults. *Nutr J.* 2010;9:26.

11. Beezhold BL, Johnston CS, Daigle DR. Vegetarian diets are associated with healthy mood states: a cross-sectional study in Seventh Day Adventist adults. *Nutr J.* 2010;9:26.

12. Knutsen SF. Lifestyle and the use of health services. *Am J Clin Nutr.* 1994;59(5 Suppl):1171S–1175S.

13. Beezhold BL, Johnston CS, Daigle DR. Vegetarian diets are associated with healthy mood states: a cross-sectional study in Seventh Day Adventist adults. *Nutr J.* 2010;9:26.

14. Fisher M, Levine PH, Weiner B, et al. The effect of vegetarian diets on plasma lipid and platelet levels. *Arch Intern Med.* 1986;146(6):1193–7.

15. Institute of Medicine. *Dietary Reference Intakes: The Essential Guide to Nutrient Requirements.* Washington, D.C.: National Academies Press; 2006.

16. Vaz JS, Kac G, Nardi AE, Hibbeln JR. Omega-6 fatty acids and greater likelihood of suicide risk and major depression in early pregnancy. *J Affect Disord.* 2014;152–154:76–82.

17. National Cancer Institute. Table 4: Food Sources of Arachidonic Acid. http://appliedresearch.cancer.gov/diet/foodsources/fatty_acids/table4.html. Modified October 18, 2013. Accessed March 11, 2015.

18. Hirota S, Adachi N, Gomyo T, Kawashima H, Kiso Y, Kawabata T. Low-dose arachidonic acid intake increases erythrocytes and plasma arachidonic acid in young women. *Prostaglandins Leukot Essent Fatty Acids.* 2010;83(2):83–8.

19. Beezhold BL, Johnston CS, Daigle DR. Vegetarian diets are associated with healthy mood states: a cross-sectional study in Seventh Day Adventist adults. *Nutr J.* 2010;9:26.

20. Beezhold BL, Johnston CS. Restriction of meat, fish, and poultry in omnivores improves mood: a pilot randomized controlled trial. *Nutr J.* 2012;11:9.

21. Beezhold BL, Johnston CS, Daigle DR. Restriction of flesh foods in omnivores improves mood: a pilot randomized controlled trial. American Public Health Association Annual Conference, November 7–11, 2009. Philadelphia, PA.

22. Katcher HI, Ferdowsian HR, Hoover VJ, Cohen JL, Barnard ND. A worksite vegan nutrition program is well-accepted and improves health-related quality of life and work productivity. *Ann Nutr Metab.* 2010;56(4):245–52.

23. Katcher HI, Ferdowsian HR, Hoover VJ, Cohen JL, Barnard ND. A worksite vegan nutrition program is well-accepted and improves health-related quality of life and work productivity. *Ann Nutr Metab.* 2010;56(4):245–52.

24. Mishra S, Xu J, Agarwal U, Gonzales J, Levin S, Barnard ND. A multicenter randomized controlled trial of a plant-based nutrition program to reduce body weight and cardiovascular risk in the corporate setting: the GEICO study. *Eur J Clin Nutr.* 2013;67(7):718–24.

25. Agarwal U, Mishra S, Xu J, Levin S, Gonzales J, Barnard ND. A multicenter randomized controlled trial of a nutrition intervention program in a multiethnic adult population in the corporate setting reduces depression and anxiety and improves quality of life: The GEICO Study. *Am J Health Promot.* 2015;29(4):245–54.

26. Tsai AC, Chang T-L, Chi S-H. Frequent consumption of vegetables predicts lower risk of depression in older Taiwanese—results of a prospective population-based study. *Public Health Nutr.* 2012;15(6):1087–92.

27. Gomez-Pinilla F, Nguyen TTJ. Natural mood foods: the actions of polyphenols against psychiatric and cognitive disorders. *Nutr Neurosci.* 2012;15(3):127–33.

28. Meyer JH, Ginovart N, Boovariwala A, et al. Elevated monoamine oxidase A levels in the brain: an explanation for the monoamine imbalance of major depression. *Arch Gen Psychiatry.* 2006; 63(11):1209–16.

29. de Villiers JC. Intracranial haemorrhage in patients treated with monoamineoxidase inhibitors. *Br J Psychiatry.* 1966;112(483):109–18.

30. Dixon Clarke SE, Ramsay RR. Dietary inhibitors of monoamine oxidase A. *J Neural Transm.* 2011;118(7):1031–41.

31. Lai JS, Hiles S, Bisquera A, Hure AJ, McEvoy M, Attia J. A systematic review and meta-analysis of dietary patterns and depression in community-dwelling adults. *Am J Clin Nutr.* 2014;99(1): 181–97.

32. White BA, Horwath CC, Conner TS. Many apples a day keep the blues away—daily experiences of negative and positive affect and food consumption in young adults. *Br J Health Psychol.* 2013;18(4):782–98.

33. Odjakova M, Hadjiivanova C. Animal neurotransmitter substances in plants. *Bulg J Plant Physiol.* 1997;23:94–102.

34. Ghirri A, Cannella C, Bignetti E. The psychoactive effects of aromatic amino acids. *Curr Nutr Food Science.* 2011;7(1):21–32.

35. Allen JA, Peterson A, Sufit R, et al. Post-epidemic eosinophilia-myalgia syndrome associated with L-tryptophan. *Arthritis Rheum.* 2011;63(11):3633–9.

36. Fernstrom JD, Faller DV. Neutral amino acids in the brain: changes in response to food ingestion. *J Neurochem.* 1978;30(6):1531–8.

37. Wurtman RJ, Wurtman JJ, Regan MM, McDermott JM, Tsay RH, Breu JJ. Effects of normal meals rich in carbohydrates or proteins on plasma tryptophan and tyrosine ratios. *Am J Clin Nutr.* 2003;77(1):128–32.

38. Wurtman JJ, Brzezinski A, Wurtman RJ, Laferrere B. Effect of nutrient intake on premenstrual depression. *Am J Obstet Gynecol.* 1989;161(5):1228–34.

39. Brinkworth GD, Buckley JD, Noakes M, Clifton PM, Wilson CJ. Long-term effects of a very low-carbohydrate diet and a low-fat diet on mood and cognitive function. *Arch Intern Med.* 2009;169(20):1873–80.

40. Fernstrom JD, Wurtman RJ. Brain serotonin content: physiological regulation by plasma neutral amino acids. *Science.* 1972;178(4059):414–6.

41. Hudson C, Hudson S, MacKenzie J. Protein-source tryptophan as an efficacious treatment for social anxiety disorder: a pilot study. *Can J Physiol Pharmacol.* 2007;85(9):928–32.

42. Schweiger U, Laessle R, Kittl S, Dickhaut B, Schweiger M, Pirke KM. Macronutrient intake, plasma large neutral amino acids and mood during weight-reducing diets. *J Neural Transm.* 1986;67(1–2):77–86.

43. Ferrence SC, Bendersky G. Therapy with saffron and the goddess at Thera. *Perspect Biol Med.* 2004;47(2):199–226.

44. Noorbala AA, Akhondzadeh S, Tahmacebi-Pour N, Jamshidi AH. Hydro-alcoholic extract of Crocus sativus L. versus fluoxetine in the treatment of mild to moderate depression: a double-blind, randomized pilot trial. *J Ethnopharmacol.* 2005;97(2):281–4.

45. Gohari AR, Saeidnia S, Mahmoodabadi MK. An overview on saffron, phytochemicals, and medicinal properties. *Pharmacogn Rev.* 2013;7(13):61–6.

46. Fukui H, Toyoshima K, Komaki R. Psychological and neuroendocrinological effects of odor of saffron (Crocus sativus). *Phytomedicine*. 2011;18(8–9):726–30.

47. Lucas M, O'Reilly EJ, Pan A, et al. Coffee, caffeine, and risk of completed suicide: results from three prospective cohorts of American adults. *World J Biol Psychiatry*. 2014;15(5): 377–86.

48. Klatsky AL, Armstrong MA, Friedman GD. Coffee, tea, and mortality. *Ann Epidemiol*. 1993; 3(4):375–81.

49. Tanskanen A, Tuomilehto J, Viinamnen H, Vartiainen E, Lehtonen J, Puska P. Heavy coffee drinking and the risk of suicide. *Eur J Epidemiol*. 2000;16(9):789–91.

50. Guo X, Park Y, Freedman ND, et al. Sweetened beverages, coffee, and tea and depression risk among older US adults. *PLoS One*. 2014;9(4):e94715.

51. Maher TJ, Wurtman RJ. Possible neurologic effects of aspartame, a widely used food additive. *Environ Health Perspect*. 1987;75:53–7.

52. Walton RG, Hudak R, Green-Waite RJ. Adverse reactions to aspartame: double-blind challenge in patients from a vulnerable population. *Biol Psychiatry*. 1993;34(1–2):13–7.

53. Lindseth GN, Coolahan SE, Petros TV, Lindseth PD. Neurobehavioral effects of aspartame consumption. *Res Nurs Health*. 2014;37(3):185–93.

54. U.S. Food and Drug Administration. Aspartame: Commissioner's final decision. *Fed Reg*. 1981;46: 38285–308.

55. Lindseth GN, Coolahan SE, Petros TV, Lindseth PD. Neurobehavioral effects of aspartame consumption. *Res Nurs Health*. 2014;37(3):185–93.

56. Whitehouse CR, Boullata J, McCauley LA. The potential toxicity of artificial sweeteners. *AAOHN J*. 2008;56(6):251–9.

57. Aspartame Information Center: Consumer Products. Aspartame website. http://www .aspartame.org/about/consumer-products/#.VF_cyr74tSU. Updated 2015. Accessed March 11, 2015.

58. Whitehouse CR, Boullata J, McCauley LA. The potential toxicity of artificial sweeteners. *AAOHN J*. 2008;56(6):251–9.

59. Yeung RR. The acute effects of exercise on mood state. *J Psychosom Res*. 1996;40(2):123–41.

60. Goodwin RD. Association between physical activity and mental disorders among adults in the United States. *Prev Med*. 2003;36(6):698–703.

61. Blumenthal JA, Babyak MA, Moore KA, et al. Effects of exercise training on older patients with major depression. *Arch Intern Med*. 1999;159(19):2349–56.

62. Blumenthal JA, Babyak MA, Doraiswamy PM, et al. Exercise and pharmacotherapy in the treatment of major depressive disorder. *Psychosom Med*. 2007;69(7):587–96.

63. Pandya CD, Howell KR, Pillai A. Antioxidants as potential therapeutics for neuropsychiatric disorders. *Prog Neuropsychopharmacol Biol Psychiatry*. 2013;46:214–23.

64. Michel TM, Pülschen D, Thome J. The role of oxidative stress in depressive disorders. *Curr Pharm Des*. 2012;18(36):5890–9.

65. McMartin SE, Jacka FN, Colman I. The association between fruit and vegetable consumption and mental health disorders: evidence from five waves of a national survey of Canadians. *Prev Med*. 2013;56(3–4):225–30.

66. Beydoun MA, Beydoun HA, Boueiz A, Shroff MR, Zonderman AB. Antioxidant status and its association with elevated depressive symptoms among US adults: National Health and Nutrition Examination Surveys 2005–6. *Br J Nutr*. 2013;109(9):1714–29.

67. Niu K, Guo H, Kakizaki M, et al. A tomato-rich diet is related to depressive symptoms among an elderly population aged 70 years and over: a population-based, cross-sectional analysis. *J Affect Disord*. 2013;144(1–2):165–70.

68. Payne ME, Steck SE, George RR, Steffens DC. Fruit, vegetable, and antioxidant intakes are lower in older adults with depression. *J Acad Nutr Diet*. 2012;112(12):2022–7.

69. Gilbody S, Lightfoot T, Sheldon T. Is low folate a risk factor for depression? A meta-analysis and exploration of heterogeneity. *J Epidemiol Community Health*. 2007;61(7):631–7.

70. Tolmunen T, Hintikka J, Ruusunen A, et al. Dietary folate and the risk of depression in Finnish middle-aged men. A prospective follow-up study. *Psychother Psychosom*. 2004;73(6):334–9.

71. Sharpley AL, Hockney R, McPeake L, Geddes JR, Cowen PJ. Folic acid supplementation for prevention of mood disorders in young people at familial risk: a randomised, double blind, placebo controlled trial. *J Affect Disord*. 2014;167:306–11.

72. Penn E, Tracy DK. The drugs don't work? Antidepressants and the current and future pharmacological management of depression. *Ther Adv Psychopharmacol*. 2012;2(5):179–88.

73. Turner EH, Matthews AM, Linardatos E, Tell RA, Rosenthal R. Selective publication of antidepressant trials and its influence on apparent efficacy. *N Engl J Med*. 2008;358(3):252–60.

74. Kirsch I. Antidepressants and the placebo effect. *Z Psychol*. 2014;222(3):128–34.

75. Kirsch I. Antidepressants and the placebo response. *Epidemiol Psichiatr Soc*. 2009;18(4):318–22.

76. Spence D. Are antidepressants overprescribed? Yes. *BMJ*. 2013;346:f191.

77. Sugarman MA, Loree AM, Baltes BB, Grekin ER, Kirsch I. The efficacy of paroxetine and placebo in treating anxiety and depression: a meta-analysis of change on the Hamilton Rating Scales. *PLoS ONE*. 2014;9(8):e106337.

78. Kirsch I. Antidepressants and the placebo effect. *Z Psychol*. 2014;222(3):128–34.

79. Blease C. Deception as treatment: the case of depression. *J Med Ethics*. 2011;37(1):13–6.

80. Kirsch I. Antidepressants and the placebo effect. *Z Psychol*. 2014;222(3):128–34.

81. Kirsch I. Antidepressants and the placebo effect. *Z Psychol*. 2014;222(3):128–34.

13. How Not to Die from Prostate Cancer

1. Jahn JL, Giovannucci EL, Stampfer MJ. The high prevalence of undiagnosed prostate cancer at autopsy: implications for epidemiology and treatment of prostate cancer in the Prostate-specific Antigen-era. *Int J Cancer*. 2014;Dec 29.

2. Draisma G, Etzioni R, Tsodikov A, et al. Lead time and overdiagnosis in prostate-specific antigen screening: importance of methods and context. *J Natl Cancer Inst*. 2009;101(6):374–83.

3. Centers for Disease Control and Prevention. Prostate Cancer Statistics. http://www.cdc.gov/cancer/prostate/statistics/index.htm. Updated September 2, 2014. Accessed March 11, 2015.

4. Maruyama K, Oshima T, Ohyama K. Exposure to exogenous estrogen through intake of commercial milk produced from pregnant cows. *Pediatr Int*. 2010;52(1):33–8.

5. Danby FW. Acne and milk, the diet myth, and beyond. *J Am Acad Dermatol*. 2005;52(2):360–2.

6. Afeiche M, Williams PL, Mendiola J, et al. Dairy food intake in relation to semen quality and reproductive hormone levels among physically active young men. *Hum Reprod*. 2013;28(8):2265–75.

7. Maruyama K, Oshima T, Ohyama K. Exposure to exogenous estrogen through intake of commercial milk produced from pregnant cows. *Pediatr Int*. 2010;52(1):33–8.

8. Steinman G. Mechanisms of twinning: VII. Effect of diet and heredity on the human twinning rate. *J Reprod Med*. 2006;51(5):405–10.

9. Melnik BC, John SM, Schmitz G. Milk is not just food but most likely a genetic transfection system activating mTORC1 signaling for postnatal growth. *Nutr J*. 2013;12:103.

10. Ludwig DS, Willett WC. Three daily servings of reduced-fat milk: an evidence-based recommendation? *JAMA Pediatr.* 2013;167(9):788–9.

11. Ludwig DS, Willett WC. Three daily servings of reduced-fat milk: an evidence-based recommendation? *JAMA Pediatr.* 2013;167(9):788–9.

12. Tate PL, Bibb R, Larcom LL. Milk stimulates growth of prostate cancer cells in culture. *Nutr Cancer.* 2011;63(8):1361–6.

13. Ganmaa D, Li XM, Qin LQ, Wang PY, Takeda M, Sato A. The experience of Japan as a clue to the etiology of testicular and prostatic cancers. *Med Hypotheses.* 2003;60(5):724–30.

14. Ganmaa D, Li XM, Wang J, Qin LQ, Wang PY, Sato A. Incidence and mortality of testicular and prostatic cancers in relation to world dietary practices. *Int J Cancer.* 2002;98(2):262–7.

15. Epstein SS. Unlabeled milk from cows treated with biosynthetic growth hormones: a case of regulatory abdication. *Int J Health Serv.* 1996;26(1):173–85.

16. Tate PL, Bibb R, Larcom LL. Milk stimulates growth of prostate cancer cells in culture. *Nutr Cancer.* 2011;63(8):1361–6.

17. Qin LQ, Xu JY, Wang PY, Kaneko T, Hoshi K, Sato A. Milk consumption is a risk factor for prostate cancer: meta-analysis of case-control studies. *Nutr Cancer.* 2004;48(1):22–7.

18. Qin LQ, Xu JY, Wang PY, Tong J, Hoshi K. Milk consumption is a risk factor for prostate cancer in Western countries: evidence from cohort studies. *Asia Pac J Clin Nutr.* 2007;16(3): 467–76.

19. Aune D, Navarro Rosenblatt DA, Chan DS, et al. Dairy products, calcium, and prostate cancer risk: a systematic review and meta-analysis of cohort studies. *Am J Clin Nutr.* 2015;101(1): 87–117.

20. Bischoff-Ferrari HA, Dawson-Hughes B, Baron JA, et al. Milk intake and risk of hip fracture in men and women: a meta-analysis of prospective cohort studies. *J Bone Miner Res.* 2011;26(4): 833–9.

21. Feskanich D, Bischoff-Ferrari HA, Frazier AL, Willett WC. Milk consumption during teenage years and risk of hip fractures in older adults. *JAMA Pediatr.* 2014;168(1):54–60.

22. Michaëlsson K, Wolk A, Langenskiöld S, et al. Milk intake and risk of mortality and fractures in women and men: cohort studies. *BMJ.* 2014;349:g6015.

23. Batey LA, Welt CK, Rohr F, et al. Skeletal health in adult patients with classic galactosemia. *Osteoporos Int.* 2013;24(2):501–9.

24. Michaëlsson K, Wolk A, Langenskiöld S, et al. Milk intake and risk of mortality and fractures in women and men: cohort studies. *BMJ.* 2014;349:g6015.

25. Cui X, Wang L, Zuo P, et al. D-galactose-caused life shortening in Drosophila melanogaster and Musca domestica is associated with oxidative stress. *Biogerontology.* 2004;5(5):317–25.

26. Cui X, Zuo P, Zhang Q, et al. Chronic systemic D-galactose exposure induces memory loss, neurodegeneration, and oxidative damage in mice: protective effects of R-alpha-lipoic acid. *J Neurosci Res.* 2006;84(3):647–54.

27. Michaëlsson K, Wolk A, Langenskiöld S, et al. Milk intake and risk of mortality and fractures in women and men: cohort studies. *BMJ.* 2014;349:g6015.

28. Michaëlsson K, Wolk A, Langenskiöld S, et al. Milk intake and risk of mortality and fractures in women and men: cohort studies. *BMJ.* 2014;349:g6015.

29. Michaëlsson K, Wolk A, Langenskiöld S, et al. Milk intake and risk of mortality and fractures in women and men: cohort studies. *BMJ.* 2014;349:g6015.

30. Michaëlsson K, Wolk A, Langenskiöld S, et al. Milk intake and risk of mortality and fractures in women and men: cohort studies. *BMJ.* 2014;349:g6015.

31. Schooling CM. Milk and mortality. *BMJ.* 2014;349:g6205.

32. Richman EL, Stampfer MJ, Paciorek A, Broering JM, Carroll PR, Chan JM. Intakes of meat, fish, poultry, and eggs and risk of prostate cancer progression. *Am J Clin Nutr.* 2010;91(3): 712–21.

33. Richman EL, Stampfer MJ, Paciorek A, Broering JM, Carroll PR, Chan JM. Intakes of meat, fish, poultry, and eggs and risk of prostate cancer progression. *Am J Clin Nutr.* 2010;91(3): 712–21.

34. Richman EL, Stampfer MJ, Paciorek A, Broering JM, Carroll PR, Chan JM. Intakes of meat, fish, poultry, and eggs and risk of prostate cancer progression. *Am J Clin Nutr.* 2010;91(3): 712–21.

35. Richman EL, Stampfer MJ, Paciorek A, Broering JM, Carroll PR, Chan JM. Intakes of meat, fish, poultry, and eggs and risk of prostate cancer progression. *Am J Clin Nutr.* 2010;91(3): 712–21.

36. Johansson M, Van Guelpen B, Vollset SE, et al. One-carbon metabolism and prostate cancer risk: prospective investigation of seven circulating B vitamins and metabolites. *Cancer Epidemiol Biomarkers Prev.* 2009;18(5):1538–43.

37. Richman EL, Stampfer MJ, Paciorek A, Broering JM, Carroll PR, Chan JM. Intakes of meat, fish, poultry, and eggs and risk of prostate cancer progression. *Am J Clin Nutr.* 2010;91(3): 712–21.

38. Richman EL, Kenfield SA, Stampfer MJ, et al. Choline intake and risk of lethal prostate cancer: incidence and survival. *Am J Clin Nutr.* 2012;96(4):855–63.

39. Richman EL, Kenfield SA, Stampfer MJ, Giovannucci EL, Chan JM. Egg, red meat, and poultry intake and risk of lethal prostate cancer in the prostate-specific antigen-era: incidence and survival. *Cancer Prev Res* (Phila). 2011;4(12):2110–21.

40. Tang WH, Wang Z, Levison BS, et al. Intestinal microbial metabolism of phosphatidylcholine and cardiovascular risk. *N Engl J Med.* 2013;368(17):1575–84.

41. Koeth RA, Wang Z, Levison BS, et al. Intestinal microbiota metabolism of L-carnitine, a nutrient in red meat, promotes atherosclerosis. *Nat Med.* 2013;19:576–85.

42. Tang WH, Wang Z, Levison BS, et al. Intestinal microbial metabolism of phosphatidylcholine and cardiovascular risk. *N Engl J Med.* 2013;368(17):1575–84.

43. Choline: there's something fishy about this vitamin. *Harv Health Lett.* 2004;30(1):3.

44. Mitch Kanter, Ph.D., e-mail communication, January 6, 2010.

45. Hubbard JD, Inkeles S, Barnard RJ. Nathan Pritikin's heart. *N Engl J Med.* 1985;313(1):52.

46. Ornish D, Weidner G, Fair WR, et al. Intensive lifestyle changes may affect the progression of prostate cancer. *J Urol.* 2005;174(3):1065–9.

47. Ornish D, Weidner G, Fair WR, et al. Intensive lifestyle changes may affect the progression of prostate cancer. *J Urol.* 2005;174(3):1065–9.

48. Barnard RJ, Gonzalez JH, Liva ME, Ngo TH. Effects of a low-fat, high-fiber diet and exercise program on breast cancer risk factors in vivo and tumor cell growth and apoptosis in vitro. *Nutr Cancer.* 2006;55(1):28–34.

49. Barnard RJ, Ngo TH, Leung PS, Aronson WJ, Golding LA. A low-fat diet and/or strenuous exercise alters the IGF axis in vivo and reduces prostate tumor cell growth in vitro. *Prostate.* 2003;56(3):201–6.

50. Barnard RJ, Ngo TH, Leung PS, Aronson WJ, Golding LA. A low-fat diet and/or strenuous exercise alters the IGF axis in vivo and reduces prostate tumor cell growth in vitro. *Prostate.* 2003;56(3):201–6.

51. Barnard RJ, Ngo TH, Leung PS, Aronson WJ, Golding LA. A low-fat diet and/or strenuous exercise alters the IGF axis in vivo and reduces prostate tumor cell growth in vitro. *Prostate.* 2003;56(3):201–6.

52. Ornish D, Weidner G, Fair WR, et al. Intensive lifestyle changes may affect the progression of prostate cancer. *J Urol*. 2005;174(3):1065–9.

53. Ornish D, Weidner G, Fair WR, et al. Intensive lifestyle changes may affect the progression of prostate cancer. *J Urol*. 2005;174(3):1065–9.

54. Ornish D, Magbanua MJ, Weidner G, et al. Changes in prostate gene expression in men undergoing an intensive nutrition and lifestyle intervention. *Proc Natl Acad Sci USA*. 2008;105(24): 8369–74.

55. Frattaroli J, Weidner G, Dnistrian AM, et al. Clinical events in prostate cancer lifestyle trial: results from two years of follow-up. *Urology*. 2008;72(6):1319–23.

56. Frey AU, Sønksen J, Fode M. Neglected side effects after radical prostatectomy: a systematic review. *J Sex Med*. 2014;11(2):374–85.

57. Carmody JF, Olendzki BC, Merriam PA, Liu Q, Qiao Y, Ma Y. A novel measure of dietary change in a prostate cancer dietary program incorporating mindfulness training. *J Acad Nutr Diet*. 2012;112(11):1822–7.

58. Blanchard CM, Courneya KS, Stein K. Cancer survivors' adherence to lifestyle behavior recommendations and associations with health-related quality of life: results from the American Cancer Society's SCS-II. *J Clin Oncol*. 2008;26(13):2198–204.

59. Carmody JF, Olendzki BC, Merriam PA, Liu Q, Qiao Y, Ma Y. A novel measure of dietary change in a prostate cancer dietary program incorporating mindfulness training. *J Acad Nutr Diet*. 2012;112(11):1822–7.

60. Carmody JF, Olendzki BC, Merriam PA, Liu Q, Qiao Y, Ma Y. A novel measure of dietary change in a prostate cancer dietary program incorporating mindfulness training. *J Acad Nutr Diet*. 2012;112(11):1822–7.

61. Carmody JF, Olendzki BC, Merriam PA, Liu Q, Qiao Y, Ma Y. A novel measure of dietary change in a prostate cancer dietary program incorporating mindfulness training. *J Acad Nutr Diet*. 2012;112(11):1822–7.

62. Richman EL, Stampfer MJ, Paciorek A, Broering JM, Carroll PR, Chan JM. Intakes of meat, fish, poultry, and eggs and risk of prostate cancer progression. *Am J Clin Nutr*. 2010;91(3): 712–21.

63. Richman EL, Carroll PR, Chan JM. Vegetable and fruit intake after diagnosis and risk of prostate cancer progression. *Int J Cancer*. 2012;131(1):201–10.

64. Allen NE, Appleby PN, Key TJ, et al. Macronutrient intake and risk of urothelial cell carcinoma in the European prospective investigation into cancer and nutrition. *Int J Cancer*. 2013; 132(3):635–44.

65. Morton MS, Chan PS, Cheng C, et al. Lignans and isoflavonoids in plasma and prostatic fluid in men: samples from Portugal, Hong Kong, and the United Kingdom. *Prostate*. 1997;32(2): 122–8.

66. van Die MD, Bone KM, Williams SG, Pirotta MV. Soy and soy isoflavones in prostate cancer: a systematic review and meta-analysis of randomized controlled trials. *BJU Int*. 2014; 113(5b):E119–30.

67. Morton MS, Chan PS, Cheng C, et al. Lignans and isoflavonoids in plasma and prostatic fluid in men: samples from Portugal, Hong Kong, and the United Kingdom. *Prostate*. 1997;32(2):122–8.

68. Lin X, Switzer BR, Demark-Wahnefried W. Effect of mammalian lignans on the growth of prostate cancer cell lines. *Anticancer Res*. 2001;21(6A):3995–9.

69. Demark-Wahnefried W, Price DT, Polascik TJ, et al. Pilot study of dietary fat restriction and flaxseed supplementation in men with prostate cancer before surgery: exploring the effects on hormonal levels, prostate-specific antigen, and histopathologic features. *Urology*. 2001;58(1): 47–52.

70. Leite KR, Camara-Lopes LH, Cury J, Dall'oglio MF, Sañudo A, Srougi M. Prostate cancer detection at rebiopsy after an initial benign diagnosis: results using sextant extended prostate biopsy. *Clinics* (Sao Paulo). 2008;63(3):339–42.

71. Demark-Wahnefried W, Robertson CN, Walther PJ, Polascik TJ, Paulson DF, Vollmer RT. Pilot study to explore effects of low-fat, flaxseed-supplemented diet on proliferation of benign prostatic epithelium and prostate-specific antigen. *Urology*. 2004;63(5):900–4.

72. Demark-Wahnefried W, Polascik TJ, George SL, et al. Flaxseed supplementation (not dietary fat restriction) reduces prostate cancer proliferation rates in men presurgery. *Cancer Epidemiol Biomarkers Prev*. 2008;17(12):3577–87.

73. Wei JT, Calhoun E, Jacobsen SJ. Urologic Diseases in America Project: benign prostatic hyperplasia. *J Urol*. 2008;179(5 Suppl):S75–80.

74. Burnett AL, Wein AJ. Benign prostatic hyperplasia in primary care: what you need to know. *J Urol*. 2006;175(3 Pt 2):S19–24.

75. Taub DA, Wei JT. The economics of benign prostatic hyperplasia and lower urinary tract symptoms in the United States. *Curr Urol Rep*. 2006;7(4):272–81.

76. Metcalfe C, Poon KS. Long-term results of surgical techniques and procedures in men with benign prostatic hyperplasia. *Curr Urol Rep*. 2011;12(4):265–73.

77. Burnett AL, Wein AJ. Benign prostatic hyperplasia in primary care: what you need to know. *J Urol*. 2006;175(3 Pt 2):S19–24.

78. Burnett AL, Wein AJ. Benign prostatic hyperplasia in primary care: what you need to know. *J Urol*. 2006;175(3 Pt 2):S19–24.

79. Gu F. Epidemiological survey of benign prostatic hyperplasia and prostatic cancer in China. *Chin Med J*. 2000;113(4):299–302.

80. Barnard RJ, Kobayashi N, Aronson WJ. Effect of diet and exercise intervention on the growth of prostate epithelial cells. *Prostate Cancer Prostatic Dis*. 2008;11(4):362–6.

81. Zhang W, Wang X, Liu Y, et al. Effects of dietary flaxseed lignan extract on symptoms of benign prostatic hyperplasia. *J Med Food*. 2008;11(2):207–14.

82. Galeone C, Pelucchi C, Talamini R, et al. Onion and garlic intake and the odds of benign prostatic hyperplasia. *Urology*. 2007;70(4):672–6.

83. Bravi F, Bosetti C, Dal Maso L, et al. Food groups and risk of benign prostatic hyperplasia. *Urology*. 2006;67(1):73–9.

84. Zhou Z, Wang Z, Chen C, et al. Transurethral prostate vaporization using an oval electrode in 82 cases of benign prostatic hyperplasia. *Chin Med J*. 1998;111(1):52–5.

85. Piantanelli L. Cancer and aging: from the kinetics of biological parameters to the kinetics of cancer incidence and mortality. *Ann N Y Acad Sci*. 1988;521:99–109.

86. Salvioli S, Capri M, Bucci L, et al. Why do centenarians escape or postpone cancer? The role of IGF-1, inflammation and p53. *Cancer Immunol Immunother*. 2009;58(12):1909–17.

87. Reed JC. Dysregulation of apoptosis in cancer. *J Clin Oncol*. 1999;17(9):2941–53.

88. Rowlands MA, Gunnell D, Harris R, Vatten LJ, Holly JM, Martin RM. Circulating insulin-like growth factor peptides and prostate cancer risk: a systematic review and meta-analysis. *Int J Cancer*. 2009;124(10):2416–29.

89. Guevara-Aguirre J, Balasubramanian P, Guevara-Aguirre M, et al. Growth hormone receptor deficiency is associated with a major reduction in pro-aging signaling, cancer, and diabetes in humans. *Sci Transl Med*. 2011;3(70):70ra13.

90. Allen NE, Appleby PN, Davey GK, Kaaks R, Rinaldi S, Key TJ. The associations of diet with serum insulin-like growth factor I and its main binding proteins in 292 women meat-eaters, vegetarians, and vegans. *Cancer Epidemiol Biomarkers Prev*. 2002;11(11):1441–8.

91. Soliman S, Aronson WJ, Barnard RJ. Analyzing serum-stimulated prostate cancer cell lines after low-fat, high-fiber diet and exercise intervention. *Evid Based Complement Alternat Med.* 2011;2011:529053.

92. Ngo TH, Barnard RJ, Tymchuk CN, Cohen P, Aronson WJ. Effect of diet and exercise on serum insulin, IGF-I, and IGFBP-1 levels and growth of LNCaP cells in vitro (United States). *Cancer Causes Control.* 2002;13(10):929–35.

93. Allen NE, Appleby PN, Davey GK, Key TJ. Hormones and diet: low insulin-like growth factor-I but normal bioavailable androgens in vegan men. *Br J Cancer.* 2000;83(1):95–7.

94. Allen NE, Appleby PN, Davey GK, Kaaks R, Rinaldi S, Key TJ. The associations of diet with serum insulin-like growth factor I and Its main binding proteins in 292 women meat-eaters, vegetarians, and vegans. *Cancer Epidemiol Biomarkers Prev.* 2002;11(11):1441–8.

14. How Not to Die from Parkinson's Disease

1. Jafari S, Etminan M, Aminzadeh F, Samii A. Head injury and risk of Parkinson disease: a systematic review and meta-analysis. *Mov Disord.* 2013;28(9):1222–9.

2. National Cancer Institute. President's Cancer Panel. Reducing environmental cancer risk: what we can do now. http://deainfo.nci.nih.gov/advisory/pcp/annualReports/pcp08-09rpt/PCP_Report_08-09_508.pdf. April 2010. Accessed March 12, 2015.

3. Zeliger HI. Exposure to lipophilic chemicals as a cause of neurological impairments, neurodevelopmental disorders and neurodegenerative diseases. *Interdiscip Toxicol.* 2013;6(3):103–10.

4. Woodruff TJ, Zota AR, Schwartz JM. Environmental chemicals in pregnant women in the United States: NHANES 2003–2004. *Environ Health Perspect.* 2011;119(6):878–85.

5. Woodruff TJ, Zota AR, Schwartz JM. Environmental chemicals in pregnant women in the United States: NHANES 2003–2004. *Environ Health Perspect.* 2011;119(6):878–85.

6. Mariscal-Arcas M, Lopez-Martinez C, Granada A, Olea N, Lorenzo-Tovar ML, Olea-Serrano F. Organochlorine pesticides in umbilical cord blood serum of women from Southern Spain and adherence to the Mediterranean diet. *Food Chem Toxicol.* 2010;48(5):1311–5.

7. Bjermo H, Darnerud PO, Lignell S, et al. Fish intake and breastfeeding time are associated with serum concentrations of organochlorines in a Swedish population. *Environ Int.* 2013;51:88–96.

8. Glynn A, Larsdotter M, Aune M, Darnerud PO, Bjerselius R, Bergman A. Changes in serum concentrations of polychlorinated biphenyls (PCBs), hydroxylated PCB metabolites and pentachlorophenol during pregnancy. *Chemosphere.* 2011;83(2):144–51.

9. Soechitram SD, Athanasiadou M, Hovander L, Bergman A, Sauer PJ. Fetal exposure to PCBs and their hydroxylated metabolites in a Dutch cohort. *Environ Health Perspect.* 2004;112(11):1208–12.

10. Ulaszewska MM, Zuccato E, Davoli E. PCDD/Fs and dioxin-like PCBs in human milk and estimation of infants' daily intake: a review. *Chemosphere.* 2011;83(6):774–82.

11. Gallo MV, Schell LM, Decaprio AP, Jacobs A. Levels of persistent organic pollutant and their predictors among young adults. *Chemosphere.* 2011;83(10):1374–82.

12. Ulaszewska MM, Zuccato E, Davoli E. PCDD/Fs and dioxin-like PCBs in human milk and estimation of infants' daily intake: a review. *Chemosphere.* 2011;83(6):774–82.

13. Aliyu MH, Alio AP, Salihu HM. To breastfeed or not to breastfeed: a review of the impact of lactational exposure to polychlorinated biphenyls (PCBs) on infants. *J Environ Health.* 2010;73(3):8–14.

14. Vogt R, Bennett D, Cassady D, Frost J, Ritz B, Hertz-Picciotto I. Cancer and non-cancer health

effects from food contaminant exposures for children and adults in California: a risk assessment. *Environ Health*. 2012;11:83.

15. Vogt R, Bennett D, Cassady D, Frost J, Ritz B, Hertz-Picciotto I. Cancer and non-cancer health effects from food contaminant exposures for children and adults in California: a risk assessment. *Environ Health*. 2012;11:Table S3. http://www.ncbi.nlm.nih.gov/pmc/articles/PMC3551655 /bin/1476-069X-11-83-S3.doc. Accessed March 28, 2015.

16. Vogt R, Bennett D, Cassady D, Frost J, Ritz B, Hertz-Picciotto I. Cancer and non-cancer health effects from food contaminant exposures for children and adults in California: a risk assessment. *Environ Health*. 2012;11:83.

17. Dórea JG, Bezerra VL, Fajon V, Horvat M. Speciation of methyl- and ethyl-mercury in hair of breastfed infants acutely exposed to thimerosal-containing vaccines. *Clin Chim Acta*. 2011; 412(17–18):1563–6.

18. Zeilmaker MJ, Hoekstra J, van Eijkeren JC, et al. Fish consumption during child bearing age: a quantitative risk-benefit analysis on neurodevelopment. *Food Chem Toxicol*. 2013;54: 30–4.

19. Fromberg A, Granby K, Højgård A, Fagt S, Larsen JC. Estimation of dietary intake of PCB and organochlorine pesticides for children and adults. *Food Chem*. 2011;125:1179–87.

20. European Food Safety Authority. Results of the monitoring of non dioxin-like PCBs in food and feed. *EFSA Journal*. 2010;8(7):1701.

21. Fromberg A, Granby K, Højgård A, Fagt S, Larsen JC. Estimation of dietary intake of PCB and organochlorine pesticides for children and adults. *Food Chem*. 2011;125:1179–87.

22. Zhang T, Sun HW, Wu Q, Zhang XZ, Yun SH, Kannan K. Perfluorochemicals in meat, eggs and indoor dust in China: assessment of sources and pathways of human exposure to perfluorochemicals. *Environ Sci Technol*. 2010;44(9):3572–9.

23. Schecter A, Cramer P, Boggess K, et al. Intake of dioxins and related compounds from food in the U.S. population. *J Toxicol Environ Health Part A*. 2001;63(1):1–18.

24. Aune D, De Stefani E, Ronco AL, et al. Egg consumption and the risk of cancer: a multisite case-control study in Uruguay. *Asian Pac J Cancer Prev*. 2009;10(5):869–76.

25. Yaginuma-Sakurai K, Murata K, Iwai-Shimada M, et al. Hair-to-blood ratio and biological half-life of mercury: experimental study of methylmercury exposure through fish consumption in humans. *J Toxicol Sci*. 2012;37(1):123–30.

26. Wimmerová S, Lancz K, Tihányi J, et al. Half-lives of serum PCB congener concentrations in environmentally exposed early adolescents. *Chemosphere*. 2011;82(5):687–91.

27. Hageman KJ, Hafner WD, Campbell DH, Jaffe DA, Landers DH, Simonich SL. Variability in pesticide deposition and source contributions to snowpack in Western U.S. national parks. *Environ Sci Technol*. 2010;44(12):4452–8.

28. Schecter A, Startin J, Wright C, et al. Congener-specific levels of dioxins and dibenzofurans in U.S. food and estimated daily dioxin toxic equivalent intake. *Environ Health Perspect*. 1994; 102(11):962–6.

29. Fiedler H, Cooper KR, Bergek S, Hjelt M, Rappe C. Polychlorinated dibenzo-p-dioxins and polychlorinated dibenzofurans (PCDD/PCDF) in food samples collected in southern Mississippi, USA. *Chemosphere*. 1997;34(5–7):1411–9.

30. Rappe C, Bergek S, Fiedler H, Cooper KR. PCDD and PCDF contamination in catfish feed from Arkansas, USA. *Chemosphere*. 1998;36(13):2705–20.

31. Ferrario JB, Byrne CJ, Cleverly DH. 2,3,7,8-Dibenzo-p-dioxins in mined clay products from the United States: evidence for possible natural origin. *Environ Sci Technol*. 2000;34(21): 4524–32.

32. US Department of Commerce. Broiler, turkey, and egg production: 1980 to 1999, No. 1143,

p. 684. In *Statistical Abstract of the United States, 2000*. Washington, D.C.: Government Printing Office, 2000.

33. Hayward DG, Nortrup D, Gardner A, Clower M. Elevated TCDD in chicken eggs and farm-raised catfish fed a diet with ball clay from a Southern United States mine. *Environ Res*. 1999; 81(3):248–56.

34. Hayward DG, Nortrup D, Gardner A, Clower M. Elevated TCDD in chicken eggs and farm-raised catfish fed a diet with ball clay from a Southern United States mine. *Environ Res*. 1999; 81(3):248–56.

35. US Food and Drug Administration. Letter from Linda Tollefson to Producers or Users of Clay Products in Animal Feeds. https://web.archive.org/web/20081107120600/http://www.fda .gov/cvm/Documents/ballclay.pdf. October 7, 1997. Accessed March 12, 2015.

36. Hanson T, Sites D. 2012 US catfish database. Fisheries and Allied Aquacultures Department Series No. 6. http://aurora.auburn.edu/repo/bitstream/handle/11200/44174/2012%20Cat fish%20Database.pdf?sequence=1. March 2013. Accessed March 26, 2015.

37. Huwe JK, Archer JC. Dioxin congener patterns in commercial catfish from the United States and the indication of mineral clays as the potential source. *Food Addit Contam Part A Chem Anal Control Expo Risk Assess*. 2013;30(2):331–8.

38. Rappe C, Bergek S, Fiedler H, Cooper KR. PCDD and PCDF contamination in catfish feed from Arkansas, USA. *Chemosphere*. 1998;36(13):2705–20.

39. Yaktine AL, Harrison GG, Lawrence RS. Reducing exposure to dioxins and related compounds through foods in the next generation. *Nutr Rev*. 2006;64(9):403–9.

40. Schecter A, Startin J, Wright C, et al. Congener-specific levels of dioxins and dibenzofurans in U.S. food and estimated daily dioxin toxic equivalent intake. *Environ Health Perspect*. 1994; 102(11):962–6.

41. US Department of Health and Human Services. The Health Consequences of Smoking: 50 Years of Progress. A Report of the Surgeon General. Atlanta, GA: US Department of Health and Human Services, Centers for Disease Control and Prevention, National Center for Chronic Disease Prevention and Health Promotion, Office on Smoking and Health, 2014.

42. Lee PN. 1979 Surgeon General's Report. http://legacy.library.ucsf.edu/tid/zkl36b00/pdf ?search=%221979%20surgeon%20general%20s%20report%20lee%22. September 2, 1979. Accessed March 12, 2015.

43. Lee PN. 1979 Surgeon General's Report. http://legacy.library.ucsf.edu/tid/zkl36b00/pdf ?search=%221979%20surgeon%20general%20s%20report%20lee%22. September 2, 1979. Accessed March 12, 2015.

44. Hearings before the Subcommittee on Public Buildings and Grounds of the Committee on Public Works and Transportation to Prohibit Smoking in Federal Buildings. http://legacy.library .ucsf.edu/tid/fzt08h00/pdf?search=%22to%20prohibit%20smoking%20in%20federal%20 buildings%20hearings%20jd%20047710%22. March 11; April 22, 1993. Accessed March 12, 2015.

45. Noyce AJ, Bestwick JP, Silveira-Moriyama L, et al. Meta-analysis of early nonmotor features and risk factors for Parkinson disease. *Ann Neurol*. 2012;72(6):893–901.

46. Morens DM, Grandinetti A, Davis JW, Ross GW, White LR, Reed D. Evidence against the operation of selective mortality in explaining the association between cigarette smoking and reduced occurrence of idiopathic Parkinson disease. *Am J Epidemiol*. 1996;144(4):400–4.

47. Noyce AJ, Bestwick JP, Silveira-Moriyama L, et al. Meta-analysis of early nonmotor features and risk factors for Parkinson disease. *Ann Neurol*. 2012;72(6):893–901.

48. Allam MF, Campbell MJ, Del Castillo AS, Fernández-Crehuet Navajas R. Parkinson's disease protects against smoking? *Behav Neurol*. 2004;15(3–4):65–71.

49. Tanner CM, Goldman SM, Aston DA, et al. Smoking and Parkinson's disease in twins. *Neurology*. 2002;58(4):581–8.

50. O'Reilly EJ, Chen H, Gardener H, Gao X, Schwarzschild MA, Ascherio A. Smoking and Parkinson's disease: using parental smoking as a proxy to explore causality. *Am J Epidemiol*. 2009;169(6): 678–82.

51. US Department of Health and Human Services. The Health Consequences of Smoking: 50 Yearsof Progress. A Report of the Surgeon General. Atlanta, GA: US Department of Health and Human Services, Centers for Disease Control and Prevention, National Center for Chronic Disease Prevention and Health Promotion, Office on Smoking and Health, 2014.

52. Wolf PA, D'Agostino RB, Kannel WB, Bonita R, Belanger AJ. Cigarette smoking as a risk factor for stroke. The Framingham Study. *JAMA*. 1988;259(7):1025–9.

53. Quik M, Perez XA, Bordia T. Nicotine as a potential neuroprotective agent for Parkinson's disease. *Mov Disord*. 2012;27(8):947–57.

54. Siegmund B, Leitner E, Pfannhauser W. Determination of the nicotine content of various edible nightshades (Solanaceae) and their products and estimation of the associated dietary nicotine intake. *J Agric Food Chem*. 1999;47(8):3113–20.

55. Brody AL, Mandelkern MA, London ED, et al. Cigarette smoking saturates brain alpha 4 beta 2 nicotinic acetylcholine receptors. *Arch Gen Psychiatry*. 2006;63(8):907–15.

56. Searles Nielsen S, Gallagher LG, Lundin JI, et al. Environmental tobacco smoke and Parkinson's disease. *Mov Disord*. 2012;27(2):293–6.

57. Siegmund B, Leitner E, Pfannhauser W. Determination of the nicotine content of various edible nightshades (Solanaceae) and their products and estimation of the associated dietary nicotine intake. *J Agric Food Chem*. 1999;47(8):3113–20.

58. Nielsen SS, Franklin GM, Longstreth WT, Swanson PD, Checkoway H. Nicotine from edible Solanaceae and risk of Parkinson disease. *Ann Neurol*. 2013;74(3):472–7.

59. Nielsen SS, Franklin GM, Longstreth WT, Swanson PD, Checkoway H. Nicotine from edible Solanaceae and risk of Parkinson disease. *Ann Neurol*. 2013;74(3):472–7.

60. Richardson JR, Shalat SL, Buckley B, et al. Elevated serum pesticide levels and risk of Parkinson disease. *Arch Neurol*. 2009;66(7):870–5.

61. Corrigan FM, Wienburg CL, Shore RF, Daniel SE, Mann D. Organochlorine insecticides in substantia nigra in Parkinson's disease. *J Toxicol Environ Health Part A*. 2000;59(4):229–34.

62. Hatcher-Martin JM, Gearing M, Steenland K, Levey AI, Miller GW, Pennell KD. Association between polychlorinated biphenyls and Parkinson's disease neuropathology. *Neurotoxicology*. 2012;33(5):1298–304.

63. Kanthasamy AG, Kitazawa M, Kanthasamy A, Anantharam V. Dieldrin-induced neurotoxicity: relevance to Parkinson's disease pathogenesis. *Neurotoxicology*. 2005;26(4):701–19.

64. Arguin H, Sánchez M, Bray GA, et al. Impact of adopting a vegan diet or an olestra supplementation on plasma organochlorine concentrations: results from two pilot studies. *Br J Nutr*. 2010; 103(10):1433–41.

65. Jiang W, Ju C, Jiang H, Zhang D. Dairy foods intake and risk of Parkinson's disease: a dose-response meta-analysis of prospective cohort studies. *Eur J Epidemiol*. 2014;29(9):613–9.

66. Park M, Ross GW, Petrovitch H, et al. Consumption of milk and calcium in midlife and the future risk of Parkinson disease. *Neurology*. 2005;64(6):1047–51.

67. Kotake Y, Yoshida M, Ogawa M, Tasaki Y, Hirobe M, Ohta S. Chronic administration of 1-benzyl-1,2,3,4-tetrahydroisoquinoline, an endogenous amine in the brain, induces parkinsonism in a primate. *Neurosci Lett*. 1996;217(1):69–71.

68. Niwa T, Yoshizumi H, Takeda N, Tatematsu A, Matsuura S, Nagatsu T. Detection of tetrahy-

droisoquinoline, a parkinsonism-related compound, in parkinsonian brains and foods by gas chromatography-mass spectrometry. *Advances in Behavioral Biology*. 1990;38A:313–6.

69. Niwa T, Yoshizumi H, Tatematsu A, Matsuura S, Nagatsu T. Presence of tetrahydroisoquinoline, a parkinsonism-related compound, in foods. *J Chromatogr*. 1989;493(2):347–52.

70. Niwa T, Takeda N, Kaneda N, Hashizume Y, Nagatsu T. Presence of tetrahydroisoquinoline and 2-methyl-tetrahydroquinoline in parkinsonian and normal human brains. *Biochem Biophys Res Commun*. 1987;144(2):1084–9.

71. Ułamek-Kozioł M, Bogucka-Kocka A, Kocki J, Pluta R. Good and bad sides of diet in Parkinson's disease. *Nutrition*. 2013;29(2):474–5.

72. Ułamek-Kozioł M, Bogucka-Kocka A, Kocki J, Pluta R. Good and bad sides of diet in Parkinson's disease. *Nutrition*. 2013;29(2):474–5.

73. Kistner A, Krack P. Parkinson's disease: no milk today? *Front Neurol*. 2014;5:172.

74. Chen H, Zhang SM, Hernn MA, Willett WC, Ascherio A. Diet and Parkinson's disease: a potential role of dairy products in men. *Ann Neurol*. 2002;52(6):793–801.

75. Jiang W, Ju C, Jiang H, Zhang D. Dairy foods intake and risk of Parkinson's disease: a dose-response meta-analysis of prospective cohort studies. *Eur J Epidemiol*. 2014;29(9):613–9.

76. Michaëlsson K, Wolk A, Langenskiöld S, et al. Milk intake and risk of mortality and fractures in women and men: cohort studies. *BMJ*. 2014;349:g6015.

77. Ridel KR, Leslie ND, Gilbert DL. An updated review of the long-term neurological effects of galactosemia. *Pediatr Neurol*. 2005;33(3):153–61.

78. Marder K, Gu Y, Eberly S, et al. Relationship of Mediterranean diet and caloric intake to phenoconversion in Huntington disease. *JAMA Neurol*. 2013;70(11):1382–8.

79. Ames BN, Cathcart R, Schwiers E, Hochstein P. Uric acid provides an antioxidant defense in humans against oxidant- and radical-caused aging and cancer: a hypothesis. *Proc Natl Acad Sci USA*. 1981;78(11):6858–62.

80. Duan W, Ladenheim B, Cutler RG, Kruman II, Cadet JL, Mattson MP. Dietary folate deficiency and elevated homocysteine levels endanger dopaminergic neurons in models of Parkinson's disease. *J Neurochem*. 2002;80(1):101–10.

81. Auinger P, Kieburtz K, McDermott MP. The relationship between uric acid levels and Huntington's disease progression. *Mov Disord*. 2010;25(2):224–8.

82. Schwarzschild MA, Schwid SR, Marek K, et al. Serum urate as a predictor of clinical and radiographic progression in Parkinson disease. *Arch Neurol*. 2008;65(6):716–23.

83. Shen C, Guo Y, Luo W, Lin C, Ding M. Serum urate and the risk of Parkinson's disease: results from a meta-analysis. *Can J Neurol Sci*. 2013;40(1):73–9.

84. Fang P, Li X, Luo JJ, Wang H, Yang X. A double-edged sword: uric acid and neurological disorders. *Brain Disord Ther*. 2013;2(2):109.

85. Kutzing MK, Firestein BL. Altered uric acid levels and disease states. *J Pharmacol Exp Ther*. 2008;324(1):1–7.

86. Schmidt JA, Crowe FL, Appleby PN, Key TJ, Travis RC. Serum uric acid concentrations in meat eaters, fish eaters, vegetarians and vegans: a cross-sectional analysis in the EPIC-Oxford cohort. *PLoS ONE*. 2013;8(2):e56339.

87. Kuo CF, See LC, Yu KH, Chou IJ, Chiou MJ, Luo SF. Significance of serum uric acid levels on the risk of all-cause and cardiovascular mortality. *Rheumatology* (Oxford). 2013;52(1):127–34.

88. Arguin H, Sánchez M, Bray GA, et al. Impact of adopting a vegan diet or an olestra supplementation on plasma organochlorine concentrations: results from two pilot studies. *Br J Nutr*. 2010;103(10):1433–41.

89. Siddiqui MK, Saxena MC, Krishna Murti CR. Storage of DDT and BHC in adipose tissue of Indian males. *Int J Environ Anal Chem*. 1981;10(3–4):197–204.

90. Norén K. Levels of organochlorine contaminants in human milk in relation to the dietary habits of the mothers. *Acta Paediatr Scand*. 1983;72(6):811–6.

91. Schecter A, Papke O. Comparison of blood dioxin, dibenzofuran and coplanar PCB levels in strict vegetarians (vegans) and the general United States population. *Org Comps*. 1998;38:179–82.

92. Schecter A, Harris TR, Päpke O, Tunga KC, Musumba A. Polybrominated diphenyl ether (PBDE) levels in the blood of pure vegetarians (vegans). *Tox Env Chem*. 2006;88(1):107–12.

93. Eskenazi B, Chevrier J, Rauch SA, et al. In utero and childhood polybrominated diphenyl ether (PBDE) exposures and neurodevelopment in the CHAMACOS study. *Environ Health Perspect*. 2013;121(2):257–62.

94. Schecter A, Päpke O, Harris TR, et al. Polybrominated diphenyl ether (PBDE) levels in an expanded market basket survey of U.S. food and estimated PBDE dietary intake by age and sex. *Environ Health Perspect*. 2006;114(10):1515–20.

95. Fraser AJ, Webster TF, McClean MD. Diet contributes significantly to the body burden of PBDEs in the general U.S. population. *Environ Health Perspect*. 2009;117(10):1520–5.

96. Schecter A, Harris TR, Päpke O, Tunga KC, Musumba A. Polybrominated diphenyl ether (PBDE) levels in the blood of pure vegetarians (vegans). *Tox Env Chem*. 2006;88(1):107–12.

97. Huwe JK, West M. Polybrominated diphenyl ethers in U.S. meat and poultry from two statistically designed surveys showing trends and levels from 2002 to 2008. *J Agric Food Chem*. 2011;59(10):5428–34.

98. Dickman MD, Leung CK, Leong MK. Hong Kong male subfertility links to mercury in human hair and fish. *Sci Total Environ*. 1998;214:165–74.

99. Srikumar TS, Johansson GK, Ockerman PA, Gustafsson JA, Akesson B. Trace element status in healthy subjects switching from a mixed to a lactovegetarian diet for 12 mo. *Am J Clin Nutr*. 1992;55(4):885–90.

100. Wimmerová S, Lancz K, Tihányi J, et al. Half-lives of serum PCB congener concentrations in environmentally exposed early adolescents. *Chemosphere*. 2011;82(5):687–91.

101. Parkinson J. *An Essay on the Shaking Palsy*. London: Whittingham and Rowland for Sherwood, Neely and Jones, 1817:7.

102. Abbott RD, Petrovitch H, White LR, et al. Frequency of bowel movements and the future risk of Parkinson's disease. *Neurology*. 2001;57(3):456–62.

103. Ueki A, Otsuka M. Life style risks of Parkinson's disease: association between decreased water intake and constipation. *J Neurol*. 2004;251 Suppl 7:vII18–23.

104. Gao X, Chen H, Schwarzschild MA, Ascherio A. A prospective study of bowel movement frequency and risk of Parkinson's disease. *Am J Epidemiol*. 2011;174(5):546–51.

105. Kamel F. Epidemiology. Paths from pesticides to Parkinson's. *Science*. 2013;341(6147):722–3.

106. Barnhill LM, Bronstein JM. Pesticides and Parkinson's disease: is it in your genes? *Neurodegener Dis Manag*. 2014;4(3):197–200.

107. Wang A, Cockburn M, Ly TT, Bronstein JM, Ritz B. The association between ambient exposure to organophosphates and Parkinson's disease risk. *Occup Environ Med*. 2014;71(4):275–81.

108. Narayan S, Liew Z, Paul K, et al. Household organophosphorus pesticide use and Parkinson's disease. *Int J Epidemiol*. 2013;42(5):1476–85.

109. Liu X, Ma T, Qu B, Ji Y, Liu Z. Pesticide-induced gene mutations and Parkinson disease risk: a meta-analysis. *Genet Test Mol Biomarkers*. 2013;17(11):826–32.

110. Lee SJ, Lim HS, Masliah E, Lee HJ. Protein aggregate spreading in neurodegenerative diseases: problems and perspectives. *Neurosci Res.* 2011;70(4):339–48.

111. Chorfa A, Lazizzera C, Bétemps D, et al. A variety of pesticides trigger in vitro α-synuclein accumulation, a key event in Parkinson's disease. *Arch Toxicol.* 2014.

112. Dunnett SB, Björklund SBA. Prospects for new restorative and neuroprotective treatments in Parkinson's disease. *Nature.* 1999;399(6738 Suppl):A32–9.

113. Campdelacreu J. Parkinson disease and Alzheimer disease: environmental risk factors. *Neurologia.* 2014;29(9):541–9.

114. Meng X, Munishkina LA, Fink AL, Uversky VN. Effects of various flavonoids on the α-synuclein fibrillation process. *Parkinson's Dis.* 2010;2010:650794.

115. Strathearn KE, Yousef GG, Grace MH, Roy SA, et al. Neuroprotective effects of anthocyanin- and proanthocyanidin-rich extracts in cellular models of Parkinson's disease. *Brain Res.* 2014; 1555:60–77.

116. Golbe LI, Farrell TM, Davis PH. Case-control study of early life dietary factors in Parkinson's disease. *Arch Neurol.* 1988;45(12):1350–3.

117. Gao X, Cassidy A, Schwarzschild MA, Rimm EB, Ascherio A. Habitual intake of dietary flavonoids and risk of Parkinson disease. *Neurol.* 2012;78(15):1138–45.

118. Kukull WA. An apple a day to prevent Parkinson disease: reduction of risk by flavonoids. *Neurol.* 2012;78(15):1112–3.

119. Gao X, Cassidy A, Schwarzschild MA, Rimm EB, Ascherio A. Habitual intake of dietary flavonoids and risk of Parkinson disease. *Neurology.* 2012;78(15):1138–45.

120. Serafini M, Testa MF, Villain D, et al. Antioxidant activity of blueberry fruit is impaired by association with milk. *Free Radic Biol Med.* 2009;46(6):769–74.

121. Jekanowski M. Survey says: a snapshot of rendering. *Render Magazine.* 2011;April:58–61.

122. Schepens PJ, Covaci A, Jorens PG, Hens L, Scharpé S, van Larebeke N. Surprising findings following a Belgian food contamination with polychlorobiphenyls and dioxins. *Environ Health Perspect.* 2001;109(2):101–3.

123. Dórea JG. Vegetarian diets and exposure to organochlorine pollutants, lead, and mercury. *Am J Clin Nutr.* 2004;80(1):237–8.

124. Dórea JG. Fish meal in animal feed and human exposure to persistent bioaccumulative and toxic substances. *J Food Prot.* 2006;69(11):2777–85.

125. Moser GA, McLachlan MS. The influence of dietary concentration on the absorption and excretion of persistent lipophilic organic pollutants in the human intestinal tract. *Chemosphere.* 2001;45(2):201–11.

126. Dórea JG. Vegetarian diets and exposure to organochlorine pollutants, lead, and mercury. *Am J Clin Nutr.* 2004;80(1):237–8.

127. Noyce AJ, Bestwick JP, Silveira-Moriyama L, et al. Meta-analysis of early nonmotor features and risk factors for Parkinson disease. *Ann Neurol.* 2012;72(6):893–901.

128. Barranco Quintana JL, Allam MF, Del Castillo AS, Navajas RF. Parkinson's disease and tea: a quantitative review. *J Am Coll Nutr.* 2009;28(1):1–6.

129. Palacios N, Gao X, McCullough ML, et al. Caffeine and risk of Parkinson's disease in a large cohort of men and women. *Mov Disord.* 2012;27(10):1276–82.

130. Nakaso K, Ito S, Nakashima K. Caffeine activates the PI3K/Akt pathway and prevents apoptotic cell death in a Parkinson's disease model of SH-SY5Y cells. *Neurosci Lett.* 2008;432(2):146–50.

131. Postuma RB, Lang AE, Munhoz RP, et al. Caffeine for treatment of Parkinson disease: a randomized controlled trial. *Neurology.* 2012;79(7):651–8.

132. Postuma RB, Lang AE, Munhoz RP, et al. Caffeine for treatment of Parkinson disease: a randomized controlled trial. *Neurology.* 2012;79(7):651–8.

133. Grazina R, Massano J. Physical exercise and Parkinson's disease: influence on symptoms, disease course and prevention. *Rev Neurosci.* 2013;24(2):139–52.

134. Chen J, Guan Z, Wang L, Song G, Ma B, Wang Y. Meta-analysis: overweight, obesity, and Parkinson's disease. *Int J Endocrinol.* 2014;2014:203930.

15. How Not to Die from Iatrogenic Causes

1. Pereira TV, Horwitz RI, Ioannidis JPA. Empirical evaluation of very large treatment effects of medical interventions. *JAMA.* 2012;308(16):1676–84.

2. Lazarou J, Pomeranz BH, Corey PN. Incidence of adverse drug reactions in hospitalized patients: a meta-analysis of prospective studies. *JAMA.* 1998;279(15):1200–5.

3. Starfield B. Is US health really the best in the world? *JAMA.* 2000;284(4):483–5.

4. Klevens RM, Edwards JR, Richards CL, et al. Estimating health care-associated infections and deaths in U.S. hospitals, 2002. *Public Health Rep.* 2007;122(2):160–6.

5. Gilbert K, Stafford C, Crosby K, Fleming E, Gaynes R. Does hand hygiene compliance among health care workers change when patients are in contact precaution rooms in ICUs? *Am J Infect Control.* 2010;38(7):515–7.

6. Gilbert K, Stafford C, Crosby K, Fleming E, Gaynes R. Does hand hygiene compliance among health care workers change when patients are in contact precaution rooms in ICUs? *Am J Infect Control.* 2010;38(7):515–7.

7. Leape LL, Berwick DM. Five years after To Err Is Human: what have we learned? *JAMA.* 2005;293(19):2384–90.

8. Starfield B. Is US health really the best in the world? *JAMA.* 2000;284(4):483–5.

9. Institute of Medicine. To Err Is Human: building a safer health system. http://www.iom.edu/~/media/Files/Report%20Files/1999/To-Err-is-Human/To%20Err%20is%20Human%201999%20%20report%20brief.pdf. November, 1999. Accessed March 12, 2015.

10. Weingart SN, Wilson RM, Gibberd RW, Harrison B. Epidemiology of medical error. *BMJ.* 2000;320(7237):774–7.

11. Millenson ML. The silence. *Health Aff* (Millwood). 2003;22(2):103–12.

12. Mills DH. Medical insurance feasibility study. A technical summary. *West J Med.* 1978;128(4):360–5.

13. Leape LL. Error in medicine. *JAMA.* 1994 Dec 21;272(23):1851–7.

14. Millenson ML. The silence. *Health Aff* (Millwood). 2003;22(2):103–12.

15. Institute of Medicine. To Err Is Human: building a safer health system. http://www.iom.edu/~/media/Files/Report%20Files/1999/To-Err-is-Human/To%20Err%20is%20Human%201999%20%20report%20brief.pdf. November, 1999. Accessed March 12, 2015.

16. Millenson ML. The silence. *Health Aff* (Millwood). 2003;22(2):103–12.

17. Lockley SW, Barger LK, Ayas NT, Rothschild JM, Czeisler CA, Landrigan CP. Effects of health care provider work hours and sleep deprivation on safety and performance. *Jt Comm J Qual Patient Saf.* 2007;33(11 Suppl):7–18.

18. Barger LK, Ayas NT, Cade BE, et al. Impact of extended-duration shifts on medical errors, adverse events, and attentional failures. *PLoS Med.* 2006;3(12):e487.

19. Millenson ML. The silence. *Health Aff* (Millwood). 2003;22(2):103–12.

20. Egger GJ, Binns AF, Rossner SR. The emergence of "lifestyle medicine" as a structured approach for management of chronic disease. *Med J Aust.* 2009;190(3):143–5.

21. Malone J, Guleria R, Craven C, et al. Justification of diagnostic medical exposures: some practical

issues. Report of an International Atomic Energy Agency Consultation. *Br J Radiol.* 2012;85(1013):523–38.

22. Pierce DA, Shimizu Y, Preston DL, Vaeth M, Mabuchi K. Studies of the mortality of atomic bomb survivors. Report 12, part I. Cancer: 1950–1990. 1996. *Radiat Res.* 2012;178(2):AV61–87.

23. Brenner D, Elliston C, Hall E, Berdon WE. Estimated risks of radiation-induced fatal cancer from pediatric CT. *AJR Am J Roentgenol.* 2001;176(2):289–96.

24. Rogers LF. Taking care of children: check out the parameters used for helical CT. *AJR Am J Roentgenol.* 2001;176(2):287.

25. Berrington de Gonzingt A, Mahesh M, Kim KP, et al. Projected cancer risks from computed tomographic scans performed in the United States in 2007. *Arch Intern Med.* 2009;169(22):2071–7.

26. Institute of Medicine. *Breast cancer and the environment: a life course approach.* Washington, D.C.: The National Academies Press; 2012.

27. Picano E. Informed consent and communication of risk from radiological and nuclear medicine examinations: how to escape from a communication inferno. *BMJ.* 2004;329(7470):849–51.

28. Schmidt CW. CT scans: balancing health risks and medical benefits. *Environ Health Perspect.* 2012;120(3):A118–21.

29. Pearce MS, Salotti JA, Little MP, et al. Radiation exposure from CT scans in childhood and subsequent risk of leukaemia and brain tumours: a retrospective cohort study. *Lancet.* 2012;380(9840):499–505.

30. Limaye MR, Severance H. Pandora's boxes: questions unleashed in airport scanner debate. *J Am Osteopath Assoc.* 2011;111(2):87–8, 119.

31. Friedberg W, Copeland K, Duke FE, O'Brien K, Darden EB. Radiation exposure during air travel: guidance provided by the Federal Aviation Administration for air carrier crews. *Health Phys.* 2000;79(5):591–5.

32. Yong LC, Petersen MR, Sigurdson AJ, Sampson LA, Ward EM. High dietary antioxidant intakes are associated with decreased chromosome translocation frequency in airline pilots. *Am J Clin Nutr.* 2009;90(5):1402–10.

33. Podmore ID, Griffiths HR, Herbert KE, Mistry N, Mistry P, Lunec J. Vitamin C exhibits pro-oxidant properties. *Nature.* 1998;392(6676):559.

34. Yong LC, Petersen MR, Sigurdson AJ, Sampson LA, Ward EM. High dietary antioxidant intakes are associated with decreased chromosome translocation frequency in airline pilots. *Am J Clin Nutr.* 2009;90(5):1402–10.

35. Yong LC, Petersen MR, Sigurdson AJ, Sampson LA, Ward EM. High dietary antioxidant intakes are associated with decreased chromosome translocation frequency in airline pilots. *Am J Clin Nutr.* 2009;90(5):1402–10.

36. Sauvaget C, Kasagi F, Waldren CA. Dietary factors and cancer mortality among atomic-bomb survivors. *Mutat Res.* 2004;551(1–2):145–52.

37. Kordysh EA, Emerit I, Goldsmith JR, et al. Dietary and clastogenic factors in children who immigrated to Israel from regions contaminated by the Chernobyl accident. *Arch Environ Health.* 2001;56(4):320–6.

38. Langham WH, Bassett H, Harris PS, Carter RE. Distribution and excretion of plutonium administered intravenously to man. Los Alamos: Los Alamos Scientific Laboratory, LAB1151. *Health Physics.* 1980;38:1,031B1,060.

39. Loscialpo MJ. Nontherapeutic human research experiments on institutionalized mentally retarded children: civil rights and remedies. *23 New Eng J on Crim & Civ Confinement.* 1997;139:143–5.

40. Assistant to the Secretary of Defense for Nuclear and Chemical and Biological Defense Programs, Department of Defense. Report on search for human radiation experiment records

1944–1994. http://www.defense.gov/pubs/dodhre/. June 1997. Accessed March 12, 2015.

41. Kouvaris JR, Kouloulias VE, Vlahos IJ. Amifostine: the first selective-target and broad-spectrum radioprotector. *Oncologist*. 2007;12(6):738–47.

42. Rao BN, Archana PR, Aithal BK, Rao BSS. Protective effect of zingerone, a dietary compound against radiation induced genetic damage and apoptosis in human lymphocytes. *Eur J Pharmacol*. 2011;657(1–3):59–66.

43. Arora R, Gupta D, Chawla R, et al. Radioprotection by plant products: present status and future prospects. *Phytother Res*. 2005;19(1):1–22.

44. Malekirad AA, Ranjbar A, Rahzani K, et al. Oxidative stress in radiology staff. *Environ Toxicol Pharmacol*. 2005;20(1):215–8.

45. Zeraatpishe A, Oryan S, Bagheri MH, et al. Effects of Melissa officinalis L. on oxidative status and DNA damage in subjects exposed to long-term low-dose ionizing radiation. *Toxicol Ind Health*. 2011;27(3):205–12.

46. Zhong W, Maradit-Kremers H, St Sauver JL, et al. Age and sex patterns of drug prescribing in a defined American population. *Mayo Clin Proc*. 2013;88(7):697–707.

47. Lindsley CW. The top prescription drugs of 2011 in the United States: antipsychotics and antidepressants once again lead CNS therapeutics. *ACS Chem Neurosci*. 2012;3(8):630–1.

48. Centers for Disease Control National Center for Health Statistics. National Ambulatory Medical Care Survey: 2010 Summary Tables. http://www.cdc.gov/nchs/data/ahcd/namcs_summary /2010_namcs_web_tables.pdf. 2010. Accessed March 12, 2015.

49. Hudson B, Zarifeh A, Young L, Wells JE. Patients' expectations of screening and preventive treatments. *Ann Fam Med*. 2012;10(6):495–502.

50. Lytsy P, Westerling R. Patient expectations on lipid-lowering drugs. *Patient Educ Couns*. 2007;67(1–2):143–50.

51. Trewby PN, Reddy AV, Trewby CS, Ashton VJ, Brennan G, Inglis J. Are preventive drugs preventive enough? A study of patients' expectation of benefit from preventive drugs. *Clin Med*. 2002;2(6):527–33.

52. Trewby PN, Reddy AV, Trewby CS, Ashton VJ, Brennan G, Inglis J. Are preventive drugs preventive enough? A study of patients' expectation of benefit from preventive drugs. *Clin Med*. 2002;2(6):527–33.

53. Trewby PN, Reddy AV, Trewby CS, Ashton VJ, Brennan G, Inglis J. Are preventive drugs preventive enough? A study of patients' expectation of benefit from preventive drugs. *Clin Med*. 2002;2(6):527–33.

54. Trewby PN, Reddy AV, Trewby CS, Ashton VJ, Brennan G, Inglis J. Are preventive drugs preventive enough? A study of patients' expectation of benefit from preventive drugs. *Clin Med*. 2002;2(6):527–33.

55. Esselstyn CB Jr, Gendy G, Doyle J, Golubic M, Roizen MF. A way to reverse CAD? *J Fam Pract*. 2014;63(7):356–364b.

56. Esselstyn CB Jr, Gendy G, Doyle J, Golubic M, Roizen MF. A way to reverse CAD? *J Fam Pract*. 2014;63(7):356–364b.

57. Duthie GG, Wood AD. Natural salicylates: foods, functions and disease prevention. *Food Funct*. 2011;2(9):515–20.

58. Fuster V, Sweeny JM. Aspirin: a historical and contemporary therapeutic overview. *Circulation*. 2011;123(7):768–78.

59. Pasche B, Wang M, Pennison M, Jimenez H. Prevention and treatment of cancer with aspirin: where do we stand? *Semin Oncol*. 2014;41(3):397–401.

60. Karnezis T, Shayan R, Fox S, Achen MG, Stacker SA. The connection between lymphangiogenic signalling and prostaglandin biology: a missing link in the metastatic pathway. *Oncotarget*. 2012;3(8):893–906.

61. Macdonald S. Aspirin use to be banned in under 16 year olds. *BMJ*. 2002;325(7371):988.

62. Siller-Matula JM. Hemorrhagic complications associated with aspirin: an underestimated hazard in clinical practice? *JAMA*. 2012;307(21):2318–20.

63. Sutcliffe P, Connock M, Gurung T, et al. Aspirin in primary prevention of cardiovascular disease and cancer: a systematic review of the balance of evidence from reviews of randomized trials. *PLoS ONE*. 2013;8(12):e81970.

64. Thun MJ, Jacobs EJ, Patrono C. The role of aspirin in cancer prevention. *Nat Rev Clin Oncol*. 2012;9(5):259–67.

65. McCarty MF. Minimizing the cancer-promotional activity of cox-2 as a central strategy in cancer prevention. Med *Hypotheses*. 2012;78(1):45–57.

66. Duthie GG, Wood AD. Natural salicylates: foods, functions and disease prevention. *Food Funct*. 2011;2(9):515–20.

67. Paterson JR, Blacklock C, Campbell G, Wiles D, Lawrence JR. The identification of salicylates as normal constituents of serum: a link between diet and health? *J Clin Pathol*. 1998;51(7): 502–5.

68. Rinelli S, Spadafranca A, Fiorillo G, Cocucci M, Bertoli S, Battezzati A. Circulating salicylic acid and metabolic and inflammatory responses after fruit ingestion. *Plant Foods Hum Nutr*. 2012;67(1):100–4.

69. Blacklock CJ, Lawrence JR, Wiles D, et al. Salicylic acid in the serum of subjects not taking aspirin. Comparison of salicylic acid concentrations in the serum of vegetarians, non-vegetarians, and patients taking low dose aspirin. *J Clin Pathol*. 2001;54(7):553–5.

70. Knutsen SF. Lifestyle and the use of health services. *Am J Clin Nutr*. 1994;59(5 Suppl):1171S–1175S.

71. McCarty MF. Dietary nitrate and reductive polyphenols may potentiate the vascular benefit and alleviate the ulcerative risk of low-dose aspirin. *Med Hypotheses*. 2013;80(2):186–90.

72. Willcox BJ, Willcox DC, Todoriki H, et al. Caloric restriction, the traditional Okinawan diet, and healthy aging: the diet of the world's longest-lived people and its potential impact on morbidity and life span. *Ann N Y Acad Sci*. 2007;1114:434–55.

73. McCarty MF. Minimizing the cancer-promotional activity of cox-2 as a central strategy in cancer prevention. *Med Hypotheses*. 2012;78(1):45–57.

74. Paterson JR, Srivastava R, Baxter GJ, Graham AB, Lawrence JR. Salicylic acid content of spices and its implications. *J Agric Food Chem*. 2006;54(8):2891–6.

75. Paterson JR, Srivastava R, Baxter GJ, Graham AB, Lawrence JR. Salicylic acid content of spices and its implications. *J Agric Food Chem*. 2006;54(8):2891–6.

76. Pasche B, Wang M, Pennison M, Jimenez H. Prevention and treatment of cancer with aspirin: where do we stand? *Semin Oncol*. 2014;41(3):397–401.

77. Paterson JR, Srivastava R, Baxter GJ, Graham AB, Lawrence JR. Salicylic acid content of spices and its implications. *J Agric Food Chem*. 2006;54(8):2891–6.

78. Baxter GJ, Graham AB, Lawrence JR, Wiles D, Paterson JR. Salicylic acid in soups prepared from organically and non-organically grown vegetables. *Eur J Nutr*. 2001;40(6):289–92.

79. Scheier L. Salicylic acid: one more reason to eat your fruits and vegetables. *J Am Diet Assoc*. 2001;101(12):1406–8.

80. Duthie GG, Wood AD. Natural salicylates: foods, functions and disease prevention. *Food Funct*. 2011;2(9):515–20.

81. Seeff LC, Richards TB, Shapiro JA, et al. How many endoscopies are performed for colorectal cancer screening? Results from CDC's survey of endoscopic capacity. *Gastroenterology*. 2004;127(6):1670–7.

82. McLachlan SA, Clements A, Austoker J. Patients' experiences and reported barriers to colonoscopy in the screening context—a systematic review of the literature. *Patient Educ Couns*. 2012;86(2):137–46.

83. Lobel EZ, Korelitz BI. Postendoscopy syndrome: "the doctor never talked to me." *J Clin Gastroenterol*. 2001;33(5):353–4.

84. McLachlan SA, Clements A, Austoker J. Patients' experiences and reported barriers to colonoscopy in the screening context—a systematic review of the literature. *Patient Educ Couns*. 2012;86(2):137–46.

85. Whitlock EP, Lin JS, Liles E, Beil TL, Fu R. Screening for colorectal cancer: a targeted, updated systematic review for the U.S. Preventive Services Task Force. *Ann Intern Med*. 2008; 149(9):638–58.

86. Manner H, Plum N, Pech O, Ell C, Enderle MD. Colon explosion during argon plasma coagulation. *Gastrointest Endosc*. 2008;67(7):1123–7.

87. Ko CW, Dominitz JA. Complications of colonoscopy: magnitude and management. *Gastrointest Endosc Clin N Am*. 2010;20(4):659–71.

88. Whitlock EP, Lin JS, Liles E, Beil TL, Fu R. Screening for colorectal cancer: a targeted, updated systematic review for the U.S. Preventive Services Task Force. *Ann Intern Med*. 2008; 149(9):638–58.

89. van Hees F, Habbema JD, Meester RG, Lansdorp-Vogelaar I, van Ballegooijen M, Zauber AG. Should colorectal cancer screening be considered in elderly persons without previous screening? A cost-effectiveness analysis. *Ann Intern Med*. 2014;160(11):750–9.

90. Whitlock EP, Lin JS, Liles E, Beil TL, Fu R. Screening for colorectal cancer: a targeted, updated systematic review for the U.S. Preventive Services Task Force. *Ann Intern Med*. 2008; 149(9):638–58.

91. Brenner H, Stock C, Hoffmeister M. Effect of screening sigmoidoscopy and screening colonoscopy on colorectal cancer incidence and mortality: systematic review and meta-analysis of randomised controlled trials and observational studies. *BMJ*. 2014;348:g2467.

92. Swan H, Siddiqui AA, Myers RE. International colorectal cancer screening programs: population contact strategies, testing methods and screening rates. *Pract Gastroenter*. 2012;36(8): 20–9.

93. Ling BS, Trauth JM, Fine MJ, et al. Informed decision-making and colorectal cancer screening: is it occurring in primary care? *Med Care*. 2008;46(9 Suppl 1):S23–9.

94. Ling BS, Trauth JM, Fine MJ, et al. Informed decision-making and colorectal cancer screening: is it occurring in primary care? *Med Care*. 2008;46(9 Suppl 1):S23–9.

95. Brett AS. Flexible sigmoidoscopy for colorectal cancer screening: more evidence, persistent ironies. *JAMA*. 2014;312(6):601–2.

96. Yabroff KR, Klabunde CN, Yuan G, et al. Are physicians' recommendations for colorectal cancer screening guideline-consistent? *J Gen Intern Med*. 2011;26(2):177–84.

97. Swan H, Siddiqui AA, Myers RE. International colorectal cancer screening programs: population contact strategies, testing methods and screening rates. *Pract Gastroenter*. 2012;36(8):20–9.

98. Swan H, Siddiqui AA, Myers RE. International colorectal cancer screening programs: population contact strategies, testing methods and screening rates. *Pract Gastroenter*. 2012;36(8): 20–9.

99. Butterfield S. Changes coming for colon cancer screening. *ACP Internist*. 2014;34(7):10–11.

100. Rosenthal E. The $2.7 trillion medical bill: colonoscopies explain why U.S. leads the world

in health expenditures. *New York Times*. http://www.nytimes.com/2013/06/02/health/colonoscopies-explain-why-us-leads-the-world-in-health-expenditures.html. June 1, 2013. Accessed March 12, 2015.

101. Whoriskey P, Keating D. How a secretive panel uses data that distorts doctors' pay. *Washington Post*. http://www.washingtonpost.com/business/economy/how-a-secretive-panel-uses-data-that-distorts-doctors-pay/2013/07/20/ee134e3a-eda8-11e2-9008-61e94a7ea20d_story.html. July 20, 2013. Accessed March 12, 2015.

102. US Government Accountability Office. Medicare: action needed to address higher use of anatomic pathology services by providers who self-refer. GAO-13-445. http://www.gao.gov/products/GAO-13-445. June 24, 2013. Accessed March 12, 2015.

103. Spirling LI, Daniels IR. Botanical perspectives on health peppermint: more than just an after-dinner mint. *J R Soc Promot Health*. 2001;121(1):62–3.

104. Amato A, Liotta R, Mulè F. Effects of menthol on circular smooth muscle of human colon: analysis of the mechanism of action. *Eur J Pharmacol*. 2014;740:295–301.

105. Leicester RJ, Hunt RH. Peppermint oil to reduce colonic spasm during endoscopy. *Lancet*. 1982;2(8305):989.

106. Asao T, Mochiki E, Suzuki H, et al. An easy method for the intraluminal administration of peppermint oil before colonoscopy and its effectiveness in reducing colonic spasm. *Gastrointest Endosc*. 2001;53(2):172–7.

107. Shavakhi A, Ardestani SK, Taki M, Goli M, Keshteli AH. Premedication with peppermint oil capsules in colonoscopy: a double blind placebo-controlled randomized trial study. *Acta Gastroenterol Belg*. 2012;75(3):349–53.

108. Stange KC. Barbara Starfield: passage of the pathfinder of primary care. *Ann Fam Med*. 2011;9(4):292–6.

109. Starfield B. Is US health really the best in the world? *JAMA*. 2000;284(4):483–5.

110. Rappoport J. An exclusive interview with Dr. Barbara Starfield: medically caused death in America. Jon Rappoport's Blog. https://jonrappoport.wordpress.com/2009/12/09/an-exclusive-interview-with-dr-barbara-starfield-medically-caused-death-in-america/. December 9, 2009. Accessed March 12, 2015.

111. Millenson ML. The silence. *Health Aff* (Millwood). 2003;22(2):103–12.

112. Holtzman NA. Chronicle of an unforetold death. *Arch Intern Med*. 2012;172(15):1174–7.

113. Anand SS, Islam S, Rosengren A, et al. Risk factors for myocardial infarction in women and men: insights from the INTERHEART study. *Eur Heart J*. 2008;29(7):932–40.

PART 2

Introduction

1. Mozaffarian D, Willet WC, Hu FB. The authors reply. *N Engl J Med*. 2011;365(11):1059.

2. Bernstein AM, Bloom DE, Rosner BA, Franz M, Willett WC. Relation of food cost to healthfulness of diet among US women. *Am J Clin Nutr*. 2010;92(5):1197–203.

3. Atwater WO. Foods: nutritive value and cost. *U.S. Department of Agriculture Farmers' Bulletin*. 1894;23:1–30.

4. Connell CL, Zoellner JM, Yadrick MK, Chekuri SC, Crook LB, Bogle ML. Energy density, nutrient adequacy, and cost per serving can provide insight into food choices in the lower Mississippi Delta. *J Nutr Educ Behav*. 2012;44(2):148–53.

5. Lo YT, Chang YH, Wahlqvist ML, Huang HB, Lee MS. Spending on vegetable and fruit consumption could reduce all-cause mortality among older adults. *Nutr J.* 2012;11:113.

6. U.S. Department of Agriculture, U.S. Department of Health and Human Services. Dietary guidelines for Americans, 2010. Washington, D.C.: U.S. Government Printing Office; 2010.

7. Dietary Guidelines Advisory Committee. The Report of the Dietary Guidelines Advisory Committee on Dietary Guidelines for Americans, 2010. Washington, D.C.: U.S. Government Printing Office; 2010.

8. U.S. Department of Agriculture, U.S. Department of Health and Human Services. Dietary guidelines for Americans, 2005. Washington, D.C.: U.S. Government Printing Office; 2005.

9. U.S. Department of Agriculture, U.S. Department of Health and Human Services. Dietary guidelines for Americans, 2010. Washington, D.C.: U.S. Government Printing Office; 2010.

10. U.S. Department of Agriculture, U.S. Department of Health and Human Services. Dietary guidelines for Americans, 2010. Washington, D.C.: U.S. Government Printing Office; 2010.

11. World Cancer Research Fund / American Institute for Cancer Research. Food, Nutrition, Physical Activity, and the Prevention of Cancer: a Global Perspective. Washington, D.C.: AICR, 2007.

12. Pork Information Gateway. Quick facts—the pork industry at a glance. http://www.porkgateway.org/FileLibrary/PIGLibrary/References/NPB%20Quick%20%20Facts%20book.pdf. Accessed April 7, 2015.

13. Green D. *McDonald's Corporation v. Steel & Morris* [1997] EWHC QB 366.

14. U.S. Department of Agriculture. Mission statement. http://www.usda.gov/wps/portal/usda/usdahome?navid=MISSION_STATEMENT. Accessed April 6, 2015.

15. U.S. Department of Agriculture, U.S. Department of Health and Human Services. Dietary guidelines for Americans, 2010. Washington, D.C.: U.S. Government Printing Office; 2010.

16. U.S. Department of Agriculture. Mission statement. http://www.usda.gov/wps/portal/usda/usdahome?navid=MISSION_STATEMENT. Accessed April 6, 2015.

17. U.S. Department of Agriculture. Greening Headquarters Update. http://www.moran.senate.gov/public/index.cfm/files/serve?File_id=668d6da1-314c-4647-9f17-25edb67bb2f2. July 23, 2012. Accessed May 20, 2015.

18. USDA Retracts Meatless Monday Recommendation. http://www.meatlessmonday.com/articles/usda-misses-mark-on-meatless-monday/. July 26, 2012. Accessed April 6, 2015.

19. Herman J. 2010. Saving U.S. dietary advice from conflicts of interest. *Food and Drug Law Journal.* 65(20):285–316.

20. Institute of Medicine. Dietary Reference Intakes for Energy, Carbohydrate, Fiber, Fat, Fatty Acids, Cholesterol, Protein, and Amino Acids. Washington, D.C.: National Academies Press, 2003.

21. Institute of Medicine. Dietary Reference Intakes for Energy, Carbohydrate, Fiber, Fat, Fatty Acids, Cholesterol, Protein, and Amino Acids. Washington, D.C.: National Academies Press, 2003.

22. U.S. Department of Agriculture. Fat and fatty acid content of selected foods containing trans-fatty acids. ARS Nutrient Data Laboratory. http://www.ars.usda.gov/SP2UserFiles/Place/12354500/Data/Classics/trans_fa.pdf. Accessed April 6, 2015.

23. Institute of Medicine. Dietary Reference Intakes for Energy, Carbohydrate, Fiber, Fat, Fatty Acids, Cholesterol, Protein, and Amino Acids. Washington, D.C.: National Academies Press, 2003.

24. Fox M. Report recommends limiting trans-fats in diet. Reuters, July 10, 2002.

25. Krebs-Smith SM, Guenther PM, Subar AF, Kirkpatrick SI, Dodd KW. Americans do not meet federal dietary recommendations. *J Nutr.* 2010;140(10):1832–8.

26. Krebs-Smith SM, Guenther PM, Subar AF, Kirkpatrick SI, Dodd KW. Americans do not meet federal dietary recommendations. *J Nutr.* 2010;140(10):1832–8.

27. Krebs-Smith SM, Guenther PM, Subar AF, Kirkpatrick SI, Dodd KW. Americans do not meet federal dietary recommendations. *J Nutr.* 2010;140(10):1832–8.

28. Stuckler D, McKee M, Ebrahim S, Basu S. Manufacturing epidemics: the role of global producers in increased consumption of unhealthy commodities including processed foods, alcohol, and tobacco. *PLoS Med.* 2012;9(6):e1001235.

29. Brownell KD. Thinking forward: the quicksand of appeasing the food industry. *PLoS Med.* 2012;9(7):e1001254.

30. Freedhoff Y, Hébert PC. Partnerships between health organizations and the food industry risk derailing public health nutrition. *CMAJ.* 2011;183(3):291–2.

31. Neuman W. Save the Children breaks with soda tax effort. *New York Times.* December 14, 2010. http://www.nytimes.com/2010/12/15/business/15soda.html. Accessed April 8, 2015.

32. Murray CJ, Atkinson C, Bhalla K, et al. The state of US health, 1990–2010: burden of diseases, injuries, and risk factors. *JAMA.* 2013;310(6):591–608.

33. Neal B. Fat chance for physical activity. *Popul Health Metr.* 2013;11(1):9.

34. Gilroy DJ, Kauffman KW, Hall RA, Huang X, Chu FS. Assessing potential health risks from microcystin toxins in blue-green algae dietary supplements. *Environ Health Perspect.* 2000; 108(5):435–9.

35. Parker-Pope T. Michael Pollan offers 64 ways to eat food. *New York Times,* January 8, 2010.

36. Arnold D. British India and the "beriberi problem," 1798–1942. *Med Hist.* 2010;54(3):295–314.

37. Freeman BB, Reimers K. Tomato consumption and health: emerging benefits. *Am J Lifestyle Med.* 2010; 5(2):182–91.

38. Denke MA. Effects of cocoa butter on serum lipids in humans: historical highlights. *Am J Clin Nutr.* 1994;60(6 Suppl):1014S–1016S.

39. Feingold Association of the United States. Regulations re 36 Colorants Covering 80 Countries. http://www.feingold.org/Research/PDFstudies/List-of-Colorants.pdf. Accessed June 30, 2015.

40. Galloway D. DIY bacon fat candle. http://lifehacker.com/5929854/diy-bacon-fat-candle. July 28, 2012. Accessed April 10, 2015.

41. Orlich MJ, Singh PN, Sabaté J, et al. Vegetarian dietary patterns and mortality in Adventist Health Study 2. *JAMA Intern Med.* 2013;173(13):1230–8.

42. Willcox BJ, Willcox DC, Todoriki H, et al. Caloric restriction, the traditional Okinawan diet, and healthy aging: the diet of the world's longest-lived people and its potential impact on morbidity and life span. *Ann NY Acad Sci.* 2007;1114:434–55.

43. Kaiser Permanente. The plant-based diet: a healthier way to eat. http://mydoctor.kaiser permanente.org/ncal/Images/New%20Plant%20Based%20Booklet%201214_tcm28-781815 .pdf. 2013. Accessed April 10, 2015.

44. Campbell TC, Parpia B, Chen J. Diet, lifestyle, and the etiology of coronary artery disease: the Cornell China study. *Am J Cardiol.* 1998;82(10B):18T–21T.

45. Schane RE, Glantz SA, Ling PM. Social smoking implications for public health, clinical practice, and intervention research. *Am J Prev Med.* 2009;37(2):124–31.

46. Willard Bishop. Supermarket facts. The future of food retailing, 2014. http://www.fmi.org /research-resources/supermarket-facts. Accessed April 7, 2015.

47. Vohs KD, Heatherton TF. Self-regulatory failure: a resource-depletion approach. *Psychol Sci.* 2000;11(3):249–54.

48. Kaiser Permanente. The plant-based diet: a healthier way to eat. http://mydoctor.kaiser permanente.org/ncal/Images/New%20Plant%20Based%20Booklet%201214_tcm28-781815 .pdf. 2013. Accessed April 10, 2015.
49. Barnard N, Scialli AR, Bertron P, Hurlick D, Edmondset K. Acceptability of a therapeutic low-fat, vegan diet in premenopausal women. *J Nutr Educ.* 2000;32(6):314–9.
50. Miller KB, Hurst WJ, Payne MJ, et al. Impact of alkalization on the antioxidant and flavanol content of commercial cocoa powders. *J Agric Food Chem.* 2008;56(18):8527–33.

Dr. Greger's Daily Dozen

1. Kon SK, Klein A. The value of whole potato in human nutrition. *Biochem J.* 1928;22(1):258–60.
2. Cheah IK, Halliwell B. Ergothioneine; antioxidant potential, physiological function and role in disease. *Biochim Biophys Acta.* 2012;1822(5):784–93.
3. United States Supreme Court. *Nix v. Hedden*, 149 U.S. 304 (1893).
4. Arkansas Code Title 1, Chapter 4, Section 1-4-115. http://archive.org/stream/govlawarcode 012008/govlawarcode012008_djvu.txt. Accessed April 8, 2015.

Beans

1. World Cancer Research Fund / American Institute for Cancer Research. Food, Nutrition, Physical Activity, and the Prevention of Cancer: a Global Perspective. Washington, D.C.: AICR, 2007.
2. U.S. Department of Agriculture. National Nutrient Database for Standard Reference Release 27. Basic Report: 16426, Tofu, raw, firm, prepared with calcium sulfate. http://ndb.nal.usda .gov/ndb/foods/show/4995. Accessed April 4, 2015.
3. Fields of gold. *Nature.* 2013;497(7447):5–6.
4. Bøhn T, Cuhra M, Traavik T, Sanden M, Fagan J, Primicerio R. Compositional differences in soybeans on the market: glyphosate accumulates in Roundup Ready GM soybeans. *Food Chem.* 2014;153:207–15.
5. Aris A, Leblanc S. Maternal and fetal exposure to pesticides associated to genetically modified foods in Eastern Townships of Quebec, Canada. *Reprod Toxicol.* 2011;31(4):528–33.
6. Bøhn T, Cuhra M, Traavik T, Sanden M, Fagan J, Primicerio R. Compositional differences in soybeans on the market: glyphosate accumulates in Roundup Ready GM soybeans. *Food Chem.* 2014;153:207–15.
7. Marc J, Mulner-Lorillon O, Boulben S, Hureau D, Durand G, Bellé R. Pesticide Roundup provokes cell division dysfunction at the level of CDK1/cyclin B activation. *Chem Res Toxicol.* 2002;15(3):326–31.
8. Walsh LP, McCormick C, Martin C, Stocco DM. Roundup inhibits steroidogenesis by disrupting steroidogenic acute regulatory (StAR) protein expression. *Environ Health Perspect.* 2000;108(8):769–76.
9. Vaughan E. Men! Save your testicles (and humanity): avoid Roundup® and GMO/GE Roundup Ready® foods. http://www.drvaughan.com/2013/07/men-save-your-testicles-and-humanity .html, July 29,2013. Accessed April 9, 2015.
10. Romano RM, Romano MA, Bernardi MM, Furtado PV, Oliveira CA. Prepubertal exposure to commercial formulation of the herbicide glyphosate alters testosterone levels and testicular morphology. *Arch Toxicol.* 2010;84(4):309–17.
11. Richard S, Moslemi S, Sipahutar H, Benachour N, Seralini GE. Differential effects of glyphosate

and Roundup on human placental cells and aromatase. *Environ Health Perspect.* 2005;113(6): 716–20.

12. De Roos AJ, Blair A, Rusiecki JA, et al. Cancer incidence among glyphosate-exposed pesticide applicators in the Agricultural Health Study. *Environ Health Perspect.* 2005;113(1):49–54.

13. De Roos AJ, Zahm SH, Cantor KP, et al. Integrative assessment of multiple pesticides as risk factors for non-Hodgkin's lymphoma among men. *Occup Environ Med.* 2003;60(9):E11.

14. Garry VF, Harkins ME, Erickson LL, Long-Simpson LK, Holland SE, Burroughs BL. Birth defects, season of conception, and sex of children born to pesticide applicators living in the Red River Valley of Minnesota, USA. *Environ Health Perspect.* 2002;110 Suppl 3:441–9.

15. Thongprakaisang S, Thiantanawat A, Rangkadilok N, Suriyo T, Satayavivad J. Glyphosate induces human breast cancer cells growth via estrogen receptors. *Food Chem Toxicol.* 2013;59: 129–36.

16. Butler D, Reichhardt T. Long-term effect of GM crops serves up food for thought. *Nature.* 1999;398(6729):651–6.

17. Smyth S. International considerations of food biotechnology regulatory frameworks. http://regulation.upf.edu/exeter-12-papers/Paper%20260%20-%20Smyth%202012%20-%20International%20Considerations%20of%20Food%20Biotechnology%20Regulatory%20Frameworks.pdf. June 29, 2012. Accessed April 9, 2015.

18. Kramkowska M, Grzelak T, Czyżewska K. Benefits and risks associated with genetically modified food products. *Ann Agric Environ Med.* 2013;20(3):413–9.

19. Murooka Y, Yamshita M. Traditional healthful fermented products of Japan. *J Ind Microbiol Biotechnol.* 2008;35(8):791–8.

20. World Cancer Research Fund / American Institute for Cancer Research. Food, Nutrition, Physical Activity, and the Prevention of Cancer: a Global Perspective. Washington, D.C.: AICR, 2007.

21. Parkin DM. 7. Cancers attributable to dietary factors in the UK in 2010. IV. Salt. *Br J Cancer.* 2011;105 Suppl 2:S31–3.

22. Lee YY, Derakhshan MH. Environmental and lifestyle risk factors of gastric cancer. *Arch Iran Med.* 2013;16(6):358–65.

23. González CA, Jakszyn P, Pera G, et al. Meat intake and risk of stomach and esophageal adenocarcinoma within the European Prospective Investigation into Cancer and Nutrition (EPIC). *J Natl Cancer Inst.* 2006;98(5):345–54.

24. Key TJ, Appleby PN, Crowe FL, Bradbury KE, Schmidt JA, Travis RC. Cancer in British vegetarians: updated analyses of 4998 incident cancers in a cohort of 32,491 meat eaters, 8612 fish eaters, 18,298 vegetarians, and 2246 vegans. *Am J Clin Nutr.* 2014;100 Suppl 1:378S–85S.

25. D'Elia L, Rossi G, Ippolito R, Cappuccio FP, Strazzullo P. Habitual salt intake and risk of gastric cancer: a meta-analysis of prospective studies. *Clin Nutr.* 2012;31(4):489–98.

26. Joossens JV, Hill MJ, Elliott P, et al. Dietary salt, nitrate and stomach cancer mortality in 24 countries. European Cancer Prevention (ECP) and the INTERSALT Cooperative Research Group. *Int J Epidemiol.* 1996;25(3):494–504.

27. D'Elia L, Rossi G, Ippolito R, Cappuccio FP, Strazzullo P. Habitual salt intake and risk of gastric cancer: a meta-analysis of prospective studies. *Clin Nutr.* 2012;31(4):489–98.

28. Ko KP, Park SK, Yang JJ, et al. Intake of soy products and other foods and gastric cancer risk: a prospective study. *J Epidemiol.* 2013;23(5):337–43.

29. D'Elia L, Rossi G, Ippolito R, Cappuccio FP, Strazzullo P. Habitual salt intake and risk of gastric cancer: a meta-analysis of prospective studies. *Clin Nutr.* 2012;31(4):489–98.

30. Turati F, Pelucchi C, Guercio V, La Vecchia C, Galeone C. Allium vegetable intake and gastric cancer: a case-control study and meta-analysis. *Mol Nutr Food Res.* 2015;59(1):171–9.

31. He J, Gu D, Wu X, et al. Effect of soybean protein on blood pressure: a randomized, controlled trial. *Ann Intern Med.* 2005;143(1):1–9.

32. Rivas M, Garay RP, Escanero JF, Cia P, Cia P, Alda JO. Soy milk lowers blood pressure in men and women with mild to moderate essential hypertension. *J Nutr.* 2002;132(7):1900–2.

33. Kanda A, Hoshiyama Y, Kawaguchi T. Association of lifestyle parameters with the prevention of hypertension in elderly Japanese men and women: a four-year follow-up of normotensive subjects. *Asia Pac J Public Health.* 1999;11(2):77–81.

34. Jenkins DJ, Wolever TM, Taylor RH, et al. Slow release dietary carbohydrate improves second meal tolerance. *Am J Clin Nutr.* 1982;35(6):1339–46.

35. Ropert A, Cherbut C, Rozé C, et al. Colonic fermentation and proximal gastric tone in humans. *Gastroenterology.* 1996;111(2):289–96.

36. Mollard RC, Wong CL, Luhovyy BL, Anderson GH. First and second meal effects of pulses on blood glucose, appetite, and food intake at a later meal. *Appl Physiol Nutr Metab.* 2011;36(5):634–42.

37. Yashin YI, Nemzer BV, Ryzhnev VY, Yashin AY, Chernousova NI, Fedina PA. Creation of a databank for content of antioxidants in food products by an amperometric method. *Molecules.* 2010;15(10):7450–66.

38. Zanovec M, O'Neil CE, Nicklas TA. Comparison of nutrient density and nutrient-to-cost between cooked and canned beans. *Food Nutr Sci.* 2011;2(2):66–73.

39. Zanovec M, O'Neil CE, Nicklas TA. Comparison of nutrient density and nutrient-to-cost between cooked and canned beans. *Food Nutr Sci.* 2011;2(2):66–73.

40. Kid Tested Firefighter Approved. Buffalo ranch roasted chickpeas. http://kidtestedfirefighter approved.com/2012/08/05/buffalo-ranch-roasted-chickpeas/. August 5, 2012. Accessed April 9, 2015.

41. Bazzano LA, Thompson AM, Tees MT, Nguyen CH, Winham DM. Non-soy legume consumption lowers cholesterol levels: a meta-analysis of randomized controlled trials. *Nutr Metab Cardiovasc Dis.* 2011;21(2):94–103.

42. Anderson JW, Bush HM. Soy protein effects on serum lipoproteins: a quality assessment and meta-analysis of randomized, controlled studies. *J Am Coll Nutr.* 2011;30(2):79–91.

43. Winham DM, Hutchins AM, Johnston CS. Pinto bean consumption reduces biomarkers for heart disease risk. *J Am Coll Nutr.* 2007;26(3):243–9.

44. Fuhrman J. Fudgy black bean brownies. *The Dr. Oz Show.* http://www.doctoroz.com/recipe /fudgy-black-bean-brownies. November 12, 2014. Accessed April 9, 2015.

45. U.S. Department of Agriculture. Oxygen Radical Absorbance Capacity (ORAC) of Selected Foods—2007. http://www.orac-info-portal.de/download/ORAC_R2.pdf. November 2007. Accessed April 10, 2015.

46. Darmadi-Blackberry I, Wahlqvist ML, Kouris-Blazos A, et al. Legumes: the most important dietary predictor of survival in older people of different ethnicities. *Asia Pac J Clin Nutr.* 2004;13(2):217–20.

47. Darmadi-Blackberry I, Wahlqvist ML, Kouris-Blazos A, et al. Legumes: the most important dietary predictor of survival in older people of different ethnicities. *Asia Pac J Clin Nutr.* 2004;13(2):217–20.

48. Desrochers N, Brauer PM. Legume promotion in counselling: an e-mail survey of dietitians. *Can J Diet Pract Res.* 2001;62(4):193–8.

49. Winham DM, Hutchins AM. Perceptions of flatulence from bean consumption among adults in 3 feeding studies. *Nutr J.* 2011;10:128.

50. Levitt MD, Lasser RB, Schwartz JS, Bond JH. Studies of a flatulent patient. *N Engl J Med.* 1976;295(5):260–2.

51. Levitt MD, Furne J, Olsson S. The relation of passage of gas and abdominal bloating to colonic gas production. *Ann Intern Med.* 1996;124(4):422–4.

52. Price KR, Lewis J, Wyatt GM, Fenwick GR. Flatulence—causes, relation to diet and remedies. *Nahrung.* 1988;32(6):609–26.

53. Matthews SB, Waud JP, Roberts AG, Campbell AK. Systemic lactose intolerance: a new perspective on an old problem. *Postgrad Med J.* 2005;81(953):167–73.

54. Levitt MD, Lasser RB, Schwartz JS, Bond JH. Studies of a flatulent patient. *N Engl J Med.* 1976;295(5):260–2.

55. McEligot AJ, Gilpin EA, Rock CL, et al. High dietary fiber consumption is not associated with gastrointestinal discomfort in a diet intervention trial. *J Am Diet Assoc.* 2002;102(4):549–51.

56. Price KR, Lewis J, Wyatt GM, Fenwick GR. Flatulence—causes, relation to diet and remedies. *Nahrung.* 1988;32(6):609–26.

57. Jood S, Mehta U, Singh R, Bhat CM. Effect of processing on flatus producing factors in legumes. *J Agric Food Chem.* 1985;3:268–71.

58. Savitri A, Bhavanishankar TN, Desikachar HSR. Effect of spices on in vitro gas production by Clostridium perfringens. *Food Microbiol.* 1986;3:195–9.

59. Di Stefano M, Miceli E, Gotti S, Missanelli A, Mazzocchi S, Corazza GR. The effect of oral alpha-galactosidase on intestinal gas production and gas-related symptoms. *Dig Dis Sci.* 2007;52(1):78–83.

60. How you can limit your gas production. 12 tips for dealing with flatulence. *Harv Health Lett.* 2007;32(12):3.

61. Magee EA, Richardson CJ, Hughes R, Cummings JH. Contribution of dietary protein to sulfide production in the large intestine: an in vitro and a controlled feeding study in humans. *Am J Clin Nutr.* 2000;72(6):1488–94.

62. Gorbach SL. Bismuth therapy in gastrointestinal diseases. *Gastroenterology.* 1990;99(3):863–75.

63. Suarez FL, Springfield J, Levitt MD. Identification of gases responsible for the odour of human flatus and evaluation of a device purported to reduce this odour. *Gut.* 1998;43(1):100–4.

64. Bouchier IA. Flatulence. *Practitioner.* 1980;224(1342):373–7.

65. Fardy J, Sullivan S. Gastrointestinal gas. *CMAJ.* 1988;139(12):1137–42.

Berries

1. McCullough ML, Peterson JJ, Patel R, Jacques PF, Shah R, Dwyer JT. Flavonoid intake and cardiovascular disease mortality in a prospective cohort of US adults. *Am J Clin Nutr.* 2012;95(2):454–64.

2. Hernandez-Marin E, Galano A, Martínez A. Cis carotenoids: colorful molecules and free radical quenchers. *J Phys Chem B.* 2013;117(15):4050–61.

3. U.S. Department of Agriculture. Oxygen Radical Absorbance Capacity (ORAC) of Selected Foods—2007. http://www.orac-info-portal.de/download/ORAC_R2.pdf. November 2007. Accessed April 10, 2015.

4. Carlsen MH, Halvorsen BL, Holte K, et al. The total antioxidant content of more than 3100 foods, beverages, spices, herbs and supplements used worldwide. *Nutr J.* 2010;9:3.

5. Carlsen MH, Halvorsen BL, Holte K, et al. The total antioxidant content of more than 3100 foods, beverages, spices, herbs and supplements used worldwide. *Nutr J.* 2010;9:3.

6. Carlsen MH, Halvorsen BL, Holte K, et al. The total antioxidant content of more than 3100 foods, beverages, spices, herbs and supplements used worldwide. *Nutr J.* 2010;9:3.

7. Dinstel RR, Cascio J, Koukel S. The antioxidant level of Alaska's wild berries: high, higher and highest. *Int J Circumpolar Health.* 2013;72.

8. Carlsen MH, Halvorsen BL, Holte K, et al. The total antioxidant content of more than 3100 foods, beverages, spices, herbs and supplements used worldwide. *Nutr J.* 2010;9:3.

9. Petta S, Marchesini G, Caracausi L, et al. Industrial, not fruit fructose intake is associated with the severity of liver fibrosis in genotype 1 chronic hepatitis C patients. *J Hepatol.* 2013;59(6): 1169–76.

10. Madero M, Arriaga JC, Jalal D, et al. The effect of two energy-restricted diets, a low-fructose diet versus a moderate natural fructose diet, on weight loss and metabolic syndrome parameters: a randomized controlled trial. *Metab Clin Exp.* 2011;60(11):1551–9.

11. U.S. Department of Agriculture Economic Research Service. U.S. sugar production. http://www.ers.usda.gov/topics/crops/sugar-sweeteners/background.aspx. November 14, 2014. Accessed April 11, 2015.

12. Petta S, Marchesini G, Caracausi L, et al. Industrial, not fruit fructose intake is associated with the severity of liver fibrosis in genotype 1 chronic hepatitis C patients. *J Hepatol.* 2013;59(6):1169–76.

13. Törrönen R, Kolehmainen M, Sarkkinen E, Mykkänen H, Niskanen L. Postprandial glucose, insulin, and free fatty acid responses to sucrose consumed with blackcurrants and lingonberries in healthy women. *Am J Clin Nutr.* 2012;96(3):527–33.

14. Törrönen R, Kolehmainen M, Sarkkinen E, Mykkänen H, Niskanen L. Postprandial glucose, insulin, and free fatty acid responses to sucrose consumed with blackcurrants and lingonberries in healthy women. *Am J Clin Nutr.* 2012;96(3):527–33.

15. Törrönen R, Kolehmainen M, Sarkkinen E, Poutanen K, Mykkänen H, Niskanen L. Berries reduce postprandial insulin responses to wheat and rye breads in healthy women. *J Nutr.* 2013; 143(4):430–6.

16. Törrönen R, Kolehmainen M, Sarkkinen E, Mykkänen H, Niskanen L. Postprandial glucose, insulin, and free fatty acid responses to sucrose consumed with blackcurrants and lingonberries in healthy women. *Am J Clin Nutr.* 2012;96(3):527–33.

17. Manzano S, Williamson G. Polyphenols and phenolic acids from strawberry and apple decrease glucose uptake and transport by human intestinal Caco-2 cells. *Mol Nutr Food Res.* 2010; 54(12):1773–80.

18. Sievenpiper JL, Chiavaroli L, de Souza RJ, et al. "Catalytic" doses of fructose may benefit glycaemic control without harming cardiometabolic risk factors: a small meta-analysis of randomised controlled feeding trials. *Br J Nutr.* 2012;108(3):418–23.

19. Christensen AS, Viggers L, Hasselström K, Gregersen S. Effect of fruit restriction on glycemic control in patients with type 2 diabetes—a randomized trial. *Nutr J.* 2013;12:29.

20. Meyer BJ, van der Merwe M, du Plessis DG, de Bruin EJ, Meyer AC. Some physiological effects of a mainly fruit diet in man. *S Afr Med J.* 1971;45(8):191–5.

21. Meyer BJ, de Bruin EJ, du Plessis DG, van der Merwe M, Meyer AC. Some biochemical effects of a mainly fruit diet in man. *S Afr Med J.* 1971;45(10):253–61.

22. Jenkins DJ, Kendall CW, Popovich DG, et al. Effect of a very-high-fiber vegetable, fruit, and nut diet on serum lipids and colonic function. *Metab Clin Exp.* 2001;50(4):494–503.

23. Jenkins DJ, Kendall CW, Popovich DG, et al. Effect of a very-high-fiber vegetable, fruit, and nut diet on serum lipids and colonic function. *Metab Clin Exp.* 2001;50(4):494–503.

24. Ou B, Bosak KN, Brickner PR, Iezzoni DG, Seymour EM. Processed tart cherry products—comparative phytochemical content, in vitro antioxidant capacity and in vitro anti-inflammatory activity. *J Food Sci.* 2012;77(5):H105–12.

25. Mullen W, Stewart AJ, Lean ME, Gardner P, Duthie GG, Crozier A. Effect of freezing and storage on the phenolics, ellagitannins, flavonoids, and antioxidant capacity of red raspberries. *J Agric Food Chem.* 2002;50(18):5197–201.

26. Marques KK, Renfroe MH, Brevard PB, Lee RE, Gloeckner JW. Differences in antioxidant

levels of fresh, frozen and freeze-dried strawberries and strawberry jam. *Int J Food Sci Nutr.* 2010;61(8):759–69.

27. Blau LW. Cherry diet control for gout and arthritis. *Tex Rep Biol Med.* 1950;8(3):309–11.

28. Overman T. Pegloticase: a new treatment for gout. *Cleveland Clinic Pharmacotherapy Update.* 2011;14(2):1–3.

29. Finkelstein Y, Aks SE, Hutson JR, et al. Colchicine poisoning: the dark side of an ancient drug. *Clin Toxicol* (Phila). 2010;48(5):407–14.

30. Fritsch PO, Sidoroff A. Drug-induced Stevens-Johnson syndrome/toxic epidermal necrolysis. *Am J Clin Dermatol.* 2000;1(6):349–60.

31. Zhang Y, Chen C, Choi H, et al. Purine-rich foods intake and recurrent gout attacks. *Ann Rheum Dis.* 2012;71(9):1448–53.

32. Kelley DS, Rasooly R, Jacob RA, Kader AA, Mackey BE. Consumption of Bing sweet cherries lowers circulating concentrations of inflammation markers in healthy men and women. *J Nutr.* 2006;136(4):981–6.

33. Zielinsky P, Busato S. Prenatal effects of maternal consumption of polyphenol-rich foods in late pregnancy upon fetal ductus arteriosus. *Birth Defects Res C.* 2013;99(4):256–74.

34. Howatson G, Bell PG, Tallent J, Middleton B, McHugh MP, Ellis J. Effect of tart cherry juice (Prunus cerasus) on melatonin levels and enhanced sleep quality. *Eur J Nutr.* 2012;51(8): 909–16.

35. Huang X, Mazza G. Application of LC and LC-MS to the analysis of melatonin and serotonin in edible plants. *Crit Rev Food Sci Nutr.* 2011;51(4):269–84.

36. Carlsen MH, Halvorsen BL, Holte K, et al. The total antioxidant content of more than 3100 foods, beverages, spices, herbs and supplements used worldwide. *Nutr J.* 2010;9:3.

37. Beatty S, Murray IJ, Henson DB, Carden D, Koh H, Boulton ME. Macular pigment and risk for age-related macular degeneration in subjects from a Northern European population. *Invest Ophthalmol Vis Sci.* 2001;42(2):439–46.

38. Cheng CY, Chung WY, Szeto YT, Benzie IF. Fasting plasma zeaxanthin response to Fructus barbarum L. (wolfberry; Kei Tze) in a food-based human supplementation trial. *Br J Nutr.* 2005;93(1):123–30.

39. Bucheli P, Vidal K, Shen L, et al. Goji berry effects on macular characteristics and plasma antioxidant levels. *Optom Vis Sci.* 2011;88(2):257–62.

40. Nakaishi H, Matsumoto H, Tominaga S, Hirayama M. Effects of black currant anthocyanoside intake on dark adaptation and VDT work-induced transient refractive alteration in healthy humans. *Altern Med Rev.* 2000;5(6):553–62.

41. Wu X, Beecher GR, Holden JM, Haytowitz DB, Gebhardt SE, Prior RL. Concentrations of anthocyanins in common foods in the United States and estimation of normal consumption. *J Agric Food Chem.* 2006;54(11):4069–75.

42. Muth ER, Laurent JM, Jasper P. The effect of bilberry nutritional supplementation on night visual acuity and contrast sensitivity. *Altern Med Rev.* 2000;5(2):164–73.

43. Rababah TM, Al-Mahasneh MA, Kilani I, et al. Effect of jam processing and storage on total phenolics, antioxidant activity, and anthocyanins of different fruits. *J Sci Food Agric.* 2011;91(6): 1096–102.

44. Marques KK, Renfroe MH, Brevard PB, Lee RE, Gloeckner JW. Differences in antioxidant levels of fresh, frozen and freeze-dried strawberries and strawberry jam. *Int J Food Sci Nutr.* 2010;61(8):759–69.

45. Vivian J. Foraging for edible wild plants: a field guide to wild berries. Mother Earth News, October/November 1999. http://www.motherearthnews.com/organic-gardening/edible-wild-plants.aspx. Accessed April 11, 2015.

Other Fruits

1. Horton R. GBD 2010: understanding disease, injury, and risk. *Lancet.* 2012;380(9859): 2053–4.

2. Murray CJ, Atkinson C, Bhalla K, et al. The state of US health, 1990–2010: burden of diseases, injuries, and risk factors. *JAMA.* 2013;310(6):591–608.

3. Lim SS, Vos T, Flaxman AD, et al. A comparative risk assessment of burden of disease and injury attributable to 67 risk factors and risk factor clusters in 21 regions, 1990–2010: a systematic analysis for the Global Burden of Disease Study 2010. *Lancet.* 2012;380(9859): 2224–60.

4. Arranz S, Silván JM, Saura-Calixto F. Nonextractable polyphenols, usually ignored, are the major part of dietary polyphenols: a study on the Spanish diet. *Mol Nutr Food Res.* 2010;54(11): 1646–58.

5. Mullen W, Marks SC, Crozier A. Evaluation of phenolic compounds in commercial fruit juices and fruit drinks. *J Agric Food Chem.* 2007;55(8):3148–57.

6. Muraki I, Imamura F, Manson JE, et al. Fruit consumption and risk of type 2 diabetes: results from three prospective longitudinal cohort studies. *BMJ.* 2013;347:f5001.

7. Li N, Shi J, Wang K. Profile and antioxidant activity of phenolic extracts from 10 crabapples (Malus wild species). *J Agric Food Chem.* 2014;62(3):574–81.

8. Vogel RA. Brachial artery ultrasound: a noninvasive tool in the assessment of triglyceride-rich lipoproteins. *Clin Cardiol.* 1999;22(6 Suppl):II34–9.

9. Rueda-Clausen CF, Silva FA, Lindarte MA, et al. Olive, soybean and palm oils intake have a similar acute detrimental effect over the endothelial function in healthy young subjects. *Nutr Metab Cardiovasc Dis.* 2007;17(1):50–7.

10. Casas-Agustench P, López-Uriarte P, Ros E, Bulló M, Salas-Salvadó J. Nuts, hypertension and endothelial function. *Nutr Metab Cardiovasc Dis.* 2011;21 Suppl 1:S21–33.

11. Vogel RA, Corretti MC, Plotnick GD. The postprandial effect of components of the Mediterranean diet on endothelial function. *J Am Coll Cardiol.* 2000;36(5):1455–60.

12. Carlsen MH, Halvorsen BL, Holte K, et al. The total antioxidant content of more than 3100 foods, beverages, spices, herbs and supplements used worldwide. *Nutr J.* 2010;9:3.

13. Cormio L, De Siati M, Lorusso F, et al. Oral L-citrulline supplementation improves erection hardness in men with mild erectile dysfunction. *Urology.* 2011;77(1):119–22.

14. Rimando AM, Perkins-Veazie PM. Determination of citrulline in watermelon rind. *J Chromatogr A.* 2005;1078(1–2):196–200.

15. Pfizer Annual Meeting of Shareholders 2014 Financial Report. http://www.pfizer.com/system/files/presentation/2014_Pfizer_Financial_Report.pdf. Accessed May 16, 2015.

16. Johnson G. Watermelon board approves officers, budget, marketing plan. The Packer. http://www.thepacker.com/news/watermelon-board-approves-officers-budget-marketing-plan. February 24, 2015. Accessed May 16, 2015.

17. Chai SC, Hooshmand S, Saadat RL, Payton ME, Brummel-Smith K, Arjmandi BH. Daily apple versus dried plum: impact on cardiovascular disease risk factors in postmenopausal women. *J Acad Nutr Diet.* 2012;112(8):1158–68.

18. Magee E. A nutritional component to inflammatory bowel disease: the contribution of meat to fecal sulfide excretion. *Nutrition.* 1999;15(3):244–6.

19. Ananthakrishnan AN, Khalili H, Konijeti GG, et al. A prospective study of long-term intake of dietary fiber and risk of Crohn's disease and ulcerative colitis. *Gastroenterology.* 2013;145(5): 970–7.

20. Lin HH, Tsai PS, Fang SC, Liu JF. Effect of kiwifruit consumption on sleep quality in adults with sleep problems. *Asia Pac J Clin Nutr.* 2011;20(2):169–74.

21. U.S. Food and Drug Administration. FDA announces discontinued marketing of GI drug, Zelnorm, for safety reasons. http://www.fda.gov/NewsEvents/Newsroom/PressAnnouncements/2007/ucm108879.htm. March 30, 2007. Accessed April 11, 2015.

22. Skinner MA. Gold kiwifruit for immune support and reducing symptoms of cold and influenza. *J Food Drug Anal.* 2012;20:261–4.

23. Hunter DC, Skinner MA, Wolber FM, et al. Consumption of gold kiwifruit reduces severity and duration of selected upper respiratory tract infection symptoms and increases plasma vitamin C concentration in healthy older adults. *Br J Nutr.* 2012;108(7):1235 45.

24. Orhan F, Karakas T, Cakir M, Aksoy A, Baki A, Gedik Y. Prevalence of immunoglobulin E–mediated food allergy in 6–9-year-old urban schoolchildren in the eastern Black Sea region of Turkey. *Clin Exp Allergy.* 2009;39(7):1027–35.

25. Rancé F, Grandmottet X, Grandjean H. Prevalence and main characteristics of schoolchildren diagnosed with food allergies in France. *Clin Exp Allergy.* 2005;35(2):167–72.

26. Szeto YT, To TL, Pak SC, Kalle W. A study of DNA protective effect of orange juice supplementation. *Appl Physiol Nutr Metab.* 2013;38(5):533–6.

27. Slyskova J, Lorenzo Y, Karlsen A, et al. Both genetic and dietary factors underlie individual differences in DNA damage levels and DNA repair capacity. *DNA Repair (Amst).* 2014;16:66–73.

28. Szeto YT, Chu WK, Benzie IF. Antioxidants in fruits and vegetables: a study of cellular availability and direct effects on human DNA. *Biosci Biotechnol Biochem.* 2006;70(10):2551–5.

29. Szeto YT, To TL, Pak SC, Kalle W. A study of DNA protective effect of orange juice supplementation. *Appl Physiol Nutr Metab.* 2013;38(5):533–6.

30. Song JK, Bae JM. Citrus fruit intake and breast cancer risk: a quantitative systematic review. *J Breast Cancer.* 2013;16(1):72–6.

31. Miller JA, Lang JE, Ley M, et al. Human breast tissue disposition and bioactivity of limonene in women with early-stage breast cancer. *Cancer Prev Res* (Phila). 2013;6(6):577–84.

32. Lorenzo Y, Azqueta A, Luna L, Bonilla F, Domínguez G, Collins AR. The carotenoid beta-cryptoxanthin stimulates the repair of DNA oxidation damage in addition to acting as an antioxidant in human cells. *Carcinogenesis.* 2009;30(2):308–14.

33. Hakim IA, Harris RB, Ritenbaugh C. Citrus peel use is associated with reduced risk of squamous cell carcinoma of the skin. *Nutr Cancer.* 2000;37(2):161–8.

34. Astley SB, Elliott RM, Archer DB, Southon S. Evidence that dietary supplementation with carotenoids and carotenoid-rich foods modulates the DNA damage: repair balance in human lymphocytes. *Br J Nutr.* 2004;91(1):63–72.

35. Feskanich D, Willett WC, Hunter DJ, Colditz GA. Dietary intakes of vitamins A, C, and E and risk of melanoma in two cohorts of women. *Br J Cancer.* 2003;88(9):1381–7.

36. Owira PM, Ojewole JA. The grapefruit: an old wine in a new glass? Metabolic and cardiovascular perspectives. *Cardiovasc J Afr.* 2010;21(5):280–5.

37. Fuhr U, Klittich K, Staib AH. Inhibitory effect of grapefruit juice and its bitter principal, naringenin, on CYP1A2 dependent metabolism of caffeine in man. *Br J Clin Pharmacol.* 1993;35(4):431–6.

38. Ratain MJ, Cohen EE. The value meal: how to save $1,700 per month or more on lapatinib. *J Clin Oncol.* 2007;25(23):3397–8.

39. Aziz S, Asokumaran T, Intan G. Penetrating ocular injury by durian fruit. *Med J Malaysia.* 2009;64(3):244–5.

40. Winokur J. *The Traveling Curmudgeon.* Seattle: Sasquatch Books, 2003.

Cruciferous Vegetables

1. Lenzi M, Fimognari C, Hrelia P. Sulforaphane as a promising molecule for fighting cancer. *Cancer Treat Res.* 2014;159:207–23.
2. Tarozzi A, Angeloni C, Malaguti M, Morroni F, Hrelia S, Hrelia P. Sulforaphane as a potential protective phytochemical against neurodegenerative diseases. *Oxid Med Cell Longev.* 2013; 2013:415078.
3. Liu H, Smith AJ, Lott MC, et al. Sulforaphane can protect lens cells against oxidative stress: implications for cataract prevention. *Invest Ophthalmol Vis Sci.* 2013;54(8):5236–48.
4. Heber D, Li Z, Garcia-Lloret M, et al. Sulforaphane-rich broccoli sprout extract attenuates nasal allergic response to diesel exhaust particles. *Food Funct.* 2014;5(1):35–41.
5. Bahadoran Z, Mirmiran P, Azizi F. Potential efficacy of broccoli sprouts as a unique supplement for management of type 2 diabetes and its complications. *J Med Food.* 2013;16(5):375–82.
6. Matusheski NV, Juvik JA, Jeffery EH. Heating decreases epithiospecifier protein activity and increases sulforaphane formation in broccoli. *Phytochemistry.* 2004;65(9):1273–81.
7. Singh K, Connors SL, Macklin EA, et al. Sulforaphane treatment of autism spectrum disorder (ASD). *Proc Natl Acad Sci USA.* 2014;111(43):15550–5.
8. Vermeulen M, Klöpping-Ketelaars IW, van den Berg R, Vaes WH. Bioavailability and kinetics of sulforaphane in humans after consumption of cooked versus raw broccoli. *J Agric Food Chem.* 2008;56(22):10505–9.
9. Ferrarini L, Pellegrini N, Mazzeo T, et al. Anti-proliferative activity and chemoprotective effects towards DNA oxidative damage of fresh and cooked Brassicaceae. *Br J Nutr.* 2012;107(9): 1324–32.
10. Collins PJ, Horowitz M, Chatterton BE. Proximal, distal and total stomach emptying of a digestible solid meal in normal subjects. *Br J Radiol.* 1988;61(721):12–8.
11. Dosz EB, Jeffery EH. Modifying the processing and handling of frozen broccoli for increased sulforaphane formation. *J Food Sci.* 2013;78(9):H1459–63.
12. Olsen H, Grimmer S, Aaby K, Saha S, Borge GI. Antiproliferative effects of fresh and thermal processed green and red cultivars of curly kale (Brassica oleracea L. convar. acephala var. sabellica). *J Agric Food Chem.* 2012;60(30):7375–83.
13. Dosz EB, Jeffery EH. Commercially produced frozen broccoli lacks the ability to form sulforaphane. *Journal of Functional Foods.* 2013;(5)2:987–90.
14. Ghawi SK, Methven L, Niranjan K. The potential to intensify sulforaphane formation in cooked broccoli (Brassica oleracea var. italica) using mustard seeds (Sinapis alba). *Food Chem.* 2013; 138(2–3):1734–41.
15. Dosz EB, Jeffery EH. Modifying the processing and handling of frozen broccoli for increased sulforaphane formation. *J Food Sci.* 2013;78(9):H1459–63.
16. Nolan C. Kale is a noun. http://engine2diet.com/the-daily-beet/kale-is-a-noun/. Accessed April 12, 2015.
17. U.S. Department of Agriculture Economic Research Service. Cabbage—average retail price per pound and per cup equivalent, 2013. http://www.ers.usda.gov/datafiles/Fruit_and _Vegetable_Prices/Vegetables/cabbage.xlsx. Accessed May 21, 2015.
18. U.S. Department of Agriculture. Oxygen Radical Absorbance Capacity (ORAC) of Selected Foods—2007. http://www.orac-info-portal.de/download/ORAC_R2.pdf. November 2007. Accessed April 10, 2015.
19. U.S. Department of Agriculture Economic Research Service. Cabbage—average retail price per pound and per cup equivalent, 2013. http://www.ers.usda.gov/datafiles/Fruit_and _Vegetable_Prices/Vegetables/cabbage.xlsx. Accessed May 21, 2015.

20. Gu Y, Guo Q, Zhang L, Chen Z, Han Y, Gu Z. Physiological and biochemical metabolism of germinating broccoli seeds and sprouts. *J Agric Food Chem.* 2012;60(1):209–13.
21. Clarke JD, Hsu A, Riedl K, et al. Bioavailability and inter-conversion of sulforaphane and erucin in human subjects consuming broccoli sprouts or broccoli supplement in a cross-over study design. *Pharmacol Res.* 2011;64(5):456–63.
22. Shapiro TA, Fahey JW, Dinkova-Kostova AT, et al. Safety, tolerance, and metabolism of broccoli sprout glucosinolates and isothiocyanates: a clinical phase I study. *Nutr Cancer.* 2006;55(1):53–62.
23. Sestili P, Paolillo M, Lenzi M, et al. Sulforaphane induces DNA single strand breaks in cultured human cells. *Mutat Res.* 2010;689(1–2):65–73.

Greens

1. Kwak CS, Moon SC, Lee MS. Antioxidant, antimutagenic, and antitumor effects of pine needles (Pinus densiflora). *Nutr Cancer.* 2006;56(2):162–71.
2. Grivetti LE, Corlett JL, Gordon BM, Lockett GT. Food in American history: Part 10. Greens: Part 1. Vegetable greens in a historical context. *Nutr Today.* 2008;42(2):88–94.
3. Krebs-Smith SM, Guenther PM, Subar AF, Kirkpatrick SI, Dodd KW. Americans do not meet federal dietary recommendations. *J Nutr.* 2010;140(10):1832–8.
4. Walker FB. Myocardial infarction after diet-induced warfarin resistance. *Arch Intern Med.* 1984;144(10):2089–90.
5. Tamakoshi A, Tamakoshi K, Lin Y, Yagyu K, Kikuchi S. Healthy lifestyle and preventable death: findings from the Japan Collaborative Cohort (JACC) Study. *Prev Med.* 2009;48(5):486–92.
6. Hung HC, Joshipura KJ, Jiang R, et al. Fruit and vegetable intake and risk of major chronic disease. *J Natl Cancer Inst.* 2004;96(21):1577–84.
7. Joshipura KJ, Hu FB, Manson JE, et al. The effect of fruit and vegetable intake on risk for coronary heart disease. *Ann Intern Med.* 2001;134(12):1106–14.
8. Joshipura KJ, Ascherio A, Manson JE, et al. Fruit and vegetable intake in relation to risk of ischemic stroke. *JAMA.* 1999;282(13):1233–9.
9. Patent publication number EP 1069819 B1. Method for selective increase of the anticarcinogenic glucosinolates in brassica species. http://www.google.com/patents/EP1069819B1?cl=en. July 24, 2002. Accessed April 13, 2015.
10. Archetti M, Döring TF, Hagen SB, et al. Unravelling the evolution of autumn colours: an interdisciplinary approach. *Trends Ecol Evol (Amst).* 2009;24(3):166–73.
11. Benaron DA, Cheong WF, Stevenson DK. Tissue optics. *Science.* 1997;276(5321):2002–3.
12. Pietrzak M, Halicka HD, Wieczorek Z, Wieczorek J, Darzynkiewicz Z. Attenuation of acridine mutagen ICR-191—DNA interactions and DNA damage by the mutagen interceptor chlorophyllin. *Biophys Chem.* 2008;135(1–3):69–75.
13. Jubert C, Mata J, Bench G, et al. Effects of chlorophyll and chlorophyllin on low-dose aflatoxin B(1) pharmacokinetics in human volunteers. *Cancer Prev Res (Phila).* 2009;2(12):1015–22.
14. Bachem A. Reed CI. The penetration of light through human skin. *Am J Physiol.* 1931;97:86–91.
15. Benaron DA, Cheong WF, Stevenson DK. Tissue optics. *Science.* 1997;276(5321):2002–3.
16. Xu C, Zhang J, Mihai DM, Washington I. Light-harvesting chlorophyll pigments enable mammalian mitochondria to capture photonic energy and produce ATP. *J Cell Sci.* 2014;127(Pt 2):388–99.
17. Qu J, Ma L, Zhang J, Jockusch S, Washington I. Dietary chlorophyll metabolites catalyze the photoreduction of plasma ubiquinone. *Photochem Photobiol.* 2013;89(2):310–3.

18. Olsen H, Grimmer S, Aaby K, Saha S, Borge GI. Antiproliferative effects of fresh and thermal processed green and red cultivars of curly kale (Brassica oleracea L. convar. acephala var. sabellica). *J Agric Food Chem.* 2012;60(30):7375-83.

19. De Nicola GR, Bagatta M, Pagnotta E, et al. Comparison of bioactive phytochemical content and release of isothiocyanates in selected brassica sprouts. *Food Chem.* 2013;141(1):297-303.

20. Capaldi ED, Privitera GJ. Decreasing dislike for sour and bitter in children and adults. *Appetite.* 2008;50(1):139-45.

21. Capaldi ED, Privitera GJ. Decreasing dislike for sour and bitter in children and adults. *Appetite.* 2008;50(1):139-45.

22. Sharafi M, Hayes JE, Duffy VB. Masking vegetable bitterness to improve palatability depends on vegetable type and taste phenotype. *Chemosens Percept.* 2013;6(1):8-19.

23. Brown MJ, Ferruzzi MG, Nguyen ML, et al. Carotenoid bioavailability is higher from salads ingested with full-fat than with fat-reduced salad dressings as measured with electrochemical detection. *Am J Clin Nutr.* 2004;80(2):396-403.

24. Unlu NZ, Bohn T, Clinton SK, Schwartz SJ. Carotenoid absorption from salad and salsa by humans is enhanced by the addition of avocado or avocado oil. *J Nutr.* 2005;135(3):431-6.

25. Roodenburg AJ, Leenen R, van het Hof KH, Weststrate JA, Tijburg LB. Amount of fat in the diet affects bioavailability of lutein esters but not of alpha-carotene, beta-carotene, and vitamin E in humans. *Am J Clin Nutr.* 2000;71(5):1187-93.

26. Bongoni R, Verkerk R, Steenbekkers B, Dekker M, Stieger M. Evaluation of different cooking conditions on broccoli (Brassica oleracea var. italica) to improve the nutritional value and consumer acceptance. *Plant Foods Hum Nutr.* 2014;69(3):228-34.

27. Johnston CS, Steplewska I, Long CA, Harris LN, Ryals RH. Examination of the antiglycemic properties of vinegar in healthy adults. *Ann Nutr Metab.* 2010;56(1):74-9.

28. Johnston CS, Gaas CA. Vinegar: medicinal uses and antiglycemic effect. *MedGenMed.* 2006; 8(2):61.

29. White AM, Johnston CS. Vinegar ingestion at bedtime moderates waking glucose concentrations in adults with well-controlled type 2 diabetes. *Diabetes Care.* 2007;30(11):2814-5.

30. Johnston CS, White AM, Kent SM. Preliminary evidence that regular vinegar ingestion favorably influences hemoglobin A1c values in individuals with type 2 diabetes mellitus. *Diabetes Res Clin Pract.* 2009;84(2):e15-7.

31. Chung CH. Corrosive oesophageal injury following vinegar ingestion. *Hong Kong Med J.* 2002;8(5):365-6.

32. Lhotta K, Höfle G, Gasser R, Finkenstedt G. Hypokalemia, hyperreninemia and osteoporosis in a patient ingesting large amounts of cider vinegar. *Nephron.* 1998;80(2):242-3.

33. Wu D, Kimura F, Takashima A, et al. Intake of vinegar beverage is associated with restoration of ovulatory function in women with polycystic ovary syndrome. *Tohoku J Exp Med.* 2013;230(1):17-23.

34. Sakakibara S, Murakami R, Takahashi M, et al. Vinegar intake enhances flow-mediated vasodilatation via upregulation of endothelial nitric oxide synthase activity. *Biosci Biotechnol Biochem.* 2010;74(5):1055-61.

35. Kajimoto O, Ohshima Y, Tayama K, Hirata H, Nishimura A, Tsukamoto Y. Hypotensive effects of drinks containing vinegar on high normal blood pressure and mild hypertensive subjects. *J Nutr Food.* 2003;6:51-68.

36. Takano-Lee M, Edman JD, Mullens BA, Clark JM. Home remedies to control head lice: assessment of home remedies to control the human head louse, Pediculus humanus capitis (Anoplura: Pediculidae). *J Pediatr Nurs.* 2004;19(6):393-8.

37. Kondo T, Kishi M, Fushimi T, Ugajin S, Kaga T. Vinegar intake reduces body weight, body fat mass, and serum triglyceride levels in obese Japanese subjects. *Biosci Biotechnol Biochem.* 2009;73(8):1837–43.

38. Bergquist SA, Gertsson UE, Knuthsen P, Olsson ME. Flavonoids in baby spinach (Spinacia oleracea L.): changes during plant growth and storage. *J Agric Food Chem.* 2005;53(24):9459–64.

39. Xiao Z, Lester GE, Luo Y, Wang Q. Assessment of vitamin and carotenoid concentrations of emerging food products: edible microgreens. *J Agric Food Chem.* 2012;60(31):7644–51.

40. Dechet AM, Herman KM, Chen Parker C, et al. Outbreaks caused by sprouts, United States, 1998–2010: lessons learned and solutions needed. *Foodborne Pathog Dis.* 2014;11(8): 635–44.

41. U.S. Food and Drug Administration. Playing it safe with eggs. http://www.fda.gov/Food/ ResourcesForYou/Consumers/ucm077342.htm. Updated March 30, 2015. Accessed April 14, 2015.

Other Vegetables

1. Murray CJ, Atkinson C, Bhalla K, et al. The state of US health, 1990–2010: burden of diseases, injuries, and risk factors. *JAMA.* 2013;310(6):591–608.

2. Lim SS, Vos T, Flaxman AD, et al. A comparative risk assessment of burden of disease and injury attributable to 67 risk factors and risk factor clusters in 21 regions, 1990–2010: a systematic analysis for the Global Burden of Disease Study 2010. *Lancet.* 2012;380(9859):2224–60.

3. O'Hara JK. The $11 trillion reward: how simple dietary changes can save lives and money, and how we get there. http://www.ucsusa.org/assets/documents/food_and_agriculture/11 -trillion-reward.pdf. August 2013. Accessed April 15, 2015.

4. Murakami A, Ohnishi K. Target molecules of food phytochemicals: food science bound for the next dimension. *Food Funct.* 2012;3(5):462–76.

5. Watzl B, Bub A, Brandstetter BR, Rechkemmer G. Modulation of human T-lymphocyte functions by the consumption of carotenoid-rich vegetables. *Br J Nutr.* 1999;82(5):383–9.

6. Willcox JK, Catignani GL, Lazarus S. Tomatoes and cardiovascular health. *Crit Rev Food Sci Nutr.* 2003;43(1):1–18.

7. Dutta-Roy AK, Crosbie L, Gordon MJ. Effects of tomato extract on human platelet aggregation in vitro. *Platelets.* 2001;12(4):218–27.

8. O'Kennedy N, Crosbie L, Whelan S, et al. Effects of tomato extract on platelet function: a double-blinded crossover study in healthy humans. *Am J Clin Nutr.* 2006;84(3):561–9.

9. O'Kennedy N, Crosbie L, van Lieshout M, Broom JI, Webb DJ, Duttaroy AK. Effects of antiplatelet components of tomato extract on platelet function in vitro and ex vivo: a time-course cannulation study in healthy humans. *Am J Clin Nutr.* 2006;84(3):570–9.

10. Fuentes E, Forero-Doria O, Carrasco G, et al. Effect of tomato industrial processing on phenolic profile and antiplatelet activity. *Molecules.* 2013;18(9):11526–36.

11. Nurk E, Refsum H, Drevon CA, et al. Cognitive performance among the elderly in relation to the intake of plant foods. The Hordaland Health Study. *Br J Nutr.* 2010;104(8):1190–201.

12. Putnam J, Allshouse J, Kantor LS. U.S. per capita food supply trends: more calories, refined carbohydrates, and fats. *FoodReview.* 2002;25:2–15.

13. Bhupathiraju SN, Tucker KL. Greater variety in fruit and vegetable intake is associated with lower inflammation in Puerto Rican adults. *Am J Clin Nutr.* 2011;93(1):37–46.

14. Cooper AJ, Sharp SJ, Lentjes MA, et al. A prospective study of the association between quantity

and variety of fruit and vegetable intake and incident type 2 diabetes. *Diabetes Care*. 2012;35(6): 1293–300.

15. Lichtenstein AH, Appel LJ, Brands M, et al. Diet and lifestyle recommendations revision 2006: a scientific statement from the American Heart Association Nutrition Committee. *Circulation*. 2006;114(1):82–96.

16. Büchner FL, Bueno-de-Mesquita HB, Ros MM, et al. Variety in fruit and vegetable consumption and the risk of lung cancer in the European prospective investigation into cancer and nutrition. *Cancer Epidemiol Biomarkers Prev*. 2010;19(9):2278–86.

17. Dias JS. Nutritional quality and health benefits of vegetables: a review. *Food and Nutrition Sciences*. 2012;3(10):1354–74.

18. Sillanpää S, Salminen J-P, Eeva T. Breeding success and lutein availability in great tit (Parus major). *Acta Oecologica*. 2009;35(6):805–10.

19. Whitehead RD, Coetzee V, Ozakinci G, Perrett DI. Cross-cultural effects of fruit and vegetable consumption on skin color. *Am J Public Health*. 2012;102(2):212–3.

20. Stephen ID, Law Smith MJ, Stirrat MR, Perrett DI. Facial skin coloration affects perceived health of human faces. *Int J Primatol*. 2009;30(6):845–57.

21. Whitehead RD, Re D, Xiao D, Ozakinci G, Perrett DI. You are what you eat: within-subject increases in fruit and vegetable consumption confer beneficial skin-color changes. *PLoS ONE*. 2012;7(3):e32988.

22. Whitehead RD, Ozakinci G, Stephen ID, Perrett DI. Appealing to vanity: could potential appearance improvement motivate fruit and vegetable consumption? *Am J Public Health*. 2012; 102(2):207–11.

23. Nagata C, Nakamura K, Wada K, et al. Association of dietary fat, vegetables and antioxidant micronutrients with skin ageing in Japanese women. *Br J Nutr*. 2010;103(10):1493–8.

24. Greens to be gorgeous: Why eating your five fruit and veg a day makes you sexy. *Daily Mail*. http://www.dailymail.co.uk/health/article-1228348/Eating-fruit-veg-makes-attractive-opposite-sex.html. November 17, 2009. Accessed April 14, 2015.

25. Paul BD, Snyder SH. The unusual amino acid L-ergothioneine is a physiologic cytoprotectant. *Cell Death Differ*. 2010;17(7):1134–40.

26. Paul BD, Snyder SH. The unusual amino acid L-ergothioneine is a physiologic cytoprotectant. *Cell Death Differ*. 2010;17(7):1134–40.

27. Berk L, Castle WB. Observations on the etiologic relationship of achylia gastrica to pernicious anemia; activity of vitamin B12 as food, extrinsic factor. *N Engl J Med*. 1948;239(24):911–3.

28. Ey J, Schömig E, Taubert D. Dietary sources and antioxidant effects of ergothioneine. *J Agric Food Chem*. 2007;55(16):6466–74.

29. Nguyen TH, Nagasaka R, Ohshima T. Effects of extraction solvents, cooking procedures and storage conditions on the contents of ergothioneine and phenolic compounds and antioxidative capacity of the cultivated mushroom Flammulina velutipes. *Int J Food Sci Tech*. 2012;47(6): 1193–205.

30. Schulzová V, Hajslová J, Peroutka R, Gry J, Andersson HC. Influence of storage and household processing on the agaritine content of the cultivated Agaricus mushroom. *Food Addit Contam*. 2002;19(9):853–62.

31. Gry J. Mushrooms traded as food. Vol II sec 2. http://norden.diva-portal.org/smash/get /diva2:733528/FULLTEXT01.pdf. July 18, 2012. Accessed April 15, 2015.

32. Mitchell SC. Food idiosyncrasies: beetroot and asparagus. *Drug Metab Dispos*. 2001;29(4 Pt 2): 539–43.

33. Donado-Pestana CM, Mastrodi Salgado J, de Oliveira Rios A, dos Santos PR, Jablonski A. Stability of carotenoids, total phenolics and in vitro antioxidant capacity in the thermal processing

of orange-fleshed sweet potato (Ipomoea batatas Lam) cultivars grown in Brazil. *Plant Foods Hum Nutr.* 2012;67(3):262–70.

34. Padda MS, Picha DH. Phenolic composition and antioxidant capacity of different heat-processed forms of sweetpotato cv. "Beauregard." *Int J Food Sci Tech.* 2008;43(8):1404–9.

35. Bovell-Benjamin AC. Sweet potato: a review of its past, present, and future role in human nutrition. *Adv Food Nutr Res.* 2007;52:1–59.

36. Center for Science in the Public Interest. 10 best foods. http://www.nutritionaction.com/free-downloads/what-to-eat-10-best-foods/. Accessed April 15, 2015.

37. Wilson CD, Pace RD, Bromfield E, Jones G, Lu JY. Consumer acceptance of vegetarian sweet potato products intended for space missions. *Life Support Biosph Sci.* 1998;5(3):339–46.

38. Drewnowski A. New metrics of affordable nutrition: which vegetables provide most nutrients for least cost? *J Acad Nutr Diet.* 2013;113(9):1182–7.

39. Ameny MA, Wilson PW. Relationship between hunter color values and b-carotene contents in white-fleshed African sweet potatoes (Ipomoea batatas Lam). *J Sci Food Agric.* 1997;73:301–6.

40. Kaspar KL, Park JS, Brown CR, Mathison BD, Navarre DA, Chew BP. Pigmented potato consumption alters oxidative stress and inflammatory damage in men. *J Nutr.* 2011;141(1):108–11.

41. Vinson JA, Demkosky CA, Navarre DA, Smyda MA. High-antioxidant potatoes: acute in vivo antioxidant source and hypotensive agent in humans after supplementation to hypertensive subjects. *J Agric Food Chem.* 2012;60(27):6749–54.

42. Carlsen MH, Halvorsen BL, Holte K, et al. The total antioxidant content of more than 3100 foods, beverages, spices, herbs and supplements used worldwide. *Nutr J.* 2010;9:3.

43. Vinson JA, Demkosky CA, Navarre DA, Smyda MA. High-antioxidant potatoes: acute in vivo antioxidant source and hypotensive agent in humans after supplementation to hypertensive subjects. *J Agric Food Chem.* 2012;60(27):6749–54.

44. Lim S, Xu J, Kim J, et al. Role of anthocyanin-enriched purple-fleshed sweet potato p40 in colorectal cancer prevention. *Mol Nutr Food Res.* 2013;57(11):1908–17.

45. Olsen A, Ritz C, Kramer L, Møller P. Serving styles of raw snack vegetables. What do children want? *Appetite.* 2012;59(2):556–62.

46. Sesame Workshop. "If Elmo eats broccoli, will kids eat it too?" Atkins Foundation grant to fund further research. https://web.archive.org/web/20130125205947/http://archive.sesameworkshop.org/aboutus/inside_press.php?contentId=15092302. September 20, 2005. Accessed June 30, 2015.

47. Kros W, Paulis WD, van der Wouden JC. Increasing vegetable intake in Mexican-American youth: design and analysis issues. *J Am Diet Assoc.* 2011;111(11):1657.

48. Fisher JO, Mennella JA, Hughes SO, Liu Y, Mendoza PM, Patrick H. Offering "dip" promotes intake of a moderately-liked raw vegetable among preschoolers with genetic sensitivity to bitterness. *J Acad Nutr Diet.* 2012;112(2):235–45.

49. Isoldi KK, Dalton S, Rodriguez DP, Nestle M. Classroom "cupcake" celebrations: observations of foods offered and consumed. *J Nutr Educ Behav.* 2012;44(1):71–5.

50. Wansink B, Just DR, Payne CR, Klinger MZ. Attractive names sustain increased vegetable intake in schools. *Prev Med.* 2012;55(4):330–2.

51. Wansink B, van Ittersum K, Painter JE. How descriptive food names bias sensory perceptions in restaurants. *Food Qual Prefer.* 2005;16(5):393–400.

52. Wansink B, Just DR, Payne CR, Klinger MZ. Attractive names sustain increased vegetable intake in schools. *Prev Med.* 2012;55(4):330–2.

53. Wansink B, Just DR, Payne CR, Klinger MZ. Attractive names sustain increased vegetable intake in schools. *Prev Med.* 2012;55(4):330–2.

54. Spill MK, Birch LL, Roe LS, Rolls BJ. Hiding vegetables to reduce energy density: an effective strategy to increase children's vegetable intake and reduce energy intake. *Am J Clin Nutr.* 2011; 94(3):735–41.

55. Blatt AD, Roe LS, Rolls BJ. Hidden vegetables: an effective strategy to reduce energy intake and increase vegetable intake in adults. *Am J Clin Nutr.* 2011;93(4):756–63.

56. Vereecken C, Rovner A, Maes L. Associations of parenting styles, parental feeding practices and child characteristics with young children's fruit and vegetable consumption. *Appetite.* 2010; 55(3):589–96.

57. World Cancer Research Fund / American Institute for Cancer Research. Food, Nutrition, Physical Activity, and the Prevention of Cancer: a Global Perspective. Washington, D.C.: AICR, 2007.

58. Annema N, Heyworth JS, McNaughton SA, Iacopetta B, Fritschi L. Fruit and vegetable consumption and the risk of proximal colon, distal colon, and rectal cancers in a case-control study in Western Australia. *J Am Diet Assoc.* 2011;111(10):1479–90.

59. Boivin D, Lamy S, Lord-Dufour S, et al. Antiproliferative and antioxidant activities of common vegetables: a comparative study. *Food Chem.* 2009;112:374–80.

60. Boivin D, Lamy S, Lord-Dufour S, et al. Antiproliferative and antioxidant activities of common vegetables: a comparative study. *Food Chem.* 2009;112:374–80.

61. Boivin D, Lamy S, Lord-Dufour S, et al. Antiproliferative and antioxidant activities of common vegetables: a comparative study. *Food Chem.* 2009;112:374–80.

62. Boivin D, Lamy S, Lord-Dufour S, et al. Antiproliferative and antioxidant activities of common vegetables: a comparative study. *Food Chem.* 2009;112:374–80.

63. Boivin D, Lamy S, Lord-Dufour S, et al. Antiproliferative and antioxidant activities of common vegetables: a comparative study. *Food Chem.* 2009;112:374–80.

64. Abdull Razis AF, Noor NM. Cruciferous vegetables: dietary phytochemicals for cancer prevention. *Asian Pac J Cancer Prev.* 2013;14(3):1565–70.

65. Nicastro HL, Ross SA, Milner JA. Garlic and onions: their cancer prevention properties. *Cancer Prev Res* (Phila). 2015;8(3):181–9.

66. Oude Griep LM, Geleijnse JM, Kromhout D, Ocké MC, Verschuren WM. Raw and processed fruit and vegetable consumption and 10-year coronary heart disease incidence in a population-based cohort study in the Netherlands. *PLoS ONE.* 2010;5(10):e13609.

67. Gliszczyńska-Swigło A, Ciska E, Pawlak-Lemańska K, Chmielewski J, Borkowski T, Tyrakowska B. Changes in the content of health-promoting compounds and antioxidant activity of broccoli after domestic processing. *Food Addit Contam.* 2006;23(11):1088–98.

68. Ghavami A, Coward WA, Bluck LJ. The effect of food preparation on the bioavailability of carotenoids from carrots using intrinsic labelling. *Br J Nutr.* 2012;107(9):1350–66.

69. Garcia AL, Koebnick C, Dagnelie PC, et al. Long-term strict raw food diet is associated with favourable plasma beta-carotene and low plasma lycopene concentrations in Germans. *Br J Nutr.* 2008;99(6):1293–300.

70. Bohm V, Bitsch R. Intestinal absorption of lycopene from different matrices and interactions to other carotenoids, the lipid status, and the antioxidant capacity of human plasma. *Eur J Nutr.* 1999;38:118–25.

71. Kahlon TS, Chiu MM, Chapman MH. Steam cooking significantly improves in vitro bile acid binding of collard greens, kale, mustard greens, broccoli, green bell pepper and cabbage. *Nutr Res.* 2008;28:351–7.

72. Javitt NB, Budai K, Miller DG, Cahan AC, Raju U, Levitz M. Breast-gut connection: origin of chenodeoxycholic acid in breast cyst fluid. *Lancet.* 1994;343(8898):633–5.

73. Stott-Miller M, Neuhouser ML, Stanford JL. Consumption of deep-fried foods and risk of prostate cancer. *Prostate.* 2013;73(9):960–9.

74. Chen MJ, Hsu HT, Lin CL, Ju WY. A statistical regression model for the estimation of acrylamide concentrations in French fries for excess lifetime cancer risk assessment. *Food Chem Toxicol.* 2012;50(10):3867–76.

75. Lineback DR, Coughlin JR, Stadler RH. Acrylamide in foods: a review of the science and future considerations. *Annu Rev Food Sci Technol.* 2012;3:15–35.

76. Jiménez-Monreal AM, García-Diz L, Martínez-Tomé M, Mariscal M, Murcia MA. Influence of cooking methods on antioxidant activity of vegetables. *J Food Sci.* 2009;74(3):H97–H103.

77. Jiménez-Monreal AM, García-Diz L, Martínez-Tomé M, Mariscal M, Murcia MA. Influence of cooking methods on antioxidant activity of vegetables. *J Food Sci.* 2009;74(3):H97–H103.

78. Jiménez-Monreal AM, García-Diz L, Martínez-Tomé M, Mariscal M, Murcia MA. Influence of cooking methods on antioxidant activity of vegetables. *J Food Sci.* 2009;74(3):H97–H103.

79. Barański M, Srednicka-Tober D, Volakakis N, et al. Higher antioxidant and lower cadmium concentrations and lower incidence of pesticide residues in organically grown crops: a systematic literature review and meta-analyses. *Br J Nutr.* 2014;112(5):794–811.

80. Krol WJ. Removal of trace pesticide residues from produce. Connecticut Agricultural Experiment Station. http://www.ct.gov/caes/cwp/view.asp?a=2815&q=376676. June 28, 2012. Accessed April 16, 2015.

81. Krieger RI, Brutsche-Keiper P, Crosby HR, Krieger AD. Reduction of pesticide residues of fruit using water only or Plus Fit Fruit and Vegetable Wash. *Bull Environ Contam Toxicol.* 2003; 70(2):213–8.

82. Krol WJ, Arsenault TL, Pylypiw HM, Incorvia Mattina MJ. Reduction of pesticide residues on produce by rinsing. *J Agric Food Chem.* 2000;48(10):4666–70.

83. Wang Z, Huang J, Chen J, Li F. Effectiveness of dishwashing liquids in removing chlorothalonil and chlorpyrifos residues from cherry tomatoes. *Chemosphere.* 2013;92(8):1022–8.

84. Zohair A. Behaviour of some organophosphorus and organochlorine pesticides in potatoes during soaking in different solutions. *Food Chem Toxicol.* 2001;39(7):751–5.

85. Zhang ZY, Liu XJ, Hong XY. Effects of home preparation on pesticide residues in cabbage. *Food Control.* 2007;18(12):1484–7.

86. Zohair A. Behaviour of some organophosphorus and organochlorine pesticides in potatoes during soaking in different solutions. *Food Chem Toxicol.* 2001;39(7):751–5.

87. U.S. Department of Agriculture. Organic Agriculture. http://www.usda.gov/wps/portal/usda/usdahome?contentidonly=true&contentid=organic-agriculture.html. Modified January 9, 2015. Accessed March 30, 2015.

88. Monette M. The science of pesticide-free potato chips. *CMAJ.* 2012;184(14):E741–2.

89. Smith-Spangler C, Brandeau ML, Hunter GE, et al. Are organic foods safer or healthier than conventional alternatives?: a systematic review. *Ann Intern Med.* 2012;157(5):348–66.

90. Barański M, Srednicka-Tober D, Volakakis N, et al. Higher antioxidant and lower cadmium concentrations and lower incidence of pesticide residues in organically grown crops: a systematic literature review and meta-analyses. *Br J Nutr.* 2014;112(5):794–811.

91. Forman J, Silverstein J. Organic foods: health and environmental advantages and disadvantages. *Pediatrics.* 2012;130(5):e1406–15.

92. Barański M, Srednicka-Tober D, Volakakis N, et al. Higher antioxidant and lower cadmium concentrations and lower incidence of pesticide residues in organically grown crops: a systematic literature review and meta-analyses. *Br J Nutr.* 2014;112(5):794–811.

93. Lindén A, Andersson K, Oskarsson A. Cadmium in organic and conventional pig production. *Arch Environ Contam Toxicol.* 2001;40(3):425–31.

94. Lee WCJ, Shimizu M, Kniffin KM, Wansink B. You taste what you see: do organic labels bias taste perceptions? *Food Qual Prefer.* 2013;29(1):33–9.

95. Williams PR, Hammitt JK. Perceived risks of conventional and organic produce: pesticides, pathogens, and natural toxins. *Risk Anal.* 2001;21(2):319–30.
96. Hammitt JK. Risk perceptions and food choice: an exploratory analysis of organic- versus conventional-produce buyers. *Risk Anal.* 1990;10(3):367–74.
97. Reiss R, Johnston J, Tucker K, Desesso JM, Keen CL. Estimation of cancer risks and benefits associated with a potential increased consumption of fruits and vegetables. *Food Chem Toxicol.* 2012;50(12):4421–7.
98. Winter CK. Pesticide residues in imported, organic, and "suspect" fruits and vegetables. *J Agric Food Chem.* 2012;60(18):4425–9.

Flaxseeds

1. Singh KK, Mridula D, Rehal J, Barnwal P. Flaxseed: a potential source of food, feed and fiber. *Crit Rev Food Sci Nutr.* 2011;51(3):210–22.
2. Hyvärinen HK, Pihlava JM, Hiidenhovi JA, Hietaniemi V, Korhonen HJ, Ryhänen EL. Effect of processing and storage on the stability of flaxseed lignan added to bakery products. *J Agric Food Chem.* 2006;54(1):48–53.
3. Cunnane SC, Hamadeh MJ, Liede AC, Thompson LU, Wolever TM, Jenkins DJ. Nutritional attributes of traditional flaxseed in healthy young adults. *Am J Clin Nutr.* 1995;61(1):62–8.
4. Davidi A, Reynolds J, Njike VY, Ma Y, Doughty K, Katz DL. The effect of the addition of daily fruit and nut bars to diet on weight, and cardiac risk profile, in overweight adults. *J Hum Nutr Diet.* 2011;24(6):543–51.
5. Chai SC, Hooshmand S, Saadat RL, Payton ME, Brummel-Smith K, Arjmandi BH. Daily apple versus dried plum: impact on cardiovascular disease risk factors in postmenopausal women. *J Acad Nutr Diet.* 2012;112(8):1158–68.
6. Peterson JM, Montgomery S, Haddad E, Kearney L, Tonstad S. Effect of consumption of dried California mission figs on lipid concentrations. *Ann Nutr Metab.* 2011;58(3):232–8.
7. Chai SC, Hooshmand S, Saadat RL, Payton ME, Brummel-Smith K, Arjmandi BH. Daily apple versus dried plum: impact on cardiovascular disease risk factors in postmenopausal women. *J Acad Nutr Diet.* 2012;112(8):1158–68.
8. Puglisi MJ, Vaishnav U, Shrestha S, et al. Raisins and additional walking have distinct effects on plasma lipids and inflammatory cytokines. *Lipids Health Dis.* 2008;7:14.
9. Chai SC, Hooshmand S, Saadat RL, Arjmandi BH. Daily apple consumption promotes cardio-vascular health in postmenopausal women. *The FASEB Journal.* 2011;25:971.10.
10. Keast DR, O'Neil CE, Jones JM. Dried fruit consumption is associated with improved diet quality and reduced obesity in US adults: National Health and Nutrition Examination Survey, 1999–2004. *Nutr Res.* 2011;31(6):460–7.
11. Edel AL, Rodriguez-Leyva D, Maddaford TG, et al. Dietary flaxseed independently lowers circulating cholesterol and lowers it beyond the effects of cholesterol-lowering medications alone in patients with peripheral artery disease. *J Nutr.* 2015;145(4):749–57.

Nuts and Seeds

1. Fraser GE, Shavlik DJ. Ten years of life: is it a matter of choice? *Arch Intern Med.* 2001;161(13):1645–52.
2. Lim SS, Vos T, Flaxman AD, et al. A comparative risk assessment of burden of disease and

injury attributable to 67 risk factors and risk factor clusters in 21 regions, 1990–2010: a systematic analysis for the Global Burden of Disease Study 2010. *Lancet.* 2012;380(9859):2224–60.

3. U.S. Department of Agriculture. Oxygen Radical Absorbance Capacity (ORAC) of Selected Foods—2007. http://www.orac-info-portal.de/download/ORAC_R2.pdf. November 2007. Accessed April 10, 2015.

4. Ros E, Mataix J. Fatty acid composition of nuts—implications for cardiovascular health. *Br J Nutr.* 2006;96 Suppl 2:S29–35.

5. Yang J, Liu RH, Halim L. Antioxidant and antiproliferative activities of common edible nut seeds. *Food Sci Tech.* 2009;42(1):1–8.

6. Bao Y, Han J, Hu FB, et al. Association of nut consumption with total and cause-specific mortality. *N Engl J Med.* 2013;369(21):2001–11.

7. Luu HN, Blot WJ, Xiang YB, et al. Prospective evaluation of the association of nut/peanut consumption with total and cause-specific mortality. *JAMA Intern Med.* 2015;175(5):755–66.

8. Fernández-Montero A, Bes-Rastrollo M, Barrio-López MT, et al. Nut consumption and 5-y all-cause mortality in a Mediterranean cohort: the SUN project. *Nutrition.* 2014;30(9):1022–7.

9. Estruch R, Ros E, Salas-Salvadó J, et al. Primary prevention of cardiovascular disease with a Mediterranean diet. *N Engl J Med.* 2013;368(14):1279–90.

10. Supplement to: Estruch R, Ros E, Salas-Salvadó J, et al. Primary prevention of cardiovascular disease with a Mediterranean diet. N Engl J Med 2013;368:1279–90. DOI: 10.1056/NEJMoa1200303

11. Estruch R, Ros E, Salas-Salvadó J, et al. Primary prevention of cardiovascular disease with a Mediterranean diet. *N Engl J Med.* 2013;368(14):1279–90.

12. Guasch-Ferré M, Bulló M, Martínez-González MA, et al. Frequency of nut consumption and mortality risk in the PREDIMED nutrition intervention trial. *BMC Med.* 2013;11:164.

13. Guasch-Ferré M, Hu FB, Martínez-González MA, et al. Olive oil intake and risk of cardiovascular disease and mortality in the PREDIMED Study. *BMC Med.* 2014;12:78.

14. Keys A. Olive oil and coronary heart disease. *Lancet.* 1987;1(8539):983–4.

15. Guasch-Ferré M, Bulló M, Martínez-González MA, et al. Frequency of nut consumption and mortality risk in the PREDIMED nutrition intervention trial. *BMC Med.* 2013;11:164.

16. Toner CD. Communicating clinical research to reduce cancer risk through diet: walnuts as a case example. *Nutr Res Pract.* 2014;8(4):347–51.

17. Li TY, Brennan AM, Wedick NM, Mantzoros C, Rifai N, Hu FB. Regular consumption of nuts is associated with a lower risk of cardiovascular disease in women with type 2 diabetes. *J Nutr.* 2009;139(7):1333–8.

18. Su X, Tamimi RM, Collins LC, et al. Intake of fiber and nuts during adolescence and incidence of proliferative benign breast disease. *Cancer Causes Control.* 2010;21(7):1033–46.

19. Natoli S, McCoy P. A review of the evidence: nuts and body weight. *Asia Pac J Clin Nutr.* 2007;16(4):588–97.

20. Martínez-González MA, Bes-Rastrollo M. Nut consumption, weight gain and obesity: Epidemiological evidence. *Nutr Metab Cardiovasc Dis.* 2011;21 Suppl 1:S40–5.

21. Wang X, Li Z, Liu Y, Lv X, Yang W. Effects of pistachios on body weight in Chinese subjects with metabolic syndrome. *Nutr J.* 2012;11:20.

22. Painter, J. The pistachio principle: calorie reduction without calorie restriction. *Weight Management Matters.* 2008;6:8.

23. Murakami K, Sasaki S, Takahashi Y, et al. Hardness (difficulty of chewing) of the habitual diet in relation to body mass index and waist circumference in free-living Japanese women aged 18–22 y. *Am J Clin Nutr.* 2007;86(1):206–13.

24. McKiernan F, Lokko P, Kuevi A, et al. Effects of peanut processing on body weight and fasting plasma lipids. *Br J Nutr.* 2010;104(3):418–26.

25. Brennan AM, Sweeney LL, Liu X, Mantzoros CS. Walnut consumption increases satiation but has no effect on insulin resistance or the metabolic profile over a 4-day period. *Obesity* (Silver Spring). 2010;18(6):1176–82.

26. Mattes RD, Kris-Etherton PM, Foster GD. Impact of peanuts and tree nuts on body weight and healthy weight loss in adults. *J Nutr.* 2008;138(9):1741S–5S.

27. Tapsell L, Batterham M, Tan SY, Warensjö E. The effect of a calorie controlled diet containing walnuts on substrate oxidation during 8-hours in a room calorimeter. *J Am Coll Nutr.* 2009; 28(5):611–7.

28. Chiurlia E, D'Amico R, Ratti C, Granata AR, Romagnoli R, Modena MG. Subclinical coronary artery atherosclerosis in patients with erectile dysfunction. *J Am Coll Cardiol.* 2005;46(8): 1503–6.

29. Montorsi P, Ravagnani PM, Galli S, et al. The artery size hypothesis: a macrovascular link between erectile dysfunction and coronary artery disease. *Am J Cardiol.* 2005;96(12B): 19M–23M.

30. Montorsi P, Montorsi F, Schulman CC. Is erectile dysfunction the "tip of the iceberg" of a systemic vascular disorder? *Eur Urol.* 2003;44(3):352–4.

31. Montorsi F, Briganti A, Salonia A, et al. Erectile dysfunction prevalence, time of onset and association with risk factors in 300 consecutive patients with acute chest pain and angiographically documented coronary artery disease. *Eur Urol.* 2003;44(3):360–4.

32. Montorsi P, Ravagnani PM, Galli S, et al. The artery size hypothesis: a macrovascular link between erectile dysfunction and coronary artery disease. *Am J Cardiol.* 2005;96(12B):19M–23M.

33. Meldrum DR, Gambone JC, Morris MA, Meldrum DA, Esposito K, Ignarro LJ. The link between erectile and cardiovascular health: the canary in the coal mine. *Am J Cardiol.* 2011;108(4): 599–606.

34. Corona G, Fagioli G, Mannucci E, et al. Penile doppler ultrasound in patients with erectile dysfunction (ED): role of peak systolic velocity measured in the flaccid state in predicting arteriogenic ED and silent coronary artery disease. *J Sex Med.* 2008;5(11):2623–34.

35. Schwartz BG, Kloner RA. How to save a life during a clinic visit for erectile dysfunction by modifying cardiovascular risk factors. *Int J Impot Res.* 2009;21(6):327–35.

36. Inman BA, Sauver JL, Jacobson DJ, et al. A population-based, longitudinal study of erectile dysfunction and future coronary artery disease. *Mayo Clin Proc.* 2009;84(2):108–13.

37. Jackson G. Erectile dysfunction and coronary disease: evaluating the link. *Maturitas.* 2012; 72(3):263–4.

38. Fung MM, Bettencourt R, Barrett-Connor E. Heart disease risk factors predict erectile dysfunction 25 years later: the Rancho Bernardo Study. *J Am Coll Cardiol.* 2004;43(8):1405–11.

39. Gupta BP, Murad MH, Clifton MM, Prokop L, Nehra A, Kopecky SL. The effect of lifestyle modification and cardiovascular risk factor reduction on erectile dysfunction: a systematic review and meta-analysis. *Arch Intern Med.* 2011;171(20):1797–803.

40. Jackson G. Problem solved: erectile dysfunction (ED) = early death (ED). *Int J Clin Pract.* 2010;64(7):831–2.

41. Aldemir M, Okulu E, Neşelioğlu S, Erel O, Kayıgil O. Pistachio diet improves erectile function parameters and serum lipid profiles in patients with erectile dysfunction. *Int J Impot Res.* 2011; 23(1):32–8.

42. Esposito K, Ciotola M, Maiorino MI, et al. Hyperlipidemia and sexual function in premenopausal women. *J Sex Med.* 2009;6(6):1696–703.

43. Baer HJ, Glynn RJ, Hu FB, et al. Risk factors for mortality in the Nurses' Health Study: a competing risks analysis. *Am J Epidemiol.* 2011;173(3):319–29.

44. Ros E, Hu FB. Consumption of plant seeds and cardiovascular health: epidemiological and clinical trial evidence. *Circulation.* 2013;128(5):553–65

45. Strate LL, Liu YL, Syngal S, Aldoori WH, Giovannucci EL. Nut, corn, and popcorn consumption and the incidence of diverticular disease. *JAMA.* 2008;300(8):907–14.

Herbs and Spices

1. Srinivasan K. Antioxidant potential of spices and their active constituents. *Crit Rev Food Sci Nutr.* 2014;54(3):352–72.

2. Carlsen MH, Halvorsen BL, Holte K, et al. The total antioxidant content of more than 3100 foods, beverages, spices, herbs and supplements used worldwide. *Nutr J.* 2010;9:3.

3. Tapsell LC, Hemphill I, Cobiac L, et al. Health benefits of herbs and spices: the past, the present, the future. *Med J Aust.* 2006;185(4 Suppl):S4–24.

4. Shishodia S, Sethi G, Aggarwal BB. Curcumin: getting back to the roots. *Ann NY Acad Sci.* 2005;1056:206–17.

5. Gupta SC, Patchva S, Aggarwal BB. Therapeutic roles of curcumin: lessons learned from clinical trials. *AAPS J.* 2013;15(1):195–218.

6. Agarwal KA, Tripathi CD, Agarwal BB, Saluja S. Efficacy of turmeric (curcumin) in pain and postoperative fatigue after laparoscopic cholecystectomy: a double-blind, randomized placebo-controlled study. *Surg Endosc.* 2011;25(12):3805–10.

7. Chandran B, Goel A. A randomized, pilot study to assess the efficacy and safety of curcumin in patients with active rheumatoid arthritis. *Phytother Res.* 2012;26(11):1719–25.

8. Kuptniratsaikul V, Dajpratham P, Taechaarpornkul W, et al. Efficacy and safety of Curcuma domestica extracts compared with ibuprofen in patients with knee osteoarthritis: a multicenter study. *Clin Interv Aging.* 2014;9:451–8.

9. Khajehdehi P, Zanjaninejad B, Aflaki E, et al. Oral supplementation of turmeric decreases proteinuria, hematuria, and systolic blood pressure in patients suffering from relapsing or refractory lupus nephritis: a randomized and placebo-controlled study. *J Ren Nutr.* 2012;22(1):50–7.

10. Vecchi Brumatti L, Marcuzzi A, Tricarico PM, Zanin V, Girardelli M, Bianco AM. Curcumin and inflammatory bowel disease: potential and limits of innovative treatments. *Molecules.* 2014;19(12):21127–53.

11. Lang A, Salomon N, Wu JC, et al. Curcumin in combination with mesalamine induces remission in patients with mild-to-moderate ulcerative colitis in a randomized controlled trial. *Clin Gastroenterol Hepatol.* 2015;13(8):1444–49.e1.

12. Percival SS, Vanden Heuvel JP, Nieves CJ, Montero C, Migliaccio AJ, Meadors J. Bioavailability of herbs and spices in humans as determined by ex vivo inflammatory suppression and DNA strand breaks. *J Am Coll Nutr.* 2012;31(4):288–94.

13. Gupta SC, Sung B, Kim JH, Prasad S, Li S, Aggarwal BB. Multitargeting by turmeric, the golden spice: from kitchen to clinic. *Mol Nutr Food Res.* 2013;57(9):1510–28.

14. Siruguri V, Bhat RV. Assessing intake of spices by pattern of spice use, frequency of consumption and portion size of spices consumed from routinely prepared dishes in southern India. *Nutr J.* 2015;14:7.

15. Gilani AH, Rahman AU. Trends in ethnopharmacology. *J Ethnopharmacol.* 2005;100(1–2):43–9.

16. Newman DJ, Cragg GM. Natural products as sources of new drugs over the last 25 years. *J Nat Prod.* 2007;70(3):461–77.

17. Atal CK, Dubey RK, Singh J. Biochemical basis of enhanced drug bioavailability by piperine: evidence that piperine is a potent inhibitor of drug metabolism. *J Pharmacol Exp Ther*. 1985; 232(1):258–62.

18. Shoba G, Joy D, Joseph T, Majeed M, Rajendran R, Srinivas PS. Influence of piperine on the pharmacokinetics of curcumin in animals and human volunteers. *Planta Med*. 1998;64(4):353–6.

19. Anand P, Kunnumakkara AB, Newman RA, Aggarwal BB. Bioavailability of curcumin: problems and promises. *Mol Pharm*. 2007;4(6):807–18.

20. Anand P, Kunnumakkara AB, Newman RA, Aggarwal BB. Bioavailability of curcumin: problems and promises. *Mol Pharm*. 2007;4(6):807–18.

21. Jacobson MS. Cholesterol oxides in Indian ghee: possible cause of unexplained high risk of atherosclerosis in Indian immigrant populations. *Lancet*. 1987;2(8560):656–8.

22. Percival SS, Vanden Heuvel JP, Nieves CJ, Montero C, Migliaccio AJ, Meadors J. Bioavailability of herbs and spices in humans as determined by ex vivo inflammatory suppression and DNA strand breaks. *J Am Coll Nutr*. 2012;31(4):288–94.

23. Arjmandi BH, Khalil DA, Lucas EA, et al. Soy protein may alleviate osteoarthritis symptoms. *Phytomedicine*. 2004;11(7–8):567–75.

24. Agarwal KA, Tripathi CD, Agarwal BB, Saluja S. Efficacy of turmeric (curcumin) in pain and postoperative fatigue after laparoscopic cholecystectomy: a double-blind, randomized placebo-controlled study. *Surg Endosc*. 2011;25(12):3805–10.

25. Aggarwal BB, Yuan W, Li S, Gupta SC. Curcumin-free turmeric exhibits anti-inflammatory and anticancer activities: identification of novel components of turmeric. *Mol Nutr Food Res*. 2013;57(9):1529–42.

26. Kim JH, Gupta SC, Park B, Yadav VR, Aggarwal BB. Turmeric (Curcuma longa) inhibits inflammatory nuclear factor (NF)-κB and NF-κB-regulated gene products and induces death receptors leading to suppressed proliferation, induced chemosensitization, and suppressed osteoclastogenesis. *Mol Nutr Food Res*. 2012;56(3):454–65.

27. Aggarwal BB, Yuan W, Li S, Gupta SC. Curcumin-free turmeric exhibits anti-inflammatory and anticancer activities: identification of novel components of turmeric. *Mol Nutr Food Res*. 2013;57(9):1529–42.

28. Bengmark S, Mesa MD, Gil A. Plant-derived health: the effects of turmeric and curcuminoids. *Nutr Hosp*. 2009;24(3):273–81.

29. Cao J, Jia L, Zhou HM, Liu Y, Zhong LF. Mitochondrial and nuclear DNA damage induced by curcumin in human hepatoma G2 cells. *Toxicol Sci*. 2006;91(2):476–83.

30. Turmeric and curcumin supplements and spices. https://www.consumerlab.com/reviews/turmeric-curcumin-supplements-spice-review/turmeric/. March 3, 2015. Accessed April 17, 2015.

31. Rasyid A, Lelo A. The effect of curcumin and placebo on human gall-bladder function: an ultrasound study. *Aliment Pharmacol Ther*. 1999;13(2):245–9.

32. Rasyid A, Rahman AR, Jaalam K, Lelo A. Effect of different curcumin dosages on human gall bladder. *Asia Pac J Clin Nutr*. 2002;11(4):314–8.

33. Asher GN, Spelman K. Clinical utility of curcumin extract. *Altern Ther Health Med*. 2013; 19(2):20–2.

34. Goel A, Kunnumakkara AB, Aggarwal BB. Curcumin as "curecumin": from kitchen to clinic. *Biochem Pharmacol*. 2008;75(4):787–809.

35. Ghosh Das S, Savage GP. Total and soluble oxalate content of some Indian spices. *Plant Foods Hum Nutr*. 2012;67(2):186–90.

36. Asher GN, Spelman K. Clinical utility of curcumin extract. *Altern Ther Health Med*. 2013; 19(2):20–2.

37. Poole C, Bushey B, Foster C, et al. The effects of a commercially available botanical supplement on strength, body composition, power output, and hormonal profiles in resistance-trained males. *J Int Soc Sports Nutr.* 2010;7:34.

38. Shabbeer S, Sobolewski M, Anchoori RK, et al. Fenugreek: a naturally occurring edible spice as an anticancer agent. *Cancer Biol Ther.* 2009;8(3):272–8.

39. Mebazaa R, Rega B, Camel V. Analysis of human male armpit sweat after fenugreek ingestion: characterisation of odour active compounds by gas chromatography coupled to mass spectrometry and olfactometry. *Food Chem.* 2011;128(1):227–35.

40. Korman SH, Cohen E, Preminger A. Pseudo-maple syrup urine disease due to maternal prenatal ingestion of fenugreek. *J Paediatr Child Health.* 2001;37(4):403–4.

41. Marsh TL, Arriola PE. The science of salsa: antimicrobial properties of salsa components to learn scientific methodology. *J Microbiol Biol Educ.* 2009;10(1):3–8.

42. Mauer L, El-Sohemy A. Prevalence of cilantro (Coriandrum sativum) disliking among different ethnocultural groups. *Flavour.* 2012;1:8.

43. Eriksson N, Wu S, Do CB, et al. A genetic variant near olfactory receptor genes influences cilantro preference. *Flavour.* 2012;1:22.

44. Knaapila A, Hwang LD, Lysenko A, et al. Genetic analysis of chemosensory traits in human twins. *Chem Senses.* 2012;37(9):869–81.

45. Eriksson N, Wu S, Do CB, et al. A genetic variant near olfactory receptor genes influences cilantro preference. *Flavour.* 2012;1:22.

46. Sahib NG, Anwar F, Gilani AH, Hamid AA, Saari N, Alkharfy KM. Coriander (Coriandrum sativum L.): a potential source of high-value components for functional foods and nutraceuticals—a review. *Phytother Res.* 2013;27(10):1439–56.

47. Rajeshwari CU, Siri S, Andallu B. Antioxidant and antiarthritic potential of coriander (Coriandrum sativum L.) leaves. *e-SPEN J.* 2012;7(6):e223–8.

48. Geppetti P, Fusco BM, Marabini S, Maggi CA, Fanciullacci M, Sicuteri F. Secretion, pain and sneezing induced by the application of capsaicin to the nasal mucosa in man. *Br J Pharmacol.* 1988;93(3):509–14.

49. Nesbitt AD, Goadsby PJ. Cluster headache. *BMJ.* 2012;344:e2407.

50. Fusco BM, Marabini S, Maggi CA, Fiore G, Geppetti P. Preventative effect of repeated nasal applications of capsaicin in cluster headache. *Pain.* 1994;59(3):321–5.

51. Nozu T, Kudaira M. Altered rectal sensory response induced by balloon distention in patients with functional abdominal pain syndrome. *Biopsychosoc Med.* 2009;3:13.

52. Bortolotti M, Porta S. Effect of red pepper on symptoms of irritable bowel syndrome: preliminary study. *Dig Dis Sci.* 2011;56(11):3288–95.

53. Bortolotti M, Coccia G, Grossi G. Red pepper and functional dyspepsia. *N Engl J Med.* 2002;346(12):947–8.

54. Hennessy S, Leonard CE, Newcomb C, Kimmel SE, Bilker WB. Cisapride and ventricular arrhythmia. *Br J Clin Pharmacol.* 2008;66(3):375–85.

55. Mustafa T, Srivastava KC. Ginger (Zingiber officinale) in migraine headache. *J Ethnopharmacol.* 1990;29(3):267–73.

56. Gottlieb MS. Discovering AIDS. *Epidemiology.* 1998;9(4):365–7.

57. Ghofrani HA, Osterloh IH, Grimminger F. Sildenafil: from angina to erectile dysfunction to pulmonary hypertension and beyond. *Nat Rev Drug Discov.* 2006;5(8):689–702.

58. Vandenbroucke JP. In defense of case reports and case series. *Ann Intern Med.* 2001;134(4):330–4.

59. Maghbooli M, Golipour F, Moghimi Esfandabadi A, Yousefi M. Comparison between the efficacy of ginger and sumatriptan in the ablative treatment of the common migraine. *Phytother Res.* 2014;28(3):412–5.

60. Desai HG, Kalro RH, Choksi AP. Effect of ginger & garlic on DNA content of gastric aspirate. *Indian J Med Res*. 1990;92:139–41.

61. Wasson S, Jayam VK. Coronary vasospasm and myocardial infarction induced by oral sumatriptan. *Clin Neuropharmacol*. 2004;27(4):198–200.

62. Laine K, Raasakka T, Mäntynen J, Saukko P. Fatal cardiac arrhythmia after oral sumatriptan. *Headache*. 1999;39(7):511–2.

63. Maghbooli M, Golipour F, Moghimi Esfandabadi A, Yousefi M. Comparison between the efficacy of ginger and sumatriptan in the ablative treatment of the common migraine. *Phytother Res*. 2014;28(3):412–5.

64. Coco AS. Primary dysmenorrhea. *Am Fam Physician*. 1999;60(2):489–96.

65. Kashefi F, Khajehei M, Tabatabaeichehr M, Alavinia M, Asili J. Comparison of the effect of ginger and zinc sulfate on primary dysmenorrhea: a placebo-controlled randomized trial. *Pain Manag Nurs*. 2014;15(4):826–33.

66. Rahnama P, Montazeri A, Huseini HF, Kianbakht S, Naseri M. Effect of Zingiber officinale R. rhizomes (ginger) on pain relief in primary dysmenorrhea: a placebo randomized trial. *BMC Complement Altern Med*. 2012;12:92.

67. Ozgoli G, Goli M, Moattar F. Comparison of effects of ginger, mefenamic acid, and ibuprofen on pain in women with primary dysmenorrhea. *J Altern Complement Med*. 2009;15(2):129–32.

68. Kashefi F, Khajehei M, Alavinia M, Golmakani E, Asili J. Effect of ginger (Zingiber officinale) on heavy menstrual bleeding: a placebo-controlled, randomized clinical trial. *Phytother Res*. 2015;29(1):114–9.

69. Khayat S, Kheirkhah M, Behboodi Moghadam Z, Fanaei H, Kasaeian A, Javadimehr M. Effect of treatment with ginger on the severity of premenstrual syndrome symptoms. *ISRN Obstet Gynecol*. 2014;2014:792708.

70. Mowrey DB, Clayson DE. Motion sickness, ginger, and psychophysics. *Lancet*. 1982;1(8273):655–7.

71. Palatty PL, Haniadka R, Valder B, Arora R, Baliga MS. Ginger in the prevention of nausea and vomiting: a review. *Crit Rev Food Sci Nutr*. 2013;53(7):659–69.

72. Ding M, Leach M, Bradley H. The effectiveness and safety of ginger for pregnancy-induced nausea and vomiting: a systematic review. *Women Birth*. 2013;26(1):e26–30.

73. Carlsen MH, Halvorsen BL, Holte K, et al. The total antioxidant content of more than 3100 foods, beverages, spices, herbs and supplements used worldwide. *Nutr J*. 2010;9:3.

74. American Thyroid Association Taskforce on Radioiodine Safety, Sisson JC, Freitas J, et al. Radiation safety in the treatment of patients with thyroid diseases by radioiodine 131I: practice recommendations of the American Thyroid Association. *Thyroid*. 2011;21(4):335–46.

75. Metso S, Auvinen A, Huhtala H, Salmi J, Oksala H, Jaatinen P. Increased cancer incidence after radioiodine treatment for hyperthyroidism. *Cancer*. 2007;109(10):1972–9.

76. Arami S, Ahmadi A, Haeri SA. The radioprotective effects of Origanum vulgare extract against genotoxicity induced by (131)I in human blood lymphocyte. *Cancer Biother Radiopharm*. 2013;28(3):201–6.

77. Berrington D, Lall N. Anticancer activity of certain herbs and spices on the cervical epithelial carcinoma (HeLa) cell line. *Evid Based Complement Alternat Med*. 2012;2012:564927.

78. Gunawardena D, Shanmugam K, Low M, et al. Determination of anti-inflammatory activities of standardised preparations of plant- and mushroom-based foods. *Eur J Nutr*. 2014;53(1):335–43.

79. Al Dhaheri Y, Attoub S, Arafat K, et al. Anti-metastatic and anti-tumor growth effects of Origanum majorana on highly metastatic human breast cancer cells: inhibition of NFκB signaling and reduction of nitric oxide production. *PLoS ONE*. 2013;8(7):e68808.

80. Haj-Husein I, Tukan S, Alkazaleh F. The effect of marjoram (Origanum majorana) tea on the hormonal profile of women with polycystic ovary syndrome: a randomised controlled pilot study. *J Hum Nutr Diet*. 2015; doi: 10.1111/jhn.12290.

81. Carlsen MH, Halvorsen BL, Holte K, et al. The total antioxidant content of more than 3100 foods, beverages, spices, herbs and supplements used worldwide. *Nutr J*. 2010;9:3.

82. Carlsen MH, Halvorsen BL, Holte K, et al. The total antioxidant content of more than 3100 foods, beverages, spices, herbs and supplements used worldwide. *Nutr J*. 2010;9:3.

83. Baliga MS, Dsouza JJ. Amla (Emblica officinalis Gaertn), a wonder berry in the treatment and prevention of cancer. *Eur J Cancer Prev*. 2011;20(3):225–39.

84. Carlsen MH, Halvorsen BL, Holte K, et al. The total antioxidant content of more than 3100 foods, beverages, spices, herbs and supplements used worldwide. *Nutr J*. 2010;9:3.

85. Darvin ME, Patzelt A, Knorr F, Blume-Peytavi U, Sterry W, Lademann J. One-year study on the variation of carotenoid antioxidant substances in living human skin: influence of dietary supplementation and stress factors. *J Biomed Opt*. 2008;13(4):044028.

86. Mohanty P, Hamouda W, Garg R, Aljada A, Ghanim H, Dandona P. Glucose challenge stimulates reactive oxygen species (ROS) generation by leucocytes. *J Clin Endocrinol Metab*. 2000; 85(8):2970–3.

87. Ghanim H, Mohanty P, Pathak R, Chaudhuri A, Sia CL, Dandona P. Orange juice or fructose intake does not induce oxidative and inflammatory response. *Diabetes Care*. 2007;30(6): 1406–11.

88. Prior RL, Gu L, Wu X, et al. Plasma antioxidant capacity changes following a meal as a measure of the ability of a food to alter in vivo antioxidant status. *J Am Coll Nutr*. 2007;26(2):170–81.

89. Carlsen MH, Halvorsen BL, Holte K, et al. The total antioxidant content of more than 3100 foods, beverages, spices, herbs and supplements used worldwide. *Nutr J*. 2010;9:3.

90. Saper RB, Kales SN, Paquin J, et al. Heavy metal content of Ayurvedic herbal medicine products. *JAMA*. 2004;292(23):2868–73.

91. Martena MJ, van der Wielen JC, Rietjens IM, Klerx WN, de Groot HN, Konings EJ. Monitoring of mercury, arsenic, and lead in traditional Asian herbal preparations on the Dutch market and estimation of associated risks. *Food Addit Contam Part A*. 2010;27(2):190–205.

92. Skulas-Ray AC, Kris-Etherton PM, Teeter DL, Chen CYO, Vanden Heuvel JP, West SG. A high antioxidant spice blend attenuates postprandial insulin and triglyceride responses and increases some plasma measures of antioxidant activity in healthy, overweight men. *J Nutr*. 2011;141(8): 1451–7.

93. Tomita LY, Roteli-Martins CM, Villa LL, Franco EL, Cardoso MA, BRINCA Study Team. Associations of dietary dark-green and deep-yellow vegetables and fruits with cervical intraepithelial neoplasia: modification by smoking. *Br J Nutr*. 2011;105(6):928–37.

94. Gomaa EA, Gray JI, Rabie S, Lopez-Bote C, Booren AM. Polycyclic aromatic hydrocarbons in smoked food products and commercial liquid smoke flavourings. *Food Addit Contam*. 1993; 10(5):503–21.

95. Fritschi G, Prescott WR Jr. Morphine levels in urine subsequent to poppy seed consumption. *Forensic Sci Int*. 1985;27(2):111–7.

96. Hahn A, Michalak H, Begemann K, et al. Severe health impairment of a 6-week-old infant related to the ingestion of boiled poppy seeds. *Clin Toxicol*. 2008;46:607.

97. Sproll C, Perz RC, Lachenmeier DW. Optimized LC/MS/MS analysis of morphine and codeine in poppy seed and evaluation of their fate during food processing as a basis for risk analysis. *J Agric Food Chem*. 2006;54(15):5292–8.

98. European Food Safety Authority. Scientific opinion on the risks for public health related to the presence of opium alkaloids in poppy seeds. *EFSA J*. 2011;9(11):2405.

99. Lachenmeier DW, Sproll C, Musshoff F. Poppy seed foods and opiate drug testing—where are we today? *Ther Drug Monit.* 2010;32(1):11–8.

100. Sproll C, Perz RC, Lachenmeier DW. Optimized LC/MS/MS analysis of morphine and codeine in poppy seed and evaluation of their fate during food processing as a basis for risk analysis. *J Agric Food Chem.* 2006;54(15):5292–8.

101. Lachenmeier DW, Sproll C, Musshoff F. Poppy seed foods and opiate drug testing—where are we today? *Ther Drug Monit.* 2010;32(1):11–8.

102. Idle JR. Christmas gingerbread (Lebkuchen) and Christmas cheer—review of the potential role of mood elevating amphetamine-like compounds formed in vivo and in furno. *Prague Med Rep.* 2005;106(1):27–38.

103. Payne RB. Nutmeg intoxication. *N Engl J Med.* 1963;269:36–8.

104. Cushny AR. Nutmeg poisoning. *Proc R Soc Med.* 1908;1(Ther Pharmacol Sect):39–44.

105. Williams EY, West F. The use of nutmeg as a psychotropic drug. Report of two cases. *J Natl Med Assoc.* 1968;60(4):289–90.

106. Williams EY, West F. The use of nutmeg as a psychotropic drug. Report of two cases. *J Natl Med Assoc.* 1968;60(4):289–90.

107. Scholefield JH. Nutmeg—an unusual overdose. *Arch Emerg Med.* 1986;3(2):154–5.

108. Davis PA, Yokoyama W. Cinnamon intake lowers fasting blood glucose: meta-analysis. *J Med Food.* 2011;14(9):884–9.

109. Solomon TPJ, Blannin AK. Effects of short-term cinnamon ingestion on in vivo glucose tolerance. *Diabetes Obes Metab.* 2007;9(6):895–901.

110. Solomon TPJ, Blannin AK. Changes in glucose tolerance and insulin sensitivity following 2 weeks of daily cinnamon ingestion in healthy humans. *Eur J Appl Physiol.* 2009;105(6):969–76.

111. Fotland TØ, Paulsen JE, Sanner T, Alexander J, Husøy T. Risk assessment of coumarin using the bench mark dose (BMD) approach: children in Norway which regularly eat oatmeal porridge with cinnamon may exceed the TDI for coumarin with several folds. *Food Chem Toxicol.* 2012;50(3–4):903–12.

112. Wickenberg J, Lindstedt S, Berntorp K, Nilsson J, Hlebowicz J. Ceylon cinnamon does not affect postprandial plasma glucose or insulin in subjects with impaired glucose tolerance. *Br J Nutr.* 2012;107(12):1845–9.

113. Davis PA, Yokoyama W. Cinnamon intake lowers fasting blood glucose: meta-analysis. *J Med Food.* 2011;14(9):884–9.

Whole Grains

1. World Cancer Research Fund / American Institute for Cancer Research. Food, Nutrition, Physical Activity, and the Prevention of Cancer: a Global Perspective. Washington, D.C.: AICR, 2007.

2. Eat 3 or more whole-grain foods every day. http://www.heart.org/HEARTORG/Getting Healthy/NutritionCenter/HealthyEating/Eat-3-or-More-Whole-Grain-Foods-Every-Day _UCM_320264_Article.jsp. Accessed April 18, 2015.

3. Wu H, Flint AJ, Qi Q, et al. Association between dietary whole grain intake and risk of mortality: two large prospective studies in US men and women. *JAMA Intern Med.* 2015;175(3):373–84.

4. Tang G, Wang D, Long J, Yang F, Si L. Meta-analysis of the association between whole grain intake and coronary heart disease risk. *Am J Cardiol.* 2015;115(5):625–9.

5. Aune D, Norat T, Romundstad P, Vatten LJ. Whole grain and refined grain consumption and the risk of type 2 diabetes: a systematic review and dose-response meta-analysis of cohort studies. *Eur J Epidemiol*. 2013;28(11):845–58.

6. Cho SS, Qi L, Fahey GC, Klurfeld DM. Consumption of cereal fiber, mixtures of whole grains and bran, and whole grains and risk reduction in type 2 diabetes, obesity, and cardiovascular disease. *Am J Clin Nutr*. 2013;98(2):594–619.

7. Lim SS, Vos T, Flaxman AD, et al. A comparative risk assessment of burden of disease and injury attributable to 67 risk factors and risk factor clusters in 21 regions, 1990–2010: a systematic analysis for the Global Burden of Disease Study 2010. *Lancet*. 2012;380(9859):2224–60.

8. Lefevre M, Jonnalagadda S. Effect of whole grains on markers of subclinical inflammation. *Nutr Rev*. 2012;70(7):387–96.

9. Montonen J, Boeing H, Fritsche A, et al. Consumption of red meat and whole-grain bread in relation to biomarkers of obesity, inflammation, glucose metabolism and oxidative stress. *Eur J Nutr*. 2013;52(1):337–45.

10. Goletzke J, Buyken AE, Joslowski G, et al. Increased intake of carbohydrates from sources with a higher glycemic index and lower consumption of whole grains during puberty are prospectively associated with higher IL-6 concentrations in younger adulthood among healthy individuals. *J Nutr*. 2014;144(10):1586–93.

11. Sofi F, Ghiselli L, Cesari F, et al. Effects of short-term consumption of bread obtained by an old Italian grain variety on lipid, inflammatory, and hemorheological variables: an intervention study. *J Med Food*. 2010;13(3):615–20.

12. Vitaglione P, Mennella I, Ferracane R, et al. Whole-grain wheat consumption reduces inflammation in a randomized controlled trial on overweight and obese subjects with unhealthy dietary and lifestyle behaviors: role of polyphenols bound to cereal dietary fiber. *Am J Clin Nutr*. 2015;101(2):251–61.

13. Esposito K, Nappo F, Giugliano F, et al. Meal modulation of circulating interleukin 18 and adiponectin concentrations in healthy subjects and in patients with type 2 diabetes mellitus. *Am J Clin Nutr*. 2003;78(6):1135–40.

14. Masters RC, Liese AD, Haffner SM, Wagenknecht LE, Hanley AJ. Whole and refined grain intakes are related to inflammatory protein concentrations in human plasma. *J Nutr*. 2010;140(3):587–94.

15. Vitaglione P, Mennella I, Ferracane R, et al. Whole-grain wheat consumption reduces inflammation in a randomized controlled trial on overweight and obese subjects with unhealthy dietary and lifestyle behaviors: role of polyphenols bound to cereal dietary fiber. *Am J Clin Nutr*. 2015;101(2):251–61.

16. Qi L, van Dam RM, Liu S, Franz M, Mantzoros C, Hu FB. Whole-grain, bran, and cereal fiber intakes and markers of systemic inflammation in diabetic women. *Diabetes Care*. 2006;29(2):207–11.

17. Sofi F, Ghiselli L, Cesari F, et al. Effects of short-term consumption of bread obtained by an old Italian grain variety on lipid, inflammatory, and hemorheological variables: an intervention study. *J Med Food*. 2010;13(3):615–20.

18. Esposito K, Giugliano D. Whole-grain intake cools down inflammation. *Am J Clin Nutr*. 2006;83(6):1440–1.

19. Jacobs DR Jr, Andersen LF, Blomhoff R. Whole-grain consumption is associated with a reduced risk of noncardiovascular, noncancer death attributed to inflammatory diseases in the Iowa Women's Health Study. *Am J Clin Nutr*. 2007;85(6):1606–14.

20. Rubio-Tapia A, Ludvigsson JF, Brantner TL, Murray JA, Everhart JE. The prevalence of celiac disease in the United States. *Am J Gastroenterol*. 2012;107(10):1538–44.

21. Cooper BT, Holmes GK, Ferguson R, Thompson RA, Allan RN, Cooke WT. Gluten-sensitive diarrhea without evidence of celiac disease. *Gastroenterology.* 1980;79(5 Pt 1):801–6.

22. Falchuk ZM. Gluten-sensitive diarrhea without enteropathy: fact or fancy? *Gastroenterology.* 1980;79(5 Pt 1):953–5.

23. Aziz I, Hadjivassiliou M, Sanders DS. Does gluten sensitivity in the absence of coeliac disease exist? *BMJ.* 2012;345:e7907.

24. Mansueto P, Seidita A, D'Alcamo A, Carroccio A. Non-celiac gluten sensitivity: literature review. *J Am Coll Nutr.* 2014;33(1):39–54.

25. Genuis SJ. Sensitivity-related illness: the escalating pandemic of allergy, food intolerance and chemical sensitivity. *Sci Total Environ.* 2010;408(24):6047–61.

26. Di Sabatino A, Corazza GR. Nonceliac gluten sensitivity: sense or sensibility? *Ann Intern Med.* 2012;156(4):309–11.

27. McCarter DF. Non-celiac gluten sensitivity: important diagnosis or dietary fad? *Am Fam Physician.* 2014;89(2):82–3.

28. Ferch CC, Chey WD. Irritable bowel syndrome and gluten sensitivity without celiac disease: separating the wheat from the chaff. *Gastroenterology.* 2012;142(3):664–6.

29. Carroccio A, Mansueto P, Iacono G, et al. Non-celiac wheat sensitivity diagnosed by double-blind placebo-controlled challenge: exploring a new clinical entity. *Am J Gastroenterol.* 2012; 107(12):1898–906.

30. Carroccio A, Mansueto P, Iacono G, et al. Non-celiac wheat sensitivity diagnosed by double-blind placebo-controlled challenge: exploring a new clinical entity. *Am J Gastroenterol.* 2012; 107(12):1898–906.

31. Biesiekierski JR, Peters SL, Newnham ED, Rosella O, Muir JG, Gibson PR. No effects of gluten in patients with self-reported non-celiac gluten sensitivity after dietary reduction of fermentable, poorly absorbed, short-chain carbohydrates. *Gastroenterology.* 2013;145(2):320–8.e1–3.

32. Peters SL, Biesiekierski JR, Yelland GW, Muir JG, Gibson PR. Randomised clinical trial: gluten may cause depression in subjects with non-coeliac gluten sensitivity—an exploratory clinical study. *Aliment Pharmacol Ther.* 2014;39(10):1104–12.

33. Aziz I, Hadjivassiliou M, Sanders DS. Editorial: noncoeliac gluten sensitivity—a disease of the mind or gut? *Aliment Pharmacol Ther.* 2014;40(1):113–4.

34. Picarelli A, Borghini R, Isonne C, Di Tola M. Reactivity to dietary gluten: new insights into differential diagnosis among gluten-related gastrointestinal disorders. *Pol Arch Med Wewn.* 2013;123(12):708–12.

35. Rubio-Tapia A, Ludvigsson JF, Brantner TL, Murray JA, Everhart JE. The prevalence of celiac disease in the United States. *Am J Gastroenterol.* 2012;107(10):1538–44.

36. Riddle MS, Murray JA, Porter CK. The incidence and risk of celiac disease in a healthy US adult population. *Am J Gastroenterol.* 2012;107(8):1248–55.

37. Volta U, Bardella MT, Calabrò A, Troncone R, Corazza GR. An Italian prospective multicenter survey on patients suspected of having non-celiac gluten sensitivity. *BMC Med.* 2014;12:85.

38. Holmes G. Non coeliac gluten sensitivity. *Gastroenterol Hepatol Bed Bench.* 2013;6(3):115–9.

39. Gaesser GA, Angadi SS. Gluten-free diet: imprudent dietary advice for the general population? *J Acad Nutr Diet.* 2012;112(9):1330–3.

40. De Palma G, Nadal I, Collado MC, Sanz Y. Effects of a gluten-free diet on gut microbiota and immune function in healthy adult human subjects. *Br J Nutr.* 2009;102(8):1154–60.

41. Gaesser GA, Angadi SS. Gluten-free diet: imprudent dietary advice for the general population? *J Acad Nutr Diet.* 2012;112(9):1330–3.

42. Horiguchi N, Horiguchi H, Suzuki Y. Effect of wheat gluten hydrolysate on the immune system in healthy human subjects. *Biosci Biotechnol Biochem.* 2005;69(12):2445–9.

43. Di Sabatino A, Corazza GR. Nonceliac gluten sensitivity: sense or sensibility? *Ann Intern Med.* 2012;156(4):309–11.

44. Koerner TB, Cleroux C, Poirier C, et al. Gluten contamination of naturally gluten-free flours and starches used by Canadians with celiac disease. *Food Addit Contam Part A.* 2013;30(12):2017–21.

45. McCarter DF. Non-celiac gluten sensitivity: important diagnosis or dietary fad? *Am Fam Physician.* 2014;89(2):82–3.

46. Tavakkoli A, Lewis SK, Tennyson CA, Lebwohl B, Green PH. Characteristics of patients who avoid wheat and/or gluten in the absence of celiac disease. *Dig Dis Sci.* 2014;59(6):1255–61.

47. Pietzak M. Celiac disease, wheat allergy, and gluten sensitivity: when gluten free is not a fad. *JPEN J Parenter Enteral Nutr.* 2012;36(1 Suppl):68S–75S.

48. Goufo P, Trindade H. Rice antioxidants: phenolic acids, flavonoids, anthocyanins, proanthocyanidins, tocopherols, tocotrienols, γ-oryzanol, and phytic acid. *Food Sci Nutr.* 2014;2(2): 75–104.

49. Choi SP, Kang MY, Koh HJ, Nam SH, Friedman M. Antiallergic activities of pigmented rice bran extracts in cell assays. *J Food Sci.* 2007;72(9):S719–26.

50. Pintha K, Yodkeeree S, Limtrakul P. Proanthocyanidin in red rice inhibits MDA-MB-231 breast cancer cell invasion via the expression control of invasive proteins. *Biol Pharm Bull.* 2015;38(4):571–81.

51. Suttiarporn P, Chumpolsri W, Mahatheeranont S, Luangkamin S, Teepsawang S, Leardkamolkarn V. Structures of phytosterols and triterpenoids with potential anti-cancer activity in bran of black non-glutinous rice. *Nutrients.* 2015;7(3):1672–87.

52. Egilman D, Mailloux C, Valentin C. Popcorn-worker lung caused by corporate and regulatory negligence: an avoidable tragedy. *Int J Occup Environ Health.* 2007;13(1):85–98.

53. Egilman DS, Schilling JH. Bronchiolitis obliterans and consumer exposure to butter-flavored microwave popcorn: a case series. *Int J Occup Environ Health.* 2012;18(1):29–42.

54. Nelson K, Stojanovska L, Vasiljevic T, Mathai M. Germinated grains: a superior whole grain functional food? *Can J Physiol Pharmacol.* 2013;91(6):429–41.

55. Hovey AL, Jones GP, Devereux HM, Walker KZ. Whole cereal and legume seeds increase faecal short chain fatty acids compared to ground seeds. *Asia Pac J Clin Nutr.* 2003;12(4): 477–82.

56. Stephen AM, Cummings JH. The microbial contribution to human faecal mass. *J Med Microbiol.* 1980;13(1):45–56.

57. Fechner A, Fenske K, Jahreis G. Effects of legume kernel fibres and citrus fibre on putative risk factors for colorectal cancer: a randomised, double-blind, crossover human intervention trial. *Nutr J.* 2013;12:101.

58. Hovey AL, Jones GP, Devereux HM, Walker KZ. Whole cereal and legume seeds increase faecal short chain fatty acids compared to ground seeds. *Asia Pac J Clin Nutr.* 2003;12(4):477–82.

59. Tan J, McKenzie C, Potamitis M, Thorburn AN, Mackay CR, Macia L. The role of short-chain fatty acids in health and disease. *Adv Immunol.* 2014;121:91–119.

60. Molteberg EL, Solheim R, Dimberg LH, Frølich W. Variation in oat groats due to variety, storage and heat treatment. II: sensory quality. *J Cereal Sci.* 1996;24(3):273–82.

61. Cerio R, Dohil M, Downie J, et al. Mechanism of action and clinical benefits of colloidal oatmeal for dermatologic practice. *J Drugs Dermatol.* 2010;9(9):1116–20.

62. Boisnic S, Branchet-Gumila MC, Coutanceau C. Inhibitory effect of oatmeal extract oligomer on vasoactive intestinal peptide-induced inflammation in surviving human skin. *Int J Tissue React.* 2003;25(2):41–6.

63. Alexandrescu DT, Vaillant JG, Dasanu CA. Effect of treatment with a colloidal oatmeal lotion

on the acneform eruption induced by epidermal growth factor receptor and multiple tyrosine-kinase inhibitors. *Clin Exp Dermatol.* 2007;32(1):71–4.

64. Wild R, Fager K, Flefleh C, et al. Cetuximab preclinical antitumor activity (monotherapy and combination based) is not predicted by relative total or activated epidermal growth factor receptor tumor expression levels. *Mol Cancer Ther.* 2006;5(1):104–13.

65. Guo W, Nie L, Wu D, et al. Avenanthramides inhibit proliferation of human colon cancer cell lines in vitro. *Nutr Cancer.* 2010;62(8):1007–16.

66. Clemens R, van Klinken BJW. Oats, more than just a whole grain: an introduction. *Br J Nutr.* 2014;112 Suppl 2:S1–3.

67. Eidson M, Saenz B. Average portion sizes of pasta from Italian casual dining restaurants in Tarrant County. http://www.srs.tcu.edu/previous_posters/Nutritional_Sciences/2010/148-Eidson-Gorman.pdf. 2010. Accessed May 21, 2015.

Beverages

1. Popkin BM, Armstrong LE, Bray GM, Caballero B, Frei B, Willett WC. A new proposed guidance system for beverage consumption in the United States. *Am J Clin Nutr.* 2006;83(3):529–42.

2. Rush EC. Water: neglected, unappreciated and under researched. *Eur J Clin Nutr.* 2013;67(5):492–5.

3. Rush EC. Water: neglected, unappreciated and under researched. *Eur J Clin Nutr.* 2013;67(5):492–5.

4. Jéquier E, Constant F. Water as an essential nutrient: the physiological basis of hydration. *Eur J Clin Nutr.* 2010;64(2):115–23.

5. Vivanti AP. Origins for the estimations of water requirements in adults. *Eur J Clin Nutr.* 2012;66(12):1282–9.

6. Adolph EF. The regulation of the water content of the human organism. *J Physiol* (Lond). 1921;55(1–2):114–32.

7. Walsh NP, Fortes MB, Purslow C, Esmaeelpour M. Author response: is whole body hydration an important consideration in dry eye? *Invest Ophthalmol Vis Sci.* 2013;54(3):1713–4.

8. Goodman AB, Blanck HM, Sherry B, Park S, Nebeling L, Yaroch AL. Behaviors and attitudes associated with low drinking water intake among US adults, Food Attitudes and Behaviors Survey, 2007. *Prev Chronic Dis.* 2013;10:E51.

9. Negoianu D, Goldfarb S. Just add water. *J Am Soc Nephrol.* 2008;19(6):1041–3.

10. Michaud DS, Spiegelman D, Clinton SK, et al. Fluid intake and the risk of bladder cancer in men. *N Engl J Med.* 1999;340(18):1390–7.

11. Chan J, Knutsen SF, Blix GG, Lee JW, Fraser GE. Water, other fluids, and fatal coronary heart disease: the Adventist Health Study. *Am J Epidemiol.* 2002;155(9):827–33.

12. Guest S, Essick GK, Mehrabyan A, Dessirier JM, McGlone F. Effect of hydration on the tactile and thermal sensitivity of the lip. *Physiol Behav.* 2014;123:127–35.

13. Benelam B, Wyness L. Hydration and health: a review. *Nutr Bull.* 2010;35:3–25.

14. Vivanti AP. Origins for the estimations of water requirements in adults. *Eur J Clin Nutr.* 2012;66(12):1282–9.

15. Benelam B, Wyness L. Hydration and health: a review. *Nutr Bull.* 2010;35:3–25.

16. Killer SC, Blannin AK, Jeukendrup AE. No evidence of dehydration with moderate daily coffee intake: a counterbalanced cross-over study in a free-living population. *PLoS ONE.* 2014;9(1):e84154.

17. Ruxton CH, Hart VA. Black tea is not significantly different from water in the maintenance of

normal hydration in human subjects: results from a randomised controlled trial. *Br J Nutr.* 2011;106(4):588–95.

18. Benelam B, Wyness L. Hydration and health: a review. *Nutr Bull.* 2010;35:3–25.

19. Saleh MA, Abdel-Rahman FH, Woodard BB, et al. Chemical, microbial and physical evaluation of commercial bottled waters in greater Houston area of Texas. *J Environ Sci Health A Tox Hazard Subst Environ Eng.* 2008;43(4):335–47.

20. Valtin H. "Drink at least eight glasses of water a day." Really? Is there scientific evidence for "8 x 8"? *Am J Physiol Regul Integr Comp Physiol.* 2002;283(5):R993–1004.

21. Kempton MJ, Ettinger U, Foster R, et al. Dehydration affects brain structure and function in healthy adolescents. *Hum Brain Mapp.* 2011;32(1):71–9.

22. Stookey JD, Brass B, Holliday A, Arieff A. What is the cell hydration status of healthy children in the USA? Preliminary data on urine osmolality and water intake. *Public Health Nutr.* 2012; 15(11):2148–56.

23. Edmonds CJ, Burford D. Should children drink more water?: the effects of drinking water on cognition in children. *Appetite.* 2009;52(3):776–9.

24. Pross N, Demazières A, Girard N, et al. Influence of progressive fluid restriction on mood and physiological markers of dehydration in women. *Br J Nutr.* 2013;109(2):313–21.

25. Péronnet F, Mignault D, du Souich P, et al. Pharmacokinetic analysis of absorption, distribution and disappearance of ingested water labeled with D_2O in humans. *Eur J Appl Physiol.* 2012;112(6):2213–22.

26. Bateman DN. Effects of meal temperature and volume on the emptying of liquid from the human stomach. *J Physiol* (Lond). 1982;331:461–7.

27. Armstrong LE, Ganio MS, Klau JF, Johnson EC, Casa DJ, Maresh CM. Novel hydration assessment techniques employing thirst and a water intake challenge in healthy men. *Appl Physiol Nutr Metab.* 2014;39(2):138–44.

28. Cuomo R, Grasso R, Sarnelli G, et al. Effects of carbonated water on functional dyspepsia and constipation. *Eur J Gastroenterol Hepatol.* 2002;14(9):991–9.

29. Freedman ND, Park Y, Abnet CC, Hollenbeck AR, Sinha R. Association of coffee drinking with total and cause-specific mortality. *N Engl J Med.* 2012;366(20):1891–904.

30. Liu J, Sui X, Lavie CJ, et al. Association of coffee consumption with all-cause and cardiovascular disease mortality. *Mayo Clin Proc.* 2013;88(10):1066–74.

31. O'Keefe JH, Bhatti SK, Patil HR, DiNicolantonio JJ, Lucan SC, Lavie CJ. Effects of habitual coffee consumption on cardiometabolic disease, cardiovascular health, and all-cause mortality. *J Am Coll Cardiol.* 2013;62(12):1043–51.

32. Malerba S, Turati F, Galeone C, et al. A meta-analysis of prospective studies of coffee consumption and mortality for all causes, cancers and cardiovascular diseases. *Eur J Epidemiol.* 2013; 28(7):527–39.

33. Shimamoto T, Yamamichi N, Kodashima S, et al. No association of coffee consumption with gastric ulcer, duodenal ulcer, reflux esophagitis, and non-erosive reflux disease: a cross-sectional study of 8,013 healthy subjects in Japan. *PLoS ONE.* 2013;8(6):e65996.

34. Wendl B, Pfeiffer A, Pehl C, Schmidt T, Kaess H. Effect of decaffeination of coffee or tea on gastro-oesophageal reflux. *Aliment Pharmacol Ther.* 1994;8(3):283–7.

35. Lee DR, Lee J, Rota M, et al. Coffee consumption and risk of fractures: a systematic review and dose-response meta-analysis. *Bone.* 2014;63:20–8.

36. Sheng J, Qu X, Zhang X, et al. Coffee, tea, and the risk of hip fracture: a meta-analysis. *Osteoporos Int.* 2014;25(1):141–50.

37. Chen B, Shi HF, Wu SC. Tea consumption didn't modify the risk of fracture: a dose-response meta-analysis of observational studies. *Diagn Pathol.* 2014;9:44.

38. Nazrun AS, Tzar MN, Mokhtar SA, Mohamed IN. A systematic review of the outcomes of osteoporotic fracture patients after hospital discharge: morbidity, subsequent fractures, and mortality. *Ther Clin Risk Manag.* 2014;10:937–48.

39. Li M, Wang M, Guo W, Wang J, Sun X. The effect of caffeine on intraocular pressure: a systematic review and meta-analysis. *Graefes Arch Clin Exp Ophthalmol.* 2011;249(3):435–42.

40. Kang JH, Willett WC, Rosner BA, Hankinson SE, Pasquale LR. Caffeine consumption and the risk of primary open-angle glaucoma: a prospective cohort study. *Invest Ophthalmol Vis Sci.* 2008;49(5):1924–31.

41. Gleason JL, Richter HE, Redden DT, Goode PS, Burgio KL, Markland AD. Caffeine and urinary incontinence in US women. *Int Urogynecol J.* 2013;24(2):295–302.

42. Davis NJ, Vaughan CP, Johnson TM, et al. Caffeine intake and its association with urinary incontinence in United States men: results from National Health and Nutrition Examination Surveys 2005–2006 and 2007–2008. *J Urol.* 2013;189(6):2170–4.

43. Bonilha L, Li LM. Heavy coffee drinking and epilepsy. *Seizure.* 2004;13(4):284–5.

44. Lloret-Linares C, Lafuente-Lafuente C, Chassany O, et al. Does a single cup of coffee at dinner alter the sleep? A controlled cross-over randomised trial in real-life conditions. *Nutrition & Dietetics.* 2012;69(4):250–5.

45. Urgert R, Katan MB. The cholesterol-raising factor from coffee beans. *Annu Rev Nutr.* 1997; 17:305–24.

46. Corrêa TAF, Rogero MM, Mioto BM, et al. Paper-filtered coffee increases cholesterol and inflammation biomarkers independent of roasting degree: a clinical trial. *Nutrition.* 2013;29(7–8): 977–81.

47. Bhave PD, Hoffmayer K. Caffeine and atrial fibrillation: friends or foes? *Heart.* 2013;99(19): 1377–8.

48. Patanè S, Marte F, La Rosa FC, La Rocca R. Atrial fibrillation associated with chocolate intake abuse and chronic salbutamol inhalation abuse. *Int J Cardiol.* 2010;145(2):e74–6.

49. Caldeira D, Martins C, Alves LB, Pereira H, Ferreira JJ, Costa J. Caffeine does not increase the risk of atrial fibrillation: a systematic review and meta-analysis of observational studies. *Heart.* 2013;99(19):1383–9.

50. Cheng M, Hu Z, Lu X, Huang J, Gu D. Caffeine intake and atrial fibrillation incidence: dose response meta-analysis of prospective cohort studies. *Can J Cardiol.* 2014;30(4):448–54.

51. Glade MJ. Caffeine—not just a stimulant. *Nutrition.* 2010;26(10):932–8.

52. Bhave PD, Hoffmayer K. Caffeine and atrial fibrillation: friends or foes? *Heart.* 2013;99(19): 1377–8.

53. Sepkowitz KA. Energy drinks and caffeine-related adverse effects. *JAMA.* 2013;309(3): 243–4.

54. O'Keefe JH, Bhatti SK, Patil HR, DiNicolantonio JJ, Lucan SC, Lavie CJ. Effects of habitual coffee consumption on cardiometabolic disease, cardiovascular health, and all-cause mortality. *J Am Coll Cardiol.* 2013;62(12):1043–51.

55. Yu X, Bao Z, Zou J, Dong J. Coffee consumption and risk of cancers: a meta-analysis of cohort studies. *BMC Cancer.* 2011;11:96.

56. Tzellos TG, Sardeli C, Lallas A, Papazisis G, Chourdakis M, Kouvelas D. Efficacy, safety and tolerability of green tea catechins in the treatment of external anogenital warts: a systematic review and meta-analysis. *J Eur Acad Dermatol Venereol.* 2011;25(3):345–53.

57. Dunne EF, Friedman A, Datta SD, Markowitz LE, Workowski KA. Updates on human papillomavirus and genital warts and counseling messages from the 2010 Sexually Transmitted Diseases Treatment Guidelines. *Clin Infect Dis.* 2011;53 Suppl 3:S143–52.

58. Tjeerdsma F, Jonkman MF, Spoo JR. Temporary arrest of basal cell carcinoma formation in a

patient with basal cell naevus syndrome (BCNS) since treatment with a gel containing various plant extracts. *J Eur Acad Dermatol Venereol.* 2011;25(2):244–5.

59. Trudel D, Labbé DP, Bairati I, Fradet V, Bazinet L, Têtu B. Green tea for ovarian cancer prevention and treatment: a systematic review of the in vitro, in vivo and epidemiological studies. *Gynecol Oncol.* 2012;126(3):491–8.

60. Butler LM, Wu AH. Green and black tea in relation to gynecologic cancers. *Mol Nutr Food Res.* 2011;55(6):931–40.

61. Onakpoya I, Spencer E, Heneghan C, Thompson M. The effect of green tea on blood pressure and lipid profile: a systematic review and meta-analysis of randomized clinical trials. *Nutr Metab Cardiovasc Dis.* 2014;24(8):823–36.

62. Liu G, Mi XN, Zheng XX, Xu YL, Lu J, Huang XH. Effects of tea intake on blood pressure: a meta-analysis of randomised controlled trials. *Br J Nutr.* 2014;112(7):1043–54.

63. Maruyama K, Iso H, Sasaki S, Fukino Y. The association between concentrations of green tea and blood glucose levels. *J Clin Biochem Nutr.* 2009;44(1):41–5.

64. Maki KC, Reeves MS, Farmer M, et al. Green tea catechin consumption enhances exercise-induced abdominal fat loss in overweight and obese adults. *J Nutr.* 2009;139(2):264–70.

65. Arab L, Khan F, Lam H. Epidemiologic evidence of a relationship between tea, coffee, or caffeine consumption and cognitive decline. *Adv Nutr.* 2013;4(1):115–22.

66. Arab L, Liu W, Elashoff D. Green and black tea consumption and risk of stroke: a meta-analysis. *Stroke.* 2009;40(5):1786–92.

67. Yang WS, Wang WY, Fan WY, Deng Q, Wang X. Tea consumption and risk of type 2 diabetes: a dose-response meta-analysis of cohort studies. *Br J Nutr.* 2014;111(8):1329–39.

68. Koyama Y, Kuriyama S, Aida J, et al. Association between green tea consumption and tooth loss: cross-sectional results from the Ohsaki Cohort 2006 Study. *Prev Med.* 2010;50(4):173–9.

69. Watanabe I, Kuriyama S, Kakizaki M, et al. Green tea and death from pneumonia in Japan: the Ohsaki cohort study. *Am J Clin Nutr.* 2009;90(3):672–9.

70. Maeda-Yamamoto M, Ema K, Monobe M, et al. The efficacy of early treatment of seasonal allergic rhinitis with benifuuki green tea containing O-methylated catechin before pollen exposure: an open randomized study. *Allergol Int.* 2009;58(3):437–44.

71. Masuda S, Maeda-Yamamoto M, Usui S, Fujisawa T. 'Benifuuki' green tea containing O-methylated catechin reduces symptoms of Japanese cedar pollinosis: a randomized, double-blind, placebo-controlled trial. *Allergol Int.* 2014;63(2):211–7.

72. Millet D. The origins of EEG. Seventh Annual Meeting of the International Society for the History of the Neurosciences (ISHN). June 3, 2002. http://www.bri.ucla.edu/nha/ishn/ab24-2002.htm. Accessed April 21, 2015.

73. Nobre AC, Rao A, Owen GN. L-theanine, a natural constituent in tea, and its effect on mental state. *Asia Pac J Clin Nutr.* 2008;17 Suppl 1:167–8.

74. Wang ZM, Zhou B, Wang YS, et al. Black and green tea consumption and the risk of coronary artery disease: a meta-analysis. *Am J Clin Nutr.* 2011;93(3):506–15.

75. Rusak G, Komes D, Likić S, Horžić D, Kovač M. Phenolic content and antioxidative capacity of green and white tea extracts depending on extraction conditions and the solvent used. *Food Chem.* 2008;110(4):852–8.

76. Green RJ, Murphy AS, Schulz B, Watkins BA, Ferruzzi MG. Common tea formulations modulate in vitro digestive recovery of green tea catechins. *Mol Nutr Food Res.* 2007;51(9):1152–62.

77. Santana-Rios G, Orner GA, Amantana A, Provost C, Wu SY, Dashwood RH. Potent antimutagenic activity of white tea in comparison with green tea in the Salmonella assay. *Mutat Res.* 2001;495(1–2):61–74.

78. Yang DJ, Hwang LS, Lin JT. Effects of different steeping methods and storage on caffeine, catechins and gallic acid in bag tea infusions. *J Chromatogr A*. 2007;1156(1–2):312–20.

79. Venditti E, Bacchetti T, Tiano L, Carloni P, Greci L, Damiani E. Hot vs. cold water steeping of different teas: do they affect antioxidant activity? *Food Chem*. 2010;119(4):1597–1604.

80. Patel SS, Beer S, Kearney DL, Phillips G, Carter BA. Green tea extract: a potential cause of acute liver failure. *World J Gastroenterol*. 2013;19(31):5174–7.

81. Kole AS, Jones HD, Christensen R, Gladstein J. A case of kombucha tea toxicity. *J Intensive Care Med*. 2009;24(3):205–7.

82. Goenka P, Sarawgi A, Karun V, Nigam AG, Dutta S, Marwah N. Camellia sinensis (tea): implications and role in preventing dental decay. *Pharmacogn Rev*. 2013;7(14):152–6.

83. Kakumanu N, Rao SD. Images in clinical medicine. Skeletal fluorosis due to excessive tea drinking. *N Engl J Med*. 2013;368(12):1140.

84. Malinowska E, Inkielewicz I, Czarnowski W, Szefer P. Assessment of fluoride concentration and daily intake by human from tea and herbal infusions. *Food Chem Toxicol*. 2008;46(3):1055–61.

85. Malinowska E, Inkielewicz I, Czarnowski W, Szefer P. Assessment of fluoride concentration and daily intake by human from tea and herbal infusions. *Food Chem Toxicol*. 2008;46(3):1055–61.

86. Quock RL, Gao JX, Chan JT. Tea fluoride concentration and the pediatric patient. *Food Chem*. 2012;130:615–7.

87. Phillips KM, Carlsen MH, Blomhoff R. Total antioxidant content of alternatives to refined sugar. *J Am Diet Assoc*. 2009;109(1):64–71.

88. Matsui M, Matsui K, Kawasaki Y, et al. Evaluation of the genotoxicity of stevioside and steviol using six in vitro and one in vivo mutagenicity assays. *Mutagenesis*. 1996;11(6):573–9.

89. Koyama E, Kitazawa K, Ohori Y, et al. In vitro metabolism of the glycosidic sweeteners, stevia mixture and enzymatically modified stevia in human intestinal microflora. *Food Chem Toxicol*. 2003;41(3):359–74.

90. Joint FAO/WHO Expert Committee on Food Additives. Evaluation of certain food additives. *World Health Organ Tech Rep Ser*. 2009;(952):1–208.

91. Gold J. Erythritol may reduce dental caries in high-risk school children. *J Evid Based Dent Pract*. 2014;14(4):185–7.

92. Ciappuccini R, Ansemant T, Maillefert JF, Tavernier C, Ornetti P. Aspartame-induced fibromyalgia, an unusual but curable cause of chronic pain. *Clin Exp Rheumatol*. 2010;28(6 Suppl 63):S131–3.

93. Halldorsson TI, Strøm M, Petersen SB, Olsen SF. Intake of artificially sweetened soft drinks and risk of preterm delivery: a prospective cohort study in 59,334 Danish pregnant women. *Am J Clin Nutr*. 2010;92(3):626–33.

94. Jacob SE, Stechschulte S. Formaldehyde, aspartame, and migraines: a possible connection. *Dermatitis*. 2008;19(3):E10–1.

95. Roberts HJ. Overlooked aspartame-induced hypertension. *South Med J*. 2008;101(9):969.

96. Roberts HJ. Perspective on aspartame-induced pseudotumor cerebri. *South Med J*. 2009;102(8):873.

97. Roberts HJ. Aspartame-induced thrombocytopenia. *South Med J*. 2007;100(5):543.

98. Den Hartog GJM, Boots AW, Adam-Perrot A, et al. Erythritol is a sweet antioxidant. *Nutrition*. 2010;26(4):449–58.

99. Carlsen MH, Halvorsen BL, Holte K, et al. The total antioxidant content of more than 3100 foods, beverages, spices, herbs and supplements used worldwide. *Nutr J*. 2010;9:3.

100. Chu CH, Pang KKL, Lo ECM. Dietary behavior and knowledge of dental erosion among Chinese adults. *BMC Oral Health*. 2010;10:13.

101. Attin T, Siegel S, Buchalla W, Lennon AM, Hannig C, Becker K. Brushing abrasion of soft-ened and remineralised dentin: an in situ study. *Caries Res.* 2004;38(1):62–6.

102. Bassiouny MA, Yang J. Influence of drinking patterns of carbonated beverages on dental erosion. *Gen Dent.* 2005;53(3):205–10.

103. Yang Q. Gain weight by "going diet?" Artificial sweeteners and the neurobiology of sugar crav-ings: Neuroscience 2010. *Yale J Biol Med.* 2010;83(2):101–8.

104. Porikos KP, Booth G, Van Itallie TB. Effect of covert nutritive dilution on the spontaneous food intake of obese individuals: a pilot study. *Am J Clin Nutr.* 1977;30(10):1638–44.

105. Mattes R. Effects of aspartame and sucrose on hunger and energy intake in humans. *Physiol Behav.* 1990;47(6):1037–44.

106. Yang Q. Gain weight by "going diet?" Artificial sweeteners and the neurobiology of sugar crav-ings: Neuroscience 2010. *Yale J Biol Med.* 2010;83(2):101–8.

107. Yang Q. Gain weight by "going diet?" Artificial sweeteners and the neurobiology of sugar crav-ings: Neuroscience 2010. *Yale J Biol Med.* 2010;83(2):101–8.

Exercise

1. Centers for Disease Control and Prevention. Obesity and overweight. http://www.cdc.gov /nchs/fastats/obesity-overweight.htm. April 29, 2015. Accessed May 17, 2015.

2. Laskowski ER. The role of exercise in the treatment of obesity. *PMR.* 2012;4(11):840–4.

3. Olshansky SJ, Passaro DJ, Hershow RC, et al. A potential decline in life expectancy in the United States in the 21st century. *N Engl J Med.* 2005;352(11):1138–45.

4. Freedhoff Y, Hébert PC. Partnerships between health organizations and the food industry risk derailing public health nutrition. *CMAJ.* 2011;183(3):291–2.

5. Westerterp KR, Speakman JR. Physical activity energy expenditure has not declined since the 1980s and matches energy expenditures of wild mammals. *Int J Obes* (Lond). 2008;32(8): 1256–63.

6. Dwyer-Lindgren L, Freedman G, Engell RE, et al. Prevalence of physical activity and obesity in US counties, 2001–2011: a road map for action. *Popul Health Metr.* 2013;11:7.

7. Laskowski ER. The role of exercise in the treatment of obesity. *PMR.* 2012;4(11):840–4.

8. Swinburn B, Sacks G, Ravussin E. Increased food energy supply is more than sufficient to ex-plain the US epidemic of obesity. *Am J Clin Nutr.* 2009;90(6):1453–6.

9. Matthews J, International Food Information Council Foundation. Food & Health Survey: Consumer Attitudes Toward Food Safety, Nutrition & Health. http://www.foodinsight .org/2011_Food_Health_Survey_Consumer_Attitudes_Toward_Food_Safety_Nutrition _Health. August 31, 2011. Accessed March 31, 2015.

10. U.S. Department of Agriculture, Agricultural Research Service. 2014. USDA National Nutrient Database for Standard Reference, Release 27. Chicken, broilers or fryers, leg, meat only, cooked, stewed. http://www.ndb.nal.usda.gov/ndb/foods/show/882. Accessed April 23, 2015.

11. Archer E, Hand GA, Blair SN. Correction: Validity of U.S. Nutritional Surveillance: National Health and Nutrition Examination Survey Caloric Energy Intake Data, 1971–2010. http:// journals.plos.org/plosone/article?id=10.1371/annotation/c313df3a-52bd-4cbe-af14 -6676480d1a43. October 11, 2013. Accessed April 23, 2015.

12. Blair SN. Physical inactivity: the biggest public health problem of the 21st century. *Br J Sports Med.* 2009;43(1):1–2.

13. Murray CJ, Atkinson C, Bhalla K, et al. The state of US health, 1990–2010: burden of dis-eases, injuries, and risk factors. *JAMA.* 2013;310(6):591–608.

14. Lim SS, Vos T, Flaxman AD, et al. A comparative risk assessment of burden of disease and injury attributable to 67 risk factors and risk factor clusters in 21 regions, 1990–2010: a systematic analysis for the Global Burden of Disease Study 2010. *Lancet*. 2012;380(9859):2224–60.

15. Murray CJ, Atkinson C, Bhalla K, et al. The state of US health, 1990–2010: burden of diseases, injuries, and risk factors. *JAMA*. 2013;310(6):591–608.

16. Wang YC, McPherson K, Marsh T, Gortmaker SL, Brown M. Health and economic burden of the projected obesity trends in the USA and the UK. *Lancet*. 2011;378(9793):815–25.

17. Dunstan DW, Barr ELM, Healy GN, et al. Television viewing time and mortality: the Australian Diabetes, Obesity and Lifestyle Study (AusDiab). *Circulation*. 2010;121(3):384–91.

18. Stamatakis E, Hamer M, Dunstan DW. Screen-based entertainment time, all-cause mortality, and cardiovascular events: population-based study with ongoing mortality and hospital events follow-up. *J Am Coll Cardiol*. 2011;57(3):292–9.

19. Chaput JP, Klingenberg L, Sjödin A. Do all sedentary activities lead to weight gain: sleep does not. *Curr Opin Clin Nutr Metab Care*. 2010;13(6):601–7.

20. Patel AV, Bernstein L, Deka A, et al. Leisure time spent sitting in relation to total mortality in a prospective cohort of US adults. *Am J Epidemiol*. 2010;172(4):419–29.

21. Van Uffelen JG, Wong J, Chau JY, et al. Occupational sitting and health risks: a systematic review. *Am J Prev Med*. 2010;39(4):379–88.

22. Patel AV, Bernstein L, Deka A, et al. Leisure time spent sitting in relation to total mortality in a prospective cohort of US adults. *Am J Epidemiol*. 2010;172(4):419–29.

23. Mosley M. Calorie burner: how much better is standing up than sitting? *BBC News Magazine*. October 16, 2013. http://www.bbc.com/news/magazine-24532996. Accessed March 31, 2015.

24. Thosar SS, Johnson BD, Johnston JD, Wallace JP. Sitting and endothelial dysfunction: the role of shear stress. *Med Sci Monit*. 2012;18(12):RA173–80.

25. Koepp GA, Manohar CU, McCrady-Spitzer SK, et al. Treadmill desks: a 1-year prospective trial. *Obesity* (Silver Spring). 2013;21(4):705–11.

26. Healy GN, Dunstan DW, Salmon J, et al. Breaks in sedentary time: beneficial associations with metabolic risk. *Diabetes Care*. 2008;31(4):661–6.

27. Peddie MC, Bone JL, Rehrer NJ, Skeaff CM, Gray AR, Perry TL. Breaking prolonged sitting reduces postprandial glycemia in healthy, normal-weight adults: a randomized crossover trial. *Am J Clin Nutr*. 2013;98(2):358–66.

28. Esen AM, Barutcu I, Acar M, et al. Effect of smoking on endothelial function and wall thickness of brachial artery. *Circ J*. 2004;68(12):1123–6.

29. Alexopoulos N, Vlachopoulos C, Aznaouridis K, et al. The acute effect of green tea consumption on endothelial function in healthy individuals. *Eur J Cardiovasc Prev Rehabil*. 2008;15(3):300–5.

30. Akazawa N, Choi Y, Miyaki A, et al. Curcumin ingestion and exercise training improve vascular endothelial function in postmenopausal women. *Nutr Res*. 2012;32(10):795–9.

31. Sugawara J, Akazawa N, Miyaki A, et al. Effect of endurance exercise training and curcumin intake on central arterial hemodynamics in postmenopausal women: pilot study. *Am J Hypertens*. 2012;25(6):651–6.

32. McHugh M. The health benefits of cherries and potential applications in sports. *Scand J Med Sci Sports*. 2011;21(5):615–6.

33. Aptekmann NP, Cesar TB. Orange juice improved lipid profile and blood lactate of overweight middle-aged women subjected to aerobic training. *Maturitas*. 2010;67(4):343–7.

34. McAnulty LS, Nieman DC, Dumke CL, et al. Effect of blueberry ingestion on natural killer cell counts, oxidative stress, and inflammation prior to and after 2.5 h of running. *Appl Physiol Nutr Metab*. 2011;36(6):976–84.

35. Connolly DA, McHugh MP, Padilla-Zakour OI, Carlson L, Sayers SP. Efficacy of a tart cherry juice blend in preventing the symptoms of muscle damage. *Br J Sports Med.* 2006;40(8): 679–83.

36. Kuehl KS, Perrier ET, Elliot DL, Chesnutt JC. Efficacy of tart cherry juice in reducing muscle pain during running: a randomized controlled trial. *J Int Soc Sports Nutr.* 2010;7:17.

37. Howatson G, McHugh MP, Hill JA, et al. Influence of tart cherry juice on indices of recovery following marathon running. *Scand J Med Sci Sports.* 2010;20(6):843–52.

38. Tarazona-Díaz MP, Alacid F, Carrasco M, Martínez I, Aguayo E. Watermelon juice: potential functional drink for sore muscle relief in athletes. *J Agric Food Chem.* 2013;61(31):7522–8.

39. Mastaloudis A, Yu TW, O'Donnell RP, Frei B, Dashwood RH, Traber MG. Endurance exercise results in DNA damage as detected by the comet assay. *Free Radic Biol Med.* 2004;36(8):966–75.

40. Tsai K, Hsu TG, Hsu KM, et al. Oxidative DNA damage in human peripheral leukocytes induced by massive aerobic exercise. *Free Radic Biol Med.* 2001;31(11):1465–72.

41. Fogarty MC, Hughes CM, Burke G, et al. Exercise-induced lipid peroxidation: Implications for deoxyribonucleic acid damage and systemic free radical generation. *Environ Mol Mutagen.* 2011;52(1):35–42.

42. Childs A, Jacobs C, Kaminski T, Halliwell B, Leeuwenburgh C. Supplementation with vitamin C and N-acetyl-cysteine increases oxidative stress in humans after an acute muscle injury induced by eccentric exercise. *Free Radic Biol Med.* 2001;31(6):745–53.

43. Fogarty MC, Hughes CM, Burke G, Brown JC, Davison GW. Acute and chronic watercress supplementation attenuates exercise-induced peripheral mononuclear cell DNA damage and lipid peroxidation. *Br J Nutr.* 2013;109(2):293–301.

44. Trapp D, Knez W, Sinclair W. Could a vegetarian diet reduce exercise-induced oxidative stress? A review of the literature. *J Sports Sci.* 2010;28(12):1261–8.

45. U.S. Office of Disease Prevention and Health Promotion. 2008 Physical Activity Guidelines for Americans. http://www.health.gov/paguidelines/pdf/paguide.pdf. Accessed April 22, 2015.

46. U.S. Surgeon General. Physical activity and health—a report of the Surgeon General. http://www.cdc.gov/nccdphp/sgr/pdf/sgrfull.pdf. November 17, 1999. Accessed April 22, 2015.

47. Pate RR, Pratt M, Blair SN, et al. Physical activity and public health. A recommendation from the Centers for Disease Control and Prevention and the American College of Sports Medicine. *JAMA.* 1995;273(5):402–7.

48. U.S. Office of Disease Prevention and Health Promotion. 2008 Physical Activity Guidelines for Americans. http://www.health.gov/paguidelines/pdf/paguide.pdf. Accessed April 22, 2015.

49. Samitz G, Egger M, Zwahlen M. Domains of physical activity and all-cause mortality: systematic review and dose-response meta-analysis of cohort studies. *Int J Epidemiol.* 2011;40(5): 1382–400.

50. Woodcock J, Franco OH, Orsini N, Roberts I. Non-vigorous physical activity and all-cause mortality: systematic review and meta-analysis of cohort studies. *Int J Epidemiol.* 2011;40(1): 121–38.

51. Samitz G, Egger M, Zwahlen M. Domains of physical activity and all-cause mortality: systematic review and dose-response meta-analysis of cohort studies. *Int J Epidemiol.* 2011;40(5): 1382–400.

52. Samitz G, Egger M, Zwahlen M. Domains of physical activity and all-cause mortality: systematic review and dose-response meta-analysis of cohort studies. *Int J Epidemiol.* 2011;40(5): 1382–400.

53. Centers for Disease Control and Prevention (CDC). Adult participation in aerobic and muscle-strengthening physical activities—United States, 2011. *MMWR Morb Mortal Wkly Rep*. 2013; 62(17):326–30.

Conclusion

1. Shimizu N, Iwamoto M, Nakano Y, et al. Long-term electrocardiographic follow-up from childhood of an adult patient with Brugada syndrome associated with sick sinus syndrome. *Circ J*. 2009;73(3):575–9.
2. Lacunza J, San Román I, Moreno S, García-Molina E, Gimeno J, Valdés M. Heat stroke, an unusual trigger of Brugada electrocardiogram. *Am J Emerg Med*. 2009;27(5):634.e1–3.
3. Smith J, Hannah A, Birnie DH. Effect of temperature on the Brugada ECG. *Heart*. 2003; 89(3):272.
4. Dillehay TD, Rossen J, Ugent D, et al. Early Holocene coca chewing in northern Peru. *Antiquity*. 2010;84(326):939–53.
5. Iozzo P, Guiducci L, Guzzardi MA, Pagotto U. Brain PET imaging in obesity and food addiction: current evidence and hypothesis. *Obes Facts*. 2012;5(2):155–64.
6. Volkow ND, Wang GJ, Fowler JS, Tomasi D, Baler R. Food and drug reward: overlapping circuits in human obesity and addiction. *Curr Top Behav Neurosci*. 2012;11:1–24.
7. Volkow ND, Wang GJ, Tomasi D, Baler RD. Obesity and addiction: neurobiological overlaps. *Obes Rev*. 2013;14(1):2–18.
8. Frank S, Linder K, Kullmann S, et al. Fat intake modulates cerebral blood flow in homeostatic and gustatory brain areas in humans. *Am J Clin Nutr*. 2012;95(6):1342–9.
9. Smeets PA, de Graaf C, Stafleu A, van Osch MJ, van der Grond J. Functional MRI of human hypothalamic responses following glucose ingestion. *Neuroimage*. 2005;24(2):363–8.
10. Burger KS, Stice E. Frequent ice cream consumption is associated with reduced striatal response to receipt of an ice cream–based milkshake. *Am J Clin Nutr*. 2012;95(4):810–7.
11. Burger KS, Stice E. Frequent ice cream consumption is associated with reduced striatal response to receipt of an ice cream–based milkshake. *Am J Clin Nutr*. 2012;95(4):810–7.
12. Albayrak Ö, Wölfle SM, Hebebrand J. Does food addiction exist? A phenomenological discussion based on the psychiatric classification of substance-related disorders and addiction. *Obes Facts*. 2012;5(2):165–79.
13. Lisle DJ, Goldhamer A. *The Pleasure Trap: Mastering the Hidden Force That Undermines Health & Happiness*. Summertown, TN: Book Publishing Company; 2007.
14. Grosshans M, Loeber S, Kiefer F. Implications from addiction research toward the understanding and treatment of obesity. *Addict Biol*. 2011;16(2):189–98.
15. Drewnowski A, Krahn DD, Demitrack MA, Nairn K, Gosnell BA. Taste responses and preferences for sweet high-fat foods: evidence for opioid involvement. *Physiol Behav*. 1992;51(2):371–9.
16. Wang GJ, Volkow ND, Thanos PK, Fowler JS. Imaging of brain dopamine pathways: implications for understanding obesity. *J Addict Med*. 2009;3(1):8–18.
17. Garavan H, Pankiewicz J, Bloom A, et al. Cue-induced cocaine craving: neuroanatomical specificity for drug users and drug stimuli. *Am J Psychiatry*. 2000;157(11):1789–98.
18. Martin-Sölch C, Magyar S, Künig G, Missimer J, Schultz W, Leenders KL. Changes in brain activation associated with reward processing in smokers and nonsmokers. A positron emission tomography study. *Exp Brain Res*. 2001;139(3):278–86.
19. Kelly J. Heal thyself. *University of Chicago Magazine*. Jan–Feb 2015. http://mag.uchicago.edu /science-medicine/heal-thyself. Accessed March 31, 2015.

Appendix: Supplements

1. Farmer B, Larson BT, Fulgoni VL III, Rainville AJ, Liepa GU. A vegetarian dietary pattern as a nutrient-dense approach to weight management: an analysis of the National Health and Nutrition Examination Survey 1999–2004. *J Am Diet Assoc.* 2011;111(6):819–27.

2. Clarys P, Deliens T, Huybrechts I, et al. Comparison of nutritional quality of the vegan, vegetarian, semi-vegetarian, pesco-vegetarian and omnivorous diet. *Nutrients.* 2014;6(3):1318–32.

3. Pawlak R, Parrott SJ, Raj S, Cullum-Dugan D, Lucus D. How prevalent is vitamin B(12) deficiency among vegetarians? *Nutr Rev.* 2013;71(2):110–7.

4. Mądry E, Lisowska A, Grebowiec P, Walkowiak J. The impact of vegan diet on B-12 status in healthy omnivores: five-year prospective study. *Acta Sci Pol Technol Aliment.* 2012;11(2):209–13.

5. Brocadello F, Levedianos G, Piccione F, Manara R, Pesenti FF. Irreversible subacute sclerotic combined degeneration of the spinal cord in a vegan subject. *Nutrition.* 2007;23(7–8):622–4.

6. Kuo SC, Yeh CB, Yeh YWY, Tzeng NS. Schizophrenia-like psychotic episode precipitated by cobalamin deficiency. *Gen Hosp Psychiatry.* 2009;31(6):586–8.

7. Milea D, Cassoux N, LeHoang P. Blindness in a strict vegan. *N Engl J Med.* 2000;342(12):897–8.

8. Haler D. Death after vegan diet. *Lancet.* 1968;2(7560):170.

9. Roschitz B, Plecko B, Huemer M, Biebl A, Foerster H, Sperl W. Nutritional infantile vitamin B12 deficiency: pathobiochemical considerations in seven patients. *Arch Dis Child Fetal Neonatal Ed.* 2005;90(3):F281–2.

10. NutraBulk vitamin B-12 sublingual 2500mcg tablets. https://nutrabulk.com/nutrabulk-vitamin-b-12-2500mcg-sublingual-tablets-1000-count.html. Accessed September 3, 2015.

11. Pawlak R, Parrott SJ, Raj S, Cullum-Dugan D, Lucus D. How prevalent is vitamin B(12) deficiency among vegetarians? *Nutr Rev.* 2013;71(2):110–7.

12. Donaldson MS. Metabolic vitamin B12 status on a mostly raw vegan diet with follow-up using tablets, nutritional yeast, or probiotic supplements. *Ann Nutr Metab.* 2000;44(5–6):229–34.

13. Institute of Medicine. Dietary reference intakes for thiamin, riboflavin, niacin, vitamin B6, folate, vitamin B12, pantothenic acid, biotin, and choline. Washington, D.C.: National Academy Press, 1998.

14. Eussen SJ, de Groot LC, Clarke R, et al. Oral cyanocobalamin supplementation in older people with vitamin B12 deficiency: a dose-finding trial. *Arch Intern Med.* 2005;165(10):1167–72.

15. Hill MH, Flatley JE, Barker ME, et al. A vitamin B-12 supplement of 500 μg/d for eight weeks does not normalize urinary methylmalonic acid or other biomarkers of vitamin B-12 status in elderly people with moderately poor vitamin B-12 status. *J Nutr.* 2013 Feb;143(2):142–7.

16. Bor MV, von Castel-Roberts KM, Kauwell GPA, et al. Daily intake of 4 to 7 μg dietary vitamin B-12 is associated with steady concentrations of vitamin B-12-related biomarkers in a healthy young population. *Am J Clin Nutr.* 2010;91(3):571–7.

17. Heyssel RM, Bozian RC, Darby WJ, Bell MC. Vitamin B12 turnover in man. The assimilation of vitamin B12 from natural foodstuff by man and estimates of minimal daily dietary requirements. *Am J Clin Nutr.* 1966;18(3):176–84.

18. Bischoff-Ferrari HA. Optimal serum 25-hydroxyvitamin D levels for multiple health outcomes. *Adv Exp Med Biol.* 2014;810:500–25.

19. Mulligan GB, Licata A. Taking vitamin D with the largest meal improves absorption and results in higher serum levels of 25-hydroxyvitamin D. *J Bone Miner Res.* 2010;25(4):928–30.

20. Harris SS. Vitamin D and African Americans. *J Nutr.* 2006;136(4):1126–9.

21. Holick MF, Matsuoka LY, Wortsman J. Age, vitamin D, and solar ultraviolet. *Lancet.* 1989;2(8671):1104–5.

22. Wacker M, Holick MF. Sunlight and vitamin D: a global perspective for health. *Dermatoendocrinol.* 2013;5(1):51–108.

23. Wacker M, Holick MF. Sunlight and vitamin D: a global perspective for health. *Dermatoendocrinol.* 2013;5(1):51–108.

24. Langdahl JH, Schierbeck LL, Bang UC, Jensen JEB. Changes in serum 25-hydroxyvitamin D and cholecalciferol after one whole-body exposure in a commercial tanning bed: a randomized study. *Endocrine.* 2012;42(2):430–5.

25. O'Sullivan NA, Tait CP. Tanning bed and nail lamp use and the risk of cutaneous malignancy: a review of the literature. *Australas J Dermatol.* 2014;55(2):99–106.

26. Levine JA, Sorace M, Spencer J, Siegel DM. The indoor UV tanning industry: a review of skin cancer risk, health benefit claims, and regulation. *J Am Acad Dermatol.* 2005;53(6):1038–44.

27. Moan J, Grigalavicius M, Dahlback A, Baturaite Z, Juzeniene A. Ultraviolet-radiation and health: optimal time for sun exposure. *Adv Exp Med Biol.* 2014;810:423–8.

28. Dasgupta PK, Liu Y, Dyke JV. Iodine nutrition: iodine content of iodized salt in the United States. *Environ Sci Technol.* 2008;42(4):1315–23.

29. Lim SS, Vos T, Flaxman AD, et al. A comparative risk assessment of burden of disease and injury attributable to 67 risk factors and risk factor clusters in 21 regions, 1990–2010: a systematic analysis for the Global Burden of Disease Study 2010. *Lancet.* 2012;380(9859):2224–60.

30. Leung AM, Braverman LE, Pearce EN. History of U.S. iodine fortification and supplementation. *Nutrients.* 2012;4(11):1740–6.

31. Teas J, Pino S, Critchley A, Braverman LE. Variability of iodine content in common commercially available edible seaweeds. *Thyroid.* 2004;14(10):836–41.

32. Rose M, Lewis J, Langford N, et al. Arsenic in seaweed forms, concentration and dietary exposure. *Food Chem Toxicol.* 2007;45(7):1263–7.

33. Teas J, Pino S, Critchley A, Braverman LE. Variability of iodine content in common commercially available edible seaweeds. *Thyroid.* 2004;14(10):836–41.

34. Di Matola T, Zeppa P, Gasperi M, Vitale M. Thyroid dysfunction following a kelp-containing marketed diet. *BMJ Case Rep.* 2014;bcr2014206330.

35. Greger M. Do Eden beans have too much iodine? http://nutritionfacts.org/2012/07/05/do-eden-beans-have-too-much-iodine/. Published July 5, 2012. Accessed April 20, 2015.

36. Tonstad S, Nathan E, Oda K, Fraser G. Vegan diets and hypothyroidism. *Nutrients.* 2013; 5(11):4642–52.

37. Leung AM, LaMar A, He X, Braverman LE, Pearce EN. Iodine status and thyroid function of Boston-area vegetarians and vegans. *J Clin Endocrinol Metab.* 2011;96(8):E1303–7.

38. Shaikh MG, Anderson JM, Hall SK, Jackson MA. Transient neonatal hypothyroidism due to a maternal vegan diet. *J Pediatr Endocrinol Metab.* 2003;16(1):111–3.

39. Becker DV, Braverman LE, Delange F, et al. Iodine supplementation for pregnancy and lactation—United States and Canada: recommendations of the American Thyroid Association. *Thyroid.* 2006;16(10):949–51.

40. Vannice G, Rasmussen H. Position of the Academy of Nutrition and Dietetics: dietary fatty acids for healthy adults. *J Acad Nutr Diet.* 2014;114(1):136–53.

41. Harris WS. Achieving optimal n-3 fatty acid status: the vegetarian's challenge . . . or not. *Am J Clin Nutr.* 2014;100 Suppl 1:449S–52S.

42. Sarter B, Kelsey KS, Schwartz TA, Harris WS. Blood docosahexaenoic acid and eicosapentaenoic acid in vegans: associations with age and gender and effects of an algal-derived omega-3 fatty acid supplement. *Clin Nutr.* 2015;34(2):212–8.

43. Bourdon JA, Bazinet TM, Arnason TT, Kimpe LE, Blais JM, White PA. Polychlorinated biphenyls (PCBs) contamination and aryl hydrocarbon receptor (AhR) agonist activity of omega-3 poly-

unsaturated fatty acid supplements: implications for daily intake of dioxins and PCBs. *Food Chem Toxicol.* 2010;48(11):3093–7.

44. Yokoo EM, Valente JG, Grattan L, Schmidt SL, Platt I, Silbergeld EK. Low level methylmercury exposure affects neuropsychological function in adults. *Environ Health.* 2003;2(1):8.

45. Chang JW, Pai MC, Chen HL, Guo HR, Su HJ, Lee CC. Cognitive function and blood methylmercury in adults living near a deserted chloralkali factory. *Environ Res.* 2008;108(3):334–9.

46. Masley SC, Masley LV, Gualtierei T. Effect of mercury levels and seafood intake on cognitive function in middle-aged adults. *Integr Med.* 2012;11(3)32–40.

47. Arterburn LM, Oken HA, Hoffman JP, et al. Bioequivalence of docosahexaenoic acid from different algal oils in capsules and in a DHA-fortified food. *Lipids.* 2007;42(11):1011–24.

48. Greene J, Ashburn SM, Razzouk L, Smith DA. Fish oils, coronary heart disease, and the environment. *Am J Public Health.* 2013;103(9):1568–76.

49. Lane K, Derbyshire E, Li W, Brennan C. Bioavailability and potential uses of vegetarian sources of omega-3 fatty acids: a review of the literature. *Crit Rev Food Sci Nutr.* 2014;54(5):572–9.

50. Witte AV, Kerti L, Hermannstädter HM, et al. Long-chain omega-3 fatty acids improve brain function and structure in older adults. *Cereb Cortex.* 2014;24(11):3059–68.

51. Farmer B, Larson BT, Fulgoni VL, Rainville AJ, Liepa GU. A vegetarian dietary pattern as a nutrient-dense approach to weight management: an analysis of the National Health and Nutrition Examination Survey 1999–2004. *J Am Diet Assoc.* 2011;111(6):819–27.

52. Moshfegh A, Goldman J, Cleveland L. What we eat in America, NHANES 2001–2002: usual nutrient intakes from food compared to dietary reference intakes. U.S. Department of Agriculture, Agricultural Research Service 2005.

53. Cogswell ME, Zhang Z, Carriquiry AL, et al. Sodium and potassium intakes among US adults: NHANES 2003–2008. *Am J Clin Nutr.* 2012;96(3):647–57.

54. Davis B, Melina V. Becoming Vegan: *The Complete Guide to Adopting a Plant-Based Diet (Comprehensive Edition).* Summertown, TN: Book Publishing Company; 2014.

55. Craig WJ, Mangels AR. Position of the American Dietetic Association: vegetarian diets. *J Am Diet Assoc.* 2009;109(7):1266–82.

56. Spock B. Good nutrition for kids. *Good Medicine.* 1998;7(2).

Index